UNDERLYING MECHANISMS OF EPILEPSY

Edited by **Fatima Shad Kaneez**

Underlying Mechanisms of Epilepsy
Edited by Fatima Shad Kaneez

Published by InTech
Janeza Trdine 9, 51000 Rijeka, Croatia

Publishing Process Manager Dragana Manestar

Technical Editor Teodora Smiljanic

Cover Designer InTech Design Team

Additional hard copies can be obtained from orders@intechopen.com

Underlying Mechanisms of Epilepsy, Edited by Fatima Shad Kaneez
p. cm.
ISBN 978-953-307-765-9

For EU product safety concerns:
IN TECH d.o.o., Prolaz Marije Krucifikse Kozulić 3, 51000 Rijeka, Croatia,
info@intechopen.com or visit our website at intechopen.com.

Meet the editor

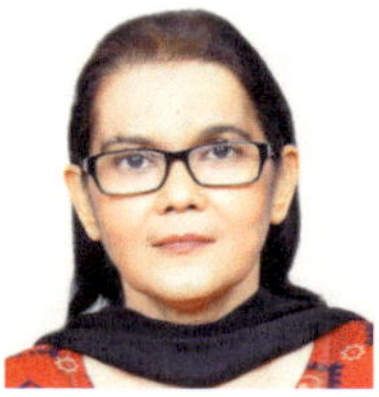

Dr. Fatima Shad Kaneez is currently working as Professor of Neurophysiology at the PAP RSB IHS, University Brunei Darussalam. She completed her PhD in 1994 in Neurosciences from the Faculty of Medicine, University of New South Wales, Sydney Australia. She has been teaching Neurosciences, General and Medical Sciences, and other Biological Sciences for the last thirty years to Science, Medical and Paramedical graduates and post-graduates in Australia, USA, UAE, Bahrain, Pakistan and Brunei Darussalam. She has also been involved in developing, writing, interacting and getting General and Medical Research grants around the world.
She completed her first post doc in Prof White's lab at Allegheny University of Health Sciences, Philadelphia, USA. There she was involved in mutating serotonin type 3 channel lumen and identifying the amino acids responsible for ionic selectivity of the channel by using site directed mutagenesis in conjunction with patch clamping. During her PhD she was the first to exhibit the presence of glycine receptor channels in postnatal hippocampal neurons. She has experience in multiple techniques including: Patch Clamp, Tissue culture, Single Cell RT PCR, Proteomics and Bioinformatics. She is a member of 14 learned societies including her role as regional representative of Women in World Neurosciences (WWN) and coordinator of the Neuroscience Program Network, IBRO (NPN). She has achieved many awards and scholarships, is the author of 20 full refereed papers published in International Tier 1 and 2 journals and 66 refereed conference and short communications. She is the editor of 3 books and 4 journals and has contributed a number of book chapters and reviews.

Contents

Preface

Approximately 1 out of 120 people have epilepsy and 2 out of every 3 new cases are found in developing countries. Young children and people over the age of 65 are more susceptible to epilepsy; however, it can occur to any one at any time in life. Although around 5% of the total world population have seizures, only 0.9% are diagnosed with epilepsy so it is very important to understand the differences between seizures and epilepsy and also to identify the factors responsible for its etiology in order to have more effective therapeutic regime. This book presents twenty chapters ranging from causes and underlying mechanisms to treatment and side effects of epilepsy. This introductory part offers merely a brief skim through some of these quite interesting multidisciplinary chapters.

The chapter entitled "Histopathological Changes in Temporal Epilepsy" is an interesting review on the etiology of drug resistant epilepsy. In this paper, authors discuss the dual pathology of epilepsy in association with other alterations due to neuronal injury and loss. Authors offer a hypothesis that the presence of an epileptogenic foci provokes a process of progressive damage of the nervous tissue and result in drug resistant epilepsy.

Next chapter, entitled "The Role of Astrocytes in Epileptogenesis" is a review about how astrocytes modulate different types of partial seizure. Authors discuss the pivotal role of astrocytes in epilepsy and their involvement in: managing the trafficking of substances between capillary vessels and neurons, homeostasis of ions, principally potassium (K+), and their role in the metabolism of the brain through the degradation of both glucose and glutamate. In addition, they discuss the release of gliotransmitters, and multiple contacts of cortical astrocytes. They also debate on how astrocytic integration can affect the function of several groups of neurons or synapses, thus working in a more coherent model. Any change in astrocytic physiology changes the equilibrium between neuronal excitation and inhibition leading to epileptogenesis.

Further on, the chapter "START proteins in Epilepsy" is based on the observations that the release of neuroactive steroids impairs neuronal survival in the hippocampus. In this chapter, various molecules including steroidogenic acute regulatory protein (StAR)-related lipid transfer domain-containing proteins (START proteins) and their relationship with neurosteroidogenesis were reviewed for further understanding of their role in epilepsy. The START domain that operates as a lipid exchange unit is suggested for further studies as to elucidate the exact nuclear roles of StarD6 on neurosteroidogenesis with StAR in the nervous system.

"Introduction of a novel molecular mechanism on epilepsy progression: roles of growth hormone signaling in a mouse model of temporal lobe epilepsy" is a chapter on epilepsy with foci and the candidate molecules involved in refractory epilepsy. Up-regulation of growth hormones found to have occurred during the process, and metabolic regulation by GH-signaling appears to be responsible for initiating the after discharge threshold during epileptogenesis.

"Role of gap junctions and connexion proteins in the mechanism of seizures" is a paper with reference to the connexion proteins, resultant hemichannels, and the association of two hemichannels on neighboring cells to form a gap junction. Literature suggested a deep and multifaceted relationship between gap junction regulation and seizure susceptibility. In this chapter authors have sought to bring together research from a wide range of disciplines encompassing electrophysiology, molecular biology and mathematical modeling, with the aim of addressing the role of gap junctions in the mechanism of seizures.

Chapter "Recombinant Laforin for Structural Studies" is about autosomal recessive Lafora disease, also known as progressive myoclonic epilepsy. This type of epilepsy is caused by the mutations in two genes: EPM2A gene, coding for the protein laforin, and NHLRC1 gene, for the protein malin. Focusing on Laforin and its involvement in Lafora disease, authors reported it as therapeutic contender for myoclonic epilepsy as well as a novel candidate for biotechnological applications of carbohydrate binding proteins.

"The Cross-talk between Mitochondria and the Nucleus in the Response to Oxidative Stress Associated with Mitochondrial Dysfunction in Mitochondrial Encephalomyopathies" is an interesting review combined with author's own work. In this review authors discussed the biochemical consequences of mitochondrial dysfunction-elicited oxidative stress, mitochondrial retrograde signaling and regulation of Ca^{2+} homoeostasis in neuronal excitability and resultant epileptic seizures. They also discussed the role of stress responsive gene, Sirt1, in the signaling pathway of the cross-talk between mitochondria and the nucleus.

"Temporal Lobe Epilepsy (TLE): molecular targets and cell death" is about TLE and other molecular mechanisms involved in the process of cell death. Authors also explored Bcl-2 gene family and their levels in the hippocampus of patients with intractable seizures. In this paper authors have nicely demonstrated that Caspase-mediated inflammatory process could be a potential mechanism for the pathogenesis of TLE and Caspase inhibitors may act as novel therapeutic agents.

"Ghrelin regulation in epilepsy" is a review discussing whether hormonal changes in relation to epilepsy are due to seizures activity per se or to consequential effects of antiepileptic drugs. Authors re-evaluate the hormones involved in epilepsy focusing on ghrelin, a 28 amino acid peptide produced by stomach. Increasing evidence indicated that ghrelin plays a role in anxiety and stress, though in vitro and in vivo experiments are still controversial. However, it is confirmed that ghrelin has anticonvulsant properties and blood ghrelin levels were shown to be decreased both in experimental epileptic rodents and in humans. Literature indicated that ghrelin can act as a neuroprotective agent due to its antiepileptic and anti-inflammatory effects on neuronal brain cells. A better understanding of ghrelin's activities may help to develop new therapeutic approaches to epilepsy.

"Regulation of GluR6-PSD95-MLK3 signalling in KA-induced rat seizure models" is a short review about the beneficial effects of the co-application of muscimol and baclofen against Kainic acid induced seizures. An experimental model based on Kainic acid (KA) injections replicates many phenomenological features of human temporal lobe epilepsy. Moreover some details are present in the article explaining how both ionotropic and metabotropic GABA agonists can inhibit the assembly of the GluR6-PSD95-MLK3 signaling responsible for KA-induced seizures.

"Biophysical Aspects of the non synaptic epileptiform Activity" is a very nicely written chapter, which demonstrates the conjoint actuation of non-synaptic mechanisms and connections, able to induce and sustain seizures. Focusing on different regions of the hippocampus, and their ability to generate or sustain non-synaptic epileptiform activities authors found them to be directly related with the reduced levels of calcium and increased level of potassium in the extracellular fluid. Authors postulated that these epileptiform activities of non-synaptic origin could be mediated by gap-junctions, ionic fluctuations, or field effect. They described the cellular mechanisms regarding epilepsy using computational simulations for membrane ionic currents, Na^+/K^+-ATPase, co-transporters, and exchangers.

"The Complex Interplay Of Epigenetics And Epilepsy" is a very well written and interesting review about the pharmacological manipulation of epigenetic factors and development of subtype-specific HDAC (Histone deacetylases) inhibitors. Evidence is emerging that epileptogenesis involves changes in the expression patterns of several classes of functionally or genomically-grouped genes that coordinate neural development, homeostasis and stress responses, and neural network formation. Abnormal activity of epigenetic mediators including DNMTs, MBDs, HDACs and repressor complexes could result in altered neuro- and gliogenesis, aberrant migration of newly born cells, and improper integration of these cells into circuits, thereby causing hyper-excitable circuits and seizures.

"Mechanisms Involved in the Pathophysiological Progression of Epilepsy" is a review about pharmacological and genetic importance in molecular signaling mechanisms underlying epileptogenesis. Authors discuss a number of ionotropic and metabotropic glutamate receptors, neurotrophin receptors, calcium regulated enzymes and non-receptor tyrosine kinases which are involved in orchestrating various biochemical events in brain, finally leading to precipitation of a multitude of severe epileptic condition. The chapter is designed to contribute novel concepts for antiepileptic drug.

"The Gingival Fibromatoses (GF)" is a review with personal observations in which authors suggested that GF can be apparent within a systemic disease, and anticonvulsant drug therapy is one of the most common causes of isolated GF. They discuss the prevalence of GF secondary to drug treatment following long term phenytoin therapy. They talk about the clinical heterogeneity and reflected genetic heterogeneity. Then they discuss different conditions which extends from the association of GF with hypertrichosis up to the multi-systemic syndromes of Zimmermann-Laband and Ramon. In addition to reviewing the literature they discuss patients with GH, tonic clonic seizures and GF unrelated to antiepileptic treatment.

"Experimental Epilepsy Models and Morphological Alterations" is a review about the different chemically and electrically induced epilepsy models. Authors conclude that there is no model for answering all questions regarding epilepsy and the studies performed by using experimental models can only explore the basic mechanisms of that particular type of epilepsy. Some chemicals can induce more than one type of epilepsy model. For example crystallized penicillin can induce simple partial, generalized myoclonic, generalized tonic-clonic and generalized absence epilepsy when given using different routes of administration. Therefore, EEG and behavioral studies should be used for analyzing the induced model.

"Two types of epilepsy models and processes of cognition" is a review in which author presents literature and her own data for the comparison of two types of epileptic activities that is the convulsive epilepsy induced by pentilenetetrazole (PTZ) kindling in Wister rats and non-convulsive absence epilepsy in WAG/Rij rats. The main difference between these two types of epilepsy was described.

Oxcarbazepine (OXC) is an antiepileptic drug (AED) of the second generation, with a chemical structure similar to carbamazepine, but with different metabolism OXC is used for the treatment of partial seizures as monotherapy or adjunctive therapy in adults, and in children aged 4 to 16 years. OXC is also sometimes used to treat acute mania in adults, bipolar disorder, and manic-depressive disorder. The neurobiological interaction between epilepsy and sleep is receiving enhanced attention. A key role for limbic monoamines in epilepsy has been established and recently some studies showed the importance of hippocampal monoamines in limbic seizures control

Medicinal herbs are a two edged sword, as discussed in the following chapter. Some herbs are often used in the treatment of the disease, including epilepsy; however, they could also induce or worsen epileptic activity. Effects of an Ethanolic extract and essential oil of *Artemisia dracunculus* L. (Tarragon) were explored before and after the induction of epileptiform activity in snail neurons, using intracellular recording technique. Ethanolic extract and essential oil of Tarragon produce different electrophysiological changes in Pentylenetetrazole (PTZ)-induced epilepsy model.

Tarragon extract results in the complete disappearance of paroxysmal depolarization shift (PDS)-induced by PTZ, while its essential oil potentiate the epileptic activities in the presence of PTZ. Based on their electrophysiological findings, authors suggested that a certain caution is needed when medicinal herbs are used for treating patients suffering from epilepsy.

"In situ release of anti epileptic drugs from nanostructure reservoirs" is a very informative chapter about novel drug delivery system. Author's exhibited how anticonvulsant drug phenytoin encapsulated into the sol-gel biocompatible Titania and can be successfully implanted into the temporal lobe of the brain by low invasion stereotactic surgery. The implantation process is such that the damage of the surrounding tissue is minimal. The drug release from the implants is controlled by the parameters of the matrix such as its morphology, drug-matrix interaction strength, etc. Depending on the parameters of the synthesis, the release profile may be designed according to the necessities in terms of release rate and the amount of the released drug. One of the main prospects of the study is to achieve better protection 'in vivo' for longer time. Also, one needs to find a correlation between the drug release 'in vitro' and its effect and release profile 'in vivo'.

In short, this book contains a range of proposals regarding causes mechanisms and treatment options of epilepsy which will be of interest to a number of scientists and scholars from different disciplines.

Prof. Dr. Fatima Shad Kaneez
Human Physiology, PAP RSB Institute of Health Sciences
University Brunei Darussalam
The State of Brunei Darussalam

Part 1

Causes and Types of Epilepsy

1

Histopathological Changes in Temporal Epilepsy

Assaad Fawaz and Al Khani Raydeh
Damascus University/Faculty of medicine
Syria

1. Introduction

A wide variety of lesions have been reported in the different studies of epilepsy in the literature; though the question is still raised if these observed lesions are the cause or the consequence of seizures. The lesions that might play a role in the onset, maintenance and progression of pharmacoresistance of epileptic seizures, as well as the lesions that might results in are not yet well predicted and comprehensible.

2. Histopathological findings

A confusing array of histopathological findings was reported in the studies of temporal lobe and hippocampus in chronic pharmacoresistant temporal epilepsy, in the literature. We would like to suggest that these findings could be grouped in certain categories:

2.1 Malformations

Many types of malformations were reported in epileptic series; these included the following: (Wolf et al, 1993-1995; Prayson et al, 1996; Volk et al, 1997; Armstrong et al, 2007; Al Khani & Assaad, 2008):

2.1.1 Subependymal nodular cortical heterotopias and band heterotopias [double cortex]

Congenital lesions composed of heterotopic cortical tissue in a periventricular subependymal location; they are closely associated with epilepsy (d'Orsi, 2004; Armstrong et al, 2007) (see fig. 1-2)

2.1.2 Cortical malformations

They include lissencephaly (smooth or nearly smooth cortical surface), hemimegalencephaly (enlarged hemisphere) and pachygyria-polymicrogyria (Sisodiya et al, 2004; Armstrong et al, 2007). Gyral fusion and abnormal elongation of a sulcus are other reported findings (see fig.3) (Al Khani & Assaad, 2008).

It is suggested that cortical malformations can both form epileptogenic foci and alter brain development in a manner that causes a diffuse hyperexcitability of the cortical network (chevaussus et al, 1999).

2.1.3 Neuronal and glioneuronal malformations

These malformations are composed of foci of havardous atypical neurons and Glioneuronal tissue. They overlap with neuronal and neuronal-glial tumors (Wolf et al, 1993-1995; prayson et al, 1996; Volk et al, 1997; Al Khani & Assaad, 2008), (see paragraph 2.4)

2.1.4 Microdysgenesis

This includes the following lesions of abnormal migration (Armstrong et al, 2007):

1. Ectopic neurons in the white matter in greater than normal numbers
2. Gray matter heterotopias: foci of displaced "gray matter" composed of neurons, glia, and neuropil characteristics.
3. Hamartia that are microscopic collections of small, round "oligodendroglia-like" cells. They may be observed in the cortex or in the white matter and have some staining characteristics of immature neurons
4. Perivascular glial nuclei refer to the presence of chains of bare glial nuclei in the white matter
5. Neuronal clusters

2.1.5 Vascular malformations

Vascular malformations are known to cause seizures; notably arteriovenous malformations. All vascular tumors of the central nervous system are considered as malformative lesions (Louis et al, 2007).

2.2 Cortical dysplasia/dysgenesis

The histopathology of "cortical dysplasia" or "cortical dysgenesis" as described by the authors (Taylor et al, 1971; Prayson et al, 1995-1996; Frater et al, 2000; Wang et al, 2006; Armstrong et al, 2007; Bernasconi et al, 2011) includes a variety of structural changes which could be focal, multifocal, or diffuse, resulting in changes in the neuronal network inciting seizures attacks: neuronal migration abnormalities, diffuse architectural disorganization of the cortex with cortical laminar disruption, gyral fusion, clusters of atypical neurons and glial cells within the cortex, malalignment of neurons, neuronal cytomegaly, increased numbers of molecular layer neurons, the presence of large neurons displaying a pyramidal or round shape, ballooned cells, and a high concentration of neurofilaments in giant neurons and of glial intermediate filaments in ballooned cells, evoking disruption of cell differentiation and maturation and an impairment of synaptogenesis (Garbelli et al, 1999). The term "cortical dysgenesis or disorganization" might be more appropriate.

Classification schemes were described; the widely adopted is that described by palmini et al. This classification distinguished two types of cortical dysplasia based of the presence or absence of dysmorphic neurons or balloon cells, as follows (palmini et al, 2004):

Type I:

IA: Isolated architectural abnormalities, usually laminar or columnar disorganization, but no dysmorphic neurons

IB: Architectural abnormalities, giant cells or immature neurons can be found

Type II:

IIA: Architectural abnormalities with dysmorphic cells are found, but no balloon cells

IIB: Architectural abnormalities with both dysmorphic cells and balloon cells

Changes of the above described "cortical dysplasia" are observed in all cases of epilepsy in some studied series (Al Khani & Assaad, 2008) (fig 3&4). Irregular brain surface and

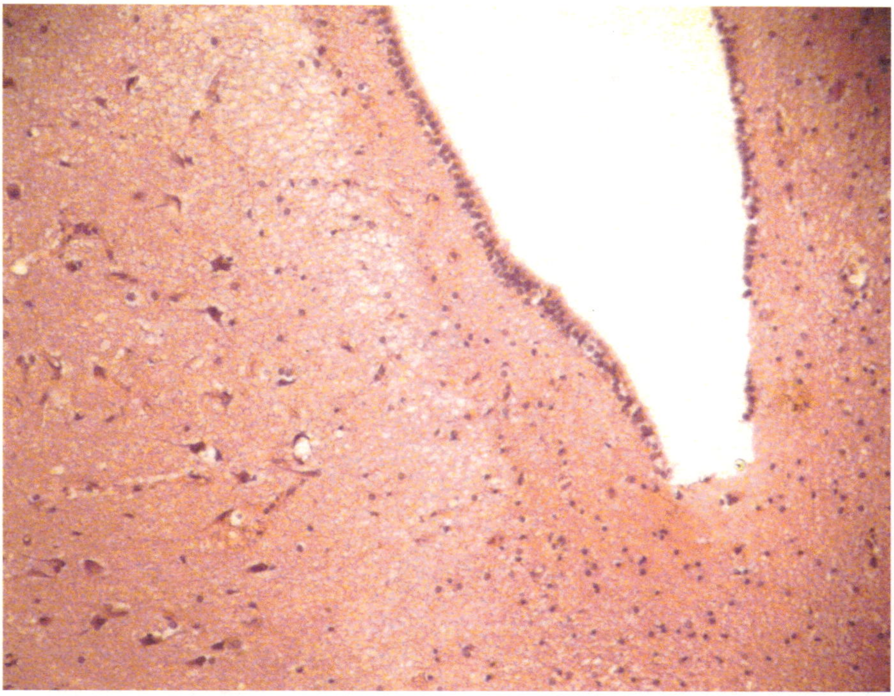

Fig. 1. Subependymal nodular cortical heterotopia observed at the left side of the figure. The columnar ependymal cells are clearly seen (HE stain).

irregular cortical thickness were also described; that might be the consequence of neuronal reorganization associated with glial cell reaction.
Cortical dysgenesis might begin as an *in utero* migrational abnormality (Sprifeafico et al, 1998) so some authors put these lesions under the category of malformations (Armstrong et al, 2007), or as an acquired cortical dysplasia in response to perinatal brain damage (Marin-Padilla et al, 1999). This alteration becomes an ongoing process that affects the structural and functional differentiation of neurons, synaptic profiles, fiber distribution, glial elements, and vasculature. Cortical dysplasia/disorganization becomes worse with the recurrence of seizures and exacerbates neuronal damage.

2.3 Signs of neuronal injury, neuronal lysis, apoptosis and neuronal loss

Neuronal damage and loss have been well documented in studies of epilepsy. Neuron loss is mainly observed in CA2& CA1 sectors of ammon horn (fig 5) and it might be observed in the other sectors in the advanced cases; it is found to be followed by axonal and mossy fibers sprouting and reorganizing (El Bahh et al, 1999; Armsrong et al, 2007). Neuron injury and loss was evident in many series, affecting especially the pyramidal cells in the cortex and the granular cells in the dentate gyrus (dentate nucleus) (Proper et al, 2000; Al Khani and Assaad, 2008) (fig.6-9). The survived cells showed variability in size and shape, edema and vacuolization, and disorganization. Unexplained PAS+ material was also described in some observations in the cytoplasm of the injured neurons. Neuronal lysis and apoptosis were noted in our study adjacent to injured neurons. Neuronal damage especially affecting these neurons was well documented in animal experimental models.(Bouilleret et al, 2000)

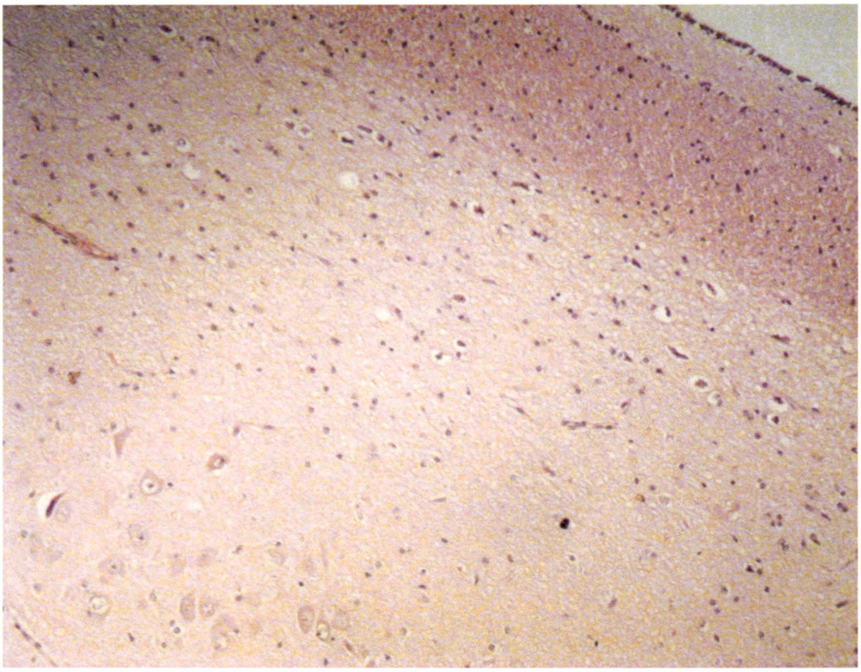

Fig. 2. Subependymal nodular cortical heterotopia showing cluster of atypical neurons at the left lower side (HE stain).

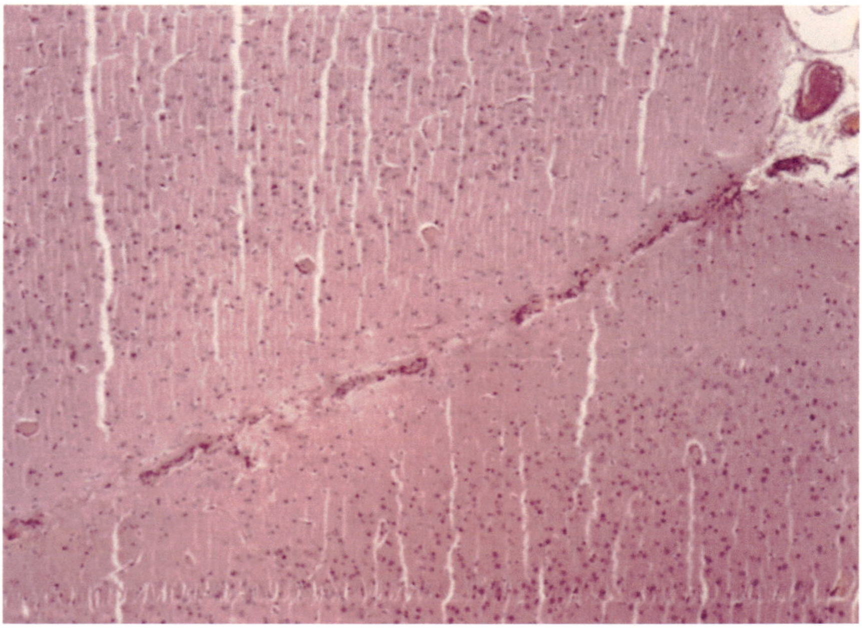

Fig. 3. Gyral fusion in the temporal lobe showing focal complete adhesion of the nervous tissue in "slits-shape"(HE stain). Cortical dysplasia is also noted at both sides of the sulcus (HE stain).

The loss of a critical number of interneurons in the dentate gyrus was suggested as a possible cause of seizure initiation (Fritschy et al, 1999) It was suggested that childhood seizures can damage or alter the postnatally developing granule cells of the human hippocampus, and that early neuron loss and aberrant axon circuits may contribute to chronic hippocampal seizures (Mathern et al, 1996). The role of apoptosis-related genes and the activation of the programmed death pathway were well documented by some authors, explaining that neuronal loss (Uysal et al, 2003; d'Orsi et al, 2004; Niquet et al, 2004;). Apoptotic neurons were noted beside neuron lysis; these two forms of cell death in histopathological findings might contribute to neuron loss (Becker et al, 1999; Al Khani & Assaad 2008) (fig 7).

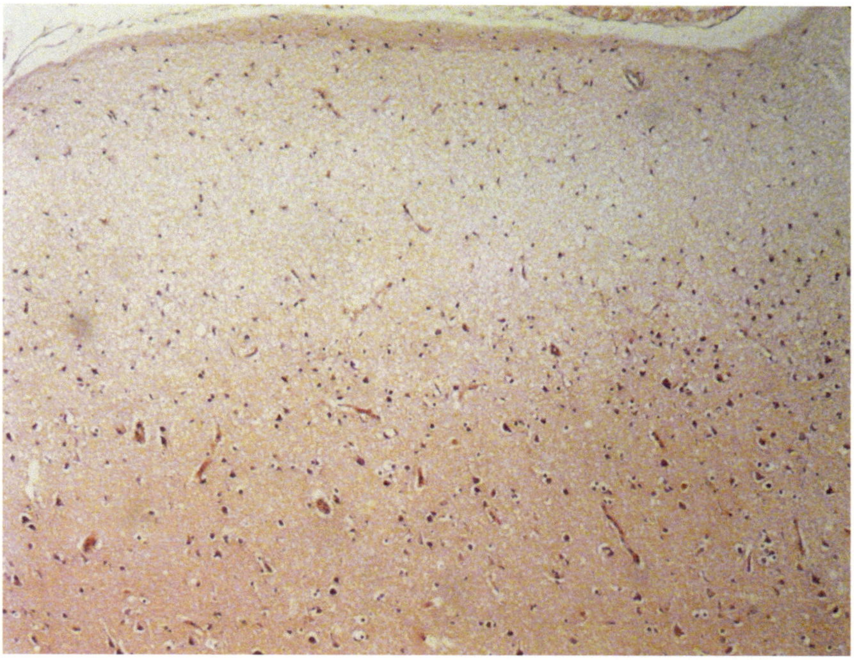

Fig. 4. Cortical dysplasia showing architectural abnormalities (HE stain). Note the subpial gliosis in this figure.

2.4 Tumors and hamartomatous tumors

Some tumors are known to be frequently associated with epilepsy, such as dysembryoplastic neuroepithelial tumors (DNETs), ganglioneuromas and gangliogliomas, which can be either bilateral or multifocal (Barbosa et al, 1999; Whittle et al, 1999; Rosemberg et al, 1998; Al Khani and Assaad, 2008; Louis et al, 2007) (fig. 10). The hamartomatous origin of these tumors is suggested by some authors, as they are composed of mature multiple cell types (Gyure et al, 2000; Louis et al, 2007) Other low-grade tumors were reported in some cases of pharmacoresistant temporal epilepsy, such as xanthoastrocytomas (fig.11), low-grade astrocytomas, oligodendrogliomas, oligoastrocytomas, vascular tumors (Oda et al, 1998) and mixed or composite tumors (Hirose et al, 1998) Their incidences varies widely from one series to another; they were found with high percentages in some series, where most of the glioneuronal tumors were

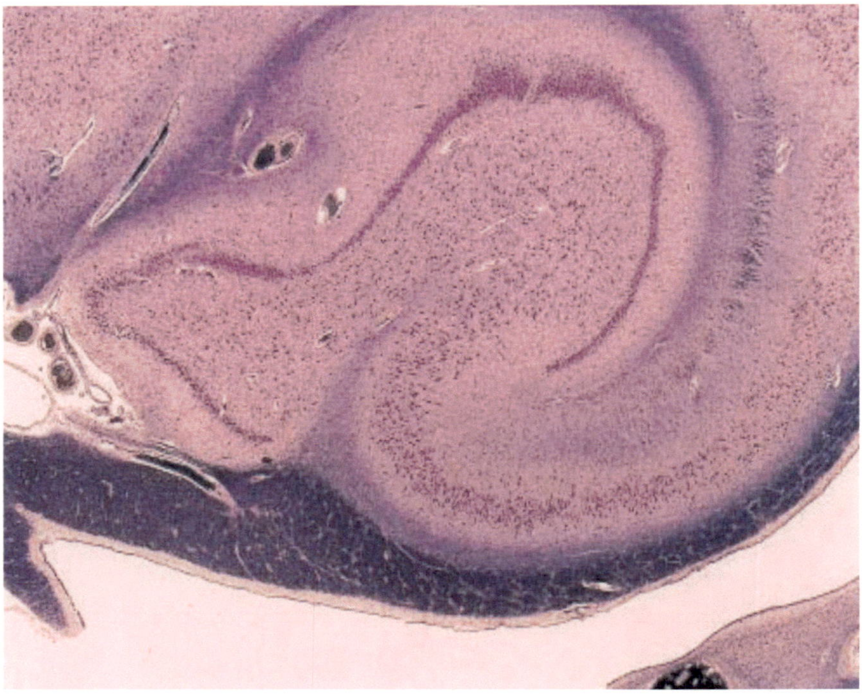

Fig. 5. The dentate gyrus and the four sectors of ammon's horn (cresyl violet stain; Armstrong et al, 2007).

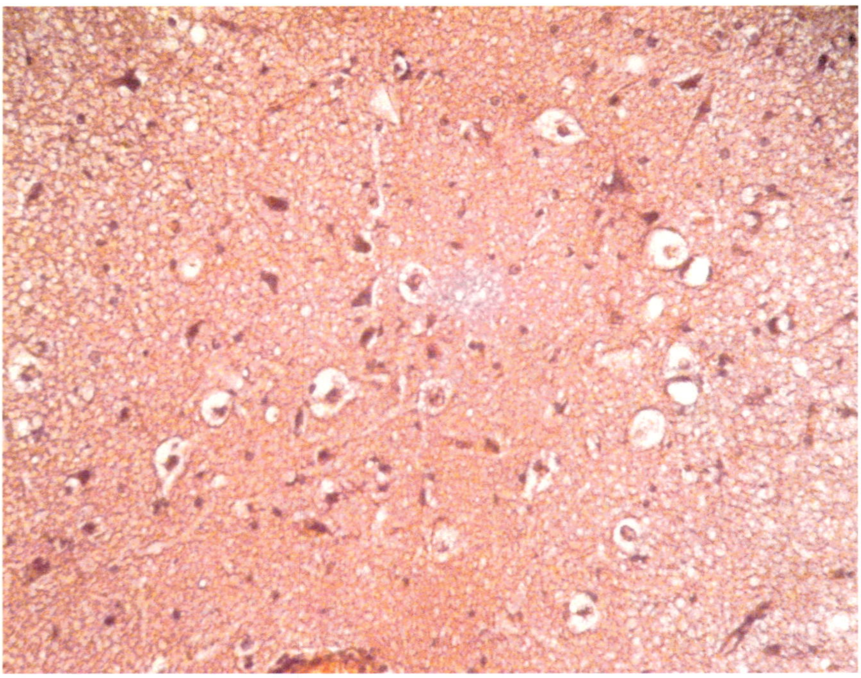

Fig. 6. Cluster of injured vacuolated neurons (HE stain).

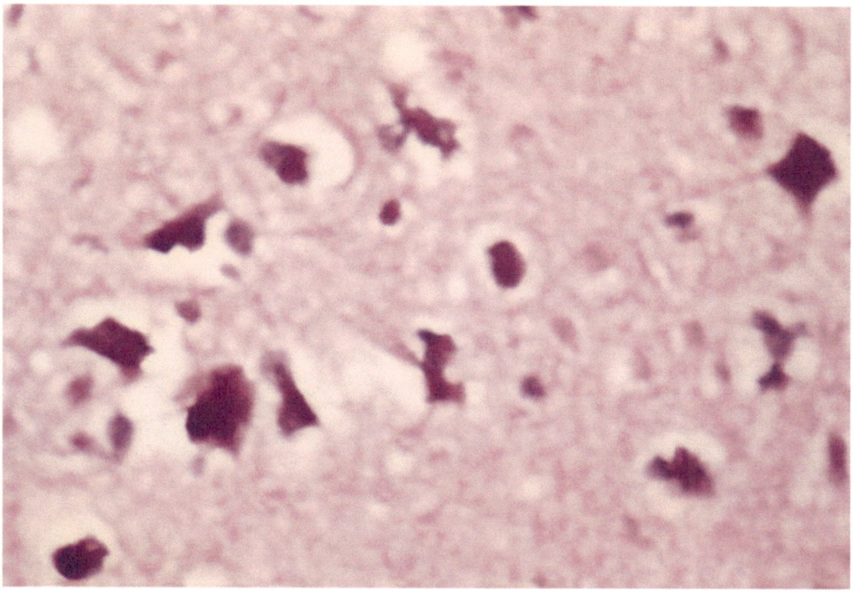

Fig. 7. Cluster of injured neurons revealing variation in sizes, vacuolization, shrinking, apoptosis, lysis, and intracytoplasmic PAS^+ material (PAS stain)

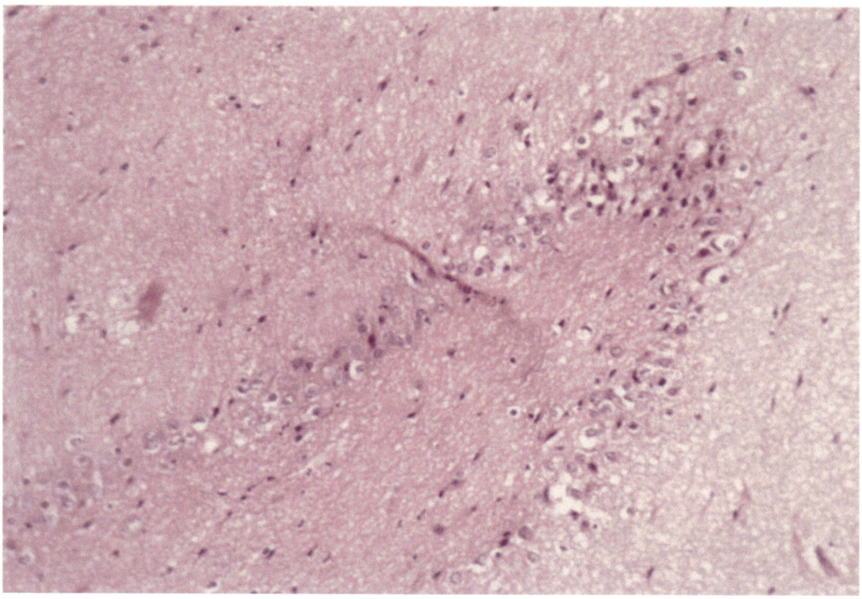

Fig. 8. Quasi complete loss of pyramidal cells in CA1 sector, with signs of neuron injury in the dentate gyrus (CA2 sector) with vacuolization, balloonization and loss of the granular neurons (HE stain).

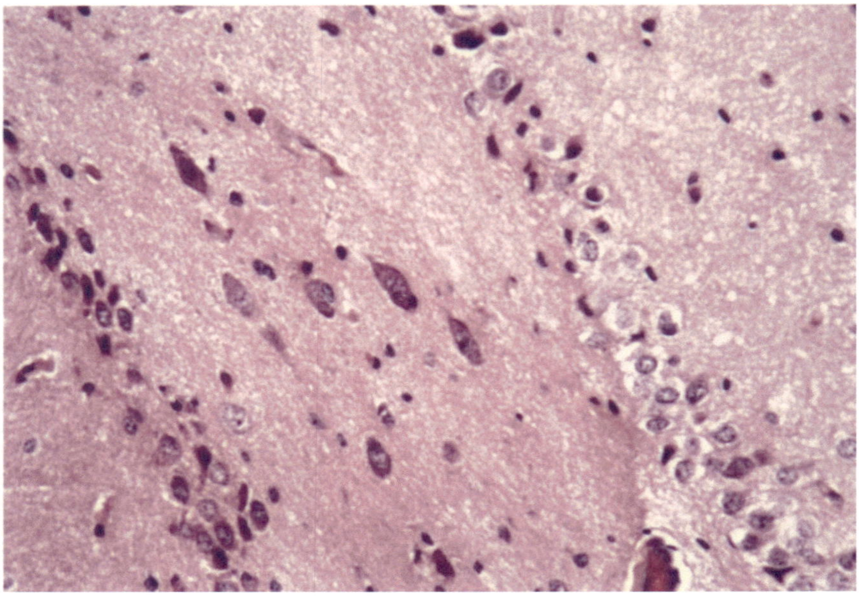

Fig. 9. Neuronal injury in the granular cells of the dentate gyrus (CA2 sector) with atypical and giant pyramidal neurons in CA1 sector. Abnormal intracytoplasmic inclusions are also noted (HE stain).

bifocal, multifocal, or associated with each other, with transitional zones or "composite tumors" as described by some other authors (Prayson et al, 1999; Al Khani & Assaad, 2008) (fig.12). The juxtaposition of these tumors, and the transition between DNETs, gangliogliomas, or hamartomatous glioneuronal lesions might support the hypothesis that all these tumors are of hamartomatous origin. The relationship and the transition between these lesions have also been reported other authors (Hirose et al, 1998; Moreno et al, 2001).

2.5 Inflammation

Different causes of inflammatory changes are described in the cases of epilepsy; the most famous is Rasmussen's encephalitis that is frequently reported in series of epilepsy (Frater et al, 2000; Prayson et al, 1999; Al Khani & Assaad, 2008) It is defined by lymphoid infiltration of the cerebrocortical perivascular compartment and neuropil, microglial nodule formation, astrogliosis, and variable neuronal loss. Cytomegalovirus and herpes virus HSV1 are found in some cases.(Jay et al, 1995).

Inflammation caused by protozoan, parasites, and brain abscess was sometimes accompanied by seizures (Armstrong et al, 2007). Chronic encephalitis without evidence of pathogenic agent is sometimes reported (Prayson et al, 1999; Al Khani & Assaad, 2008) .

2.6 Ischemic and hemorrhagic disorders

Ischemic changes and infarct were reported in some series; this might results in severe atrophy (fig. 13). Abnormal blood supply was noted by some authors (Al Khani & Assaad, 2008; Fratel et al, 2000; Li et al, 1999; Prayson et al, 1999; Bernhardt et al, 2009). Hematomas were associated in some series with chronic epilepsy (Hisada et al, 1999; Al Khani & Assad, 2008).

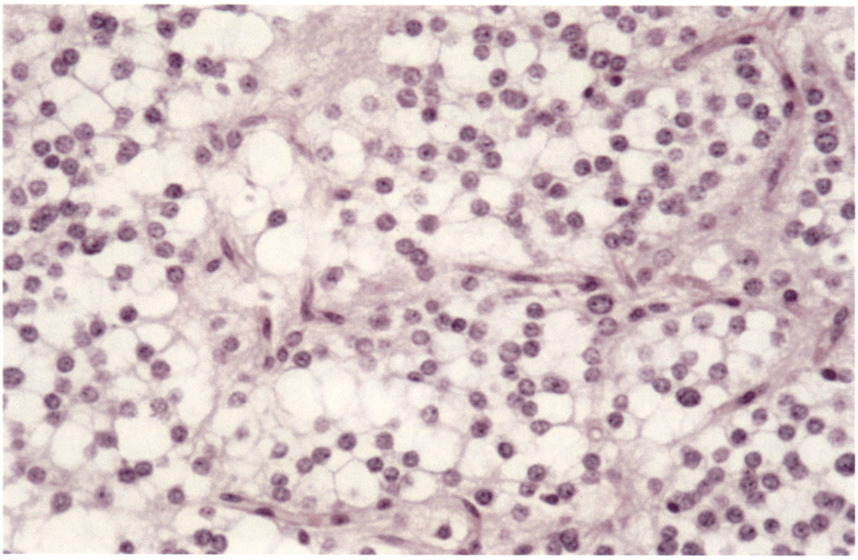

Fig. 10. Dysembryoplastic neuroepithelial tumor is a common tumor found in epileptic cases.

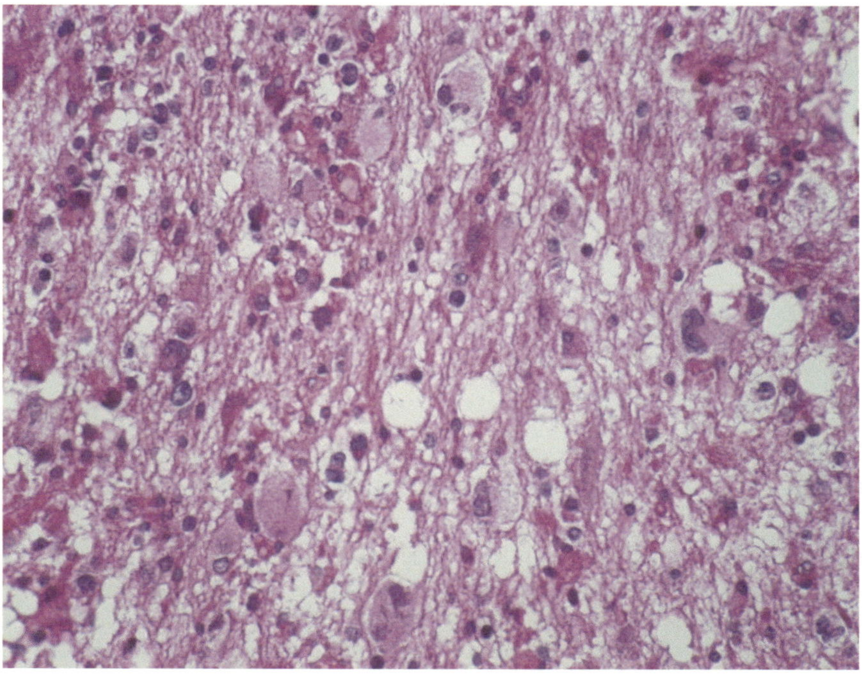

Fig. 11. Xanthoastrocytoma is a rare low-grade glial tumor that can constitute an epileptogenic focus.

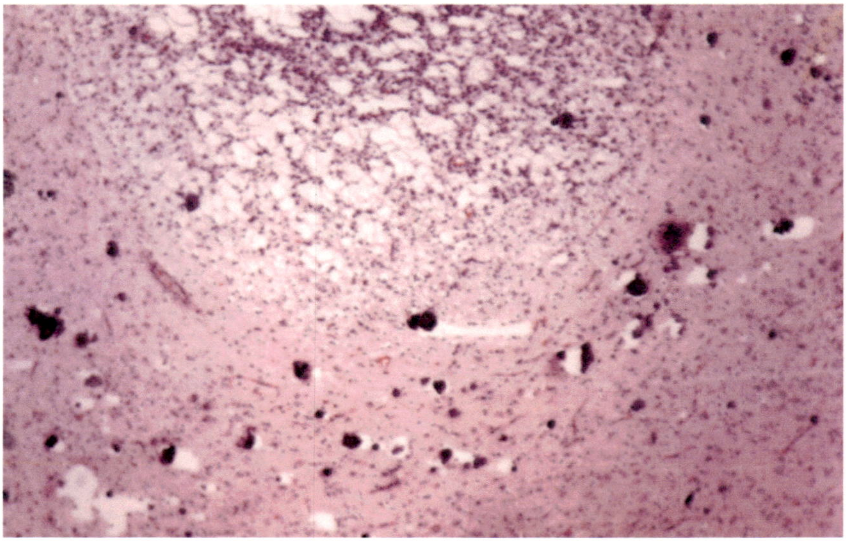

Fig. 12. Dysembryoplastic neuroepithelial tumor at the upper side of the figure, showing transition to ganglioglioma; reinforcing the malformative nature of these tumors.

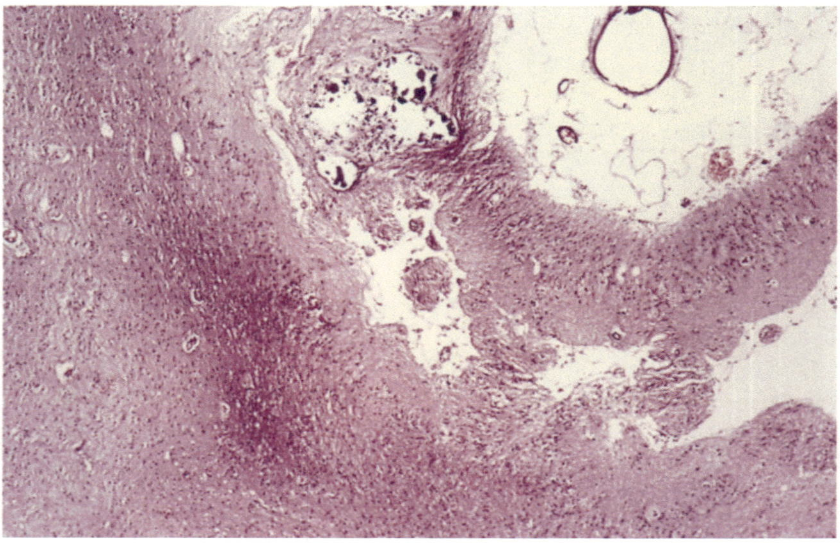

Fig. 13. Severe atrophy of the temporal lobe and the hippocampus due to atypical vascularization. Focal calcification is noted at the middle upper part of the figure (HE stain).

2.7 Metabolic disorders, vacuolization, and cystic changes

This was represented by vacuolar degeneration of neurons and glial cells (fig. 14), and cystic changes of the cortical, subcortical or glial tissue, reaching many centimeters in some cases where they could be detected on the macroscopic examination of the cut section; otherwise, they were microscopic findings. Cystic changes of the nervous tissue were constant observations in some refractory epilepsy series; thought they are considered as non-specific findings. These cysts were not alcianophilic, PAS stain was also negative (Al Khani &

Assaad, 2008). Progressive metabolic changes were noted, occurring during the development of hippocampal sclerosis in a model of mesial temporal lobe epilepsy (Bouilleret et al, 2000) The progress of metabolic or pathologic abnormalities of temporal lobe epilepsy may not be altered by adequate seizure control, as the presence of an epileptogenic focus might be associated with progressive neuronal injury even in clinically well-controlled patients (Spanaki et al, 2000) This might explain the exacerbation of neuronal damage and nervous tissue injuries with all the pathological changes constantly observed. Some authors found that hippocampal cell loss results in decreased efferent synaptic activity and neuronal activity in the thalamus and basal ganglia, and subcortical hypometabolism, which may reinforce the epileptogenic potential of the mesial temporal lobe discharge (Dlugos et al, 1999). In a studied series of refractory epilepsy, signs of metabolic disorders were noted in all of the cases (Al Khani & Assaad, 2008).

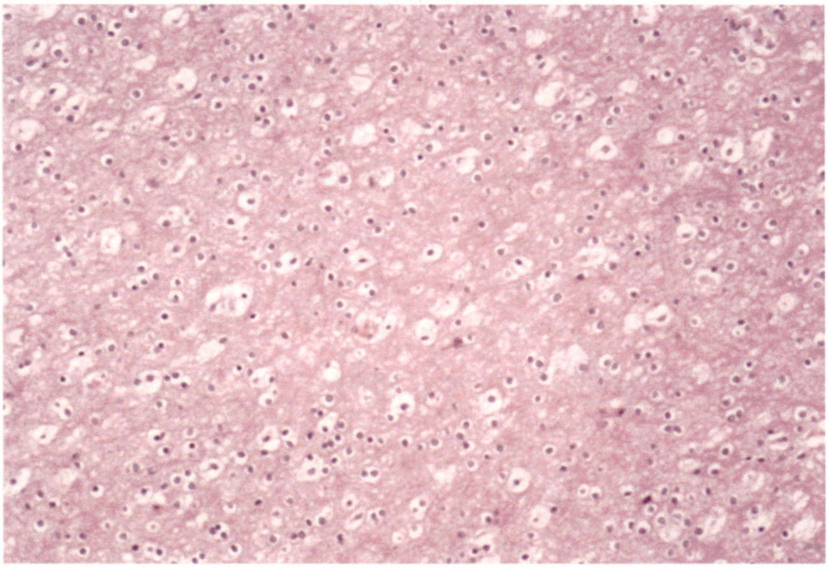

Fig. 14. Vacuolization of the glial cells in the temporal lobe and hippocampus (HE stain).

2.8 Northern epilepsy

Other authors found intraneuronal accumulation of cytoplasmic autofluorescent granules in which is called as northern epilepsy (Herva et al, 2000).

2.9 Sclerosis/gliosis

Gliosis is noted in all of the reported series of epilepsy with various degrees. Some investigators view hippocampal sclerosis as the primary cause of temporal lobe epilepsy, whereas others interpret the changes to be the result of chronic seizure activity. The macroscopic and radiological term of hippocampal sclerosis is interpreted, on histopathological examination, as astrogliosis associated with neuronal loss (Rushing et al, 1997; Prayson et al, 1999). Astrogliosis or oligoastrogliosis (fig 15) was observed, in varying degrees, in the temporal lobe and hippocampus in all cases of drug resistant epilepsy in some series (Al Khani & Assaad, 2008), even in patients with no remarkable abnormalities on MRI in the temporal lobe, but with an irregular hippocampal signal on MRI. Cortical gliosis, especially subpial gliosis (fig 4) was always accompanied by advanced cortical dysplasia; this leads to believe that progressive gliosis might be a reactive process induced by neuronal injury and loss, seizure attacks, and metabolic disorders. Sclerosis/gliosis might be considered as the end-stage of the all modifications. Focal oligogliosis is sometimes noted (fig 16).

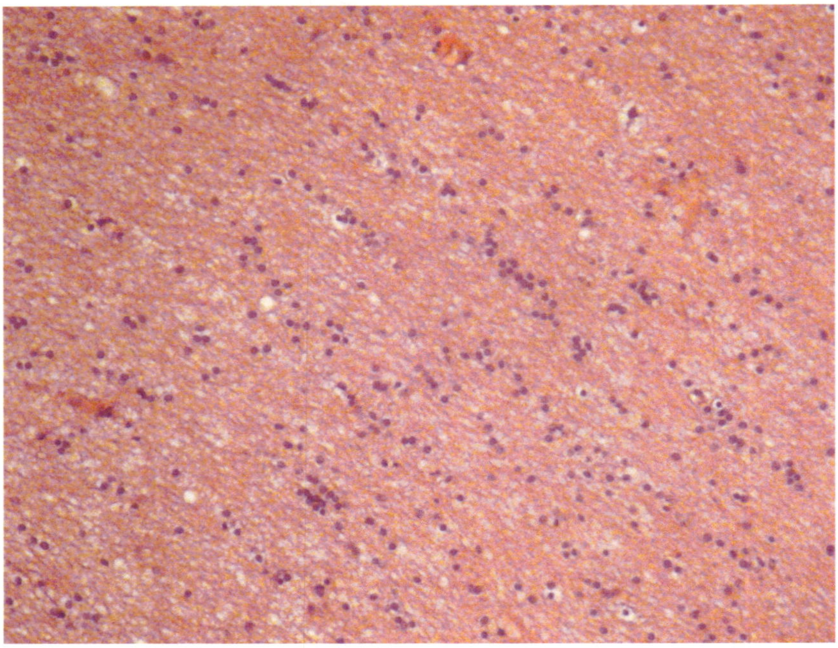

Fig. 15. Oligoastrogliosis in the white matter (HE stain).

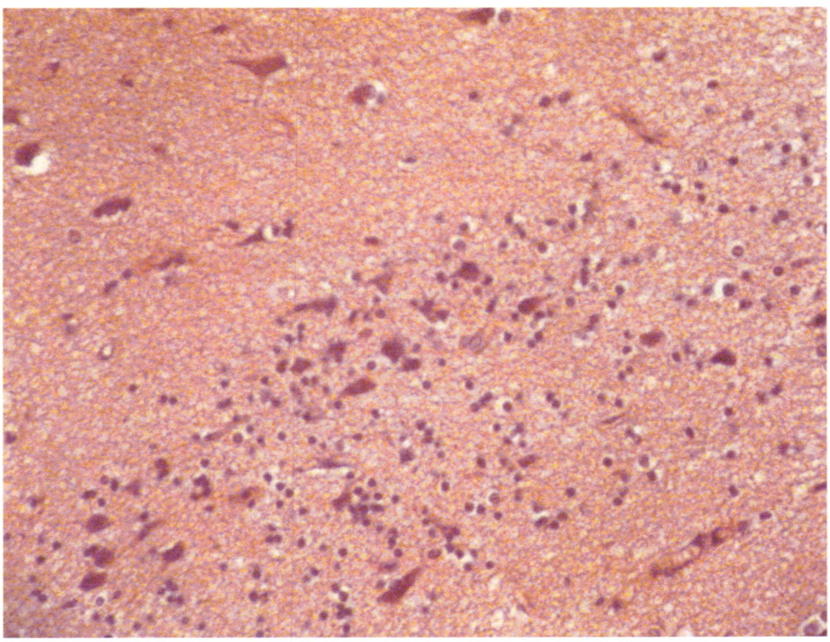

Fig. 16. Focal oligogliosis in a heterotopic subependymal cortical nodule (HE stain).

3. Combinations of lesions: "Dual pathology"

Some authors mentioned that seizure attacks require dual pathology, as several observations revealed combinations of lesions (Jay et al, 1994; Oda et al, 1998; Juhsz et al, 1999; Li et al, 1999; Prayson et al, 2010); for example, the coexistence of brain tumors and cortical dysplasia, neuronal migration disorders and low grade gliomas, lesions having both neoplastic and malformed foci, extrahippocampal lesion plus hippocampal atrophy, and coexistence of hippocampal sclerosis and a potentially epileptogenic cortical lesion. It was also reported that bilateral hippocampal atrophy was found frequently in patients with temporal lobe developmental malformations, and that the presence of bilateral amygdala or amygdalo-hippocampal atrophy was associated with a higher risk of seizure recurrence (Kuzniescky et al, 1999). The multifocality of malformative lesions was well reported by some authors (Wolf et al, 1995; Moreno et al, 2001; Armstrong et al, 2007). In our series (Al Khani & Assaad, 2008) dual pathology was well documented as tumors were always present in association with other changes, that were almost always seen: cortical dysplasia, astrogliosis, cystic changes, and neuron injury and loss. The presence of bifocal or multifocal tumors and/or hamartomas was another observation to be noted.

4. Conclusion

A wide variety of lesions is documented in histopathological study of the temporal lobe and the hippocampus in temporal epilepsy, especially pharmacoresistant epilepsy. Some lesions were constantly present; cortical disorganization, neuron injury and loss, and gliosis. A presumable epileptogenic focus as hamartoma or tumoral lesion is frequently observed. Multiplicity and multifocality of lesions are well documented, reinforcing the hypothesis that the presence of an epileptogenic focus provokes a process of progressive damage of the nervous tissue. The good understanding of these processes and their sequencing, especially those leading to neuron death and loss, might contribute in the prevention of progression of epileptic seizure and the damage of nervous tissue in previously susceptible patients.

5. References

Al Khani, R., Assaad, F., (2008). Histopathological findings in chronic pharmacoresistant temporal epilepsy: A pathognomonic combination of lesions maintaining neuron injury? *Pan Arab Journal of Neurosurgery*, Vol.12, No.2, (October), pp. 86-93, ISSN 1319-6995

Armstrong, D., Halliday, W., Hawkins, C., & Takashima, S., (2007). Epilepsy, *Pediatric Neuropathology: A Text Atlas*, pp. 376-384, Springer, ISBN 978-4-431-70246-7, Tokyo, Berlin, Heidlberg, New York

Barbosa Coutinho, L.M., Hilbig, A, Calcagnotto, M.E., et al., (1999). Neuropathology of hard to control epilepsy. Study of 300 consecutive cases. *Arqivos de Neuro-psiquiatria, Vol.57, No.2B,* (June), pp. 405-14, ISSN 0004-282X

Becker, A.J., Gillardon, F., Blümcke. I, Langendrfer, D., Beck, H., Wiestler, O.D., (1999). Differential regulation of apoptosis-related genes in resistant and vulnerable subfields of the rat epileptic hippocampus. *Brain Research and Molecular Brain Research, Vol 67, No.1,* (April), pp. 172-6, ISSN 0165-0173

Bernasconi, A., Bernasconi, N, Bernhardt B.C., Schrader, D., (2011). Advances in MRI for 'Cryptogenic' Epilepsy: Histopathology of cortical dysplasia. *Nature Reviews.*

Neurology, Vol.7, No.2, pp. 99-108. Accessed on 20 March, 2011. Available from http://www.medscape.com/viewarticle/737007_2

Bernhardt, B.C., Rozen, D.A., Worsley, K.J., et al., (2009). Longitudinal and cross-sectional analysis of atrophy in pharmacoresistant temporal lobe epilepsy. *Neurology,* Vol.72, No.20, pp. 1747-54, ISSN 0028-3878

Bouilleret, V., Boyet, S., Marescaux, C., Nehlig, A., (2000). Mapping of the progressive metabolic changes occurring during the development of hippocampal sclerosis in a model of mesial temporal lobe epilepsy. *Brain Research,* No. 852, (January), pp. 255-62, ISSN 0006-8993

Chevassus au Louis, N., Baraban, SC., Gaïarsa J.L., Ben Ari, Y., (1999). Cortical Malformations and epilepsy: new insights from animal models. *Epilepsia,* Vol. 40. No.7, (July), pp. 811-21, ISSN 0013-9580

Dlugos, D.J., Jaggi, J., O'Connor, W.M., et al., (1999). Hippocampal cell density and subcortical metabolism in temporal lobe epilepsy. *Epilepsia,* Vol.40., No.4, (April), pp. 408-13, ISSN 0013-9580

d'Orsi, G., Tinuper, P., Bisulli, F., et al., (2004). A. Clinical features and long term outcome of epilepsy in periventricular nodular heterotopia. Simple compared with plus forms. *Journal of Neurology, Neurosurgery, and Psychiatry,* Vol.75, No.6, (June), pp. 873-8, ISSN 0022-3050

El Bahh, B., Lespinet, V., Lurton, D., Coussemacq, M., Le Gal La Salle, G., Rougier, A., (1999). Correlations between granule cell dispersion, mossy fiber sprouting, and hippocampal cell loss in temporal lobe epilepsy. *Epilepsia,* Vol.40, No.10, (October), pp. 1393-401, ISSN 0013-9580

Frater, J.L., Prayson, R.A., Morris III, H.H., Bingaman, W.E., (2000). Surgical pathologic findings of extratemporal-based intractable epilepsy: a study of 133 consecutive resections. *Archives of Pathology & Laboratory Medecine,* Vol.142, No.4, (April), pp. 545-9, ISSN 0003-9985

Fritschy, J.M., Kiener, T., Bouilleret, V., Loup, F., (1999). GABAergic neurons and GABA(A)-receptors in temporal lobe epilepsy. *Neurochemistry International, Vol.34, No.5,* (May), pp. 435-45, ISSN 0197-0186

Garbelli, R., Munari, C., De Biasi, S., et al., (1999). Taylor's cortical dysplasia: a confocal and ultrastructural immunohistochemical study. *Brain Pathololgy, Vol.9, No.3,* (July), pp. 445-61, ISSN 1015-6305

Gyure, K.A., Sandberg, G.D., Prayson, R.A., Morrison, A.L., Armstrong, R.C., Wong, K., (2000). Dysembryoplastic neuroepithelial tumor: an immunohistochemical study with myelin oligodendrocyte glycoprotein. *Archives of Pathology & Laboratory Medecine,* Vol. 124. No.1, (January),pp. 123-6, ISSN 0003-9985

Henshall, D.C., Schindler, C.K., So, N.K., et al., (2004). Death-associated protein kinase expression in human temporal lobe epilepsy. *Annals of Neurology,* Vo.55, No.4, (April), pp. 485-94, ISSN 0364-5134

Herva, R., Tyynel, J., Hirvasniemi, A., Syrjkallio Ylitalo, M., Haltia, M., (2000). Northern epilepsy: a novel form of neuronal ceroid-lipofuscinosis. *Brain Pathology,* Vol.10, No.2, (April), pp. 215-22, ISSN 1015-6305

Hirose, T., Scheithauer, B.W., (1998). Mixed dysembryoplastic neuroepithelial tumor and ganglioglioma. *Acta Neuropathologica (Berl),* Vol. 95, No.6, (June), pp. 650-54, ISSN 0001-6322

Hisada K., Morioka, T., Nishio, S., Amano, T., Iwaki, T., Fukui, M., (1999). Temporal lobe epilepsy associated with old intracerebral hemorrhage due to capillary telangiectasis in the temporal lobe: case report. *No To Shinkei,* Vol.51, No.8, (August), pp. 729-35, ISSN 0006-8969

Jay, V., Becker, L.E., Otsubo, I.H., et al., (1995). Chronic encephalitis and epilepsy (Rasmussen's encephalitis): detection of cytomegalovirus and herpes simplex I by polymerase chain reaction and in-situ hybridization. *Journal of Neurology,* No.45, pp. 108, ISSN 0340-5354

Jay, V. & Becker, L.E., (1994). Surgical pathology of epilepsy: a review. *Pediatric Pathology & Molecular Medicine, Vol.14, No.4,* (July), pp. 731-50, ISSN 1522-7952

Juhsz, C., Nagy, F., Muzik, O., Watson, C., Shah J., Chugani H.T., (1999). [11C]Flumazenil PET in patients with epilepsy with dual pathology. *Epilepsia,* Vol.40, No.5, (May), pp. 566-74, ISSN 0013-9580

Kuzniecky, R., Ho, S.S., Martin, R., et al., (1999). Temporal lobe developmental Malformations and hippocampal sclerosis: epilepsy surgical outcome. *Neurology,* Vol.52, No.3, (February), pp. 479-84, ISSN 0028-3878

Li, L.M., Cendes, F., Andermann F., et al., (1999). Surgical outcome in patients with epilepsy and dual pathology. *Brain,* No.122, (Pt 5), (May), pp. 799-805, ISSN 0006-8950

Louis, D.N., Ohgaki, H., Wiestler, O.D., Cavenee, W.K., (Eds.), (2007). *WHO Classification of Tumors of the Central Nervous System,* 4th edition., IARC, ISBN 978-92-832-2430-2, Lyon, France

Marin-Padilla, M., (1999). Developmental neuropathology and impact of perinatal brain damage. III: gray matter lesions in the neocortex. *Journal of Neuropathology and Exp Neurology,* May, 58(5):407-29, ISSN 0022-3069

Mathern, G.W., Babb, T.L., Mischel, P.S., et al., (1996). Childhood generalized and mesial temporal epilepsies demonstrate different amounts and patterns of hippocampal neuron loss and mossy fiber synaptic reorganization. *Brain,* No.119, (Pt.3), (June), pp. 965-87, ISSN 0006-8950

Moreno, A., de Felipe, J., Garcia Sola, R., Navarro, A., Ramon, y., Cajal, S., (2001). Neuronal and mixed neuronal glial tumors associated to epilepsy. A heterogeneous and related group of tumours. *Histology and Histopathology, Vol.16, No.2, (*April), pp. 613-22, ISSN 0213-3911

Niquet J., Wasterlain, C.G., (2004). Bim, Bad, and Bax: a deadly combination in epileptic seizures. *The Journal of Clinical Investigation,* Vol.113, No.7, (April), pp. 960-2, ISSN 0021-9738

15. Oda, M., Arai, N., Maehara, T., Shimizu, H., Kojima, H., Yagishita, A., (1998). Brain tumors in surgical neuropathology of intractable epilepsies, with special reference to cerebral dysplasias. *Brain Tumor Pathology,* Vol.15, No.1, pp. 41-51, ISSN 1433-7398

Palmini, A., Najm, I., Avanzini, G., et al., (2004). Terminology and classification of the cortical dysplasias. Neurology, No.62, pp. S2-S8, ISSN 0028-3878

Prayson, R.A., Estes, M.L., (1995). Cortical dysplasia: a histopathologic study of 52 cases of partial lobectomy in patients with epilepsy. *Human Pathology, Vol.26, No.5, (*May), pp. 503-500, ISSN 0046-8177

Prayson, R.A., Reith, J.D., Najm, I.M., (1996). Mesial temporal sclerosis. A clinicopathologic study of 27 patients, including 5 with coexistent cortical dysplasia. *Archives of Pathology & Laboratory Medecine,* Vol.120, *No.6,* (June), pp. 532-6, ISSN 0003-9985

Prayson, R.A., Bingaman, W., Frater, J.L., Wyllie, E., (1999). Histopathologic findings in 37 cases of functional hemispherectomy. *Annals of Diagnostic Pathology, Vol.3, No.4, (*August), pp. 205-12, ISSN 1092-9134

Prayson, R.A., (1999) Composite ganglioglioma and dysembryoplastic neuroepithelial tumor. *Archives of Pathology & Laboratory Medicine,* Vol.123, *No.3,* (March), pp. 247-50, ISSN 0003-9985

Prayson, R.A., Fong, J., Najm, I., (2010). Coexistent pathology in chronic epilepsy patients with neoplasms. *Modern pathology, No.*23, pp. 1097-1103, ISSN 0893-3952

Proper, E.A., Oestreicher, A.B., Jansen, G.H., et al., (2000). Immunohistochemical characterization of mossy fiber sprouting in the hippocampus of patients with pharmaco-resistant temporal lobe epilepsy. *Brain,* No.123, (Pt 1), (January), pp. 19-30, ISSN 0006-8950

Rosemberg, S., & Vieira, G.S., (1998). Dysembryoplastic neuroepithelial tumor. An epidemiological study from a single institution. *Arqivos de Neuro-psiquiatria, Vol.56, No.2,* (June), pp. 232-6, ISSN 0004-282X

Rushing, E.J., Barnard, J.J., Bigio, E.H., Eagan, K.P., & White, C.L. 3rd, (1997). Frequency of unilateral and bilateral mesial temporal sclerosis in primary and secondary epilepsy: a forensic autopsy study. *The American Journal of Forensic Medicine and Pathology, Vol.18, No.4,* (December), pp. 335-41, ISSN 0195-7910

Sisodiya, S.M., (2004). Malformations of cortical development: burdens and insights from important causes of human epilepsy. *The Lancet Neurology,* Vol.3, No.1, (January), pp. 29-38, ISSN 1474-4422

Spreafico R, Pasquier B, Minotti L, et al., (1998). Immunocytochemical investigation on dysplastic human tissue from epileptic patients. *Epilepsy Research, Vol.32, No.1-2,* (September), pp. 34-48, ISSN 0920-1211

Spanaki, M.V., Kopylev, L., Liow, K., DeCarli, C., et al., (2000). Relationship of seizure frequency to hippocampus volume and metabolism in temporal lobe epilepsy. *Epilepsia,* Vol.41, No.9, (September), pp. 1227-9, ISSN 0013-9580

Uysal H, Cevik IU, Soylemezoglu F, et al., (2003) Is the cell death in mesial temporal sclerosis apoptotic? *Epilepsia,* Vol.44, No.6, (June), pp. 778-84, ISSN 0013-9580

Volk, E.E, Prayson, R.A. (1997). Hamartomas in the setting of chronic epilepsy: a clinicopathologic study of 13 cases. *Human Pathology, Vol.28, No.2,* (February), pp. 227-32, ISSN 0046-8177

Wang, V.Y., Chang, E.F., Barbaro, & N.M., (2006). Focal cortical dysplasia: A review of pathological features, Genetics, and surgical outcome. Neurosurgery Focus, Vol.20, No.1, ISSN 1092-0684. Accessed on 21 Mar 2011. Available from: www.medscape.com/viewarticle/522325.

Whittle, I.R, Dow, G.R., Lammie, G.A., & Wardlaw J., (1999). Dsyembryoplastic neuroepithelial tumour with discrete bilateral multifocality: further evidence for a germinal origin. *British Journal of Neurosurgery, Vol.13, No.5,* (October), pp. 508-11, ISSN 0268-8697

Wolf HK., Wellmer J., Muller M.B., Wiestler O.D., Hufnagel A., & Pietsch, T., (1995). Glioneuronal malformative lesions and dysembryoplastic neuroepithelial tumors in patients with chronic pharmacoresistant epilepsies. *Journal of Neuropathology and Experimental Neurology,* Vol.54, No.2, (March), pp. 245-54, ISSN 0022-3069

Wolf, H.K.& Wiestler, O.D., (1993) Surgical pathology of chronic epileptic seizure disorders. *Brain Pathology, No.4,* (October 3), pp. 371-80, ISSN 1015-6305

Wolf, H.K., Birkholz, T., Wellmer, J., Blumcke, I., Pietsch, T., Wiestler, O.D., (1995) Neurochemical profile of glioneuronal lesions from patients with pharmacoresistant focal epilepsies. *Journal of Neuropathology and Experimental Neurology,* Vol.54, No.5, (September), pp. 689-97, ISSN 0022-3069

Zix, C., Billard, C., Motte, J., (1999) Epilepsy due to mesiotemporal sclerosis in children: 10 cases. *Archives de Pediatrie, Vol.6, No.*4, (April), pp. 398-405, ISSN 0929-693X

2

The Role of Astrocytes in Epileptogenesis

Jesús Pastor[1,2] and Rafael G. Sola[1,3]
[1]*Epilepsy Unit, Hospital Universitario La Princesa*
[2]*Faculty of Medicine, Universidad San Pablo-CEU*
[3]*Faculty of Medicine, UAM, Madrid*
Spain

1. Introduction

Epilepsy is a major neurological disorder that affects 0.5-2.0% of the global population (Hauser, 1998; Picot et al.; 2008). The term "epilepsy" likely encompasses a number of various etiological and pathophysiological processes. The International League Against Epilepsy (ILAE) has classified the epilepsies as being either focal or generalized. In all likelihood, this classification implies different causes and anatomical/functional substrates. Epileptogenesis (the processes by which epilepsy develops within an otherwise normal brain) probably differs for the various types of epilepsy (Lüders, 2008). In this sense, epileptogenesis of (for example) temporal lobe epilepsy (TLE) with hippocampal sclerosis (HS), would be different from that observed in patients with cortical dysplasia; this would hold true for other cryptogenic or idiopathic focal epilepsies as well. Therefore, to date, it has not been possible to establish a unique underlying cause or mechanism that is involved in the transition from normal to epileptic cortical tissue, although there are several hypotheses to explain the different types of seizures and epilepsies.

From a therapeutic point of view, the epilepsies in humans can be divided into pharmaco sensitive and pharmaco resistant. In the former, the patient is successfully treated by one or more anti-epileptic drugs (AED). Nearly two-thirds of patients respond to anticonvulsant therapy. However, in a significant percentage of patients, the seizures cannot be controlled by drugs, despite verifying both maximal dosage and an adequate treatment duration. The percentages of medical intractability among epileptic patients are: focal epilepsy, 24%; idiopathic epilepsy, 9.3%; and catastrophic epilepsy, 66.7% (Lardizabal, 2008). In some cases, a viable therapeutic option is surgery. Generally, the candidates for this treatment are patients who suffer from focal or partial epilepsy. In these patients, it is possible—at least in theory—to identify a well-defined area of the cortex that is responsible for the seizures; this is known as the epileptic zone (EZ). From an operational point of view, the EZ is defined as the region in which excision or disconnection relieves the patient from seizures. This option frequently involves removing the brain section where the EZ is located, and this possibility offers a unique opportunity to gain access to the real processes (the neural networks, membrane properties and synaptic dynamics) underlying partial epilepsy in human patients.

TLE is the most common form of partial epilepsy in adults and is usually drug-resistant (Engel 2001; Wieser, 2004). This type of pathology is frequently associated with a salient pathological condition called hippocampal sclerosis (see Figure 1 -Kuzniecky et al.; 1987).

For several decades, HS has been considered the source of the electrical events that cause spontaneous seizures (Falconer, 1974; Spencer 1998). However, HS is found in approximately 40-65% of patients who undergo surgery for TLE (de Lanerolle et al.; 2003), and whether hippocampal sclerosis is the cause or the consequence of repeated seizures is still a matter of debate (Jefferys, 1999; Boison, 2008). The progression of epileptogenesis to chronic epilepsy often leads to pharmacoresistance and affects up to 30% of all patients with epilepsy, particularly those with TLE (Engel, 2001).

A wide range of brain injuries and brain lesions are associated with an increased risk of epilepsy. In fact, such symptomatic etiologies account for 30-49% of all unprovoked seizures and epilepsy (Herman, 2002). The most common risk factors are cerebrovascular disease (21%), tumor (11%) and traumatic brain injury (7%) (Forsgren, 1990). A feature that is common to all of these conditions is the compromised permeability of the blood-brain barrier (BBB). Although idiopathic epilepsy accounts for up to 65% of cases, these patients likely share some pathophysiological mechanisms with injury-induced epilepsies.

Much is known regarding neuronal electrophysiology in epileptic tissues (Avoli et al.; 2005; Pastor et al.; 2006); however, there is little information regarding the transition from a normal brain to an epileptic brain. Recently, it was shown in both rats and humans that astrocytes could be involved in some types of partial seizure (de Lanerolle et al.; 2010). Astrocytes are situated in key pivotal places that may play a role in epilepsy in several ways. Indeed, astrocytes control the trafficking of substances between capillary vessels and neurons. Another important function is in the homeostasis of extracellular ions, principally potassium (K^+), which is directly involved in neuronal excitability. Finally, astrocytes are mediators of the neuron-to-neuron synapse through the tripartite synapse. In addition to astrocytes, another important factor is a change in the permeability of the BBB, which is formed by endothelial cells, although glial cells contribute yet to its function.

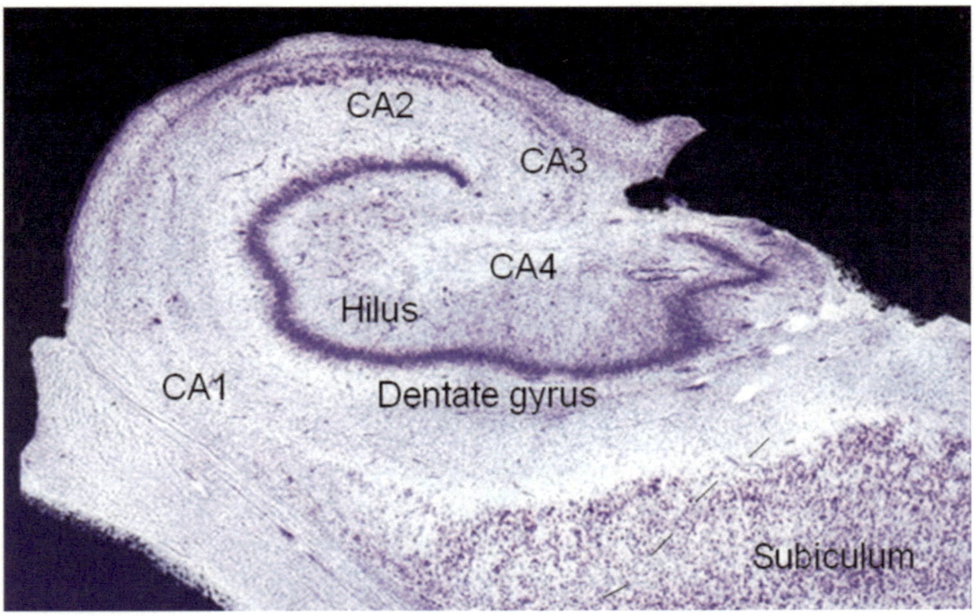

Fig. 1. Microphotograph of a Nissl-stained hippocampus obtained from a patient who underwent surgery for TLE. A loss of cells is evident in the CA1, CA3 and hilus regions.

Albumin, the most abundant protein in blood, has also been implicated in epileptogenesis (Seiffert et al.; 2004; Herrera-Peco et al.; 2008) together with changes in BBB permeability or the inflammatory cascade, although the role of these mechanisms in epilepsy are still poorly understood (de Lanerolle et al.; 2010). Although not conclusive, different results point to astrocytes as being important mediators of the mechanisms involved in epileptogenesis and the origin and spreading of seizures. In this chapter, we review some of the recent theories and results concerning these topics, with a special emphasis on results obtained from human patients. We shall analyze the role of BBB permeability in the leakage of albumin into the brain's extracellular space and the possible role of this protein in the activation of astrocytes. Although other reviews have focused on the role of the TGF-β receptor (TGF-βR) in the action of albumin, we shall review a putative role for a different albumin receptor that is currently not well characterized but clearly has different properties than TGF-βR.

2. A brief introduction to astrocyte physiology

Glial cells outnumber neurons by approximately 10-50:1. Glial cells can be divided into two major classes called microglia and macroglia.

- Microglia are phagocytes that mobilize in response to brain injury (for example, infection or disease). From a physiological and embryological point of view, they are unrelated to the others cells of the nervous system. Microglia are activated and recruited during infection, seizure and injury or disease, including multiple sclerosis, stroke, acquired immunodeficiency syndrome (AIDS)-related dementia and Parkinson's disease. In this regard, microglia serve as major antigen-presenting cells.
- Macroglia comprise three different types of cells:
  - Oligodendrocytes and Schwann cells are located in the Central Nervous System (CNS) and Peripheral Nervous System (PNS), respectively. Both cell types provide insulation for neuronal axons. Each oligodendrocyte envelops an average of 15 axonal internodes. However, each Schwann cell envelops only one internode on a single axon. The insulation provided by these cells is necessary for saltatory nerve conduction (Donaldson & Mia-Sin Wu, 2001).
  - Astrocytes are the most numerous glial cells and tend to have long processes, some of which terminate as end-feet on the surface of neurons and, among other things, supply nutrients. Some astrocytes project their end-feet to capillaries, where they help endothelial cells form the BBB. However, their exact definition and the types of astrocytes that exist remain incompletely understood (Haydon & Carmignoto, 2006; de Lanerolle et al.; 2010).

Traditionally, the main role of astrocytes has been considered to be to provide support to neurons (Barres, 1991). However, over the previous decades, astrocytes have been found to play several roles other than supportive. Seminal works showed that astrocytes express receptors for neurotransmitters (Porter & McCarthy, 1997) and can respond to a local application of glutamate with a calcium elevation that travels as a wave through a syncytium (Corner-Bell et al.; 1990). Together, these data suggest that astrocytes possess the capacity to signal using spike-like calcium transients. In fact, these calcium spikes can travel over long distances and serve as a tool for communication.

Astrocytes are normally identified by their expression of glial fibrillary acidic protein (GFAP). However, glial cells can be further categorized according to their functional properties as follows (Matthias et al.; 2003, Wallraff et al.; 2004; Jabs et al.; 2008):

- Cells with large outward K^+ current and attenuated inward K^+ current (I_{Kir}). The resting potential (V_r) of these cells is therefore relatively depolarized (~-31 mV). Most of these cells contain TTX-sensitive Na^+ currents but are unable to generate action potentials. These cells express alpha-amino-3-hydroxy-5-methyl-4-isoxazolepropionic acid (AMPA) type receptors (GluR), but not glutamate transporter currents. Finally, these cells completely lack gap junction coupling but receive spontaneous synaptic input from glutamatergic and γ-aminobutyric acid neurons (GABAergic).
- Cells that resemble protoplasmic astrocytes. These cells have a more negative V_r (~-70 mV), and I_{Kir} is present. These cells express glutamate transporter currents (GluT) but not GluR currents. Finally, these cells are extensively coupled via gap junctions.
- A third cell type closely resembles the GluR cell type described above. These are considered a third class of macroglia and have various names, including neuron glia-2 (NG2) cells, oligodendrocyte precursor cells, polydendrocytes, synantocytes and complex cells (Pauker & Bergles, 2006). These cells express chondroitin sulfate proteoglycan, do not express GFAP and lack GluT currents and gap junctions. As with GluR astrocytes, they express AMPA receptors as well as GABA receptors; moreover, they receive synaptic terminals. Current injection into these cells elicits action potentials that are reversibly blocked by TTX. To complicate matters further, two classes of NG2 cells have been recently identified (Káradóttir et al.; 2008): one class expresses voltage-gated Na^+ currents together with voltage-gated K^+ currents, whereas the other does not express Na^+ currents. Presumably, both of these cell classes additionally express voltage-gated Ca^{2+} currents.

2.1 Plasma membrane properties of astrocytes

Some astrocytes exhibit a high resting K^+ conductance and possess gap junction coupling; thus, the first major function that was assigned to these cells was the clearance of extracellular K^+ following neuronal activity. However, glial cells express a set of receptors that is similar to neurons, but at different relative densities. This suggests that astrocytes perform other functions than buffering K^+. Among their intrinsic membrane proteins are metabotropic glutamate receptors (mGluR) (Zur Nieden and Deitmer, 2006), purinergic receptors (Jeremic et al.; 2001) and GABA type-B receptors. Other ionotropic receptors, such as AMPA, are also present. An elevated amount of GluR1 in the AMPA receptors of reactive astrocytes has been reported, which suggests an increased responsiveness of these astrocytes to glutamate (Seifert et al.; 2004). This change has been observed in astrocytes that were obtained from sclerotic tissue. Moreover, in animal models, mGluR3, mGluR5 and mGluR8 up-regulation has been reported in the hippocampus (Steinhäuser & Seifert, 2002). These receptors are involved in the astrocyte's response to glial and neurotransmitter. During normal brain function activity, astrocytes play a major role in the clearance of glutamate that is released from the nerve terminal into the extracellular space.

Astrocytes achieve this through the activity of two glutamate transporter molecules, namely the excitatory amino acid transporter (EAAT) subtypes $EAAT_1$ and $EAAT_2$ (de Lanerolle et al.; 2010). The GABA transporter GAT_3 is usually only weakly expressed (if at all) in astrocytes. Aquaporin 4 (AQP4) is a water transporter molecule that is found on astrocytes. The distribution of these transporter molecules is asymmetric, being more densely expressed on the perivascular astrocytic end-feet than on the membrane that faces the neuropil (de Lanerolle et al.; 2010).

Several studies demonstrated the presence of voltage-dependent ionic channels, including Na^+, K^+ and Ca^{2+} channels (Barres et al.; 1990; Sontheimer et al.; 1991; Sontheimer & Waxman, 1993). Voltage-gated Na^+ channels are present in astrocytes in various brain regions. It has been postulated that this might serve to regulate $[Na^+]_i$ and thereby control the activity of the Na^+/glutamate transporter or Na^+/K^+ ATPase exchanger (Sontheimer et al.; 1994). Calcium channels have also been identified in both cultured astrocytes and acute astrocyte preparations (Verkhratsky & Steinhäuser, 2000). Astrocytes play a major role in K^+ homeostasis in the central nervous system. During neuronal activity, $[K^+]_o$ is temporally increased, which depolarizes nearby membranes. Astrocytes help move K^+ away from regions of high concentration to restore the normal extracellular concentration (Steinhäuser & Seifert, 2002). Inwardly rectifying potassium (Kir) channels in astrocytes play a major role in removing K^+ from the extracellular space.

2.2 Calcium signaling in astrocytes

Glial cells respond with changing $[Ca^{2+}]_i$ to various neurotransmitters, the most important of which are glutamate, ATP, adenosine and GABA (Haydon & Carmignoto, 2006). These transmitters activate metabotropic receptors that are coupled to second messenger systems.

Astrocytes not only exhibit changes in $[Ca^{2+}]_i$ after extracellular neurotransmitter release, but spontaneous calcium oscillations can also occur in the absence of neuronal activity (Nett et al.; 2002; Parri & Crunelli 2003; Zur Nieden & Deitmer, 2006). It has been established that both evoked and spontaneous astrocyte calcium increases depend on calcium release from internal stores (Fiacco & McCarthy, 2006). A neurotransmitter-induced increase in astrocytic calcium activates astrocytic metabotropic Gq-coupled receptors that drive the release of calcium from the endoplasmic reticulum (ER) upon activation of phospholipase C (PLC) and conversion of phosphotidylinositol bisphosphate to inositol triphosphate (IP_3) (Nadal et al.; 1995; Porter & McCarthy, 1996; Araque et al.; 1998a, Newman 2005; Pastor et al.; 2010).

Spontaneous $[Ca^{2+}]_i$ changes are not completely understood, but some theories that are supported by various experimental data have been postulated. These include a mechanism involving voltage-gated calcium channels and calcium induced-calcium release (Parri & Crunelli, 2003), activation of mGluR by the quantal release of small amounts of glio or neurotransmitters (possibly spillover from synaptic region) (Zur Neider & Deitmer, 2006) and a "switch" in the intrinsic activity of metabotropic receptors (Pasti et al.; 1997). Although the ryanodine receptor has been implicated in calcium changes in epilepsy (Tashiro et al.; 2002), its role has not yet been clarified because several studies failed to show any significant contribution in astrocytes that were obtained from epileptic patients (see Figure 2 and reference Pastor et al.; 2010).

In astrocytes, a local calcium increase following IP_3 receptor activation often propagates as a "calcium wave" some distance from its point of origin (Nadal et al.; 1997). The propagation of calcium waves is believed to occur via calcium diffusing locally (after its initial release) to neighboring IP_3 receptors, where it acts as a co-agonist with IP_3 to release stored calcium from adjacent compartments (Fiacco & McCarthy, 2006).

Upon stimulation, astrocytes in culture display a calcium wave that propagates intercellularly through thousands of cells (Cornell-Bell et al.; 1990). The mechanisms that are involved in the propagation of intercellular calcium waves in cultured astroglia include: (1) gap junctions between astrocytes that allow the intercellular diffusion of second messengers such as IP_3, and (2) the calcium-induced release of ATP that diffuses extracellularly to

neighboring astrocytes to activate purinergic receptors that are coupled to internal calcium stores (Cotrina et al.; 2000; Suadicani et al.; 2004). There is no evidence of the existence of intercellular astrocyte calcium waves in intact tissue, suggesting that long-range glial signaling may be an artifact of cultured astroglia; however, it has been proposed that this process might occur in pathological conditions such as epilepsy (Peters et al.; 2003). In general, these observations suggest that widespread intercellular calcium waves are not likely to occur between astrocytes under physiological conditions *in situ*. However, a recent *in vivo* study showed that "Ca^{2+} signals (...) can propagate through the cell and couple to adjacent astrocytes in the form of a Ca^{2+} wave" (Ding et al.; 2007).
These changes in $[Ca^{2+}]_i$ can act as a second messenger in various cellular process, including the release of gliotransmitters or the modification of gene expression patterns.

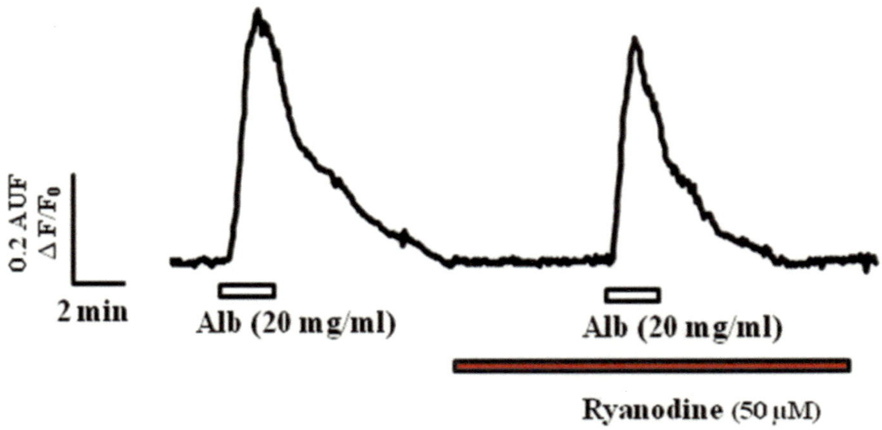

Fig. 2. Ryanodine fails to block the response to bovine plasma albumin (Alb; 20 mg/ml) in astrocytes obtained from epileptic patients (unpublished data).

2.3 Interactions between astrocytes and neurons

Astrocytes were initially considered to be supportive cells. However, during the last years of the past century, it became clear that glial cells can also contribute to information processing by neurons. Various studies have led to the proposal of the "tripartite synapse", in which the astrocyte monitors synaptic activity and provides feedback by modulating the strength of the synaptic connection (Araque et al.; 1999; 2001). This concept is based on studies showing that glial cells respond to neuronal activity with an $[Ca^{2+}]_i$ increase, which in turn triggers the release of gliotransmitters that can cause feedback regulation of neuronal activity.
Calcium increases in astrocytes are coupled to the regulated release of neuroactive molecules and classic neurotransmitters that include ATP, inflammatory cytokines, vasoactive compounds, D-serine and glutamate (Parpura et al.; 1994 ; Coco et al.; 2003 ; Zonta et al.; 2003; Mothet et al.; 2005).
Other modes of glutamate release by astrocytes are calcium-independent and include release through large pores, including gap junction hemi-channels and purinergic P2X7 receptors (Ye et al.; 2003; Fellin et al.; 2006), a reversal of glutamate transport (Anderson & Swanson, 2000) and by volume-sensitive anion channels (Takano et al.; 2005). However, calcium-independent modes of astrocytic glutamate release have only been observed under

pathological conditions, such as severe energy depletion, highly increased external K^+ and in divalent cation-free extracellular solutions. Therefore, a considerable body of data suggests that the calcium-dependent release of glutamate from astrocytes occurs via a regulated exocytotic vesicular mechanism.

It has been shown that synaptotagmin 4 is essential for Ca^{2+}-dependent glutamate release. Presumably, an excess of the synaptotagmin isoform 4 in place of isoform 1 suggests that the kiss-and-run release mechanism prevails over full vesicle fusion (Wang et al.; 2001). Moreover, several studies demonstrated the presence and participation of SNARE proteins in exocytosis (Araque et al.; 2000).

Glutamate release likely acts through NMDA receptors (NMDARs) that are composed of NR1/NR2B subunits. These receptors are located extrasynaptically, whereas in the synaptic membrane, the NR1/NR2A configuration is found (Haydon & Carmignoto, 2006). This situation of NMDAR can account for the high amplitude and slow kinetics of the slow inward currents (SIC; see Figure 3) that are recorded after astrocytic glutamate release (~100 pA), whereas synaptic currents are only around 2-3 pA in amplitude. In addition to exerting kinetic differences, synaptic and extrasynaptic NMDA receptors may accomplish different—and to some degree opposing—functional roles (Krapivinsky et al.; 2003).

It has been suggested that the release of glutamate from a single astrocyte has the potential to act synchronously on several different dendrites. Indeed, this mechanism may underlie the generation of paroxysmal depolarization shifts (PDS) that can be induced in several neurons in a rat model of epilepsy. Besides NMDARs, AMPA receptors (AMPARs) may also be activated by astrocytic glutamate release. These receptors are also present at extrasynaptic locations, and their activation may serve as a type of coincidence detector with synaptic NMDARs (Haydon & Carmignoto, 2006).

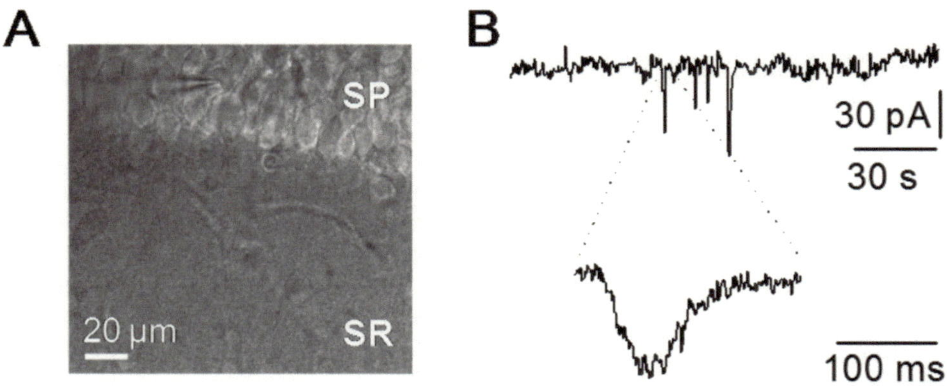

Fig. 3. Astrocytes can activate neurons by gliotransmitter release. **A)** Infrared differential interface contrast (DIC) image showing the stratum radiatum (SR) and the recorded neuron in the stratum pyramidale (SP) of a rat hippocampal slice. **B)** Whole-cell currents from a CA1 pyramidal neuron showing a neuronal slow inward current (SIC, expanded in the bottom trace). Courtesy of Dr. Alfonso Araque, Consejo Superior de Investigaciones Científicas, Madrid.

Glutamate is not the only molecule that is released from astrocytes to modulate the activity of neurons. Other molecules are functionally important as well. In fact, in addition to requiring glutamate for NMDAR activation, the co-agonist D-serine may also be important. Astrocytes are the only cells that express the enzyme serine racemase, making glial cells the only source for this molecule in the brain (Wolosker et al.; 1999). It has been suggested that vesicles might contain both D-serine and glutamate, thereby allowing their simultaneous release upon increased $[Ca^{2+}]_i$ (Haydon & Carmignoto, 2006).

Another important gliotransmitter that is released by astrocytes is ATP, and the mechanisms that are involved are the subject of debate. There is evidence that the release of both ATP and glutamate involve phospholipase C, but it has been suggested that ATP release depends on the diacylglycerol pathway (Wang et al.; 2000), although this hypothesis is still under debate. Released at micromolar concentrations ATP has powerful effects on adjacent neurons acting through purinergic receptors (P2). ATP can activate P_2 presynaptic receptors. In fact, the activation of P_2Y_1 receptors in CA1 interneurons—most likely after the release of ATP from both neurons and astrocytes—may induce action potentials in these neurons and lead to increased GABAergic synaptic inhibition of pyramidal neurons (Bowser & Khakh, 2004). However, an excitatory effect of ATP has been described in which glutamate-mediated miniature end-plate synaptic currents are increased (Gordon et al.; 2005). Once ATP has been released into the extracellular space, a variety of ectonucleotidases degrade ATP into adenosine. Adenosine is a ubiquitous modulator of synaptic transmission and neuronal activity and acts through specific receptors. Indeed, there are high-affinity inhibitory adenosine A_1 and excitatory A_{2A} receptors that are activated by nanomolar concentrations of adenosine as well as low-affinity or low-abundance A_{2B} and A_3 receptors. The most relevant function of adenosine is to induce presynaptic inhibition of transmitter release and therefore has potent anticonvulsant and neuroprotective functions (Boison, 2008). It is important to note that adenosine—either released or produced by ATP degradation—can diffuse from the synaptic cleft and act laterally to regulate the strength of neighboring synapses in a mechanism named heterosynaptic suppression, which is mediated by the accumulation of adenosine acting through A_1 receptors (Zhang et al.; 2003). We will see below in detail the effect of adenosine on seizure threshold (see 4.5 The role of adenosine kinase in epileptogenesis); however, suffice it to say that adenosine acting through A_1 receptors has a potent anticonvulsant effect.

In addition to the release of gliotransmitters, it is important to consider that one cortical astrocyte makes contacts with approximately 300-600 neuronal dendrites. These "local modules" of astrocytic integration can affect the function of several groups of neurons or synapsis, thus working in a more coherent mode (Halassa et al.; 2007).

Astrocytes play an important role in the metabolism of the brain through their exclusive role in the degradation of both glucose and glutamate. The importance of astrocytes in these processes lies in their expression of key enzymes that are not normally found in neurons. Of course, these processes are extremely important for appropriate brain function but are beyond the scope of this review. The reader is referred to Hertz et al. (1999) and Herrera-Peco et al. (2008).

2.4 Astrocytes are activated by albumin

Albumin ($C_{123}H_{193}N_{35}O_{37}$) is the most abundant protein in blood, representing more than 50% of all proteins. Its molecular weight is 2754.06 g/mol, and its concentration in plasma is around 35-55 mg/ml (Nadal et al.; 2001). Among its functions is the binding of several polar lipids, particularly lysophosphatidic acid (LPA), other fatty acids and sphingomyelins that are derived from platelet activation (Fuentes, E.t al.; 1999). Albumin is also the main component in maintaining osmotic plasma pressure. Thus far, albumin has been shown to activate various cell types, including rat astrocytes in culture (Nadal et al.; 1995; 1997) and in brain slices (Ivens et al.; 2007; Nadal et al.; 1998).

Depending on its concentration, plasma albumin—that is, albumin obtained from non-clotted blood—can have a dual effect on astrocytic $[Ca^{2+}]_i$. A low albumin concentration can induce a decrease in calcium, whereas higher doses increase $[Ca^{2+}]_i$ in a dose-dependent manner (Figure 4). These effects, which were initially studied in astrocytes obtained from rat pups, were recently demonstrated in humans (Pastor et al.; 2010).

The dual effect on cytosolic calcium in astrocytes depends on two different components of native plasma albumin that can be separated by methanol extraction (Nadal et al.; 1994; 1995). The protein component of albumin causes a reduction in $[Ca^{2+}]_i$, whereas native albumin—to which the lipid factor is normally attached—induces repetitive calcium spiking and DNA synthesis in addition to decreased $[Ca^{2+}]_i$. This factor cannot be a protein contaminant such as a growth factor because its activity can be extracted by methanol through a dialysis membrane, is sensitive to lipases but not boiling and can be reconstituted with extracted albumin to restore the full activity of native albumin. The preferential extraction by methanol suggests that the factor is a polar lipid such as a phospholipid or ganglioside (Nadal et al.; 1995). This polar lipid has not yet been identified, but it has been suggested that it might be the same substance that binds to glia cell stimulating factor (GSF) (Nuñez & García-Sancho, 1996).

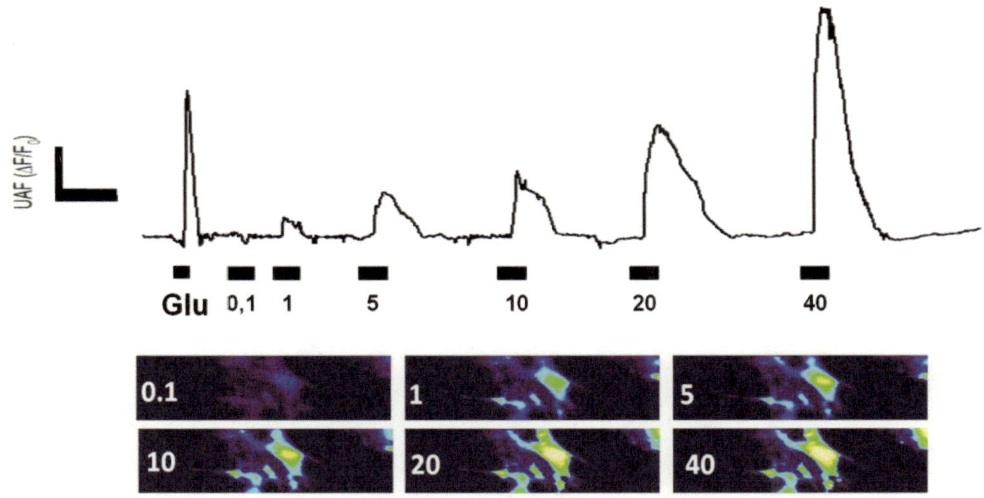

Fig. 4. Changes in $[Ca^{2+}]_i$ in human astrocytes induced by bovine plasma albumin (BPA). The bars indicate the application of glutamate (Glu 500 mM) or BPA at the indicated concentrations (in mg/ml). Note that 0.1 mg/ml BPA induced a decrease in fluorescence. The microphotographs show the changes in $[Ca^{2+}]_i$ of one human astrocyte (arrow) to BPA. The numbers at left indicate the albumin concentration. The cells were loaded with Fura-2 AM (10^{-6} mol/L). Unpublished data.

As is the case with other neurotransmitters, the change in $[Ca^{2+}]_i$ depends on the release of IP_3 after G-protein-mediated activation of PLC (Nadal et al.; 1995; 1997; Pastor et al.; 2010). The albumin receptor has not yet been identified.

In addition to its effects on cytosolic calcium, plasma albumin can also induce the synthesis of DNA. This process of synthesis is the normal precursor to mitosis, which implies that albumin can act as a mitogen in astrocytes.

In addition to the calcium pathway that is activated by albumin, this protein is also taken up by astrocytes, neurons and microglia (albeit to a lesser extent) (Ivens et al.; 2007; van Vliet et al.; 2007). This effect of albumin on glial cells is mediated by the TGF-βR (TGF-βR; Figure 5), which activates the Smad signaling pathway (Cacheux et al.; 2009). This mechanism of activation has been extensively studied in a rat model of epilepsy and is discussed below in detail.

An important question regarding the type of albumin (either plasmatic or serum) remains unanswered. In fact, both models, the albumin-receptor activated and the TGF-βR, have been described with plasma albumin (Nadal et al.; 1995; Pastor et al.; 2010) and serum albumin (Seiffert et al.; 2004; Ivens et al.; 2007) respectively. In the latter case, albumin carries different lipids that are derived from the coagulation cascade, including lysophosphatidic acid (LPA), lysophosphatidylcholine, sphingomyelin and platelet-activating factor. All of these lipids can elicit calcium signals of varying magnitude in cortical astrocytes, although only LPA-induced calcium signals are comparable in amplitude to those induced by the active physiological lipid that is bound to plasma albumin. None of these lipids, however, was found to cause cell division in astrocytes (Fuentes et al.; 1999). There is therefore no direct invariable relationship between the ability of lipids to induce calcium signals and mitogenic activity. Perhaps under pathologic conditions, coagulation plays an important role in the effect of albumin on astrocytes; nevertheless, albumin would be attached to a polar lipid that has an effect distinct from LPA.

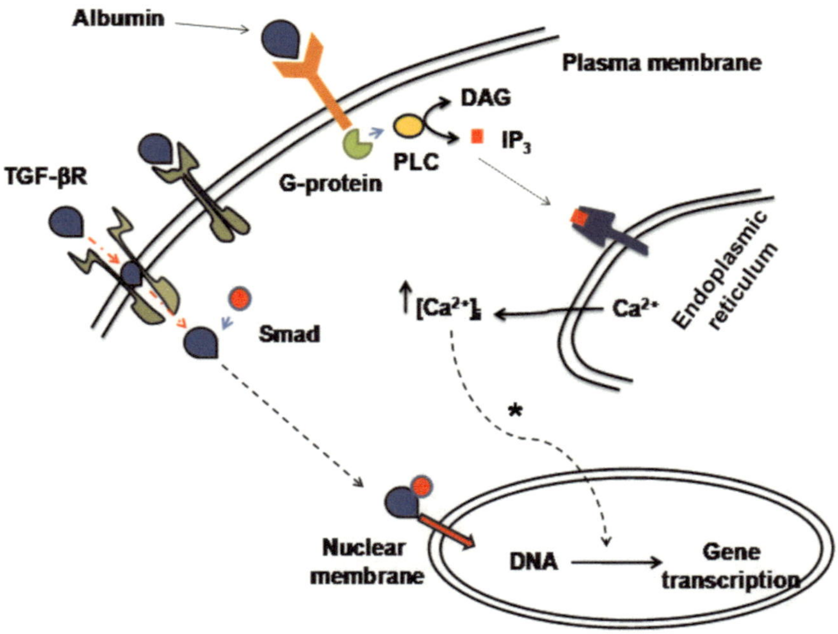

Fig. 5. Mechanisms of action of albumin in astrocytes. Depicted is the IP3-cytosolic calcium pathway with its proposed effect on gene transcription, indicated by the asterisk. TGF-βR signaling pathway is also shown. Both of these pathways are present in cultured human astrocytes. * Hypothesized action. See text for more details.

3. The structure and function of the blood-brain barrier

The BBB is a diffusion barrier that impedes the influx of most compounds between the blood and the brain, thereby isolating the brain from the external environment. Three cellular elements of the brain's microvasculature comprise the BBB and are responsible for its properties. These components are:

- Endothelial cells. Tight junctions (TJs) are special transmembrane proteins that are located between cerebral endothelial cells, where they form a diffusion barrier that selectively excludes most blood-borne substances from entering the brain. There is some evidence of cross-talk with astrocytes. Indeed, endothelial cells seem to be the primary source of leukemia inhibitory factor (LIF), which helps induce astrocyte differentiation (Mi et al.; 2001). Other molecules that are presumably released by endothelial cells to affect astrocytes include bradykinin and glutamate. Moreover, endothelial cells are involved in neurogenesis, primarily via vascular endothelial growth factor (VEGF) (Loussaint et al.; 2002).
- Astrocyte end-feet. These structures tightly ensheath the vessel wall and appear to be critical for the induction and maintenance of the TJ barrier, although astrocytes are not believed to have a role in the mammalian BBB. However, astrocytes are important because they help induce the generation of BBB structures in endothelial cells. Astrocytes can act on endothelial cells by releasing cytokines such as TGF-β and glial cell-derived neurotrophic factor (GDNF) (Utsumi et al.; 2000, Ramsauer et al.; 2002). Intracellular calcium waves mediate bidirectional astrocyte-endothelial interactions. In co-culture models, two signaling mechanisms are presumably involved: 1) astrocytes and endothelial cells can exchange calcium signals via a pathway that is dependent on intracellular IP_3 and gap junctions; and 2) diffusion of a purinergic messenger. However, *in vivo*, astrocytes and endothelial cells are not in contact, and therefore, these findings need to be confirmed. Nevertheless, the dilation of arterioles triggered by neuronal activity depends on glutamate-mediated $[Ca^{2+}]_i$ oscillations in astrocytes (Zonta et al.; 2003).
- Pericytes are undifferentiated cells that wrap around the endothelial cells of microvessels, including capillaries, venules and arterioles. Pericytes are believed to provide structural support and vasodynamic capacity to the microvasculature (Ballabh et al.; 2004). Pericytes can also help to stabilize capillaries that are recently formed by endothelial cells, thereby regulating angiogenesis (Balabanov & Dore-Duffy, 1998).

The BBB differs from endothelial cells in the rest of the body by the absence of fenestrations, extensive tight junctions (TJs) and bare pinocytic vesicular transport. The building blocks of the BBB are comprised of several molecules and subcellular structures that confer its unique properties, the most important of which are:

- Complex junctions in the BBB are formed by TJs and adherens junctions. Tight junctions are sites of apparent fusion between leaflets of the plasma membranes of adjacent cells, whereas adherens junctions are composed of cadherin-catenin complexes and their associated proteins (Matter & Balda, 2003). Cytoplasmic proteins link membrane proteins to actin, which is the principal protein of the cytoskeleton.
- Tight-junction–associated membrane proteins, including occludins, claudins and junctional adhesion molecules (Furuse et al.; 1993; Martin-Pardura et al.; 1998; Morita et al.; 1999). These proteins form the extracellular component of TJs.
- Cytoplasmic accessory proteins, including zonula occludens (ZO) proteins, cingulin and several others (Itoh et al.; 1999). Actin binds to ZO proteins, thereby providing structural support to the endothelial cells (Haskins et al.; 1998).

Dysfunction of the BBB exacerbates a number of neurologic diseases, including stroke and neuroinflammatory disorders. Under pathological conditions, different chemical mediators that increase BBB permeability are released. Among these mediators are glutamate, aspartate, taurine, ATP, endothelin-I, tumor necrosis factor (TNF)-α and interleukin-1β (IL-1β), all of which are produced by astrocytes (Kutsova et al.; 1999; Abbot 2000; 2002). Moreover, endothelial cells can release bradykinin, 5-HT, histamine, substance P, platelet activating factor and free radicals (Abbot, 2002; St'astný et al.; 2000).

The function of the BBB is to control the traffic of substances between the blood and the brain. This is achieved in three ways:

- Diffusion of lipid-soluble substances. The BBB permits the rapid exchange of lipid-soluble gases such as O_2 and CO_2, an exchange that is limited only by the surface area of the blood vessel and cerebral blood flow. Barrier vessels are impermeable to molecules that are poorly soluble in lipids. The permeability coefficient of the BBB for many substances is directly proportional to the lipid solubility of the substance, which is measured as its oil-water partition coefficient (Laterra & Goldstein, 2000).
- Facilitated and energy-dependent receptor-mediated transport of specific water-soluble substances. Most substances that must cross the BBB are not lipid soluble and therefore need a specific carrier-mediated transport system. One of the most important substances is glucose, which is transported by the glucose transporter isotype-1, or Glut1 (Guerin et al.; 1999). Amino acids are also transported by three distinct carrier systems. Another transport system is related to the multidrug resistance to chemotherapy (MDR) transporter (Schinkel et al.; 1994).
- Ion channels. Various studies support the existence of a nonselective luminal ion channel that is inhibited by both amiloride and atrial natriuretic peptide. The existence of luminal Na^+/H^+ and $Cl^-/HCO3^-$ exchangers has also been suggested. The external membrane of brain endothelial cells contains a relatively high density of Na^+/K^+-ATPase pump. In conjunction with K^+ channels in astrocytes, this abluminal endothelial pump may play an important role in removing extracellular K^+ that is released during intense neuronal activity. In addition, the nonselective luminal ion channel, a distinct abluminal K^+ channel and the abluminal Na^+/K^+-ATPase may work together to tightly regulate the entry of Na^+ and the release or recycling of K^+ (Haydon & Carmignoto, 2006). Aquaporin-4 is the major water channel expressed in brain perivascular astrocytic processes and is the principal system for regulating the traffic of water between the brain and blood. Thus, its role in cerebral edema is very important.

4. The role of astrocytes in epileptogenesis

Until recently, little was known regarding the process by which a normal brain becomes epileptic following an external or internal insult, for example following traumatic brain injury or seizures that are induced by fever or infectious disease. These symptomatic epilepsies account for a significant number of patients; however, for patients with idiopathic or cryptogenic epilepsy, the antecedents remain unknown. In general, except for well-defined etiologies (e.g.; cortical dysplasia), the brain's transition from normal to epileptic—namely, epileptogenesis—remains obscure.

However, several lines of evidence involving astrocytes have begun to emerge during the last decade, providing a somewhat coherent framework. These lines of evidence can be grouped according to the different structures that are involved.

4.1 Modification of astrocyte membrane proteins

Diverse changes have been described for the expression of intrinsic plasma membrane proteins in astrocytes at the epileptic seizure foci.

In sclerotic hippocampi, reactive astrocytes express mGluR2/3, mGluR4 and mGluR8. Similarly, mGluR3, mGluR5 and mGluR8 are up-regulated in the hippocampus in experimental animal models of TLE. Activation of these receptors may lead to an increase in $[Ca^{2+}]_i$ and Ca^{2+} wave propagation, thereby leading to the release of glutamate from astrocytes (Volterra & Meldolesi, 2005).

Using microdialysis, increased levels of *in situ* extracellular glutamate have been found in sclerotic seizure foci (During & Spencer, 1993; Cavus et al.; 2002). Moreover, the down-regulation of $EAAT_1$ and $EAAT_2$ has also been reported (Proper et al.; 2002). However, other groups were unable to confirm this observation (Tessler et al.; 1998).

In sclerotic astrocytes, the GABA transporter GAT_3 is up-regulated. In the same vein, microdialysis in epileptic patients has revealed decreased levels of extracellular GABA in the epileptic foci during the ictal state (During & Spencer 1993). The increased expression of the transporter would help to reduce extracellular GABA levels, thereby decreasing inhibitory tone during the ictal state.

Expression of the protein AQP4 is reduced on the perivascular membrane of the astrocyte in sclerotic hippocampi, whereas its expression is unchanged on the membrane that faces the neuropil. This change may cause a decrease in water extrusion from the neuropil to the vessel (Eid et al.; 2005).

In addition to changes in the expression of transport proteins in epileptic foci, ion channels in astrocytes are also modified. Cultured astrocytes obtained from patient hippocampus and entorhinal cortex[1] displayed much larger tetrodotoxin (TTX)-sensitive Na^+ currents than astrocytes from non-sclerotic hippocampi (O'connor et al.; 1998). However, as with other results, there are discrepancies regarding the increased Na^+ current (Hinterkeuser et al.; 2000). Changes in the differential expression of calcium channels have been reported in the sclerotic hippocampus, but the functional significance of this change remains unclear (de Lanerolle et al.; 2010).

Impaired K^+ buffering has been detected in sclerotic patient hippocampi, suggesting that there are defective channels in the sclerotic region, particularly in CA1 (Gabriel et al.; 1998). The buffering of K^+, which is likely performed by the GFAP+ subset of Glu-like astrocytes (and carried out by the Kir channels), depends on a parallel flux of water through the plasma membrane to avoid hyperosmolarity. Water molecules and K^+ are taken up by the astrocytic membrane of the neuropil and pushed into the blood and cerebrospinal fluid (CSF) through the end-food pole. A loss of AQP4 would impede the movement of water and contribute to increased $[K^+]_o$. Concomitantly, the down-regulation of Kir4.1 channels during a critical time window has been described in a rat model of epilepsy (Ivens et al.; 2007), as we discuss in detail below. Clearly, this process can contribute to further increase the concentration of extracellular K^+.

4.2 Changes in genes expression and metabolism

In the sclerotic hippocampus, changes in various enzymes that are involved in the metabolism of astrocytes and the interaction between astrocytes and neurons have been

---

[1]The entorhinal cortex is part of the parahippocampal gyrus and is the main source of input to the hippocampus through the perforant pathway and the collaterals of the temporoammonic pathway.

described (Herrera-Peco et al.; 2008). In this regard, a loss of glutamine synthetase in CA1 and CA3, an increase in the activity of glutamate dehydrogenase and/or a decrease in the activity of lactate dehydrogenase have all been reported. Besides, extracellular levels of lactate are elevated in the sclerotic hippocampus (de Lanerolle et al.; 2010).

On the other hand, several astrocyte-related genes are up-regulated in sclerotic regions. These changes in the pattern of gene expression are consistent with increased gliosis or immune and inflammatory responses (Lee et al.; 2007). This is discussed in detail below.

It is likely that much of these changes are a consequence of epilepsy rather than a cause. Therefore, more data are needed before we can formulate an exact picture of the genetic changes that are related to epileptogenesis.

4.3 Changes in BBB permeability

It has long been recognized that there is a proliferation of the microvasculature in the sclerotic hippocampus, an observation that has been recently confirmed (Rigau et al.; 2007). However, on the contrary, there are recent reports showing a significant loss of microvessels in the CA1 region of sclerotic hippocampi (Kastanauskaite et al.; 2009). In any case, most groups agree on the presence of blood vessel changes in TLE-associated hippocampal sclerosis.

Several molecules that are located in the perivascular end-feet exhibit changes in sclerotic regions. AQP4 and dystrophin are reduced, whereas CD44 and plectin 1 are increased. Other molecules such as the chemokines CCL2 and CCL3 are up-regulated, as are the chemokine receptors CCR1 and CCR2 (de Lanerolle, 2010).

It is believed that these glial-derived chemokines can guide circulating leukocytes through endothelial junctions and into the brain's extracellular space. These chemokines can also help mediate the extravasation of albumin (de Lanerolle et al.; 2010). Therefore, these changes can alter the permeability of the BBB, thereby allowing molecules that normally are excluded to access the brain. Indeed, it has been shown that the BBB is leakier during seizures (de Lanerolle et al.; 2010). Furthermore, immunohistochemical localization of albumin in resected hippocampi from TLE patients showed strong albumin immunoreactivity in the parenchyma throughout the hippocampus next to the blood vessels. Neurons and astrocytes located around the vessels were also albumin-positive, thus demonstrating an increase in BBB permeability. Such extravasations of albumin were not observed in control hippocampi (van Vliet et al.; 2007). In an animal model, the extravasation of serum albumin to the brain's extracellular space was associated with a prominent activation of astrocytes, but no inflammatory response or marked cell loss. This activation was associated with the development of epileptiform discharges within 4–7 days (Seiffert et al.; 2004).

Changes other than permeability have been reported in the BBB. The erythropoietin receptor is strongly expressed in the capillaries of sclerotic hippocampi, which suggests an increased uptake of erythropoietin into the hippocampus (Eid et al.; 2004).

4.4 Inflammatory and immune responses in the brain

Astrocytes contribute to the inflammatory response in the CNS. Glial cells can produce a range of immunologically relevant molecules, including class II major histocompatibility complex antigens, cytokines and chemokines. Studies have shown that glial cells—including both astrocytes and microglia—express high levels of pro-inflammatory cytokines in regions that are recruited in the generation and propagation of seizures. In astrocytes and microglia of patients with TLE and hippocampal sclerosis, the IL-1β system is activated, particularly in end-feet perivascular regions and in endothelial cells in sclerotic brain regions (Ravizza et al.; 2007). These changes can affect the permeability of the BBB, perhaps by disrupting tight-junction organization (Del Machio et al.; 1996). It has been showed that IL-1β has a pro-ictogenic role that is mediated by the receptor IL-1R1 (Vezzani et al.; 2002). Exposure to IL-1β or TNF-α exacerbates the excitotoxic neuronal damage that is induced by NMDA or AMPA, thus suggesting that cell survival depends on the tissue concentration and duration of action of cytokines. This deleterious effect is mediated by the induction of toxic mediators to affect neuronal excitability.

The damage in the brain that is induced by IL-1β can be mediated by an increase in the function of NMDA receptors or by an increase in extracellular glutamate. In this sense, IL-1β increases NMDA-mediated Ca^{2+} influx into neurons, thereby promoting excitotoxicity (Vezzani et al.; 2008). Other well-established mechanisms include the inhibition of glutamate uptake by glial cells and an increase in glutamate release via TNF-α production (Bezzi et al.; 2001). Additionally, IL-1β activates nitric oxide (NO) synthase, increasing the glutamate release. Presumably, all of these mechanisms lead to increased glutamatergic transmission and toxicity. However, GABAergic transmission is also affected by inflammation. Indeed, IL-1β has been shown to inhibit $GABA_A$ receptors, thereby contributing to hyperexcitability (Wang et al.; 2000).

Other cytokines that are produced by glial cells—such as IL-6, TNF-α and prostaglandins—have been shown to have either pro-ictogenic or inhibitory effects on seizures in a concentration-dependent manner, and this depends on the type of receptors involved and the origin of the cells (Vezzani et al.; 2008). It has been reported that TNF-α activates the rapid recruitment AMPA receptors that lack the $GluR_2$ subunit to the neuronal membrane; this molecular conformation is permissive for Ca^{2+} influx, thereby increasing neurotoxicity.

Moreover, in the sclerotic hippocampus, there is an up-regulation of the p65 subunit of the nuclear factor kappa-light-chain-enhancer of activated B cells (NF-κB) (Crespel et al.; 2002), a protein complex that control DNA transcription and is involved in the cellular responses to stress. In the sclerotic hippocampus, immunoreactivity of complement proteins was increased in regions of neuronal loss (including CA1, CA3 and the hylus of the dentate gyrus). All of these data imply a direct participation of the inflammatory pathway in epilepsy.

4.5 The participation of albumin in the activation of astrocytes

Albumin is usually not in contact with astrocytes or neurons. Indeed, its concentration in the extracellular space of the CNS (~35 ng/ml) is three orders of magnitude lower than in blood (Nadal et al.; 2001). The effect of albumin on glial cells depends on both the protein itself and the lipids to which it is attached (Nadal et al.; 1995; 1997).

Recently, it was elegantly demonstrated in rats that albumin can act directly on astrocytes, thereby facilitating epileptogenesis (Seiffert et al.; 2004, Ivens et al.; 2007; Van Vliet et al.; 2007). It has been shown that direct brain exposure to serum albumin is associated with albumin uptake into astrocytes that is mediated by TGF-βR. This uptake is followed by the down-regulation of Kir4.1 channels in astrocytes, which results in reduced buffering of extracellular potassium. This in turn leads to an increased activity-dependent accumulation of extracellular potassium, which results in facilitated NMDAR-mediated neuronal hyperexcitability and ultimately epileptiform activity (Ivens et al.; 2007). Presumably, these effects are mediated by GFAP+/GluT astrocytes. On the other hand, albumin can act on NG2/GluR astrocytes; in these cells, TGF-βR can induce the transcription factor NF-κB, which can modify the expression of cyclooxygenase 2 (COX-2).

However, albumin can act on astrocytes through a pathway that is distinct from TGF-βR. This pathway has not been extensively explored; however, changes in $[Ca^{2+}]_i$ can induce new DNA synthesis in cultured astrocytes (Pastor et al.; 2010). It is therefore reasonable to speculate that changes in gene expression that are observed during epileptogenesis in rats are induced by the calcium-dependent pathway and not only through the action of TGF-βR.

4.6 The role of adenosine kinase in epileptogenesis

Inhibitory neuromodulation by adenosine is primarily mediated by the activation of A_1 receptors that are coupled to inhibitory G_i and G_o G-proteins. As a result, the release of glutamate and others neurotransmitters is inhibited. In addition, A_1 receptor activation can decrease brain metabolism and alter astrocytic function, thereby conferring beneficial effects (Haberg et al.; 2000; van Claker & Biber, 2005). In contrast to A_1 receptors, A_{2A} receptors are coupled to excitatory G_s and G_{olf} G-proteins and both excitatory and inhibitory responses have been reported (Boison, 2008). The activity of this type of receptor is restricted to active synapses. Stimulating nerve terminals at a high frequency can release ATP, which can be degraded to adenosine, which in turn acts by binding to A_{2A} receptors. Subsequent activation of A_{2A} can lead to the down-regulation of A_1 receptors. With respect to the low-affinity A_{2B} and low-density A_3 receptors, it appears that these receptors may only be relevant under pathological conditions, for example following traumatic brain injury or during cerebral ischemia (Pearson et al.; 2006). In summary, the extracellular level of adenosine has an important role in seizure threshold.

Astrocytes play a key role in regulating the levels of extracellular adenosine (Boison 2006; Haydon & Carmignoto, 2006); this is presumably via an adenosine cycle that involves the vesicular release of ATP, extracellular degradation to adenosine, uptake of adenosine via nucleoside transporters and intracellular phosphorylation of AMP (Boison, 2008). It is known that astrocytes are the primary source of ATP under physiological conditions, thus favoring a relative tone of inhibition within the neural network.

Extracellular levels of adenosine can be regulated by reuptake through nucleoside transporters, which can be divided into three isoforms of concentrative nucleoside transporters (CNT1, 2 and 3) that are coupled to the Na^+ gradient and into four isoforms of equilibrative nucleoside transporters (ENT1 through ENT4) (Smith et al.; 2007). Under physiological conditions, ENTs appear to play a central role in controlling the extracellular level of adenosine in the brain.

Once adenosine is transported into the astrocyte, it is phosphorylated by adenosine kinase (ADK), an enzyme that is almost exclusively expressed in these glial cells in the adult brain (Studer et al.; 2006).

Adenosine kinase has a biphasic response to stress after a brain injury (Boison, 2008):

- First, ADK is rapidly down-regulated, leading to an elevated level of adenosine. This enhancement serves as a protective factor via the activation of A_1 receptors. This increase in extracellular adenosine might be a general astrocyte-based mechanism to protect the brain after stroke, ischemia, status epilepticus, or a similar condition.
- In the second phase, there is an up-regulation of ADK that leads to a significant decrease in the level of extracellular adenosine, thereby reducing the tone of the A1 receptors. This up-regulation of ADK is accompanied by parallel changes in G-protein-coupled receptors, for example, down-regulation of A_2 receptors or increased expression of $GABA_B$ receptors.

It has been shown that increased levels of adenosine may induce or trigger astrogliosis by effect that appears to be largely mediated by A_{2A} receptors. Thus, activation of this receptor type potentiates the synaptic action of brain-derived neurotrophic factor (BDNF) in the hippocampus (Diogenes et al.; 2007), stimulates glutamate outflow and leads to excessive glial activation, ultimately inducing astrocytosis. Indeed, it has been shown that stimulating A_{2A} receptors during brain injury (e.g.; hypoxia or inflammation) directly leads to gliosis (Cunha, 2005). Thus, it can be stated that astrogliosis is a consequence of acute ADK down-regulation. This state can be chronically maintained, allowing the development and persistence of chronic epilepsy and ultimately drug resistance. In summary, a common consequence of brain injury is astrogliosis, which can be considered the most prominent astroglial response to CNS damage (Pekny & Nilsson, 2005) and a hallmark of the epileptic brain, being present in up to 90% of surgically resected hippocampi (Thom et al.; 2002), and it has been proposed to be an important factor both in the development of seizures and in the persistency of seizure disorders. Moreover, neuronal cell loss and astrogliosis can propagate to other parts of the limbic system, including the amygdala and perirhinal cortex (Wieser, 2004). However, this causal relationship between astrogliosis, ADK up-regulation and epilepsy was recently discussed. A recent report presented evidence that the global expression levels of ADK are more closely related to epilepsy than to astrogliosis, per se (Li et al.; 2008).

4.7 A global portrait of the process

All of these data can be summarized as follows. Various types of injury, including bleeding, ischemia, infectious disease and traumatic injury, can alter the permeability of the BBB. In inflammatory or infectious disease, activation of leukocytes can induce the release of chemokines, thereby changing permeability. In other cases (for example, after brain trauma), the anatomical dysfunction of capillaries is the first step. As a consequence, albumin, which is physiologically excluded from the brain, might efflux from the vessels. In the processes that are associated with coagulation (e.g.; intracranial bleeding), albumin can bind to LPA or other platelet-derived lipids. However, at least in the initial steps, other processes such as mechanical disruption of the BBB are not associated with coagulation; in this case, albumin would not need to be attached to lipids that are produced after platelet activation. As a consequence of BBB breakdown, albumin will enter the extracellular space of the brain, where it can interact with cells that normally do not have contact. The interaction with NG2/GluR astrocytes will modify the expression of COX_2 and subsequently PGE_2, thereby inducing glutamate release through a Ca^{2+}-dependent mechanism. NG2 cells are present and accumulate in the sclerotic hippocampus. Neuronal activity, however, can depolarize NG2 cells, thereby allowing the influx of Ca^{2+}, thereby increasing $[Ca^{2+}]_i$ and glutamate release. Thus, it has been suggested that the presence of NG2/GluR cells in the sclerotic hippocampus can help to increase excitability and/or facilitate the propagation of a depolarization wave.

On the other hand, albumin will bind to either TGF-βR or albumin receptors in GFAP+/GluT astrocytes. In the former case, albumin will be taken into the astrocyte and transported to the nucleus, where it will induce various modifications in gene expression. We can speculate, in the second case, that albumin acting through the albumin receptor will increase $[Ca^{2+}]_i$, which in turn would act as a second messenger in affecting gene expression, including down-regulation of AQP4 in the BBB lumen, glutamine synthetase and Kir4.1 channels. As a consequence of these changes, extracellular glutamate and $[K^+]_o$ would increase These modifications in the external milieu will lead to changes in the excitability of neurons, presumably by modifying NMDA function.

In addition to changing extracellular albumin concentration, the primary injury can lead to a general protective reaction that consists of ADK down-regulation. If the injure is not too severe, general homeostatic mechanisms might control and reverse this process. However, if the damage is severe enough, the down-regulation will be followed by an up-regulation of ADK, thereby decreasing the anticonvulsant effect of adenosine and triggering the appearance of astrogliosis, followed by recurrent seizures and resistance to drugs.

5. Discussion and conclusions

We have revisited some diverse aspects related to epilepsy and astrocytes, including changes in gene expression patterns, integral membrane proteins and vasculature permeability in the brain. Presently, one cannot be certain which of these changes are causal or consequential to the epileptic process is. However, there cannot be doubt with regard to the participation of these changes in the disease.

The ultimate cause of epilepsy is most likely multifactorial and is both intrinsic (e.g.; genetics) and extrinsic (e.g.; stroke, inflammation, infection); however, for the first time we can now present an overview of many of the processes that lead from a normal brain to an epileptic brain.

There can be no doubt that considering this process is extremely important. Properly understanding the process of epileptogenesis might lead to the development of new approaches directed at preventing the appearance of a first seizure or recurrent seizures after a window period, addressing the increased permeability in the BBB or the efflux of albumin into the brain and perhaps blocking of the astrocytes with agents directed against either the TGF-β or calcium-dependent pathway. In this same vein— but perhaps a bit more delayed in the therapy cascade—new pharmacological approaches for increasing the anticonvulsant effects of adenosine can be studied.

However, therapeutics is not the only potential benefit of the emergence of this theory. Diagnosis can be improved by measuring the levels of molecules in the brain by PET or SPECT scanning. For example, the levels of adenosine or TGF-β receptors in patients may be measured in the future, which could be valuable in identifying the epileptic zone in patients who are being evaluated for epilepsy surgery.

A large body of data has been gleaned from animal models. However, animal models and the human pathology are not exactly equivalent; therefore, most of these hypothesis must be tested in humans, where the actual illness occurs. It is important to keep this point in mind if we wish to provide relief to epileptic patients. In this sense, it has been shown in humans that cortical slowing is a typical finding after a mild traumatic brain injury, and this may be associated with persistently increased BBB permeability and a regional cerebral blood flow (rCBF) deficit (Korn et al.; 2005).

The general portrait that has been outlined in this chapter likely raises as many questions as it answers. For example:

- Is this model correct in human patients? Obviously, this is the most important question. Several lines of evidence suggest that this model— or a modified model—could be responsible for partial epilepsies in humans. However, this hypothesis needs to be demonstrated definitively.

- Is there any difference between plasma and serum albumin? It is likely that not all CNS injuries will be associated with coagulation. Therefore, it is important to discern which mechanism of astrocyte activation (TGF-βR or calcium-dependent) is acting in a given pathological condition.
- Which of these pathways (TGF-βR or calcium-dependent), if any, act in humans? Do both pathways act in all epileptogenic processes, or do they act differentially depending on the etiology?
- What is the role of astrogliosis in epilepsy? Is it merely a finding or a causal process?

To summarize, we can affirm that astrocytes are undoubtedly very important players in the process of epileptogenesis, although their true role still needs to be completely uncovered.

6. Acknowledgment

This work was supported by a grant from the Plan Nacional de Investigación Científica, Desarrollo e Innovación Tecnológica (I+D+I), Instituto de Salud Carlos III, PS09/02116 and Convocatoria de ayudas internas para la investigación, Universidad San Pablo-CEU USP-PPC09/09.

7. References

Abbott, N.J. (2000). Inflammatory mediators and modulation of blood-brain barrier permeability. *Cell. Mol. Neurobiol.* 20, 131-147, ISSN 0272-4340.

Abbott, N.J. (2002). Astrocyte-endothelial interactions and blood-brain barrier permeability. *J. Anat.* 200, 629- 638, 0021-8782.

Anderson, C.M. & Swanson, R.A. (2000). Astrocyte glutamate transport: Review of properties, regulation, and physiological functions. *Glia* 32: 1-14, ISSN 0894-1491.

Araque, A.; Parpura, V.; Sanzgiri, R.P. & Haydon, P.G. (1998). Glutamate-dependent astrocyte modulation of synaptic transmission between cultured hippocampal neurons. *Eur J Neurosci* 10:2129-2142, ISSN 0953-816X.

Araque, A.; Li, N.; Doyle, R.T. & Haydon, P.G. (2000). SNARE protein dependent glutamate release from astrocytes. *J Neurosci* 20: 666-673, ISSN 0270-6474.

Araque, A.; Carmignoto, G. & Haydon, P.G. (2001). Dynamic signaling between astrocytes and neurons. *Annu Rev Physiol* 63: 795-813, ISSN 0066-4278.

Avoli M, Louvel J, Pumain R & Köhling F (2005). Cellular and molecular mechanisms of epilepsy in the human brain. *Prog Neurobiol*; 77: 166-200, ISSN 0301-0082.

Balabanov, R. & Dore-Duffy, P. (1998). Role of the CNS microvascular pericyte in the blood-brain barrier. *J. Neurosci. Res.* 53, 637- 644, ISSN 0270-6474.

Ballabh, P.; Braum, A. & Nedergaard, M. (2004). The blood-brain barrier: an overview. Structure, regulation and clinical implications. *Neurobiol Dis* 16: 1-13, ISSN 0969-9961.

Barres, B.A. (1991). Glial ion channels. *Curr. Opin. Neurobiol,* 1: 345-359, ISSN 0959-4388.

Boison, D. (2006). Adenosine kinase, epilepsy and stroke: mechanisms and therapies. *Trends Pharmacol. Sci.* 27, 652-658, ISSN 0165-6147.

Boison, D. (2008). The adenosine kinase hypothesis of epileptogenesis. *Prog Neurobiol* 84: 249-262, ISSN 0301-0082.

Bowser, D.N. & Khakh, B.S. (2004). ATP excites interneurons and astrocytes to increase synaptic inhibition in neuronal networks. *J Neurosci* 24: 8606-8620, ISSN 0270-6474.

Cacheaux, L.P.; Ivens, S.; David, Y.; Lakhter, A.J.; Bar-Klein, G.; Shapira, M.; Heinemann, U.; Friedman, A. & Kaufer, D. (2009) Transcriptome Profiling Reveals TGF-β Signaling Involvement in Epileptogenesis. *J. Neurosci.*; 29(28): 8927– 8935, ISSN 0270-6474.

Coco, S.; Calegari, F.; Pravettoni, E.; Pozzi, D.; Taverna, E.; Rosa, P.; Matteoli, M. &, Verderio, C. (2003). Storage and release of ATP from astrocytes in culture. *J Biol Chem* 278:1354–1362, ISSN 0021-9258.

Cornell-Bell, A.H.; Finkbeiner, S.M.; Cooper, M.S. & Smith, S.J. (1990). Glutamate induces calcium waves in cultured astrocytes: Long-range glial signaling. *Science* 247:470–473, ISSN 0036-8075.

Cotrina, M.L.; Lin, J.H.; Lopez-Garcia, J.C.; Naus, C.C. & Nedergaard, M. (2000). ATP-mediated glia signaling. *J Neurosci* 20:2835–2844, ISSN 0270-6474.

Crespel, A.; Coubes, P.; Rousset, M.C,, Brana. C,, Rougier, A.; Rondouin, G.; Bockaert, J.; Baldy-Moulinier, M. & Lerner-Natoli, M. (2002). Inflammatory reactions in human medial temporal lobe epilepsy with hippocampal sclerosis. *Brain Res*; 952:159 - 169, ISSN 0006-8993.

Cunha, R.A. (2005). Neuroprotection by adenosine in the brain: from A1 receptor activation to A2A receptor blockade. *Purinergic Signal.* 1, 111–134, ISSN 1573-9538.

de Lanerolle, N.C.; Lee, T-S. & Spencer, D.D. (2010) Astrocytes and epilepsy. *Neurotherapeutics* 7 (4):424-438, ISSN 1933-7213.

de Lanerolle, N.C.; Kim, J.H.; Williamson, A.; Spencer, S.S.; Zaveri, H.P.; Eid, T. & Spencer, D.D. (2003). A retrospective analysis of hippocampal pathology in human temporal lobe epilepsy: evidence for distinctive patient subcategories. *Epilepsia;* 44:677 - 687, ISSN 0013-9580.

Del Maschio, A.; Zanetti, A.; Corada, M.; Rival, Y.; Ruco, L.; Lampugnani, M.G.; Dejana, E. (1996) Polymorphonuclear leukocyte adhesion triggers the disorganization of endothelial cell-to-cell adherens junctions. *J Cell Biol* 135:497 - 510, ISSN 0021-9525.

Ding, S.; Fellin, T.; Zhu, Y.; Lee, S-Y.; Auberson, Y.P.; Meany, D.F.; Coulter, D.A.; Carmignoto, G. & Haydon, P.G. (2007). Enhanced astrocytic Ca2+ signals contribute to neuronal excitotoxicity after status epilepticus. *J Neurosci,* 27(40): 10674-10684, ISSN 0270-6474.

Diogenes, M.J.; Assaife-Lopes, N.; Pinto-Duarte, A.; Ribeiro, J.A. & Sebastiao, A.M. (2007). Influence of age on BDNF modulation of hippocampal synaptic transmission: interplay with adenosine A(2A) receptors. *Hippocampus* 17, 577–585, ISSN 1050-9631.

Eid, T.; Brines, M.; Cerami, A.; Spencer, D.D.; Kim, J.H.; Schweitzer, J.S.; Ottersen, O.P. & de Lanerolle, N.C. (2004). Increased expression of erythropoietin receptor on blood vessels in the human epileptogenic hippocampus with sclerosis. *J Neuropathol Exp Neurol;* 63:73 - 83, ISSN 0022-3069.

Engel, J Jr. (2001). Mesial temporal lobe epilepsy: what have we learned? Neuroscientist 7, 340–352.

Falconer, M.A. (1974). Mesial temporal (Ammon's horn) sclerosis as a common cause of epilepsy. Aetiology, treatment, and prevention. *Lancet* 2, 767–770, ISSN 0140-6736.

Fellin, T.; Pozzan, T. & Carmignoto, G. (2006). Purinergic receptors mediate two distinct glutamate release pathways in hippocampal astrocytes. *J Biol Chem* 281:4274–4284, ISSN 0021-9258.

Fiacco, T. & McCarthy, K.D. (2005). Astrocytes calcium elevations : properties, propagation, and effects on brain signaling. *Glia*, 54 : 676-690, ISSN 0894-1491.

Forsgren, L. (1990) Prospective incidence study and clinical characterization of seizures in newly referred adults. *Epilepsia*; 31:292–301, ISSN 0013-9580.

Fuentes, E.; Nadal, A. & McNaughton, P. (1999) Lysophospholipids Trigger Calcium Signals but Not DNASynthesis in Cortical Astrocytes. *Glia* 28:272–276, ISSN 0894-1491.

Furuse, M.; Sasaki, H. & Tsukita, S. (1999). Manner of interaction of heterogeneous claudin species within and between tight junction strands. *J. Cell Biol.* 147, 891– 903, ISSN 0021-9525.

Gordon, G.R.; Baimoukhametova, D.V.; Hewitt, S.A.; Rajapaksha, W.R.; Fisher, T.E.; & Bains, J.S. (2005). Norepinephrine triggers release of glial ATP to increase postsynaptic efficacy. *Nat Neurosci* 8: 1078–1086, ISSN 1097-6256.

Guerin, C.; Laterra, J.; Hruban, R.; Brem, H.; Drewes, L.R. & Goldstein, G.W. (1990). The glucose transporter and blood-brain barrier of human brain tumors. *Ann Neurol* 28:758–765, ISSN 0364-5134.

Haberg, A.; Qu, H.; Haraldseth, O.; Unsgard, G. & Sonnewald, U. (2000). In vivo effects of adenosine A1 receptor agonist and antagonist on neuronal and astrocytic intermediary metabolism studied with ex vivo 13C NMR spectroscopy. *J. Neurochem.* 74, 327–333, ISSN 0022-3042.

Halassa, M.M.; Fellin, T.; Takano, H.; Dong, J.H. & Haydon, P.G. (2007). Synaptic islands defined by the territory of a single astrocyte. *J. Neurosci.* 27, 6473–6477, ISSN 0270-6474.

Haskins, J.; Gu, L.; Wittchen, E.S.; Hibbard, J. & Stevenson, B.R. (1998). ZO-3, a novel member of the MAGUK protein family found at the tight junction, interacts with ZO-1 and occludin. *J. Cell Biol.* 141, 199–208, ISSN 0021-9525.

Hauser, W.A. (1998) Incidence and prevalence. In *Epilepsy. A comprehensive textbook Vol. 1.* Engel J Jr, Pedley T, pp. 47-57. Lippincott-Raven, ISBN: 0-397-51639-8, Philadelphia.

Haydon, P.G. & Carmignoto, G. (2006) Astrocyte control of synaptic transmission and neurovascular coupling. *Physiol Rev.*; 86(3):1009-31, ISSN 0031-9333.

Herman, S.T. (2002). Epilepsy after brain insult. Targeting epileptogenesis. *Neurology* 59 (supple 5); S21-S26, ISSN 0028-3878.

Herrera-Peco, I.; Sola, R.G.; Osejo, V.; Wix-Ramos, R. & Pastor, J. (2008). Role of astrocytes activated by albumin in epileptogenesis. *Rev Neurol* 47(11): 582-587, ISSN 0210-0010.

Hertz, L.; Dringen, R.; Schousboe, A. & Robinson, S.R. (1999). Astrocytes: glutamate producers for neurons. *J Neurosci Res*; 57:417 – 428, ISSN 0360-4012.

Itoh, M.; Furuse, M.; Morita, K.; Kubota, K.; Saitou, M. & Tsukita. S, (1999). Direct binding of three tight junction-associated MAGUKs, ZO-1, ZO- 2, and ZO-3, with the COOH termini of claudins. *J. Cell Biol.* 147, 1351–1363, ISSN 0021-9525.

Ivens, S.; Kaufer, D.; Flores, L.P.; Bechmann, I.; Zumsteg, D.; Tomkins, O.; Seiffert, E.; Heinemann, U. & Friedman, A. (2007) TGF-beta receptor-mediated albumin uptake into astrocytes is involved in neocortical epileptogenesis. *Brain* 130(Pt2):553-547, ISSN 0006-8950.

Jefferys, J.G. (1999). Hippocampal sclerosis and temporal lobe epilepsy: cause or consequence? *Brain* 122 (6), 1007–1008, ISSN 0006-8950.

Korn, A.; Golan, H.; Melamed, I.; Pascual-Marqui, R. & Friedman, A. (2005). Focal Cortical Dysfunction and Blood–Brain Barrier Disruption in Patients With Postconcussion Syndrome. *Journal Clin. Neurophysiol,* 22 (1): 1-9, ISSN 0736-0258.

Krapivinsky, G.; Krapivinsky, L.; Manasian, Y.; Ivanov, A.; Tyzio, R.; Pellegrino, C.; Ben-Ari, Y.; Clapham, D.E. & Medina, I. (2003). The NMDA receptor is coupled to the ERK pathway by a direct interaction between NR2B and RasGRF1. *Neuron* 40: 775–784, ISSN 0896-6273.

Kustova, Y.; Grinberg, A.; Basile, A.S.; (1999). Increased blood–brain barrier permeability in LP-BM5 infected mice is mediated by neuroexcitatory mechanisms. *Brain Res.* 839, 153–163, ISSN 0006-8993.

Kuzniecky, R.; De la Sayette, V.; Ethier, R.; Melanson, D.; Andermann, F.; Berkovic, S.; Robitaille, Y.; Olivier, A.; Peters, T. & Feindel, W. (1987) Magnetic resonance imaging in temporal lobe epilepsy: pathological correlations. *Ann Neurol* 22: 341–347, ISSN 0364-5134.

Jeremic, A.; Jeftinija, K.; Stevanovic, J.; Glavaski, A. & Jeftinija, S. (2001). ATP stimulates calcium-dependent glutamate release from cultured astrocytes. *J Neurochem* 77:664–675, ISSN 0022-3042.

Johnston, D. & Miao-Sin Wu, S, (2001). Propagation of the action potential in myelinated axons. In : Foundations of Cellular Neurophysiology, pp. 185-187, ISBN 0-262-10053-3, Bradford Book, Massachussettss.

Lardizabal, D.V. (2008) Medical intractability in epilepsy. In: *Texbook of Epilepsy Surgery.* H.O. Lüders, p: 245-248, ISBN: 1 84184 576 0, Infoma Healthcare, London.

Laterra, J. & Goldstein, G.W. (2000). Ventricular organization of cerebrospinal fluid: blood-brain barrier, brain edema and hydrocephalus. In *Principles of Neuralsciences, 4th Ed* Eds: ER Kandel, JH Schwartz, TM Jessell; pp: 1288-1295, ISBN 0-8385-7701-6; McGraw-Hill, New York,.

Lee, T-S.; Mane, S.; Eid, T.; Zhao, H.; Lin, A.; Guan, Z.; Kim, J.H.; Schweitzer, J.; King-Stevens, D.; Weber, P.; Spencer, S.S.; Spencer, D.D. & de Lanerolle, N.C. (2007). Gene expression in temporal lobe epilepsy is consistent with increased release of glutamate by astrocytes. *Mol Med;* 13:1 - 13, ISSN 1076-1551.

Li, T.; Lan, J-Q. & Boison, D. (2008). Uncoupling of astrogliosis from epileptogenesis in adenosine kinase (ADK) transgenic mice. *Neuron Glia Biology,* 4(2): 91-99, ISSN 1740-925X.

Louissaint, Jr, A.; Rao, S.; Leventhal, C. & Goldman, S.A. (2002). Coordinated interaction of neurogenesis and angiogenesis in the adult songbird brain. *Neuron* 34, 945- 960, ISSN 0896-6273.

Lüders, H.O. (2008). Classification of epileptic seizures and epilepsies. In: *Texbook of Epilepsy Surgery.* Ed H.O. Lüders, p: 245-248, ISBN: 1 84184 576 0, Infoma Healthcare, London;

Martin-Padura, I.; Lostaglio, S.; Schneemann, M.; Williams, L.; Romano, M.; Fruscella, P.; Panzeri, C.; Stoppacciaro, A.; Ruco, L.; Villa, A.; Simmons, D. & Dejana, E. (1998). Junctional adhesion molecule, a novel member of the immunoglobulin superfamily that distributes at intercellular junctions and modulates monocyte transmigration. *J. Cell Biol.* 142, 117–127, ISSN 0021-9525.

Matter, K. & Balda, M.S. (2003). Signalling to and from tight junctions. *Nat. Rev. Mol. Cell Biol.* 4, 225- 236.

Mi, H.; Haeberle, H. & Barres, B.A. (2001). Induction of astrocyte differentiation by endothelial cells. *J. Neurosci.* 21, 1538–1547, ISSN 0270-6474.

Morita, K.; Sasaki, H.; Fujimoto, K.; Furuse, M. & Tsukita, S. (1999). Claudin-11/OSP-based tight junctions of myelin sheaths in brain and Sertoli cells in testis. *J. Cell Biol.* 145, 579–588, ISSN 0021-9525.

Mothet, J.P.; Pollegioni, L.; Ouanounou, G.; Martineau, M.; Fossier, P. & Baux, G. (2005). Glutamate receptor activation triggers a calcium-dependent and SNARE protein-dependent release of the gliotransmitter D-serine. *Proc Natl Acad Sci USA* 102:5606–5611, ISSN 0027-8424.

Nadal, A.; Fuentes, E.; Pastor, J. & McNaughton, P.A. (1994). Dual effects of active serum albumin on [Ca2+]i of rat cortical astrocytes. *J Physiol* 45 P: 147-148P, ISSN 0022-3751.

Nadal, A.; Fuentes, E.; Pastor, J. & McNaughton, P.A. (1995) Albumin is a potent trigger of calcium signals and DNA synthesis in astrocytes. *Proc Natl Acad Sci USA* 92, 1426-1430, ISSN 0027-8424.

Nadal, A.; Fuentes, E.; Pastor, J. & McNaughton, P.A. (1997) Albumin induces calcium waves in cortical astrocytes. *Glia* 19: 343-351, ISSN 0894-1491.

Nadal, A.; Sul, J.Y.; Valdeolmillos, M. & McNaughton, P.A. (1998) Albumin elicits calcium signals from astrocytes in brain slices from neonatal rat cortex. *J Physiol* 509(3): 711-716, ISSN 0022-3751.

Nadal, A.; Fuentes, E. & McNaughton, P.A. (2001) Glial cell responses to lysophospholipids bound to albumin in serum and plasma. *Prog Brain Res* 132: 367-374, ISSN 0079-6123.

Nett, W.J.; Oloff, S.H. & McCarthy, K.D. (2002). Hippocampal astrocytes in situ exhibit calcium oscillations that occur independent of neuronal activity. *J Neurophysiol* 87:528–537, ISSN 0022-3077.

Newman, E.A. (2005). Calcium increases in retinal glial cells evoked by light-induced neuronal activity. *J Neurosci* 25:5502–5510, ISSN 0270-6474.

Nuñez, L. & García-Sancho, J. (1996). Two different constituents of plasma increas cytosolic calcium selectively in neurons or glia of primary rat cerebellar cultures. *J. Physiol,* 490(3): 577-583, ISSN 0022-3751.

Parpura, V.; Basarsky, T.A.; Liu, F.; Jeftinija, K.; Jeftinija, S. & Haydon, P.G, (1994). Glutamate-mediated astrocyte-neuron signalling. *Nature* 369: 744–747, ISSN 0028-0836.

Parri, H.R. & Crunelli, V. (2003). The role of Ca2+ in the generation of spontaneous astrocytic Ca2+ oscillations. *Neuroscience* 120: 979–992, ISSN 0306-4522.

Pastor, J.; Uzcátegui, Y.G.; Gal, B.; Ortega, G.J.; Sola, R.G. & Menéndez de la Prida. L, (2006). The pathophysiological foundations of temporal-lobe epilepsy: studies in humans and animals. *Rev. Neurol.;* 42(11): 663-673, ISSN 0210-0010.

Pastor, J.; Herrera, I.; Ortega, G.J. & Sola, R.G. (2010) Human astrocytes in culture respond to albumin with an increase in cytosolic calcium and DNA synthesis. *Epilepsia,* 51(Suppl. 4): 34, ISSN 0013-9580

Pearson, T.; Damian, K.; Lynas, R.E. & Frenguelli, B.G. (2006). Sustained elevation of extracellular adenosine and activation of A(1) receptors underlie the post-ischaemic inhibition of neuronal function in rat hippocampus in vitro. *J. Neurochem.* 97, 1357–1368, ISSN 0022-3042.

Pekny, M. & Nilsson, M.;(2005). Astrocyte activation and reactive gliosis. *Glia* 50, 427–434, ISSN 0894-1491.

Peters, O.; Schipke, C.G.; Hashimoto, Y. & Kettenmann, H. (2003). Different mechanisms promote astrocyte Ca21 waves and spreading depression in the mouse neocortex. *J Neurosci* 23:9888–9896, ISSN 0270-6474.

Picot, M.C.; Baldy-Moulinier, M.; Daurs, J.P.; Dujois, P. & Crespel, A. (2008). The prevalence of epilepsy and pharmacoresistant epilepsy in adults: a population-based study in a Western European country. *Epilepsia* 49:1230–1238, ISSN 0013-9580.

Porter, J.T. & McCarthy, K.D. (1997). Astrocytic neurotransmitter receptors in situ and in vivo. *Prog Neurobiol* 51:439–455, ISSN 0301-0082.

Ramsauer, M.; Krause, D. & Dermietzel, R. (2002). Angiogenesis of the blood - brain barrier in vitro and the function of cerebral pericytes. *FASEB J.* 16, 1274–1276, ISSN 0892-6638.

Ravizza, T.; Gagliardi, B.; Noè, F.; Boer, K.; Aronica, E. & Vezzani, A. (2007). Innate and adaptive immunity during epileptogenesis and spontaneous seizures: evidence from experimental models and human temporal lobe epilepsy. *Neurobiol Dis* 29:142 - 160, ISSN 0969-9961.

Rigau, V.; Morin, M.; Rousset, M.C.; de Bock, F.; Lebrun, A.; Coubes, P.; Picot, M.C.; Baldy-Moulinier, M.; Bockaert, J.; Crespel, A. & Lerner-Natoli, M. (2007). Angiogenesis is associated with blood-brain barrier permeability in temporal lobe epilepsy. *Brain,* 130:1942 - 1956, ISSN 0006-8950.

Schinkel, A.H.; Smit, J.M.; Vantellingen, O.; Beijnen, J.H.; Wagenaar, E.; Vandeemter, L.; Vandervalk, M.A.; Robanusmaandag, E.C.; Teriele, H.P.J.; Berns, A.J.M. & Borst, P. (1994). Disruption of the mouse *mdr1a* P-glycoprotein gene leads to a deficiency in the blood-brain barrier and to increased sensitivity to drugs. *Cell* 77:491–502, ISSN 0092-8674.

Seifert, G.; Hüttmann, K.; Schramm, J. & Steinhäuser, C. (2004). Enhanced relative expression of glutamate receptor 1 flip AMPA receptor subunits in hippocampal astrocytes of epilepsy patients with Ammon' s horn sclerosis. *J Neurosci*; 24: 1996–2003, ISSN 0270-6474.

Seiffert, E.; Dreier, J.P.; Ivens, S.; Bechmann, I.; Tomkins, O.; Heinemann, U. & Friedman, A. (2004). Lasting blood-brain barrier disruption induces epileptic focus in the rat somatosensory cortex. *J Neurosci.* 24(36): 7829-36, ISSN 0270-6474

Smith, K.M.; Slugoski, M.D.; Cass, C.E.; Baldwin, S.A.; Karpinski, E. & Young, J.D, (2007). Cation coupling properties of human concentrative nucleoside transporters hCNT1, hCNT2 and hCNT3. *Mol. Membr. Biol.* 24, 53–64, ISSN 0968-7688.

Spencer, S.S. (1998). Substrates of localization-related epilepsies: biological implications of localizing findings in humans. *Epilepsia* 39, 114–123, ISSN 0013-9580.

St'astný, F.; Skultetyova, I.; Pliss, L. & Jezova, D. (2000). Quinolinic acid enhances permeability of rat brain microvessels to plasma albumin. *Brain Res. Bull.* 53, 415–420, ISSN 0361-9230.

Steinhäuser, C. & Seifert, G. (2002). Glial membrane channels and receptors in epilepsy: impact for generation and spread of seizure activity. *Eur J Pharmacol,* 447: 227 - 237, ISSN 0014-2999.

Studer, F.E.; Fedele, D.E.; Marowsky, A.; Schwerdel, C.; Wernli, K.; Vogt, K.; Fritschy, J-M, & Boison, D. (2006). Shift of adenosine kinase expression from neurons to astrocytes during postnatal development suggests dual functionality of the enzyme. *Neuroscience* 142, 125–137, ISSN 0306-4522.

Suadicani, S.O.; Flores, C.E.; Urban-Maldonado, M.; Beelitz, M. & Scemes, E. (2004). Gap junction channels coordinate the propagation of intercellular Ca21 signals generated by P2Y receptor activation. *Glia* 48:217–229, ISSN 0894-1491.

Takano, T.; Kang, J.; Jaiswal, J.K.; Simon, S.M.; Lin, J.H.; Yu, Y.; Li, Y.; Yang, J.; Dienel, G.; Zielke, H.R. & Nedergaard, M. (2005). Receptor-mediated glutamate release from volume sensitive channels in astrocytes. *Proc Natl Acad Sci USA* 102:16466–16471, ISSN 0027-8424.

Thom, M.; Sisodiya, SM.; Beckett, A.; Martinian, L.; Lin, W.R.; Harkness, W.; Mitchell, T.N.; Craig, J.; Duncan, J. & Scaravilli, F. (2002). Cytoarchitectural abnormalities in hippocampal sclerosis. *J. Neuropathol. Exp. Neurol.* 61, 510–519, ISSN 0022-3069.

Tian, G.F.; Azmi, H.; Takano, T.; Xu, Q.; Peng, W.; Lin, J.; Oberheim, N.A.; Lou, N.; Wang, X.; Zielke, H.R.; Kang, J. & Nedergaard, M. (2005). An astrocytic basis of epilepsy. *Nat. Med;* 11(9): 973-981, ISSN 1078-8956.

Utsumi, H.; Chiba, H.; Kamimura, Y.; Osanai, M.; Igarashi, Y.; Tobioka, H.; Mori, M. & Sawada, N. (2000). Expression of GFRalpha-1, receptor for GDNF, in rat brain capillary during postnatal development of the BBB. *Am. J. Physiol.: Cell Physiol.* 279: 361–368, ISSN 0363-6143.

van Calker, D. & Biber, K. (2005). The role of glial adenosine receptors in neural resilience and the neurobiology of mood disorders. *Neurochem. Res.* 30, 1205–1217, ISSN 0364-3190.

van Vliet, E.A.; da Costa Araujo, S.; Redeker, S.; van Schaik, R.; Aronica, E. & Gorter, J.A. (2007). Blood-brain barrier leakage may led to progression of temporal lobe epilepsy. *Brain* 130:521–534, ISSN 0006-8950.

Vezzani, A.; Moneta, D.; Richichi, C.; Aliprandi, M.; Burrows, S.J.; Ravizza, T.; Perego, C. & De Simoni, M.G. (2002). Functional role of inflammatory cytokines and antiinflammatory molecules in seizures and epileptogenesis. *Epilepsia* 43 (Suppl 5): 30–35, ISSN 0013-9580.

Vezzani, A.; Ravizza, T.; Balosso, S. & Aronica, E. (2008). Glia as a source of cytokines: implications for neuronal excitability and survival. *Epilepsia,* 49 (Suppl.2): 24-32, ISSN 0013-9580.

Wang, S.; Cheng, Q.; Malik, S. & Yang, J. (2000). Interleukin-1beta inhibits gamma-aminobutyric acid type A (GABA(A)) receptor current in cultured hippocampal neurons. *J Pharmacol Exp Ther* 292:497 - 504, ISSN 0022-3565.

Wang, Z.; Haydon, P.G, & Yeung, E.S, (2000). Direct observation of calcium-independent intercellular ATP signaling in astrocytes. *Anal Chem* 72: 2001–2007, ISSN 3-2700

Wang, C.T.; Grishanin, R.; Earles, C.A.; Chang, P.Y.; Martin, T.F.; Chapman, E.R. & Jackson, M.B. (2001). Synaptotagmin modulation of fusion pore kinetics in regulated exocytosis of dense-core vesicles. *Science* 294: 1111–1115, ISSN 0036-8075.

Wieser, H.G. (2004). ILAE Commission on Neurosurgery of Epilepsy. ILAE Commission Report. Mesial temporal lobe epilepsy with hippocampal sclerosis. *Epilepsia* 45, 695–714, ISSN 0013-9580.

Wolosker, H.; Blackshaw, S. & Snyder, S.H. (1999). Serine racemase: a glial enzyme synthesizing D-serine to regulate glutamate-*N*-methyl-D-aspartate neurotransmission. *Proc Natl Acad Sci USA* 96: 13409–13414, ISSN 0027-8424

Ye, Z.C.; Wyeth, M.S.; Baltan-Tekkok, S. & Ransom, B.R. (2003). Functional hemichannels in astrocytes: A novel mechanism of glutamate release. *J Neurosci* 23:3588–3596, ISSN 0270-6474.

Zhang, J.M.; Wang, H.K.; Ye, C.Q.; Ge, W.; Chen, Y.; Jiang, Z.L.; Wum, C.P.; Poo, M.M.; & Duan, S. (2003). ATP released by astrocytes mediates glutamatergic activity-dependent heterosynaptic suppression. *Neuron* 40: 971–982, ISSN 0896-6273.

Zonta, M.; Angulo, M.C.; Gobbo, S.; Rosengarten, B.; Hossmann, K.A.; Pozzan, T. & Carmignoto, G. (2003). Neuron-to-astrocyte signaling is central to the dynamic control of brain microcirculation. *Nat. Neurosci.* 6, 43– 50, ISSN 1097-6256.

Zur Nieden, R. & Deitmer, J.W. (2006). The role of metabotropic glutamate receptors for the generation of calcium oscillations in rat hippocampal astrocytes in situ. *Cereb Cortex* 16:676–687, ISSN 1047-3211.

3

START Proteins in Epilepsy

Sang Pil Yoon
Jeju National University
Republic of Korea

1. Introduction

Epilepsy is a condition with seizures by abnormal, recurrent, and excessive discharges from neurons. Observations in experimental models of epilepsy are providing a better understanding of the mechanisms of seizure-induced excitotoxicity, neuroprotective responses and neurogenesis (Naegele, 2007). Excitotoxic neurodegeneration can be investigated in epilepsy models employing kainic acid or pilocarpine. Each model results in distinctive patterns of degeneration within the hippocampus through kainate subclass of glutamate receptors or cholinergic receptors, respectively. Kainic acid triggers neuronal injury directly by binding to kainate receptors on mossy fiber endings and on the principal neurons of the hippocampus. Pilocarpine causes cell death of a majority of the nonprincipal neurons of the hilus and CA1 pyramidal cells.

Intensive researches have shown that some steroids display neuroprotective properties in various diseases including epilepsy (Wojtal et al., 2006; Biagini et al., 2010). The steroids can be classified into 'neuroactive steroids' and 'neurosteroids'. The term 'neuroactive steroids' may be synthesized both in the nervous system and in the endocrine glands such as gonads, adrenal glands and placenta, and exert their effects on neural tissue. 'Neurosteroids', the concept derived from Baulieu (1997), are a family of steroid hormones including pregnenolone, dehydroepiandrosterone, progesterone and their derivatives. Neurosteroids are synthesized in the nervous system de novo from cholesterol and accumulated in the nervous system independently of classical steroidogenic gland secretion rates.

Neurosteroids act in the nervous system in an autocrine/paracrine configuration (Plassart-Schiees & Baulieu, 2001). They may regulate gene expression by binding to nuclear receptors or affect neurotransmission through action at membrane ion-gated and other neurotransmitter receptors. In addition, they affect neuronal growth, survival and differentiation, cause regression of neuritic extensions before they have established contact with other neurons or glia and protect neurons from death. Modulatory roles of neurosteroids include γ-amino-butyric acid (GABA), N-methyl-D-aspartate, nicotinic/muscarinic cholinergic, serotonin, kainite and glycine receptor functions.

Neuroprotective properties of neurosteroids have been revealed and gained particular attention in the treatment of diseases where neurodegeneration is predominant, including epilepsy (Naegele, 2007; Biagini et al., 2010). Seizures not only cause cell death, but also elicit neuroprotective responses in injured neurons and glia. Seizures trigger the release of neuroactive steroids that impair hippocampal neuron survival in excitotoxicity. Increased neurosteroid synthesis, presumably occurring in glial cells during epileptogenesis, delays the appearance of recurrent spontaneous seizures in temporal lobe epilepsy. In this chapter, various molecules connected with neurosteroidogenesis are reviewed in order to provide further understanding on epilepsy.

2. Neurosteroids and lipid/cholesterol

Lipids have broad information carrying function in the central nervous system (CNS) as both ligands and substrates for proteins (Adibhatla & Hatcher, 2008). Lipid metabolism may be important for the CNS, as this organ has the highest concentration of lipids next to adipose tissue. The crucial role of lipids in tissue physiology and cell signaling is demonstrated by the many neurological disorders, and altered lipid metabolism is also believed to be a key event which contributes to CNS injuries. Lipids serve not only structural components of the cell membrane but also precursors for various second messengers. Especially, cholesterol is an important regulator of lipid organization and the precursor for steroid biosynthesis.

The first step in the biosynthesis of neurosteroids is the conversion of cholesterol to pregnenolone (Wojtal et al., 2006; Biagini et al., 2010). This reaction is catalyzed by the cytochrome P450 cholesterol side-chain cleavage (p450scc) in successive chemical reactions. First and foremost, transport of cholesterol to the mitochondria is a prerequisite for neurosteroidogenesis. Cholesterol is not only needed for the growth and remodeling of neuronal and glial membranes, but also is an important regulator of lipid organization and the precursor for steroid biosynthesis (Adibhatla & Hatcher, 2008). The majority of cholesterol in the brain is derived from de novo synthesis in the neurons, astrocytes predominantly, and oligodendrocytes. Cholesterol is then secreted via transport molecules, taken up by lipoprotein receptors on neurons and internalized to the endosome/lysosome system.

Cholesterol is transported to mitochondria by Niemann-Pick C1 (NPC1) protein where the neurosteroids are synthesized via the rate limiting intermediate, pregnenolone (Adibhatla & Hatcher, 2008). NPC1 protein is involved in transport of lipids, particularly cholesterol, from the late endosome/lysosome. Deficiency in the protein results in lysosomal accumulation of cholesterol and other lipids. Then, proteins located in the mitochondrial membranes, such as peripheral benzodiazepine receptor (PBR) and steroidogenic acute regulatory protein (StAR), allow cholesterol to cross the hydrophilic intermembrane space (Lavaque et al., 2006). In the mitochondria, the neurosteroids are synthesized from the cholesterol via the rate limiting intermediate pregnenolone.

Observations are providing a better understanding of the transport of cholesterol by NPC1, PBR or StAR (Adibhatla & Hatcher, 2008). Niemann-Pick disease type C is due to mutations in either the NPC1 or NPC2 genes, resulting in defective cholesterol transport and cholesterol accumulation. The PBR, which might function as a cholesterol channel, is essential for the delivery of cholesterol to the inner mitochondrial membrane and the synthesis of steroids. However, it should be noted that these molecules are not the only molecules implicated in the metabolism of cholesterol and little attention has been paid to StAR-related lipid transfer (START) domain-containing proteins (START proteins).

3. START proteins

START domain is an evolutionary conserved protein module of approximately 210 amino acids (Soccio & Breslow, 2003; Alpy & Tomasetto, 2005; Lavigne et al., 2010). START domain is conserved through in plants and animals and serves as a versatile binding interface for lipids. The crystal structures of solved START domain reveal a conserved 'helix-grip' fold, in which a central antiparallel β-sheet is gripped by N-terminal and C-terminal α-helices, the latter being closely packed above the nine-strand curved β-sheet.

In humans, START domains are found in 15 distinct proteins and can be classified by 6 subfamilies (Table 1). Mammalian START proteins have diverse expression patterns and can be found free in the cytoplasm, attached to membranes or in the nucleus. START proteins implicate in intracellular lipid transport, lipid metabolism, and cell signaling events. Mutation or mis-expression of START proteins is linked to pathological processes, including genetic disorders, autoimmune diseases and cancer. Nevertheless, START proteins have not been extensively studied in the nervous system except 2 proteins, StAR and StarD6.

Group	Other names	Subcellular localization	Gene
StarD1	StarD1/StAR	Mitochondria	8p11.2
	StarD3/MLN64	Late endosomes	17q11-q12
StarD4	StarD4	Cytosol and Nucleus	5q22.1
	StarD5	Cytosol and Nucleus	15q26
	StarD6	Nucleus	18q21.2
StarD2	StarD2/PCTP	Cytosol	17q21-q24
	StarD7	?	2q11.2
	StarD10	Cytosol and Nucleus	11q13
	StarD11/CERT	Cytosol and Golgi	5q13.3
RhoGAP	StarD8	?	Xq13.1
	StarD12/DLC-1	Plasma membrane	8p22
	StarD13/DLC-2	Cytosol	13q12-q13
Thioesterase	StarD14/BFIT	?	1p32.3
	StarD15/CACH	Cytosol	5q14.1
StarD9	StarD9	?	15q15.1-q15.2

Table 1. Phylogenetic group and 15 human START proteins quoted from Alpy & Tomasetto (2005) with slight modification. BFIT, brown fat-inducible thioesterase; CACH, cytoplasmic acetyl-CoA hydrolase; CERT, Goodpasture-antigen-binding protein Δ 26; DLC, deleted in liver cancer; MLN64, metastatic lymph node 64; PCTP, phosphatidylchoine transfer protein; RhoGAP; Rho-GTPase-activating-protein-domain.

3.1 Subcellular characteristics of StAR and StarD6

StAR, the prototype of START proteins, is first characterized in murine MA-10 Leydig tumor cells that luteinizing hormone induces the expression of StAR and ultimately results in increased synthesis of pregnenolone (Clark et al., 1994). Its function has been extensively studied in classical steroidogenic tissue such as adrenal gland and ovary, and it has been shown to be involved in the intramitochondrial trafficking of cholesterol (Stocco, 2001). In steroidogenic cells, StAR-mediated delivery of cholesterol to inner mitochondrial membrane is a hormonally regulated step and StAR expression is tightly regulated (Stocco, 2001; Stocco et al., 2005).

StarD6 is originally reported in male germ cell-specific protein of StarD4 group of START proteins (Soccio et al., 2002; Gomes et al., 2005). It is immunolocalized only in the nuclei of germ cells, not in the interstitial cells of Leydig, and may have a pivotal role in spermatogenesis rather than in steroidogenesis. StarD6 is detected in the nucleus of mature sperm cells, where it could interact with transcriptional machinery in a lipid-dependent manner. Since lipids play an important role in sperm capacitation and function, StarD6 might regulate lipid movement within the sperm cell membrane.

StarD6 in the Leydig cells has also been reported under perinatal hypothyroidism while germ cell-specific immunoreactivity is delayed (Chang et al., 2007a), which means that StarD6 also might play a role in the steroidogenesis under certain conditions such as testosterone deficiency. In this context, StarD6 might interact with mitochondrial membranes just similar to that of StAR (Bose et al., 2008). StarD6 has a protease-sensitive C-terminus similar to that of StAR and exhibits a steroidogenic activity equal to StAR. Recently, this question is ascertained in the nervous system by morphometry (Chang et al., 2010).

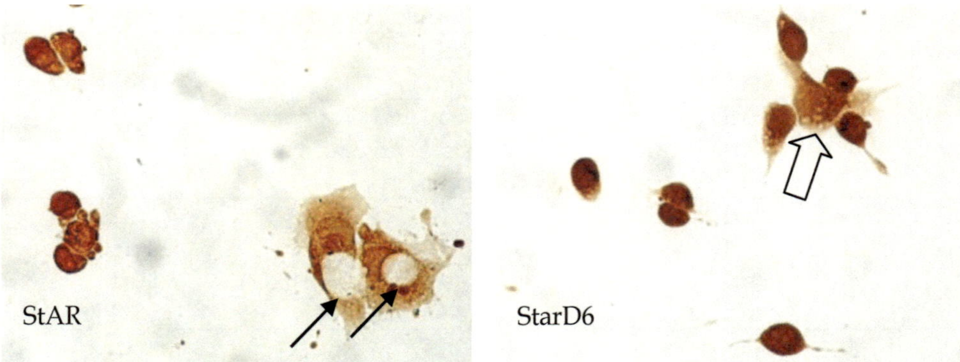

Fig. 1. Micrographs of StAR and StarD6 in cultured dopaminergic neurons (SK-N-SH cell line). StAR is localized in the cytoplasm (arrows) but StarD6 loses the localization in nucleus (open arrow) according to maturation. Original magnification X40. (quoted from Chang et al., 2010)

Morphological aspects of StarD6 are significantly different from those of StAR in cultured neuronal and glial cells. Cultured cells are dopaminergic neuronal cells (SK-N-SH) and glioma cells, M059-K and M059-J, which M059-J lack DNA-dependent protein kinase (DNA-PK) activity while M059-J express normal levels of DNA-PK. StAR tends to localize in the cytoplasm but StarD6 showed a weak intensity in the nucleus according to neuronal maturation (Fig. 1), while both are immunolocalized in the nuclei as well as the cytoplasm in glioma cells. The number of StAR and StarD6 immunopositive cells is significantly different in SK-N-SH and M059-K and M059-J, respectively. Especially, the immunoreactivities of StarD6 in glioma cells are considerably changed by the presence of DNA-PK, while there is no significance in StAR (Fig. 2).

The morphometric results with StarD6 in glioma cells have meaning, since oxidative DNA damage by excitotoxicity may activate DNA repair proteins in affected neurons (Naegele, 2007). The number of StarD6 is significantly decreased in the glioma cell line which lacks DNA-PK activity. DNA-PK plays a role in nonhomologous end joining (NHEJ) against DNA damage, which comprises of catalytic subunit of the DNA-PK (DNA-PKcs), Ku70, and Ku80 (Martin, 2008). NHEJ system is activated by severe forms of DNA damage, DNA double-stand breaks. Increasing evidences implicate DNA-PK in neuroprotective properties. Experimental DNA-PK null mice show increased excitotoxicity and result in augmented apoptosis (Culmsee et al., 2001; Neema et al., 2005). It suggests that the activity of StarD6 in the nucleus might depend on the DNA repair system in preventing DNA damage.

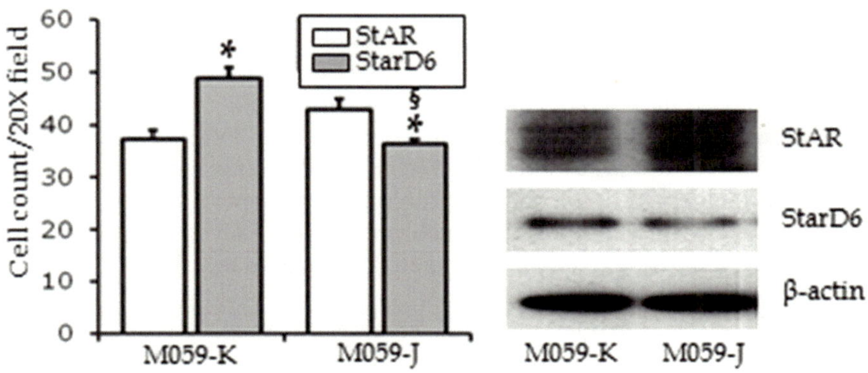

Fig. 2. Histographs of StAR and StarD6 in cultured glioma cell lines. M059-J cells lack DNA-dependent protein kinase (DNA-PK) activity, while M059-K cells express normal levels of DNA-PK (acquired from American Type Culture Collection, ATCC, Rockville, MD, USA). The number of immunopositive cells was significantly different by StAR or StarD6 in the M059-K and M059-J, respectively (*$p<0.05$). Unlike StAR, the immunoreactivities of StarD6 were considerably changed by the presence of DNA-PK (§$p<0.05$), and it was also demonstrated by Western blot analysis. Data are quoted from Chang et al., 2010 (left) and unpublished data (right).

3.2 Distribution of StAR and StarD6 in the nervous system

StAR appears to be widely distributed throughout the brain, although different levels of expression have been detected between different brain areas including human (Furukawa et al., 1998; King et al., 2002; Sierra et al., 2003; Sierra, 2004; Lavaque et al., 2006). High levels of StAR mRNA expression have been detected in the cerebral cortex, hippocampus proper, dentate gyrus, olfactory bulb, and cerebellar cortex. In general, there is a good agreement between those from in situ mRNA localization and data from immunohistochemical studies. This may implicate that steroidogenesis is a generalized process in the nervous system.

StAR immunoreactivity has been detected in several neuronal populations, in ependymocytes and in some astroglial cells in the brain (Lavaque et al., 2006). StAR expression, however, seems to be restricted to very specific neuronal and astroglial populations in each brain area. Strong StAR immunoreactivity is observed in the soma of large neurons, which are characterized by high mitochondrial content. Although StAR is predominantly expressed by neurons in the CNS, astrocytes also express STAR and is known to synthesize neurosteroids from cholesterol. StAR may contribute to the regulation of cell proliferation in the nervous system, since steroids are known to affect neuronal and glial differentiation (Lavaque et al., 2006). Important changes in the pattern and/or level of expression of StAR occur in different brain areas during postnatal development (Kim et al., 2002; Sierra et al., 2003). For instance, in the cerebellar cortex Purkinje cells express StAR as well as have an active steroidogenic activity, in particular during the developmental period (Tsutsui et al., 2003). Changes of StAR in the developing cerebellar cortex may therefore be related with the differentiation of Purkinje cells. Important changes in the expression of StAR occur as well during brain aging. In 24-month-old rats StAR immunoreactivity is increased in hippocampal and cortical neurons compared with young animals (Sierra et al., 2003), while decreased in the aged cerebellum (Lavaque et al., 2006). It is unknown what is the physiological significance of these changes in StAR expression in the brain and whether they are associated with differences in steroidogenesis.

Furthermore, StAR is colocalized in the same neural cells with p450scc and with other steroidogenic enzymes (Furukawa et al., 1998; King et al., 2002). It may implicate that StAR as a transport protein may participate in neurosteroidogenesis in the CNS. Strikingly, no deficiency in brain function or structure was reported either in StAR knockout mice or in congenital adrenal hyperplasia patients (Sierra, 2004). The brain may have StAR-independent mechanisms of mitochondrial cholesterol transport. It should be noted that other proteins that contain the START domain might be involved in steroidogenesis and that their regional patterns of expression in the brain remain to be determined.

	StAR	StarD6
Cerebrum	Neuron (layers V-VI) >>glia	Neuron (layers V-VI) >glia
Hippocampus		
Cornu ammonis	Strata oriens/radiatum	Stratum pyramidale
Dentate gyrus	Mild granular layer	Granular layer
Cerebellum	Purkinje cell (+)	Purkinje cell (±)

Table 2. Distribution of StAR and StarD6 in the nervous system. Although StAR and StarD6 can be detected in neurons and glia, they are primarily immunolocalized in the neurons of rodents. Unlike the cerebral cortex, they have compensatory distribution in the hippocampus and cerebellum. (According to Furukawa et al., 1998; King et al., 2002; Sierra et al., 2003; Sierra, 2004; Chang et al., 2007b, 2009, 2010)

Not much is known on the distribution, development and aging of StarD6 in the CNS (Table 2). StarD6 is seen in the cerebral cortex, cerebellum, hippocampus, spinal cord and dorsal root ganglia (Chang et al., 2007b, 2009), where the highest expression of StAR is reported (Sierra, 2004; Lavaque et al., 2006). Strong StarD6 immunoreactivity is observed in deeper layers of cerebral cortex, principal cell layers of hippocampus and substantia gelatinosa of spinal cord, but devoid in Purkinje cell layer of cerebellum and lower motor neurons of spinal cord. From morphological point of view StarD6 also immunolocalized in glial cells, but the characteristics are not determined properly.

StarD6 immunolocalization was mainly restricted to the nucleus, but cytoplasmic immunostaining frequently appeared in the principal neurons of hippocampus and spinal cord. This subcellular localization pattern is a distinctive feature of StarD4 group (Alpy & Tomasetto, 2005; Soccio et al., 2005). But the characteristics of the immunostaining of the StarD6 in the cytoplasm and the nucleus remain largely undetermined. The existing data (Gomes et al., 2005; Chang et al., 2007a,2007b,2009,2010; unpublished data) are obtained with the rat-specific polyclonal anti-StarD6 antibody (raised from Dr. Soh's laboratory, Chonnam National University, Republic of Korea), and it should be confirmed by the monoclonal antibody.

3.3 Changes of StAR and StarD6 in epilepsy

3.3.1 Generalized changes of StAR and StarD6 in epileptic hippocampus

Neurosteroids can interact with various neurotransmitters (Joëls, 2009; Biagini et al., 2010). In particular, neurosteroids are well known to potentiate the actions of GABA via $GABA_A$

receptors against stress. Neurosteroids not only facilitate inhibitory responses, but also reduce the slope of the field excitatory postsynaptic potential in the dentate gyrus toward more inhibition. Various neurotrophic factors, including hormones, alter cellular activity in all hippocampal subfields in a region-specific way (Joëls, 2009).

StAR has been related to neuroprotection (Sierra et al., 2003; Sierra, 2004). StAR mRNA and protein levels are transitorily increased following excitotoxic brain injury induced by the administration of kainic acid (Sierra et al., 2003). A fast and transient increase in StAR mRNA levels in the hippocampus was detected in the first 12 hours after injury. This was accompanied by an increase in StAR immunoreactivity in granular and hilar hippocampal neurons in the first 12-24 hours after the administration of kainic acid.

In addition, StAR immunostaining is more intense in neurons located in the strata oriens and radiatum of normal hippocampus. The pattern of distribution changed in the pilocarpine-induced epileptic hippocampus (Chang et al., 2010). StAR was immunolocalized in the stratum pyramidale as well as the strata oriens and radiatum 3 hours after pilocarpine treatment, while changed immunoreactivity in the dentate gyrus was not remarkable. But, the changes in distribution in the hippocampus proper did not discussed in kainic acid-induced epilepsy model (Sierra et al., 2003).

A strong increase in StAR immunoreactivity was observed in layers II and III of the pyriform cortex of kainic acid-injected animals (Sierra et al., 2003). However, in deeper cortical layers the cellular mortality was very high. Therefore, a large increment of StAR expression of hippocampal granular neurons after brain injury is especially resistant to the toxicity of kainic acid. The expression in dentate gyrus is related to neuroprotection in status epilepticus. Moreover, subgranular neurons have mitotic activity and increased StAR might affect on neurogenesis and differentiation in epileptic hippocampus.

StarD6 is acutely and transiently increased after excitotoxic brain injury also (Chang et al., 2009, 2010). The changes are seen in the granular and polymorphic layers of the dentate gyrus and the CA subfields of the hippocampus 3 hours after pilocarpine treatment. In the CA1-2 areas, StarD6 immunoreactivity was increased in the strata lacunosum-moleculare as well as stratum oriens and stratum radiatum after the lesion. This increase in immunolocalization remained until 12 hours after experiencing epilepsy, and then slightly decreased up to 24 hours after epilepsy. StarD6 immunoreactivity remained in the pyramidal layer of the CA subfields, whereas the granular layer of dentate gyrus was not very intensely stained. In agreement with the distributional changes, a significant increase in StarD6 protein is detected 3 hour after brain injury with respect to the untreated animals and 24 hours after epilepsy.

Similar results in distribution and Western blot analysis are obtained in domoic acid-induced epilepsy model (unpublished data). Domoic acid is a kainic acid analogue and characteristically damages the hippocampus since hippocampus has well developed glutamate receptors (Coulter et al., 2002; Naegele 2007). Western analysis revealed significant change in the level of StarD6 in response to domoic acid, an increase being observed 4 hours after the epilepsy compared with normal hippocampus.

3.3.2 Time-course of StAR and StarD6 after epileptic injury

Neurosteroids are potent trophic and survival factors for the nervous system and the synthesis is related to the extent of p450scc induction. The p450scc enzyme is found in neurons, astrocytes, oligodendrocytes, and in activated microglial cells (Biagini et al., 2010).

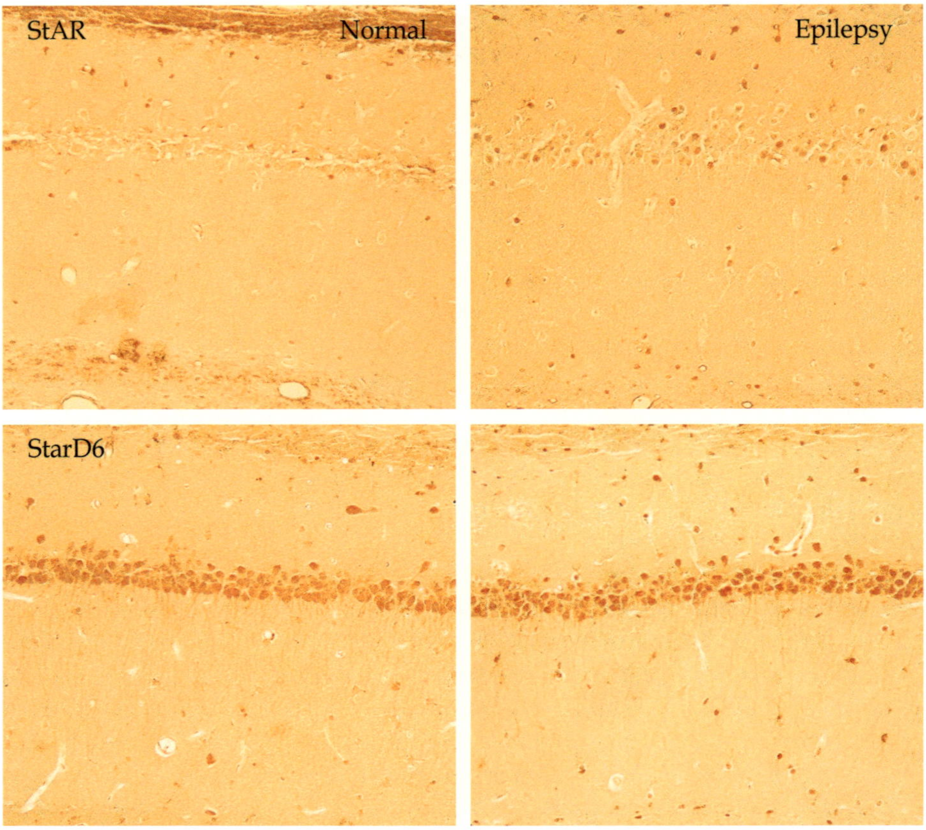

Fig. 3. Compensatory distribution of StAR and StarD6 in normal and epileptic hippocampus. StAR immunolocalization was seen in the strata oriens and radiatum while StarD6 in the stratum pyramidale in normal hippocampus. Augmented immunolocalization of StAR was observed in the stratum pyramidale and StarD6 in the strata lacunosum-moleculare after pilocarpine-induced epilepsy. Figures are aligned by stratum pyramidale. Original magnification X20.

Neurosteroid levels can be altered as consequence of neuronal damage as well as of glial cell activation. A significant increase in p450scc both in neurons and glial cells is reported, but the neuron-specific changes were limited to the first few days after status epilepticus whereas those in glial cells were long-lasting. Therefore, neurosteroidogenesis is related to the extent of p450scc induction in glial cells consequent to status epilepticus.

Activation of various molecules connected with steroidogenesis after brain injury results in a significantly increased synthesis of neurosteroids. Interestingly the increase in StAR and StarD6 was restricted to neurons in epileptic hippocampus. An urgent increase of StarD6, even compared with StAR, after excitotoxic brain injury may be the first attempt to respond to primary neurodegeneration (Figure 4). Early induction of StarD6 as well as StAR is followed by later increase in the expression of various steroidogenic enzymes including p450scc (Furukawa et al., 1998; Garcia-Ovejero et al., 2002; Biagini et al., 2006).

The induction of StAR in neurons under neurodegenerative conditions is followed by the increase in the expression of PBR in glial cells (Lavaque et al., 2006). The induction of StAR and PBR has a different time course. StAR expression is increased within the first day after lesion while the increase in PBR expression is observed from 1 to 5 weeks after lesion. Therefore, StAR and PBR may participate in different phases of steroidogenesis after brain injury. The increased expression of these molecules may be the cause of the increase in the production of neurosteroids, such as pregnenolone. Changes in the expression of StAR and PBR may also result in the production of other neuroprotective steroids.

Meanwhile, the results with StarD6 suggest another aspect on neurosteroidogenesis. On the assumption that StarD6 participate in the regulation of the production of neuroprotective steroids, the responses of StarD6 might be coincided with the hypothesis that it is the first attempt to respond to epilepsy in accordance with brain injury resulting in a significant increased synthesis of neurosteroids (Di Michele et al., 2000). As a result, nuclear immunostaining and early response of StarD6 may regulate gene expression by binding to nuclear receptors (Mellon et al., 2001; Plassart-Schiess & Baulieu, 2001). StarD6 can act as transcriptional machinery in a lipid-dependent manner and thus stimulate neurosteroidogenesis by activating StAR and other steroidogenic enzymes. But, direct relationship between StAR and StarD6 is not confirmed yet in the nervous system.

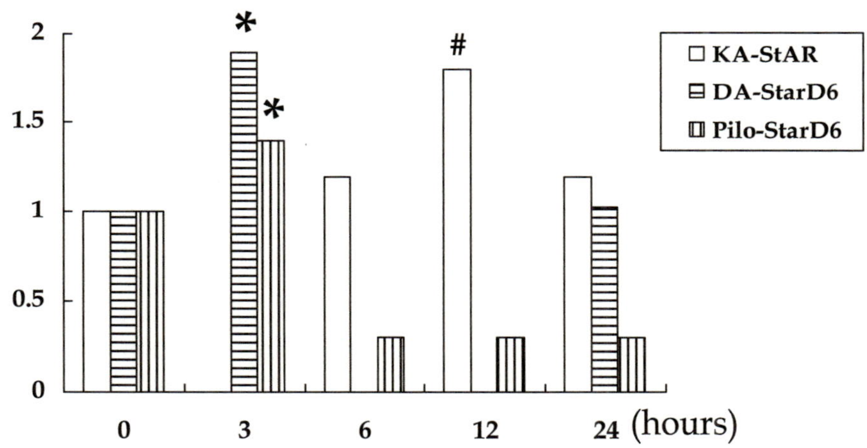

Fig. 4. Representative changes in StAR and StarD6 in the hippocampus after excitotoxic insult. The histogram shows relative densitometric values of StAR mRNA (Sierra et al., 2003) and StarD6 protein (Chang et al., 2009; unpublished data). The animals killed 12 h after kainic acid (KA) administration showed a significant increase in StAR mRNA levels. Considerable changes in StarD6 level in response to domoic acid (DA) or pilocarpine (Pilo) observed 3-4 hours after the epilepsy. (The densitometric results are modified from original manuscript)

3.3.3 Area-specific changes of StAR and StarD6 in epileptic hippocampus

Epilepsy could cause widespread neurodegeneration in CA1-3 pyramidal layers of the hippocampus (Naegele, 2007), but there is enough ground for controversy on the area-specific degeneration of hippocampus. Epilepsy-related neurodegeneration is mainly limited to CA3 area of the hippocampus (Neema et al., 2005; Kajitani et al., 2006; Ma et al., 2006; Chuang et al., 2009; Zhang et al., 2009), while the neurons in CA1 area survive in various animal models (Marti et al., 2002; Dinocourt et al., 2003; Cavazos et al., 2004; Sanon et al., 2005; Wittner et al., 2005).

When rats are treated with kainic acid, a rapid and transient increase in StAR mRNA and protein was detected 12 hours after brain injury in the hippocampus (Sierra et al., 2003). A strong increase in StAR immunostaining was observed in the granular layer of dentate gyrus while the control hippocampus was not very intensely stained. The results do not provide effective involvement of StAR for steroidogenesis, but possible role in neuroprotection in neurons against excitotoxic injury. In this context, distribution of StAR changed in the pilocarpine-induced epileptic hippocampus (Chang et al., 2010). StAR immunostaining is localized in the strata oriens and radiatum of normal hippocampus, and in the stratum pyramidale as well in epileptic hippocampus. The changes in immunolocalization are reported in CA1-2 areas, not in the dentate gyrus.

Similar results on area-specific changes are reported with StarD6 in epileptic hippocampus (Chang et al., 2009, 2010; unpublished data). The StarD6 immunolocalizations are seen in the strata lacunosum-moleculare as well as strata oriens and radiatum after excitotoxic injury with pilocarpine and domoic acid, respectively. The changes in the strata correspond with distribution of steroidogenic enzymes such as p450scc (Furukawa et al., 1998; Garcia-Ovejero et al., 2002; Biagini et al., 2006). As a result, StarD6, StAR and p450scc might act in consecutive order following excitotoxic brain injury, result in neurosteroidogenesis.

In addition, the morphometric data (Chang et al., 2010) with StarD6 in DNA-PK deficient cells are in accord with the previous reports that lack of DNA-PK promotes apoptosis (Culmsee et al., 2001; Neema et al., 2005). It can be interpreted that the activity of StarD6 in the nucleus might depend on the DNA repair proteins. To investigate whether StarD6 is related with DNA repair system in nervous system, epilepsy model was established by domoic acid (unpublished data, Fig. 5). Contrary to the hypothesis based on previous reports, there was negative correlation between StarD6 and NHEJ (data not shown).

But the levels of apurinic/apyrimidinic endonuclease (APE, also called redox factor-1) and 8-oxoguanine DNA glycosylase (Ogg1) increased considerably at 4 hours after domoic acid injection. The responses are quite similar to previous reports with kainic acid (Quach et al., 2005; Jarrett et al., 2008) and that of StarD6 (Fig. 4). The results support the notion that oxidative DNA damage in neurons is primarily removed by base excision repair (BER) pathway rather than by NHEJ (Fishel et al., 2007). Despite activation of DNA repair systems after excitotoxic injury, the repair responses may not sufficient to overcome for extensive DNA damage.

The distribution of BER proteins revealed that transient increase of APE in strata radiatum and lacunosum-moleculare and Ogg1 in stratum pyramidale. Increased immunoreactivities of APE and Ogg1 diminished in the pyramidal cells of CA3 area 24 hours after domoic acid injection compared to CA1. In case of StarD6, the immunostaining was induced in the strata radiatum and lacunosum-moleculare after epilepsy and then normalized in the stratum pyramidale in CA3 as well as CA1. Neurodegeneration in CA3 pyramidal cells may be caused by the decreased BER activity after seizure since there was no area-specific change in StarD6 especially in CA3. StarD6 in the nucleus did not respond on DNA repair system after epilepsy, but immunolocalization of StarD6 as well as APE in the strata lacunosum-moleculare may have significance where localized various steroidogenic enzymes (Furukawa et al., 1998; Patte-Mensah et al., 2003; Biagini et al., 2006; Wojtal et al., 2006; Chia et al., 2008).

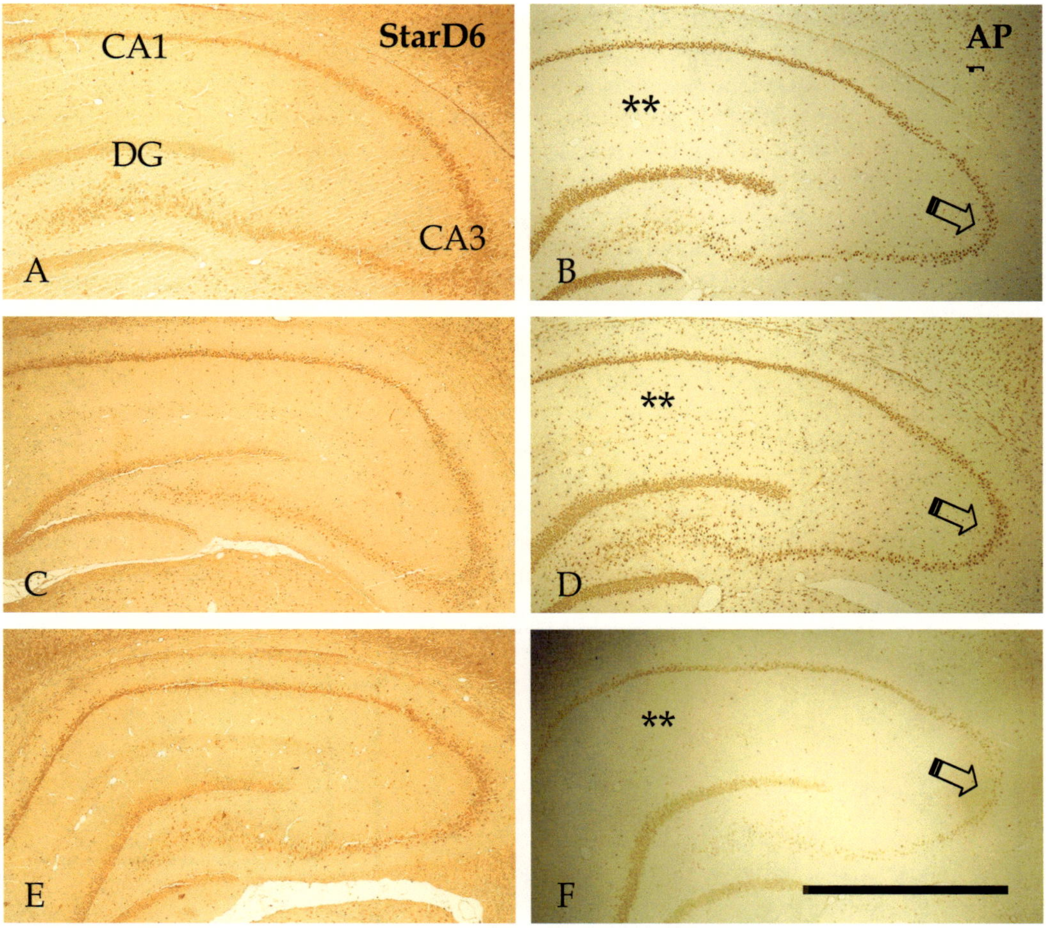

Fig. 5. Area-specific changes of StarD6 and APE in epileptic hippocampus. Immunoreactivities of StarD6 and APE increased in the strata radiatum and lacunosum-moleculare (*) 3 hours after epilepsy (C and D) compared with control hippocampus (A and B) or 5 days after epilepsy (E and F). Note the changes in stratum pyramidale. Although StarD6 immunoreactivity remained in all subfields, the intensities diminished in CA3 (arrow) while those in CA1 were maintained. Scale bar = 1mm.

3.3.4 Functional aspects of StAR and StarD6 in epileptic hippocampus

StAR has been shown to be involved in the intramitochondrial trafficking of cholesterol (Alpy & Tomasetto, 2005; Lavigne et al., 2010). Then, cholesterol is made available to the first enzyme of the steroidogenic pathway, p450scc, which transforms cholesterol into pregnenolone, the precursor for glucocorticoids, mineralocorticoids and sex steroids. StAR-mediated delivery of cholesterol to the inner mitochondrial membrane, where p450scc is located, is a hormonally regulated step, which is rate limiting in steroidogenesis.

The up-regulation of StAR expression after excitotoxic injury suggests that this protein may play a role in the adaptation of neural tissue to neurodegenerative conditions (Sierra et al., 2003; Sierra, 2004; Lavaque et al., 2006; Chang et al., 2010). That is, StAR in the dentate gyrus and hippocampus might be associated with neuroprotection and neurosteroidogenesis, respectively. Strikingly, no deficiency in brain function or structure was reported either in StAR knockout mice or in congenital adrenal hyperplasia patients (Sierra, 2004). The brain may have StAR-independent mechanisms of mitochondrial cholesterol transport.

It should be noted that StAR is not the only molecule implicated in the mitochondrial transport of cholesterol. PBR, which might function as a cholesterol channel, is essential for the delivery of cholesterol to the inner mitochondrial membrane and the synthesis of steroids. NPC1 is also involved in transport of lipids from the late endosome to mitochondria. Furthermore, there has been described a family of proteins which contain the START domain. These START domain proteins, such as StarD6, are related to steroidogenesis.

In some START proteins, the START domain probably functions in lipid sensing rather than in lipid transfer (Alpy and Tomasetto, 2005; Lavigne et al., 2010). StarD2/PCTP, StarD4, StarD5 and StarD10 are detected in the cytoplasm and nucleus, and StarD6 only in the nucleus. It is therefore possible that some START-containing proteins have nuclear roles and may even regulate transcription in a lipid-dependent manner. Structurally, the START domain contains a lipid-binding domain specific for diacylglycerol/phorbol-ester, the C1 domain (Brose and Rosenmund, 2002) and functions as a lipid-sensing domain providing a rapid way of regulating the catalytic activity, and thus modulates lipid metabolism.

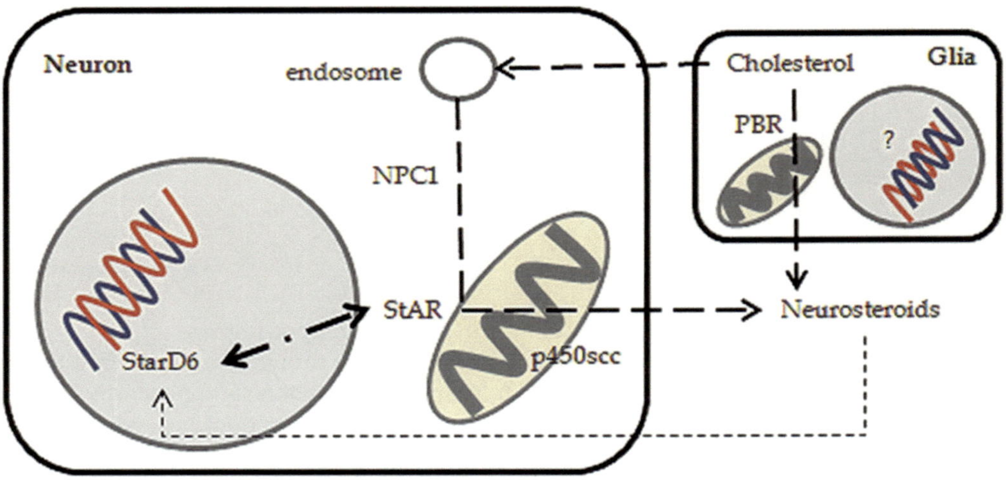

Fig. 6. Schematic representation of various molecules participating in neurosteroidogenesis. StAR and PBR is mainly localized in the outer mitochondrial membrane of neuron and glia, respectively, while p450scc acts in the inner mitochondrial membrane. Note StarD6 in the nucleus, which may interact with StAR for neurosteroidogenesis. Stimulus-dependent up-regulation of START proteins appears as follows; StarD6 in a few hours and StAR in a day, while PBR and p450scc in a few weeks.

The changed immunolocalization of StarD6 in the strata lacunosum-moleculare might suggest a role of this protein as a regulator of transcription related to the cholesterol metabolism (Chang et al., 2009, 2010, unpublished data). Although StAR is a well known protein implicated in the steroidogenesis, StarD6 changed the localization from stratum pyramidale to the strata lacunosum-moleculare after excitotoxic injury. Another important change is the time course of responsiveness after epilepsy. The response of StarD6 arises

from the nucleus with DNA repair proteins to respond to excitotoxic stimuli. StarD6 can function as a lipid-sensing domain and modulate neurosteroid synthesis.
There is growing evidence that cholesterol is of particular importance in development of Alzheimer's disease (Wojtal et al., 2006; Adibhatla & Hatcher, 2008). In the patients' brains of Alzheimer's disease, a general trend was observed towards decreased levels of all steroids. The lower levels correlated with increased amounts of β-amyloid peptides and phosphorylated tau proteins. Increased level of StAR is reported in aged rats (Sierra et al., 2003) and in patients with Alzheimer's disease (Webber et al., 2006) compared with young animals and age-matched patients without dementia, respectively. It means that the expression of StAR hormonally regulated by the level of neurosteroids in the nervous system. Although the existing knowledge on StarD6 is still incomplete, it can be expected that StarD6 is also regulated by the levels of neurosteroids, cholesterol and lipid. Furthermore, StarD6 is localized in the nucleus and appears early response than StAR in epilepsy (Chang et al., 2009, 2010, unpublished data), results in stimulus-dependent expression of StAR follows after StarD6.

4. Conclusion

The START domain operates as a lipid exchange and/or a lipid-sensing domain. There are 15 mammalian proteins that possess a START domain, an evolutionary conserved protein module and they are involved in several different biological processes: lipid transfer, lipid metabolism and signal transduction. While the role of StAR in steroid hormone production has been demonstrated, StarD6 remain largely uncharacterized. Much less is understood about how its START domain specifically recognizes cholesterol and how it affects on other molecules participating in neurosteroidogenesis. StarD6 can take precedence over other molecules such as StAR, PBR and p450scc in excitotoxic brain injury and they might be hormonally regulated. There are no reports on the brain function or structure in StarD6 knockout animal model or in patients' brain and the brain may have StarD6-independent mechanisms of lipid/cholesterol sensing. Therefore, further studies are needed to elucidate the exact nuclear roles of StarD6 on neurosteroidogenesis with StAR in the nervous system. It could suggest new therapeutic strategy for epilepsy since neurosteroids act as autocrine or paracrine neuromodulators and the regulation of neurosteroidogenesis may have profound influences in the nervous system.

5. Acknowledgment

I am indebted to In Youb Chang (Chosun University, Republic of Korea) for critical reading of the chapter; Sa Sun Cho (Professor Emeritus, Seoul National University, Republic of Korea) for his helpful discussion. Anti-StarD6 antibody was a kind gift of Jaemog Soh (Chonnam National University, Republic of Korea).

6. References

Alpy, F. & Tomasetto, C. (2005). Give lipids a START: the StAR-related lipid transfer (START) domain in mammals. *Journal of Cell Science*, Vol. 118, No. (Pt)13, (July 2005), pp. 2791-2801, ISSN 0021-9533

Adibhatla, R.M. & Hatcher, J.F. (2008). Altered lipid metabolism in brain injury and disorders. *Subcellular Biochemistry*, Vol. 49, (April 2008), pp. 241-268, ISSN 0306-0225

Baulieu, E.E. (1997). Neurosteroids: of the nervous system, by the nervous system, for the nervous system. *Recent Progress in Hormone Research*, Vol. 52, (January 1997), pp. 1-31, ISSN 0079-9963

Biagini, G.; Baldelli, E.; Longo, D.; Pradelli, L.; Zini, I.; Rogawski, M.A. & Avoli, M. (2006). Endogenous neurosteroids modulate epileptogenesis in a model of temporal lobe epilepsy. *Experimental Neurology*, Vol. 201, No. 2, (October 2006), pp. 519-524, ISSN 0014-4886

Biagini, G.; Panuccio, G. & Avoli, M. (2010). Neurosteroids and epilepsy. *Current Opinion in Neurology*, Vol. 23, No. 2, (April 2010), pp. 170-176, ISSN 1350-7540

Bose, H.S.; Whittal, R.M.; Ran, Y.; Bose, M.; Baker, B.Y. & Miller, W.L. (2008). StAR-like activity and molten globule behavior of StARD6, a male germ-line protein. *Biochemistry*, Vol. 47, No. 8, (February 2008), pp. 2277-2288, ISSN 0006-2960

Brose, N. & Rosenmund, C. (2002). Move over protein kinase C, you've got company: alternative cellular effectors of diacylglycerol and phorbol esters. *Journal of Cell Science*, Vol. 115, No. (Pt)23, (December 2002), pp. 4399-4411, ISSN 0021-9533

Cavazos, J.E.; Jones, S.M. & Cross, D.J. (2004). Sprouting and synaptic reorganization in the subiculum and CA1 region of the hippocampus in acute and chronic models of partial-onset epilepsy. *Neuroscience*, Vol. 126, No. 3, (March 2004), pp. 677-688, ISSN 0306-4522

Chang, I.Y.; Shin, S.Y.; Kim, J.W.; Yu, J.M.; Kim, J.S.; Song, P.I. & Yoon, S.P. (2007a). The changed immunolocalization of START-domain-containing 6 (StarD6) during the development of testes in rat perinatal hypothyroidism. *Acta Histochemica*, Vol. 109, No. 4, (August 2007), pp. 315-321, ISSN 0065-1281

Chang, I.Y.; Kim, J.H.; Hwang, G.; Song, P.I.; Song, R.J.; Kim, J.W. & Yoon, S.P. (2007b). Immunohistochemical detection of StarD6 in the rat nervous system. *Neuroreport*, Vol. 18, No. 15, (October 2007), pp. 1615-1619, ISSN 0959-4965

Chang, I.Y.; Kim, J.K.; Lee, S.M.; Kim, J.N.; Soh, J.; Kim, J.W. & Yoon, S.P. (2009). The changed immunoreactivity of StarD6 after pilocarpine-induced epilepsy. *Neuroreport*, Vol 20, No. 10, (July 2009), pp. 963-967, ISSN 0959-4965

Chang, I.Y.; Jeon, Y.J.; Jung, S.M.; Jang, Y.H.; Ahn, J.B.; Park, K.S. & Yoon, S.P. (2010). Does the StarD6 mark the same as the StAR in the nervous system? *Journal of Chemical Neuroanatomy*, Vol. 40, No. 3, (November 2010), pp. 239-242, ISSN 0891-0618

Chia, W.J.; Jenner, A.M.; Farooqui, A.A. & Ong, W.Y. (2008). Changes in cytochrome P4450 side chain cleavage expression in the rat hippocampus after kainite injury. *Experimental Brain Research*, Vol. 186, No. 1, (March 2008), pp. 143-149, ISSN 0014-4819

Chuang, Y.C.; Chen, S.D.; Liou, C.W.; Lin, T.K.; Chang, W.N.; Chan, S.H. & Chang, A.Y. (2009). Contribution of nitric oxide, superoxide anion, and peroxynitrite to activation of mitochondrial apoptotic signaling in hippocampal CA3 subfield following experimental temporal lobe status epilepticus. *Epilepsia*, Vol. 50, No. 4, (June 2009), pp. 731-746, ISSN 0013-9580

Clark, B.J.; Wells, J.; King, S.R. & Stocco, D.M. (1994). The purification, cloning, and expression of a novel luteinizing hormone-induced mitochondrial protein in MA-10 mouse Leydig tumor cells. Characterization of the steroidogenic acute regulatory protein (StAR). *Journal of Biological Chemistry,* Vol. 269, No. 45, (November 1994), pp. 28314-28322, ISSN 0021-9258

Coulter, D.A.; Mclntyre, D.C. & Lőöscher, W. (2002). Animal models of limbic epilepsies: what can they tell us? *Brain Pathology,* Vol. 12, No. 2, (April 2002), pp. 240-256, ISSN 1015-6305

Culmsee, C.; Bondada, S. & Mattson, M.P. (2001). Hippocampal neurons of mice deficient in DNA-dependent protein kinase exhibit increased vulnerability to DNA damage, oxidative stress and excitotoxicity. *Brain Research Molecular Brain Research,* Vol. 87, No. 2, (March 2001), pp. 257-262, ISSN 0169-328X

di Michele, F.; Lekieffre, D.; Pasini, A.; Bernardi, G.; Benavides, J. & Romeo, E. (2000). Increased neurosteroids synthesis after brain and spinal cord injury in rats. *Neuroscience Letters,* Vol. 284, No. 1-2, (April 2000), pp. 3-12, ISSN 0304-3940

Dinocourt, C.; Petanjek, Z.; Freund, T.F.; Ben-Ari, Y. & Exclapez, M. (2003). Loss of interneurons innervating pyramidal cell dendrites and axon initial segments in the CA1 region of the hippocampus following pilocarpine-induced seizures. *Journal of Comparative Neurology,* Vol. 459, No. 4, (May 2003), pp. 407-425, ISSN 0021-9967

Fishel, M.L.; Vasko, M.R. & Kelley, M.R. (2007). DNA repair in neurons: so if they don't divide what's to repair? *Mutation Research,* Vol. 614, No. 1-2, (January 2007), pp. 24-36, ISSN 0027-5107

Furukawa, A.; Miyatake, A.; Ohnishi, T. & Ichikawa, Y. (1998). Steroidogenic acute regulatory protein (StAR) transcripts constitutively expressed in adult rat central nervous system: colocalization of StAR, cytochrome P-450scc (CYP XIA1), and 3beta-hydroxysteroid dehydrogenase in the rat brain. *Journal of Neurochemistry,* Vol. 71, No. 6, (December 1998), pp. 2231-2238, ISSN 0022-3042

Garcia-Ovejero, D.; Veiga, S.; Garcia-Segura, L.M. & DonCarlos, L.L. (2002). Glial expression of estrogen and androgen receptors after rat brain injury. *Journal of Comparative Neurology,* Vol. 450, No. 3, (August 2002), pp. 256-271, ISSN 0021-9967

Gomes, C.; Oh, S.D.; Kim, J.W.; Chun, S.Y.; Lee, K.S.; Kwon, H.B. & Soh, J. (2005). Expression of the putative sterol binding protein Stard6 gene is male germ cell specific. *Biology of Reproduction,* Vol. 72, No. 3, (March 2005), pp. 651-658, ISSN 0006-3363

Jarrett, S.G.; Liang, L.P.; Hellier, J.L.; Staley, K.J. & Patel, M. (2008). Mitochondrial DNA damage and impaired base excision repair during epileptogenesis. *Neurobiology of Disease,* Vol. 30, No. 1, (April 2008), pp. 130-138, ISSN 0969-9961

Joëls, M. (2009). Stress, the hippocampus, and epilepsy. *Epilepsia,* Vol. 50, No. 4, (April 2009), pp. 586-597, ISSN 0013-9580

Kajitani, K.; Yamaguchi, H.; Dan, Y.; Furuichi, M.; Kang, D. & Nakabeppu, Y. (2006). MTH1, an oxidized purine nucleoside triphosphatase, suppresses the accumulation of oxidative damage of nucleic acids in the hippocampal microglia during kainite-induced excitotoxicity. *Journal of Neuroscience,* Vol. 26, No. 6, (February 2006), pp. 1688-1698, ISSN 0270-6474

Kim, H.J.; Park, C.H.; Roh, G.S.; Kang, S.S.; Cho, G.J. & Choi, W.S. (2002). Changes of steroidogenic acute regulatory protein mRNA expression in postnatal rat development. *Brain Research Developmental Brain Research*, Vol. 139, No. 2, (December 2002), pp. 247-254, ISSN 0165-3806

King, S.R.; Manna, P.R.; Ishii, T.; Syapin, P.J.; Ginsberg, S.D.; Wilson, K.; Walsh, L.P.; Parker, K.L.; Stocco, D.M.; Smith, R.G. & Lamb, D.J. (2002). An essential component in steroid synthesis, the steroidogenic acute regulatory protein, is expressed in discrete regions of the brain. *Journal of Neuroscience*, Vol. 22, No. 24, (December 2002), pp. 10613-10620, ISSN 0270-6474

Lavaque, E.; Sierra, A.; Azcoitia, I. & Garcia-Segura, L.M. (2006). Steroidogenic acute regulatory protein in the brain. *Neuroscience*, Vol. 138, No. 3, (March 2006), pp. 741-747, ISSN 0306-4522

Lavigne, P.; Najmanivich, R. & Lehoux, J.G. (2010). Mammalian StAR-related lipid transfer (START) domains with specificity for cholesterol: structural conservation and mechanism of reversible binding. *Subcellular Biochemistry*, Vol. 51, (April 2010), pp. 425-437, ISSN 0306-0225

Ma, D.L.; Tang, Y.C.; Chen, P.M.; Chia, S.C.; Jiang, F.L.; Burgunder, J.M.; Lee, W.L. & Tang, F.R. (2006). Reorganization of CA3 area of the mouse hippocampus after pilocarpine induced temporal lobe epilepsy with special reference to the CA3-septum pathway. *Journal of Neuroscience Research*, Vol. 83, No. 2, (February 2006), pp. 318-331, ISSN 0360-4012

Martin, L.J. (2008). DNA damage and repair: relevance to mechanisms of neurodegeneration. *Journal of Neuropathology and Experimental Neurology*, Vol. 67, No. 5, (May 2008), pp. 377-387, ISSN 0022-3069

Mellon, S.H.; Griffin, L.D. & Compagnone, N.A. (2001). Biosynthesis and action of neurosteroids. *Brain Research Reviews*, Vol. 37, No. 1-3, (November 2001), pp. 3-12, ISSN 0165-0173

Naegele, J.R. (2007). Neuroprotective strategies to avert seizure-induced neurodegeneration in epilepsy. *Epilepsia*, Vol. 48, No. Supplement s2, (April 2007), pp. 107-117, ISSN 0013-9580

Neema, M.; Navarro-Quiroga, I.; Chechlacz, M.; Gilliams-Francis, K.; Liu, J.; Lamonica, K.; Lin, S.L. & Naegele, J.R. (2005). DNA damage and nonhomologous end joining in excitotoxicity: neuroprotective role of DNA-PKcs in kainic acid-induced seizures. *Hippocampus*, Vol. 15, No. 8, (October 2005), pp. 1057-1071, ISSN 1050-9631

Patte-Mensah, C.; Kappes, V.; Freund-Mercier, M.J.; Tsutsui, K. & Mensah-Nyagan, A.G. (2003). Cellular distribution and bioactivity of the key steroidogenic enzyme, cytochrome P450 side chain cleavage, in sensory neural pathways. *Journal of Neurochemistry*, Vol. 86, No. 5, (September 2003), pp. 1233-1246, ISSN 0022-3042

Plassart-Schiess, E. & Baulieu, E.E. (2001). Neurosteroids: recent findings. *Brain Research Reveiws*, Vol. 37, No. 1-3, (November 2001), pp. 133-140, ISSN 0165-0173

Ponting, C.P. & Aravind, L. (1999). START: a lipid-binding domain in StAR, HD-ZIP and signaling proteins. *Trends in Biochemical Sciences*, Vol. 24, No. 4, (April 1999), pp. 130-132, ISSN 0968-0004

Quach, N.; Chan, T.; Lu, T.A.; Schreiber, S.S. & Tan, Z. (2005). Induction of DNA repair proteins, Ref-1 and XRCC1, in adult rat brain following kainic acid-induced seizures. *Brain Research*, Vol. 1042, No. 2, (May 2005), pp. 236-240, ISSN 0006-8993

Rune, G.M. & Frotscher, M. (2005). Neurosteroid synthesis in the hippocampus: role in synaptic plasticity. *Neuroscience*, Vol. 136, No. 3, (March 2005), pp. 833-842, ISSN 0306-4522

Sanon, N.; Carmant, L.; Emond, M.; Congar, P. & Lacaille, J.C. (2005). Short-term effects of kainic acid on CA1 hippocampal interneurons differently vulnerable to excitotoxicity. *Epilepsia*, Vol. 46, No. 6, (June 2005), pp. 837-848, ISSN 0013-9580

Sierra, A.; Lavaque, E.; Perez-Martin, M.; Azcoitia, I.; Hales, D.B. & Garcia-Segura, L.M. (2003). Steroidogenic acute regulatory protein in the rat brain: cellular distribution, developmental regulation and overexpression after injury. *European Journal of Neuroscience*, Vol. 18, No. 6, (September 2003), pp. 1458-1467, ISSN 0953-816X

Sierra, A. (2004). Neurosteroids: the StAR protein in the brain. *Journal of Neuroendocrinology*, Vol. 16, No. 9, (September 2004), pp. 787-793, ISSN 0953-8194

Soccio, R.E.; Adams, R.M.; Romanowski, M.J.; Sehayek, E.; Burley, S.K. & Breslow, J.L. (2002). The cholesterol-regulated StarD4 gene encodes a StAR-related lipid transfer protein with two closely related homologues, StarD5 and StarD6. *Proceedings of the National Academy of Sciences of the United States of America*, Vol. 99, No. 10, (May 2002), pp. 6943-6948, ISSN 0027-8424

Soccio, R.E. & Breslow, J.L. (2003). StAR-related lipid transfer (START) proteins: mediators of intracellular lipid metabolism. *Journal of Biological Chemistry*, Vol. 278, No. 25, (June 2003), pp. 22183-22186, ISSN 0021-9258

Soccio, R.E.; Adams, R.M.; Maxwell, K.N. & Breslow, J.L. (2005). Differential gene regulation of StarD4 and StarD5 cholesterol transfer proteins: activation of StarD4 by SREBP-2 and StarD5 by endoplasmic reticulum stress, *Journal of Biological Chemistry*, Vol. 280, No. 19, (May 2005), pp. 19410-19418, ISSN 0021-9258

Stocco, D.M. (2001). StAR protein and the regulation of the steroid hormone biosynthesis. *Annual Review of Physiology*, Vol. 63, (March 2001), pp. 193-213, ISSN 0066-4278

Stocco, D.M.; Wang, X.; Jo, Y. & Mann, P.R. (2005). Multiple signaling pathways regulating steroidogenesis and star expression: more complicated than we thought. *Molecular Endocrinology*, Vol. 19, No. 11, (November 2005), pp. 2647-2659, ISSN 0888-8809

Tsutsui, K.; Sakamoto, H. & Ukena, K. (2003). A novel aspect of the cerebellum: biosynthesis of neurosteroids in the Purkinje cell. *Cerebellum*, Vol. 2, No. 3, (June 2003), pp. 215-222, ISSN 1473-4222

Webber, K.M.; Stocco, D.M.; Casadesus, G.; Bowen, R.L.; Atwood, C.S.; Previll, L.A.; Harris, P.L.; Zhu, X.; Perry, G. & Smith, M.A. (2006). Steroidogenic acute regulatory protein (StAR): evidence of gonadotrophin-induced steroidogenesis in Alzheimer disease. Molecular neurodegeneration, Vol. 1, (October 2006), pp. 14, ISSN 1750-1326

Wittner, L.; Eross, L.; Czirjak, S.; Halasz, P.; Freund, T.F. & Magloczky, Z. (2005). Surviving CA1 pyramidal cells receive intact perisomatic inhibitory input in the human epileptic hippocampus. *Brain*, Vol. 128, No. (Pt)1, (January 2005), pp. 138-152, ISSN 0006-8950

Wojtal, K.; Trojnar, M.K. & Czuczwar S.J. (2006). Endogenous neuroprotective factors: neurosteroids. *Pharmacological Reports*, Vol. 58, No. 3, (May-June 2006), pp. 335-340, ISSN 1734-1140.

Zhang, S.; Khanna, S. & Tang, F.R. (2009). Patterns of hippocampal neuronal loss and axon reorganization of the dentate gyrus in the mouse pilocarpine model of temporal lobe epilepsy. *Journal of Neuroscience Research*, Vol. 87, No. 5, (April 2009), pp. 1135-1149, ISSN 0360-4012

4

Introduction of a Novel Molecular Mechanism of Epilepsy Progression: Roles of Growth Hormone Signaling in a Mouse Model of Temporal Lobe Epilepsy

Keiko Kato
Kyoto Sangyo University, Kyoto
Japan

1. Introduction

Epilepsy is a chronic neurological disease involving recurring behavioral seizures, and affects approximately 1% of the worldwide population of humans and cats, and 2-3% of dogs. Epilepsy causes recurring behavioral seizures, which are transient behavioral changes caused by disordered, synchronized, and rhythmic firings of populations of neurons in the brain that propagate to regions connected with the first insult on the neural circuits, induced by abnormal neural plasticity (Browne and Holmes 2000). The seizure expression is induced by idiopathic/cryptogenic and remote symptomatic causes, as concrete examples, febrile illness in children younger than 16 years (Besli et al., 2010) and cerebrovascular and ethanol/drug-related accidents in adults. When the seizures are prolonged, or occur in a series, there is an increased risk of status epilepticus. About 15 % of persons with epilepsy experience status epilepticus, which induces more brain damage. It is known that large populations of epilepsy patients express status epilepticus due to medication changes in both children and adults. Hence, improving the compliance of patients to take medicine appropriately is very helpful to prevent the expression of status epilepticus.

Despite the importance of medication, more than one third of patients with epilepsy are estimated to have pharmacoresistant epilepsy (Browne and Holmes 2000). Half of patients with refractory epilepsy are characterized as having mesial temporal lobe epilepsy (TLE) with foci in the amygdaloid complex, hippocampus, and surrounding cortex. To solve the problem of pharmacoresistance, it is important to clarify the molecular mechanisms involved in the development of pharmacoresistant seizures. Additionally, patients with epilepsy are at high risk of developing anxiety, depression, learning disorders, and sudden death (Dodrill, 1986; Franks, 2003; Motamedi and Meador, 2003; Sillanpää and Shinnar, 2010). To improve the quality of life of patients, it is useful to clarify the comorbidity between seizures and other neuropsychiatry disorders. Depression and anxiety have the highest incidence in patients with TLE (Perini, et al., 1996). Hence, it should be clarified how the molecular signaling system regulates the development of pharmacoresistant abnormal neural plasticity and, as a result, recurring prolonged seizures that are induced by symptomatic causes. New drugs that can respond to seizures that known drugs fail to cure should be developed based on the newly found signaling machinery. Many researchers have found molecular candidates responsible for seizure progression and the molecular mechanisms have been clarified little by little (Jia et al., 2011; Pitkänen and Lukasiuk, 2011). On the other hand, we have focused on clarification of the molecular mechanisms of epilepsy progression using a mesial TLE mouse model, amygdale kindled mice, showing epileptic seizures induced due to the development of abnormal neural plasticity in TLE regions. So far we have found three molecules responsible for epileptogenesis, a growth hormone, a sialyltransferase, and ganglioside GQ1b (Matsuhashi et al., 2003; Kato et al., 2008; Kato et al., 2009). The clarification of signaling mechanisms with these molecules will resolve the pharmacoresistancy and open a path for therapeutic intervention for cases of anxiety and depression in the near future.

2. Experimental animals

2.1 Introduction of experimental animal models

Several chronic models showing recurrent seizures have been developed as shown in Table 1.

Stimulant	Chronic recurrent seizures	References
Physical	kindling	Goddard et al., 1969; Racine et al., 1972; Kato et al., 2001
Chemical (metal)	alumina cream	Heinemann et al., 1986
	cobalt	Chang et al., 2004
	ferric iron	Willmore and Ueda, 2009
Chemical (drug)	pentylenetetrazol (Chronic schedule)	Schallier et al., 2009
	kainate	Antonucci et al., 2009
	pilocarpine	Pitkänen et al., 2011
Inherited	EL mice	Fueta et al., 1983
	DBA/2 mice (audiogenic)	Seyfried and Glaser, 1981
	SER rat	Hanaya et al., 2010
	Mongolian gerbil	Buchhalter 1993
	targeted gene-deficient mice	Puranam and McNamara, 1999; Meisleret al., 2001

Table 1. Species of epileptic model animals (especially rodents).

Physical (electro-stimulation): Kindling consists of the repeated administration of subconvulsive electrical stimulus to any of several brain regions, resulting in the development of EEG seizures (afterdischarges) and progressive behavioral seizures. When repeated stimuli are administrated into the amygdaloid complex and hippocampus, mesial temporal lobe epilepsy (MTLE), which is the cause in one-half patients with refractory epilepsy, is induced as eventual secondary generalized grand mal seizures. The kindling model provides better insights into how abnormal neural plasticity is altered and newly acquired during epileptogenesis. Furthermore, when the number of grand mal seizures increases, status epilepticus is also caused in kindled mice. We therefore focused on kindling to clarify the molecular mechanisms of epileptogenesis and the occurrence of status epilepticus.

Chemical (metal): When alumina cream is applied to the cerebral cortex of monkeys and cats, chronic spontaneous seizures are induced, however, the seizures subside after several months to years (Heinemann et al., 1986). Investigating the mechanisms of the termination of seizure expressions might provide clues to end refractory epilepsy. Implantation of cobalt into the cerebral cortex easy induces focal and secondarily generalized seizures in rodents, however, cobalt metal causes a large area of cortex to be lost, while the hippocampus containing the dentate gyrus appears intact (Chang et al., 2004). Microinjection of ferric ions into the rodent brain results in chronic recurrent seizures, which are brain injury responses induced by hemorrhage and free radical reactions observed in human posttraumatic epilepsy (Willmore and Ueda, 2009).

Chemical (drug): Status epilepticus model mice are prepared with pentylenetetrazol (PTZ), kainate, and pirocarpin. PTZ-induced seizures: injection of PTZ (43 mg/kg) into the peritoneal cavity of 4-week-old mice 3 times per week for 4 weeks induced stereotyped spontaneous seizures (unpublished procedure). Kainate-induced seizures: an infusion of kainate (1 nmol/0.5 μl) into the hippocampus of 8-week-old mice induces status epilepticus about 20 days after infusion (unpublished procedure; Antonucci et al., 2009). Pirocapine-induced seizures: pirocarpine (100 mg/kg) is injected into the peritoneal cavity every 20 min until onset of status epilepticus (Elliott et al., 2003). SE induced with kainate and pirocarpine accompanies hippocampal damage, which seems to mimic human hippocampal atrophy. Additionally, the concentration of each drug should not be over the adequate dosage, as mice die immediately following the appearance of seizures.

Spontaneous and genetic manipulation: EL mouse: tonic-chronic seizures appear when a mouse is tossed to height of 10 cm 10 times a day for 2-3 weeks (unpublished procedure; Fueta et al., 1983). Audiogenic seizure model of DBA/2: audiogenic seizures appear when a 3-week-old mouse receives one 60-sec exposure to a pure tone sound (120 db) (Seyfried and Glaser, 1981). SER rat: rats homozygous for both zitter (zi) and tremor (tm) autosomal recessive mutations shows spontaneous epileptic seizures involving hippocampal atrophy in the CA3 subfield, in addition to many vacuoles in the brain (Hanaya et al., 2010). Gerbils with hypoplasia of the basilar artery circle suffer chronic seizures by a sudden change of circumstances (Buchhalter 1993). On the other hand, many one-gene-deficient mice have been produced with epileptic seizures, in which it is suggested that several channel gene deficient-dependent seizures mimic idiopathic seizures (Puranam and McNamara, 1999; Meisleret al., 2001).

2.2 Preparation of kindled mice

Figure 1 shows the dorsal side of the head (B) and the coronal section of the brain (C) in kindled mice with a microinjection cannula. All procedures were performed according to the guidelines for animal welfare of Osaka Prefecture University and Kyoto Sangyo University, and approved protocols. Surgical procedures were conducted under anesthesia with isoflurane (Dainippon Sumitomo Pharma Co. Ltd., Osaka, Japan) and Escain (Mylan Inc., Osaka, Japan) as described previously (Kato et al., 2001). Positions of brain regions were determined according to the stereotaxic coordinates shown by Paxinos and Franklin

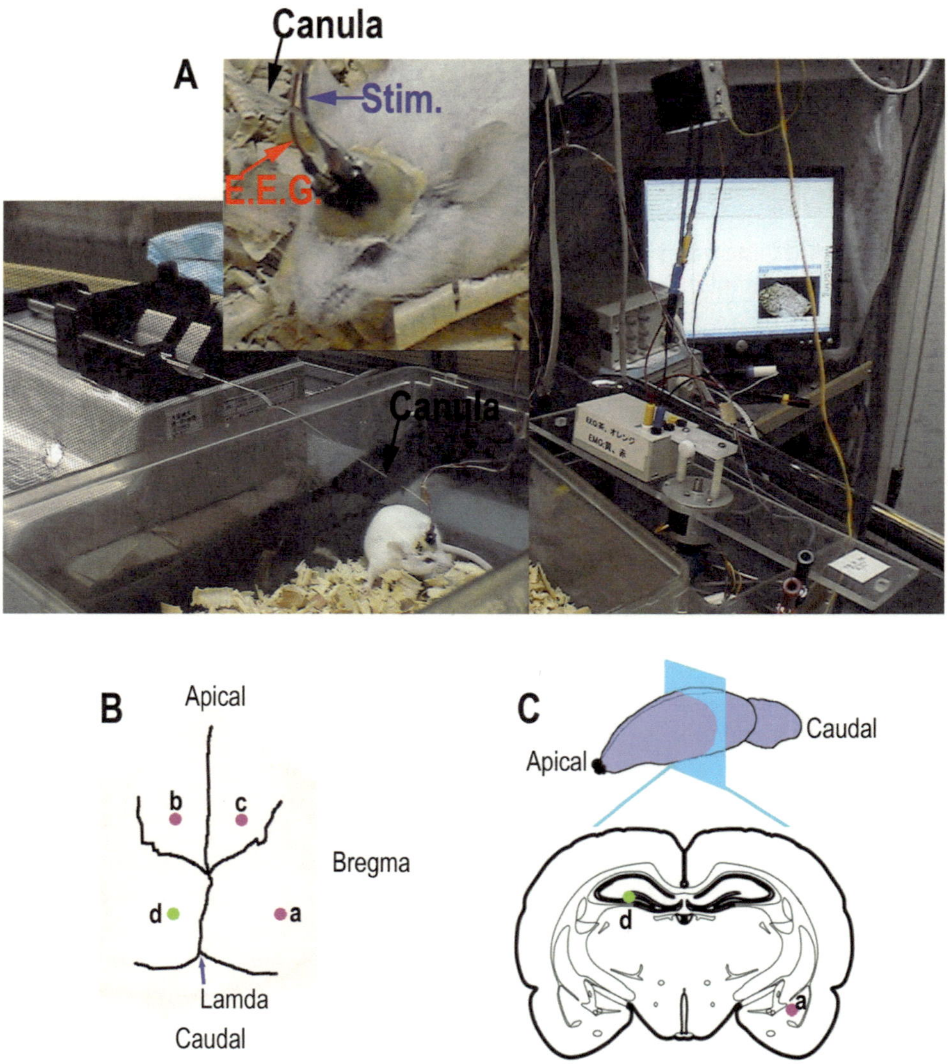

Fig. 1. Photos show free-moving mice receiving kindling stimulation, E.E.G. recording, and microinjection (A) and views showing positions of electrodes and microinjection cannula (B and C). Views showing the dorsal side of the head (left) and a coronal section of the brain (right) in kindled mice with a microinjection cannula (A). In (A), Stim., stimulation; E.E.G., electroencephalographic; cannula, microinjection cannula transplanted into the hippocampus.

(2001). Unipolar cathode electrode; made of tungsten steel and 0.1 mm in width (Inter Medical Co. Ltd., Nagoya, Japan), and an anode electrode; made of a screw and 1.0 mm in width and 3.0 mm in length (Biotex Kyoto, Japan), were implanted on the right side of the basolateral amygdaloid complex (A -2.0, L 3.0, V 4.5 mm from bregma; **a**) and on the left side of the subdural space (A 2.0, L 1.5 mm from bregma; **b**), respectively. Ten days after surgery, unrestrained conscious mice received a biphasic square wave pulse [480 μA; 60 Hz, 200 μs duration, for 2 sec] using an electrical stimulator (SEN-3301; Nihon Kohden, Tokyo,

Japan) and isolator (SS-202J) once a day. Electroencephalographic (EEG) recordings were carried out with bilateral electrodes of the subdural space (b and c) prior to and after stimulation using PreAmp and Head Amp (BEMCT-21 and BH-3, Low cut = 0.5, High cut = 30; Biotex, Kyoto, Japan) and the data acquisition program SleepSign ver.2.0 (Kissei Comtec Co. Ltd., Nagano, Japan). Seizures were monitored with a modified classification of Racine's criteria (Racine 1972) and the duration of afterdischarge and freezing was added to the behavioral criteria as described previously (Kato et al., 2001): stage 1, plus mouth and facial movement; stage 2, plus forelimb clonus and duration of afterdischarge greater than 5 sec; stage 3, plus forelimb clonus and duration of freezing greater than 15 sec; stage 4, plus tonic clonic seizures and tail up; stage 5, plus falling over. After reaching stage 5, mice were used in experiments as fully kindled mice following more stimulation for only 3 days. The brains of the mice were removed after decapitation within 2 hrs of the last kindling stimulation. The sham-operated mice were not stimulated but otherwise treated identically in all respects.

2.3 Microinjection of drugs into the brains

To observe the effect of drugs during epileptogenesis, a microinjection cannula (ID=0.2 mm; Eicom Corp., Kyoto, Japan) with a guide cannula (ID = 0.4 mm, OD = 0.5mm; Eicom Corp.) was also implanted on the left side of the hippocampus (A -2.0, L 1.5, V 2.5 mm; d in Fig. 1B and C) at the time of surgery to prepare kindled mice (Kato et al., 2009).

One microliter of genotropin (1 µl of 540 pmol/µl; Faizer, Tokyo, Japan), pegvisomant (90 pmol/µl, antagonist, Faizer) and buffer (40 mg/ml D-mannitol, 2 mg/ml glycine, and 0.02 mM sodium phosphate, pH 6.85); and 1 µl octreotide acetate (1 µl of 90 pmol/µl; Novartis, Tokyo, Japan) and buffer (45 mg/ml D-mannitol, 3.4 mg/ml lactic acid in NaHCO3, pH 4.5) were injected into the hippocampus of unrestrained conscious mice (d in Fig. 1B) at a flow rate of 0.5 µl /min using a microsyringe pump (KDS 200 series; KD Scientific) according to the schedule described in Fig. 3A, in which we administered drugs every other day 7 times in total before and during epileptogenesis, respectively. Concentrations of the drugs applied to mice were determined based on the weight of drugs per weight of human patients. Mice received a biphasic square wave pulse 30 min following the microinjection. Statistical tests were mainly performed using a combination of Excel and Statview-J 5.0. Additionally, one microliter each of genotropin octreotide acetate, and pegvisomant (antagonist, recombinant protein, 12 mg/ml; Pfizer) was injected into the hippocampus of respective mice without kindling stimulation. Pegvisomant was used to investigate whether it affected the functions of endogenous GH in the brain.

3. Differential expressions during epilepsy progression and following status epilepticus

Reports have indicated gene expression patterns during and following epileptogenesis and the development of status epilepticus induced in rodents with drugs and electro-stimulation (Nedivi et al., 1993; Tang *et al.*, 2002; Becker *et al.*, 2003; Elliott *et al.*, 2003; Lukasiuk *et al.*, 2003; Gorter *et al.*, 2006). They have found several promising new anti-epileptogenic targets, for example, previous studies have indicated common immediate early genes including SER-regulated genes (Becker *et al.*, 2003; Gorter *et al.*, 2006) and prostaglandin-endoperoxide synthase 2 (Ptgs2, Cox-2) (Gorter *et al.* 2006; Ristori *et al.* 2008) as candidates for genes causative of epileptogenesis. While inhibition of Cox-2 reduces epileptiform bursting in the hippocampus slice (Ristori *et al.*, 2008), the inhibitor had no effect on epileptogenesis or spontaneous seizures *in vivo* (Holtman et al., 2009). This contradiction suggests that the roles of Cox-2 should also be studied in epilepsy. It was also reported that the expressions of hormone genes, such as galanin (Lerner et al., 2008; Mitsukawa et al., 2008), neuropeptide Y (Shannon and Yang, 2004; El Bahh *et al.*, 2005; Silva *et al.*, 2005), leptin (Shanley et al., 2002), and somatostatin (Monno *et al.*, 1993; Buckmaster *et al.*, 2002) were up-regulated in the brain following epileptogenesis and showed anti-epileptic effects. On the other hand, candidate genes associated with human epilepsy have been nominated in the HuGE database (Jia et al., 2011). More recent experimental research has shown the effect of antiepileptic drugs on differential gene expressions and antiepileptogenic behaviors (Pitkänen and Lukasiuk, 2011).

In the present review, we introduce growth hormone signaling as a candidate molecular system associated with epileptogenesis. We have screened differential gene expressions in the brain regions during kindling epileptogenesis by genechip array. As a result, we have identified growth hormone (GH), increasing the gene expression in the brain regions that kindling stimuli propagate from the basolateral amygdala during epileptogenesis (Fig. 2). On the other hand, the present amygdala kindled mice also indicated up-regulated expressions of SER-regulated genes (Kato et al., 2009) and the Cox-2 transcript (Fig. 4) following kindled seizures.

4. Research

4.1 Growth hormone signaling system

Differential expressions of the GH transcript that increases in the brain during and following kindling epileptogenesis (Fig. 2) have been confirmed using a quantitative real-time polymerase chain reaction-based analysis of mRNA (qRT-PCR) and Western blot analysis (Kato et al., 2009). Next, we investigated the distribution of the GH transcript in the brain to know whether the transcript is expressed in regions where the kindling-stimuli propagate in amygdala-kindled mice using *in situ* hybridization (Kato et al., 2009). Neuronal cells were typically oval with cRNA signals of GH in the regions, in which GH mRNA was expressed moderately in the brain, particularly around the limbic area containing the piriform cortex, the anterior thalamic nucleus, and the hippocampus. Previous studies of neural connections have already clarified that amygdala kindling leads more easily to the propagation of stimuli to the hippocampus→anterior thalamus→apical cortex involving the cingulate through neural connections (Meibach and Siegel 1977; Amaral and Witter 1995; Price 1995; Gemmell and O'Mara 2002). Thus, it was suggested that regions of the brain that express GH could be involved in the propagation of stimuli in neural circuits during epileptogenesis.

To compare mRNA levels, total RNA was prepared from the apical part of the cerebral cortex (yellow circle), thalamus, (green circle), and the caudal part of the cerebral cortex [which includes posterior hippocampus, amygdaloid complex, temporal lobe] (red circle) of kindled, intermediate stage 3, and sham-operated mice. GeneChip array shows up-regulation of GH transcript during epileptogenesis (A). Means and S.E.M. were calculated based on raw signal intensities (MG430_Scal_Signal) compensated by signal intensity with GAPDH control probes on the Mouse Genome 430 2.0 Array of the Affymetrix Genechip. There were significant differences of GH expression using Kruskal-Wallis tests of Kyplot 4.0:

in the apical cortex (x70.6, **p<0.01), the thalamus (x54.4, **p<0.01) and caudal cortex (x23.2, *<0.05) between sham-operated and full-kindled mice.

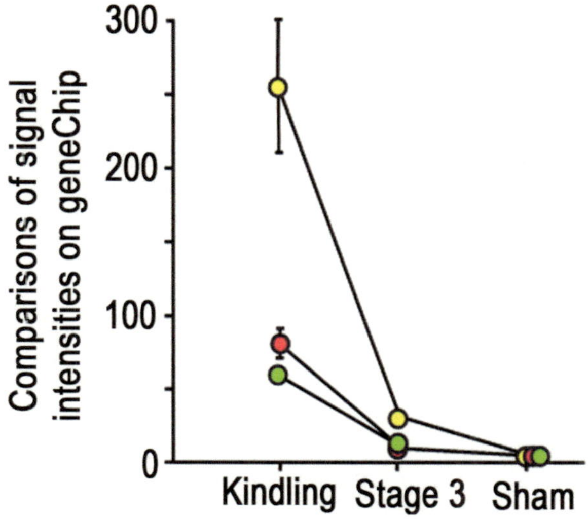

Fig. 2. Comparisons of expression levels of Gh between full-kindled, intermediate stage 3, and sham-operated mice using genechip array. To compare mRNA levels, total RNA was prepared from the apical part of the cerebral cortex (yellow circle), thalamus, (green circle), and the caudal part of the cerebral cortex [which includes posterior hippocampus, amygdaloid complex, temporal lobe] (red circle) of kindled, intermediate stage 3, and sham-operated mice. GeneChip array shows up-regulation of GH transcript during epileptogenesis (A). Means and S.E.M. were calculated based on raw signal intensities (MG430_Scal_Signal) compensated by signal intensity with GAPDH control probes on the Mouse Genome 430 2.0 Array of the Affymetrix Genechip. There were significant differences of GH expression using Kruskal-Wallis tests of Kyplot 4.0: in the apical cortex (x70.6, **p<0.01), thalamus (x54.4, **p<0.01), and caudal cortex (x23.2, *<0.05) between sham-operated and full-kindled mice.

To investigate whether GH has distinct roles in epileptogenesis, we injected genotropin (human GH recombinant, rGH) and octreotide, which is a somatostatin analog reducing secretion of GH (Lamberts 1987) into the hippocampus according to the schedule described in Fig. 3A. First, the administration of rGH resulted in a significant enhancement of epileptogenesis compared to the control as a whole (two-way factorial ANOVAs in Fig. 3C) and an increased number of spikes in afterdischarge following epileptic seizures (two-way factorial ANOVAs in Fig. 3B). Second, the progression of behavioral changes during epileptogenesis was attenuated (two-way factorial ANOVA in Fig. 3E); however, there were no differences in the number of spikes and duration of afterdischarges (Fig. 3D). This suggests that growth hormone causes the afterdischarge threshold to decrease during epileptogenesis.

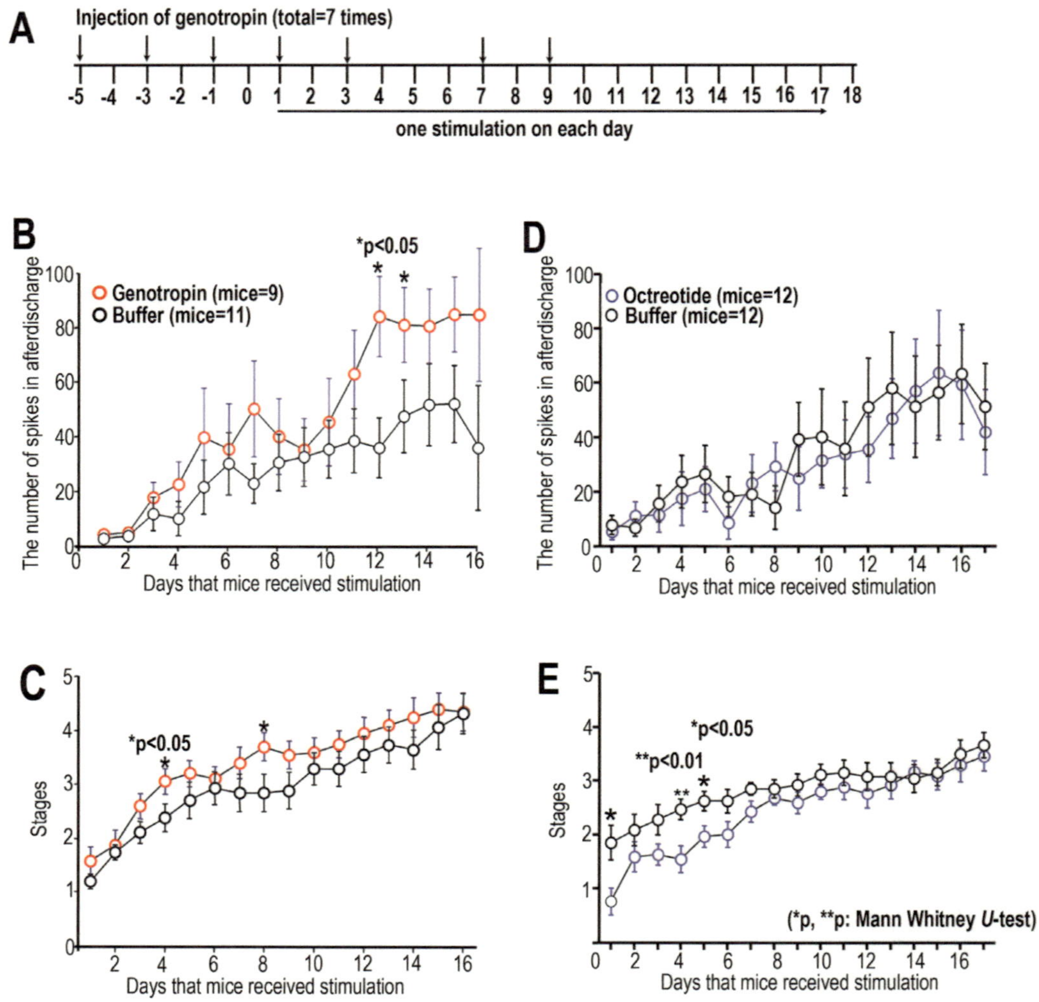

Fig. 3. Effect of genotropin and octreotide on epileptogenesis (adapted from Kato et al., 2009). Schedules of injection (A) of genotropin (1 ml of 540 pmol/ml, red circles in B and 4C), octreotide acetate (1 ml of 90 pmol/ml, blue circles in D and E), and their buffer (1 ml, black circles in B-E) or kindling stimulation are shown. Stimulation was started from number 1 and continued to the 17th day. The number of spikes in afterdischarges on electroencephalograms (EEGs) are shown (B and D). Transition of stages (C and D). Means and S.E.M. for the two characteristics of mice with or without drugs following stimulation on each day were evaluated with two-way factorial ANOVA, which showed differences in mice with or without in B to E (Kato et al., 2009). The data for days when mice received stimulation were compared between injections of drugs and the buffer (Mann-Whitney U-test: *p<0.05, **p<0.01). Administration of the hormone into the hippocampus markedly enhanced the progression of kindling, and the number of spikes during afterdischarges increased in mice following development of tonic-clonic convulsion. On the other hand, the administration of an inhibitor of its secretion into the hippocampus elicited a delay in progression.

As we have demonstrated the effect of GH on the brain during epileptogenesis, we next investigated whether the presence of GH induced GH signaling in the brain during epileptogenesis. As a method of investigation, we determined whether GH regulated the expressions of seizure-responsive genes directly in the brain. Finally, when the hippocampus was exposed to rGH for 24 hrs without kindling stimulation, rGH induced significant differential expressions of Egr1 mRNA (Kato et al., 2009), but not Cox-2 mRNA in the caudal cortex containing the hippocampus and amygdaloid complex (Fig. 4, result experimented by Mr. M. Suzuki). Both Egr1 and Cox-2 mRNAs were seizure-responsive genes in our kindling system. These relative results show that exogenous rGH induced an increase of Egr1 mRNA directly at least downstream of GH signaling, while Cox-2 transcripts were not regulated by GH signaling. It has been reported that Cox-2 inhibitor

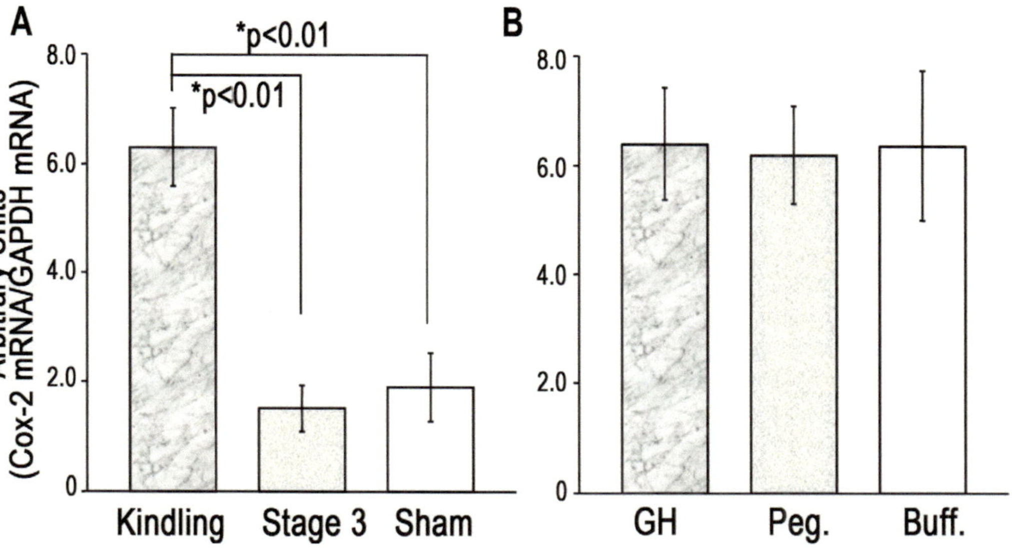

Fig. 4. Effects of kindled seizures (A) and rGH microinjections (B) on expression levels of Cox-2 (prepared by M. Suzuki). Isolation of RNA and real-time RT-PCR followed the methods described previously (Kato et al., 2009). Quantitative PCR of Cox-2 mRNA was performed with SYBR Green (Power SYBR Green PCR Master Mix, Applied Biosystems) using a 7300 Real-Time PCR system. Primer pairs used for the PCR were: 5′- GAT CAT CAA TAC TGC CTC AA -3′/5′-CAG CTC AGT TGA ACG CCT TT-3′ (Cox-2, 184 bp, 1729-1912bp in NM_011198). The bar graph (mean + S.E.M.) shows the ratio of Cox-2 mRNA relative to GAPDH mRNA between sham-operated (n=10), stage 3 (n=8), and full-kindled (n=10) mice in the cerebral cortex containing the hippocampus and amygdala using the Kruskal-Wallis test [Steel-Dwass test]: *p<0.001, [kindling/stage 3 (between kindling and stage 3), *5p<0.01; kindling/sham, *4p<0.01]. Another bar graph shows the ratio of these transcripts in the caudal part of the cerebral cortex containing the hippocampus and amygdala with the administration of rhGH (n=4), pegvisomant (n=4), and the buffer (n=4) using the Kruskal-Wallis test: p=0.981. There was no difference in Cox-2 transcripts among drug administrations.

has little effects on epileptogenesis or spontaneous seizures (Holtman et al., 2009), which also suggests that Cox-2 does not function under GH signaling.
GH regulates physiological processes, including carbohydrate and lipid metabolism as well as somatic growth and development, therefore, it is possible that epileptogenesis is correlated with the differential expression of carbohydrates and lipids. Next, we screened the differential expression of gangliosides during epileptogenesis.

4.2 Effect of ganglioside expressions

A crude ganglioside mixture was prepared with extracts of the hippocampus dissected from adult mice following kindled seizures, and high performance thin-layer chromatography (HPTLC) analysis was performed according to previous reports (Iwamori and Nagai, 1981). The signal intensity of each ganglioside developed on the HPTLC plate was calculated in individual mice (6 kindled and 6 sham-operated mice) using PDquest software (Bio-rad,Tokyo, Japan) and analyzed using a combination of Excel and Statview-J 5.0. The analysis demonstrated a decrease of GM1 and increase of GQ1b following kindled seizures (Kato et al., 2008). The increase of GQ1b in the hippocampus following kindled seizures was confirmed by immunofluorescence with anti-GQ1b antibody. Taken together, the level of endogenous GQ1b increased following seizures in amygdaloid kindled mice, suggesting that the contents of GQ1b in the hippocampus are subject to epileptogenesis regulated by GH signaling.

5. Conclusion

We first found that GH plays distinct roles in epileptogenesis in the limbic system of the brain via GH signaling. While it was reported that GH is involved in lipolysis and has an effect that opposes that of insulin in the peripheral tissues (Scacchi *et al.*, 2003), the present kindled seizures up-regulated the expressions of GQ1b in the brain. Given that 2-deoxy-D-glucose (2DG) increases the afterdischarge threshold (Garriga-Canut *et al.* 2006) and the present kindled-seizures cause up-regulation of the expressions of an enzyme related to carbohydrate transition, α2,3-sialyltransferase (ST3Gal IV), in the hippocampus and thalamus (Okabe *et al.*, 2001; Matsuhashi *et al.*, 2003). Hence, we propose that metabolic regulation by GH signaling adjusts the afterdischarge threshold during epileptogenesis. We have developed ST3Gal IV gene-deficient mice and are studying the involvement of ST3Gal IV in epileptogenesis. The relevance of GH signaling, sialylation, and lipid metabolism in the progress of epilepsy should be clarified in the near future.

6. Acknowledgements

This work was partly supported by grants from the Ministry of Education, Science, Culture, and Sports, a research fellowship of the Japan Society for the Promotion of Science (NO. 15500260 and 17580260), Senri Life Science Foundation, the Japan Epilepsy Research Foundation, and Core Research for Evolutional Science and Technology (CREST) of the Japan Science and Technology Agency (JST).

7. References

Amaral D. G. & Witter M. P. (1995) *Hippocampal formation, in The Rat Nervous System* second edition (ed. Paxinos, G.). pp. 443-493. Academic Press Inc., San Diego.

Antonucci F.; Bozzi Y. & Caleo M. (2009) Intrahippocampal infusion of botulinum neurotoxin E (BoNT/E) reduces spontaneous recurrent seizures in a mouse model of mesial temporal lobe epilepsy. Epilepsia. 50:963-966.

Becker A. J.; Chen J. ; Zien A.; Sochivko D.; Normann S.; Schramm J.; Elger C. E.; Wiestler O. D. & Blümcke I. (2003) Correlated stage- and subfield-associated hippocampal gene expression patterns in experimental and human temporal lobe epilepsy. Eur J Neurosci. 18:2792-2802.

Besli G.E.; Saltik S.; Erguven M.;, Bulut O. & Abul M.H. (2010) Status epilepticus in children: causes, clinical features and short-term outcome. Pediatr Int. 52:749-753.

Browne T.R. & Holmes G.L. (2000) Handbook of Epilepsy 2nd Ed. pp42-55, pp91-94. Philadelphia, PA, Lippincott Williams & Wilkins.

Buchhalter J. R. (1993) Animal models of inherited epilepsy. Epilepsia. 34 Suppl 3:S31-S41.

Buckmaster P. S.; Otero-Corchón V.; Rubinstein M. & Low M. J. (2002) Heightened seizure severity in somatostatin knockout mice. Epilepsy Res. 48:43-56.

Chang J.H.; Yang X.F.; Zempel J.M. & Rothman S.M. (2004) The unilateral cobalt wire model of neocortical epilepsy: a method of producing subacute focal seizures in rodents. Epilepsy Res. 61:153-160.

Dodrill C.B. (1986) Correlates of generalized tonic-clonic seizures with intellectual, neuropsychological, emotional, and social function in patients with epilepsy. Epilepsia 27:399-411.

El Bahh B.; Balosso S.; Hamilton T.; Herzog H.; Beck-Sickinger A.G.; Sperk G.; Gehlert D.R.; Vezzani A. & Colmers W.F. (2005) The anti-epileptic actions of neuropeptide Y in the hippocampus are mediated by Y_2 and not Y_5 receptors. Eur J Neurosci. 22:1417-1430.

Elliott R.C.; Miles M.F. & Lowenstein D.H. (2003) Overlapping microarray profiles of dentate gyrus gene expression during development- and epilepsy-associated neurogenesis and axon outgrowth. J Neurosci. 23:2218-2227.

Franks R.P. (2003) Psychiatric issues of childhood seizure disorders. Child Adolesc Psychiatr Clin N Am. 12:551-565.

Fueta Y.; Mita T. & Matsuoka S. (1983) Experimental animal epilepsy. A new device for the induction of epileptic seizures in the murine, El mouse. J UOEH. 5:359-364.

Garriga-Canut M.; Schoenike B.; Qazi R.; Bergendahl K.; Daley T.J.; Pfender R.M.; Morrison J.F.; Ockuly J.; Stafstrom C.; Sutula T. & Roopra A. (2006) 2-deoxy-D-glucose reduces epilepsy progression by NRSF-CtBP-dependent metabolic regulation of chromatin structure. Nat Neurosci. 9:1382-1387.

Gemmell C. & O'Mara S.M. (2002) Plasticity in the projection from the anterior thalamic nuclei to the anterior cingulate cortex in the rat *in vivo*: paired-pulse facilitation, long-term potentiation and short-term depression. Neuroscience 109:401-406.

Goddard G.V.; McIntyre D.C. & Leech C.K. (1969) A permanent change in brain function resulting from daily electrical stimulation. Exp Neurol. 25:295-330.

Gorter J.A.; van Vliet E.A.; Aronica E.; Breit T.; Rauwerda H.; Lopes da Silva F.H. & Wadman W.J. (2006) Potential new antiepileptogenic targets indicated by microarray analysis in a rat model for temporal lobe epilepsy. J Neurosci. 26:11083-11110.

Hanaya R.; Sasa M.; Sugata S.; Tokudome M.; Serikawa T.; Kurisu K. & Arita K. (2010) Hippocampal cell loss and propagation of abnormal discharges accompanied with the expression of tonic convulsion in the spontaneously epileptic rat. Brain Res. 1328:171-180.

Heinemann U.; Konnerth A.; Pumain R. & Wadman W.J. (1986) Extracellular calcium and potassium concentration changes in chronic epileptic brain tissue. Adv Neurol. 44:641-661.

Holtman L.; van Vliet E.A.; van Schaik R.; Queiroz C.M.; Aronica E. & Gorter J.A. (2009) Effects of SC58236, a selective COX-2 inhibitor, on epileptogenesis and spontaneous seizures in a rat model for temporal lobe epilepsy. Epilepsy Res. 84:56-66.

Iwamori M. & Nagai Y. (1981) Comparative study on ganglioside compositions of various rabbit tissues. Tissue-specificity in ganglioside molecular species of rabbit thymus, Biochim. Biophys. Acta 665:214-220.

Jia P.; Ewers J.M. & Zhao Z. (2011) Prioritization of epilepsy associated candidate genes by convergent analysis. PLoS One 6:e17162.

Kato K.; Iwamori M. & Hirabayashi Y. (2008) Increase of GQ1b in the hippocampus of mice following kindled-seizures. Neurosci Lett. 441:286-290.

Kato K.; Masa T.; Tawara Y.; Kobayashi K.; Oka T.; Okabe A. & Shiosaka S. (2001) Dendritic aberrations in the hippocampal granular layer and the amygdalohippocampal area following kindled-seizures. Brain Res. 901:281-295.

Kato K.; Suzuki M.; Kanno H.; Sekino S.; Kusakabe K.; Okada T.; Mori T.; Yoshida K. & Hirabayashi Y. (2009) Distinct Role of Growth Hormone on Epilepsy Progression in a Model of Temporal Lobe Epilepsy. J Neurochem. 110:509-519.

Lamberts S.W.; Verleun T.; Hofland L. & Del Pozo E. (1987) A comparison between the effects of SMS 201-995, bromocriptine and a combination of both drugs on hormone release by the cultured pituitary tumour cells of acromegalic patients. Clin Endocrinol. (Oxf) 27:11-23.

Lerner J.T.; Sankar R. & Mazarati A.M. (2008) Galanin and epilepsy. Cell Mol Life Sci. 65:1864-1871.

Lukasiuk K.; Kontula L. & Pitkänen A. (2003) cDNA profiling of epileptogenesis in the rat brain. Eur J Neurosci. 17:271-279.

Matsuhashi H.; Horii Y. & Kato K. (2003) Region-specific and epileptogenic-dependent expression of six subtypes of α2,3-sialyltransferase in the adult mouse brain. J Neurochem. 84:53-66.

Meibach R.C. & Siegel A. (1977) Thalamic projections of the hippocampal formation: evidence for an alternate pathway involving the internal capsule. Brain Res. 134:1-12.

Meisler M.H.; Kearney J.; Ottman R. & Escayg A. (2001) Identification of epilepsy genes in human and mouse. Annu Rev Genet. 35:567-588.

Mitsukawa K.; Lu X. & Bartfai T. (2008) Galanin, galanin receptors and drug targets. Cell Mol Life Sci. 65:1796-1805.

Motamedi G. & Meador K. (2003) Epilepsy and cognition. Epilepsy Behav. 4:S25-S38.

Monno A.; Rizzi M.; Samanin R. & Vezzani A. (1993) Anti-somatostatin antibody enhances the rate of hippocampal kindling in rats. Brain Res. 602:148-152.

Müller C.J.; Gröticke I.; Bankstahl M. & Löscher W. (2009) Behavioral and cognitive alterations, spontaneous seizures, and neuropathology developing after a pilocarpine-induced status epilepticus in C57BL/6 mice. Exp Neurol. 219:284-297.

Nedivi E.; Hevroni D.; Naot D.; Israell D. & Citri Y. (1993) Numerous candidate plasticity-related genes revealed by differential cDNA cloning. Nature 363:718-722.

Okabe A.; Tawara Y.; Masa T.; Oka T.; Machida A.; Tanaka T.; Matsuhashi H.; Shiosaka S. & Kato K. (2001) Differential expression of mRNAs for sialyltransferase isoenzymes induced in the hippocampus of mouse following kindled seizures. J Neurochem. 77:1185-1197.

Paxinos G. & Franklin K.B.J. (2001) *The mouse brain in Stereotaxic Coordinates second edition.* Academic Press Inc., San Diego.

Perini G.I.; Tosin C.; Carraro C.; Bernasconi G.; Canevini M.P.; Canger R.; Pellegrini A. & Testa G. (1996) Interictal mood and personality disorders in temporal lobe epilepsy and juvenile myoclonic epilepsy. J. Neurol. Neurosurg. Psychiatry 61:601-605.

Pitkänen A. & Lukasiuk K. (2011) Mechanisms of epileptogenesis and potential treatment targets. Lancet Neurol. 10:173-186.

Price J.L. (1995) *Thalamus, in The Rat Nervous System* second edition (ed. Paxinos, G.) pp. 629-648. Academic Press Inc., San Diego.

Puranam R.S. & McNamara J.O. (1999) Seizure disorders in mutant mice: relevance to human epilepsies. Curr Opin Neurobiol. 9:281-287.

Racine R.J. (1972). Modification of seizure activity by electrical stimulation. II. motor seizure. *Electroencephalography and Clinical Neurophysiology, 32*:281-294.

Ristori C.; Cammalleri M.; Martini D.; Pavan B.; Casini G.; Cervia D. & Bagnoli P. (2008) The cyclooxygenase-2/prostaglandin E2 pathway is involved in the somatostatin-induced decrease of epileptiform bursting in the mouse hippocampus.Neuropharmacology. 54:874-884.

Scacchi M.; Pincelli A.I. & Cavagnini F. (2003) Nutritional status in the neuroendocrine control of growth hormone secretion: the model of anorexia nervosa. Front Neuroendocrinol. 24:200-224.

Schallier A.; Massie A.; Loyens E.; Moechars D.; Drinkenburg W.; Michotte Y. & Smolders I. (2009) vGLUT2 heterozygous mice show more susceptibility to clonic seizures induced by pentylenetetrazol. Neurochem Int. 55:41-44.

Seyfried T.N. & Glaser G.H. (1981) Genetic linkage between the AH locus and a major gene that inhibits susceptibility to audiogenic seizures in mice. Genetics. 99:117-126.

Shanley L.J.; O'Malley D.; Irving A.J.; Ashford M.L. & Harvey J. (2002) Leptin inhibits epileptiform-like activity in rat hippocampal neurones via PI 3-kinase-driven activation of BK channels. J Physiol. 545(Pt 3):933-944.

Shannon H.E. & Yang L. (2004) Seizure susceptibility of neuropeptide-Y null mutant mice in amygdala kindling and chemical-induced seizure models. Epilepsy Res. 61:49-62.

Sillanpää M. & Shinnar S. (2010) Long-term mortality in childhood-onset epilepsy. N Engl J Med. 363:2522-2529.

Silva A.P.; Xapelli S.; Pinheiro P.S.; Ferreira R.; Lourenço J.; Cristóvão A.; Grouzmann E.; Cavadas C.; Oliveira C.R. & Malva J.O. (2005) Up-regulation of neuropeptide Y

levels and modulation of glutamate r elease through neuropeptide Y receptors in the hippocampus of kainate-induced epileptic rats. J Neurochem. 93:163-170.
Tang Y.; Lu A.; Aronow B.J.; Wagner K.R. & Sharp F.R. (2002) Genomic responses of the brain to ischemic stroke, intracerebral haemorrhage, kainate seizures, hypoglycemia, and hypoxia. Eur J Neurosci. 15:1937-1952.
Willmore L.J. & Ueda Y. (2009) Posttraumatic epilepsy: hemorrhage, free radicals and the molecular regulation of glutamate. Neurochem Res. 34:688-697.

5

Bridging the Gap – Understanding the Role of Gap Junctions in Seizures

Logan J. Voss, Gregory Jacobson and Jamie W. Sleigh
Waikato Hospital Department of Anaesthesia and Waikato University
New Zealand

1. Introduction

Epilepsy is a major cause of ongoing disability and a significant cause of hospital admission. According to the World Health Organisation, the disease affects approximately 50 million people worldwide and current pharmacological treatment regimes are ineffective in approximately 30% of cases (http://www.who.int/mediacentre/factsheets/fs999/en/index.html). Clearly, there is a need for more effective and targeted pharmacological epilepsy treatments.

In simplistic terms, seizures are said to result from an imbalance in the regulation of brain activity, such that too much excitation or too little inhibition tips the balance towards hyperexcitability (seizure). The reality is almost certainly more complicated, as evidenced by common reports of low efficacy of some currently used antiepileptic drugs, whose primary mechanisms of action are either depression or enhancement of brain excitatory and inhibitory pathways, respectively. The complexity of this area of neurobiology is further highlighted by the observation that seizures can be triggered by anaesthetic drugs, many of which are themselves effective anticonvulsants. Clearly, there are subtleties to the mechanisms of seizure generation and regulation, the complexity of which we are only beginning to understand. A greater understanding of these underlying mechanisms will inevitably lead to more targeted and effective treatment options.

One area that has become the focus of considerable amounts of research in the last 10 years is the role of gap junctions in seizure mechanisms. Gap junctions form direct cytoplasmic connections between cells, providing electrical continuity and allowing passage of low molecular weight molecules from one cell to another. Gap junctions are created from the assembly of six connexin proteins in the cell membrane into a hemichannel; and the association of two hemichannels on neighbouring cells forms a mature gap junction. Acting as electrical synapses, it has been hypothesised that gap junctions could promote seizure activity by facilitating the spread and synchronisation of electrical activity in the brain. In support of this, there are a growing number of experimental studies showing a reduction in seizure severity following pharmacological gap junction blockade (Bostanci and Bagirici 2007; Nassiri-Asl et al. 2009). Intriguingly, several studies point to gap junction blockade having the opposite effect (Voss et al. 2009; Jacobson et al. 2010), suggesting that the relationship between gap junction regulation and seizure propensity is multifaceted.

The apparent discrepancies in the literature surrounding the role of gap junctions in seizurogenesis probably reflect two main complicating factors. Firstly, there are no known drugs that selectively regulate gap junctions; all have off-target effects which could confound experiments utilising these agents (Juszczak and Swiergiel 2009). Secondly, the effect of gap junction regulation on seizure activity will almost certainly depend on the specific gap junction subtype manipulated. The reason for this is that gap junctions of a given subtype tend to be restricted to a particular class of cells; meaning that targeted modulation of a specific gap junction subtype effectively restricts the effect to a specific cell population. It should not be surprising therefore, that blockade of gap junctions linking inhibitory interneurons for example, will have a different effect to blockade of those between excitatory pyramidal cells.

The central tenet of this chapter is that we cannot begin to fully understand the role that gap junctions play in seizure mechanisms until we appreciate the need for a targeted approach to gap junction modulation; in terms of both off-target, non-gap junctional side-effects and gap junction subtype specificity. These ideas are also important for the development of more effective epilepsy treatment options based on gap junction modulation, which will depend upon the targeted modulation of gap junction subtypes (Song and Tanouye 2006). Achieving targeted gap junction modulation is a major challenge for experimental biologists; however, there are new techniques and approaches that offer some hope for future research. For example, mimetic peptides (short polymers of amino acids) have shown promise as a tool for blocking gap junction formation (Evans and Boitano 2001). The specificity of effect of mimetic peptides comes from the sequence of amino acids, which are chosen to mimic a portion of the extracellularly exposed gap junction connexin protein. The introduced peptide binds to the native protein and interferes with the cell-cell docking process required for mature gap junction formation. In this way, formation of new gap junctions of the targeted subtype is prevented. Experimental approaches can also be supplemented by mathematical modelling studies, which have the enviable advantage that model parameters can be manipulated with absolute specificity. Clearly, no computer model developed to date comes close to representing the brain in all its complexity or functionality; but when aligned with (and refined by) experimental data, computer models can provide an informative adjunct to experimental biology.

In this chapter, we provide a detailed review of the current knowledge around the aforementioned topics. Our discussion focuses on the relationship between gap junctions and seizurogenesis in the mature, adult brain. Gap junction expression is highly dynamic early in development and understanding the contribution of changing levels of different gap junction subtypes to seizures is beyond the scope of this discussion. To this end, the chapter will be structured into three sections. Firstly, we will review the neurobiology of gap junctions and the distribution of gap junction subtypes across cell populations and cerebral locations in the adult brain. Our focus will be on brain regions known to be involved in seizurogenesis; principally the hippocampus and the cerebral cortex. We will then give an overview of recent as well as potential novel approaches to manipulating gap junctions that may provide more specificity of effect, such as mimetic peptides and siRNA technologies; and may also provide the basis of new therapeutic approaches to treating epilepsy. Finally, we will discuss how differentiation between gap junction-linked astrocytic, interneuronal and pyramidal cell networks may help us to understand the nature of gap junction regulation of seizure processes. This research is in its infancy, but there are clues from recent experimental and mathematical modelling studies that provide a solid foundation from which to explore this topic.

2. Gap junction structure and subtype distribution

Gap junctions are proteinaceous structures that form connections between adjacent cells, directly linking the cytoplasm of one cell to another. The basic structural unit is the connexin protein, of which there are 21 known subtypes in the human (Sohl and Willecke 2004). Connexins associate within the cytoplasmic membrane into a hexameric structure known as a connexon, or hemichannel; the association of two hemichannels on adjacent cells forms a mature, functional gap junction (see Fig 1). The junction so-formed allows direct electrical communication between cells and the passage of small molecular weight chemicals; and also serve intracellular signalling roles independent of their channel-forming function (see (Goodenough and Paul 2003; Jiang and Gu 2005) for reviews).

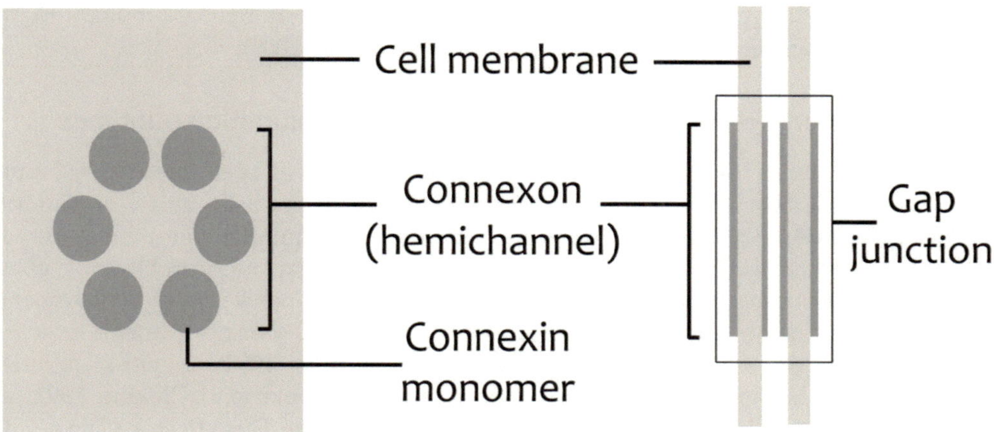

Fig. 1. Schematic representation of gap junction structural organisation

Gap junctions are found in most animal tissues and are widely expressed throughout the mammalian brain (Condorelli et al. 2003). However, expression patterns are not uniform and the distribution of different gap junction subtypes is dependent upon location and developmental maturity. For simplicity and in order to focus on the regions of greatest clinical relevance for human epilepsy (Hauser and Kurland 1975; Wiebe 2000), we will limit our discussion to the distribution of gap junction subtypes within the mature cerebral cortex and hippocampus.

2.1 Cortical and hippocampal gap junction expression

Only a limited number of connexins have been shown unequivocally to be expressed in the mature cerebral cortex. Connexin30, 32, 43, 45 and 47 gap junctions are expressed by cortical glial cells (Dermietzel et al. 1991; Dermietzel et al. 1997; Condorelli et al. 2002; Condorelli et al. 2003). The most common of these are connexin30 and connexin43, which are expressed by astrocytes (Dermietzel et al. 1991; Condorelli et al. 2002). Oligodendrocytes express connexin32 and connexin45 (Dermietzel et al. 1997), but constitute a small fraction of glial cells in the CNS (5-10% compared to 50-60% for actrocytes (Singh et al. 2003)). Connexin32 expression has also been localised to CNS neurons, but only in subcortical structures (thalamus and basal ganglia) (Dermietzel et al. 1989). Central nervous system neurons express connexin36, 45 and 57, with the latter restricted to horizontal cells of the retina (Hombach et al. 2004). Connexin36 is the most common neuronal gap junction in the mature cerebral cortex, and its expression is restricted primarily to inhibitory interneurons (Deans et al. 2001). Connexin45 is expressed neuronally (Condorelli et al. 2003; Maxeiner et al. 2003), however adult cortical expression of connexin45 is low and restricted to parieto-occipital and entorhinal cortical regions (Maxeiner et al. 2003). Thus, in the mature cerebral cortex, the most prominent gap junctions are those between inhibitory neurons (connexin36) and those between astrocytes (connexin30 and 43).

Connexin distribution patterns in the hippocampus are similar to those in the cerebral cortex; astrocytic gap junctions are formed predominantly by connexin30 (Condorelli et al. 2002; Rouach et al. 2008), and connexin43 (Rouach et al. 2008) and GABAergic interneuronal junctions by connexin36 (Deans et al. 2001). There is evidence that connexin36 may also be sparsely expressed by pyramidal cells in the hippocampus where they are thought to form axo-axonal junctions (Schmitz et al. 2001; Hamzei-Sichani et al. 2007).

3. Genetic experimental techniques for targeting gap junction subtypes

Determining the exact role of gap junctions in seizurogenesis has been challenging because all known gap junction blocking drugs lack specificity (for an excellent review see (Juszczak and Swiergiel 2009)). For example, the gap junction blockers quinine and mefloquine have anti- and pro-seizurogenic properties independent of their gap junction-blocking effects. Quinine, at modest concentrations (~20μM), is well known to block a variety of neuronal ion channels; in particular quinine's use-dependent blockade of sodium channels is a very similar action to the antiepileptic drug phenytoin (Lin et al. 1998). In vitro, quinine is convulsive at an intraperitoneal dose of 250 mg/kg (Amabeoku and Chikuni 1992) and mefloquine at 150mg/kg (Amabeoku and Farmer 2005) in mice. This effect is via a $GABA_A$ antagonist action (Thompson and Lummis 2008) and is seen in *in vitro* slices at 100μM and 400 μM for mefloquine and quinine, respectively (Thompson and Lummis 2008). Mefloquine may also enhance neuronal excitability in cultures via a disruption to calcium homeostasis at greater than 30μM (Dow et al. 2003). Mefloquine also inhibits $5\text{-}HT_3$ receptors at 10μM (Thompson and Lummis 2008). $5\text{-}HT_3$ receptors are a ligand-gated Na/K channel and blockade would tend to have an inhibitory effect on neuronal excitability.

The lack of specificity of pharmacological gap junction blockers has made it very difficult to interpret studies utilising these agents. Not only do they have non-gap-junctional off-target effects, they also affect multiple gap junction subtypes. Perhaps the exception to this is mefloquin (Cruikshank et al. 2004), which is reasonably specific for connexin36 gap junctions when delivered at an appropriately low dose (this is particularly so for cell cultures, where low doses that are more specific for connexin36 can be utilised (Cruikshank et al. 2004)). To fully understand the role of gap junctions in seizure processes, it is imperative to differentiate between gap junction subtypes. That is, it would be naïve to assume that blocking connexin43 gap junctions linking astrocytes would have the same functional effect as blocking connexin36 gap junctions linking inhibitory interneurons.

Genetic approaches to controlling connexin subtype expression and function (reviewed recently by Giaume and Theis (2010)) have potential to greatly increase our understanding of gap junction function. By targeting the subtype-specific connexin sequences at either the DNA, RNA or protein level, it may be possible to regulate gap junction function with unparalleled precision. In the section that follows we will outline the genetic techniques that offer the greatest promise as experimental tools in this regard, including mimetic peptides, transgenic manipulation and DNA/RNA interference. In section four we will look at functional studies that have utilised some of these techniques for the purpose of understanding gap junction regulation of seizure activity.

3.1 Mimetic peptides

Connexin mimetic peptides are short amino acid polymers corresponding to extracellular regions of the connexin protein. These molecules have shown promise as specific blockers of gap junction activity (Evans and Boitano 2001; Herve and Dhein 2010). It is thought that by binding to the connexin protein, connexin mimetics prevent connexon docking and block formation of the fully functional gap junction (Evans and Boitano 2001). In theory it should be possible to effect blockade of a specific gap junction subtype by designing mimetic peptide sequences specific to the connexin subtype in question. While promising in principle, there are some obstacles to the use of mimetics to effectively block gap junctions.

Firstly, there is considerable overlap in the amino acid sequences in the extracellular domains of connexin proteins. For example, GAP27 is a mimetic peptide that was developed to target the second extracellular loop of the connexin43 protein. The amino acid sequence SRPTEK within GAP27 is also present in the extracellular domains of most other connexin subtypes; thus, GAP27 may block gap junctions universally (Evans and Boitano 2001). Specificity to connexin43 can be enhanced by restricting the age range of animals used. Cortical grey matter expression of connexin30 does not develop until three weeks after birth, peaks at four weeks and remains high into adulthood (Kunzelmann et al. 1999). In contrast, connexin43 is already expressed in neonatal tissue and also remains high into adulthood (Kunzelmann et al. 1999). Thus, in one to three week old rodents, connexin43 is the predominant astrocytic gap junction. Expression of the other main cortical connexin subtype, interneuronal connexin36, develops between that of connexin43 and connexin30, peaking at two weeks after birth and declining during the third week (Belluardo et al. 2000). Expression of connexin43 and connexin30 in astrocytic cultures show similar developmental time-courses, with connexin43 present in the first days of culture and connexin30 expression not detected until the cultures are five to six weeks old (Kunzelmann et al. 1999).

Secondly, connexin mimetic peptides also block connexin hemichannels, albeit at different concentrations and over a different time course compared to their effect on gap junctions. Hemichannel effects occur at lower concentrations (5µM compared to 500-1000µM) (O'Carroll et al. 2008; Samoilova et al. 2008) and more rapidly (<30mins compared to >10 hours, cultures and hippocampal slices, respectively) (Leybaert et al. 2003; Samoilova et al. 2008). Although under normal physiological conditions the open probability of connexon hemichannels is low due to the blocking effect of divalent extracellular ions (magnesium and calcium) (Ebihara 2003; Ebihara et al. 2003), the open probability can be enhanced when extracellular magnesium and/or calcium levels are reduced (Ebihara et al. 2003). Thus, a possible effect of mimetic peptides on hemichannels must be considered likely when utilising the low-magnesium seizure model and at the higher mimetic concentrations required for gap junction blockade.

Thirdly, the brain also expresses channels formed from pannexins, a group of proteins that share basic structural similarities to the connexin family at the level of the mature protein but are otherwise unrelated. Pannexins are expressed by inhibitory neurons in the hippocampaus (Bruzzone et al. 2003); however, the specific cellular expression in the cerebral cortex is not known. Pannexins form hemichannels in vivo, not complete cell-cell gap junctions (MacVicar and Thompson 2009). Because pannexins do not share sequence homology with connexins (Baranova et al. 2004; Locovei et al. 2006), in theory they should not be blocked by connexin mimetic peptides. However, there is evidence showing that pannexin hemichannels are blocked by connexin mimetic peptides via a physical steric hindrance mechanism (Dahl 2007; Wang et al. 2007). Also, unlike connexon hemichannels, pannexin channels can be activated under normal physiological conditions (Bao et al. 2004). Thus, a possible effect of mimetic peptides on pannexin channels cannot be overlooked. Furthermore, pannexins themselves may be involved in seizurogenic processes, as shown by mimetic peptide blockade of Pannexin-1 in hippocampal slices (Thompson et al. 2008).

3.2 Connexin transgenic knockout animals

Gene knockout is a widely used technique for studying the function of a gene by removing that gene in an otherwise normal animal. This prevents the expression of the gene and its protein product. With conventional knockout techniques, embryonic stem cells are genetically manipulated by recombining a DNA cassette in place of the gene of interest to disrupt that locus. The manipulated stem cells are transferred into a developing embryo at the blastocyst stage and offspring homozygous for the altered loci are produced through a series of breeding crosses. Thus, the knockout animals develop in the absence of the gene under investigation. While this can be a powerful tool for investigating the function of the absent gene, it suffers from the limitation that developmental compensation can confound functional studies. Furthermore, because the gene is rendered non-functional in all tissues from which it would normally be expressed, it can be difficult to isolate any functional effects observed to a specific tissue or organ.

To circumvent these problems, these techniques have been refined to allow for conditional knockout of a gene of interest in a site- and time-specific manner. The most common of these techniques utilises the viral-derived Cre/loxP recombinase system (see Kuhn and Torres (2002) for review). Cre is a recombinase enzyme that catalyses the removal of DNA segments flanked by loxP; which are specific 34 base-pair DNA sequences. The technique involves crossing two transgenic strains of animals, one expressing Cre and the other engineered with LoxP sites flanking a gene of interest (i.e. a *floxed* allele) to create a new strain in which Cre-mediated recombination removes the floxed gene. Tissue-specific gene knockout is achieved by restricting Cre expression to a particular tissue, for example by placing the enzyme under the control of a tissue-specific promoter (Kuhn et al. 1995). Time-specific gene knockout can be achieved by using an inducible Cre promoter to control the expression of the Cre recombinase transgene (Kuhn et al. 1995). This conditional knockout approach thereby theoretically allows any gene of interest to be deleted in a tissue- and time-specific manner during development. An example of an application of this approach is the conditional removal of connexin36 in neurons by crossing NESTIN-Cre animals with connexin36 floxed animals (Wellershaus et al. 2008).

Deletion of various members of the connexin family has revealed some detail of the role of these proteins in regulating normal brain behaviour and thereby points to the contribution that these proteins may make to various normal and pathological neurological states. Examples include observations that Connexin36 knockout mice have reduced frequency hippocampal gamma oscillations (Buhl et al. 2003) and display an increased sensitivity to the seizures induced by the proconvulsant drug pentylenetetrazol (Jacobson et al. 2010).

3.3 Antisense oligodeoxynucleotide (AsODN)

Antisense oligonucleotide (AsODN) directed destruction of messenger RNA (mRNA) molecules is a method by which to reduce gene expression at the level of the expressed transcript. AsODNs are short DNA sequences that are complementary to a targeted single stranded mRNA. For association of an AsODN with its target sequence, mRNA binding must occur. This involves binding of matched nucleotides along the length of both the AsODN and targeted mRNA sequence - with purine bases (guanine or adenine) associating with pyrimidine bases (cytosine or thymine or uracil); accordingly, very specific binding to a matched target sequence can be achieved. The AsODN-mRNA hybrid molecule formed by this association is digested by the endogenous enzyme RNase H1, effectively eliminating the targeted AsODN-transcript hybrid and reducing levels of the associated mature protein due to lower levels of translation. There are a number of reports of AsODNs being used to experimentally reduce levels of connexin protein (e.g. Moore and Burt (1994); Law et al. (2006)) although none of these studies have addressed the effects of connexin depletion on seizure phenotype.

3.4 Small interfering RNA (siRNA) targeting of connexin gene expression

Another approach to studying the function of a protein is to reduce levels (knockdown) of its messenger RNA (mRNA) transcripts by the use of small interfering RNA. The effect on phenotype (the physical manifestation) of such a knockdown provides clues as to the role of the targeted transcript, and thereby its protein product, in normal physiology.

Small interfering RNA are short RNA duplexes (i.e. double stranded) molecules 21-28 nucleotides long, which can recruit cellular protein machinery - i.e. the RNAi silencing complex or RISC - to detect a specific transcript and to degrade it in the cytoplasm. As a result, the mRNA transcript is no longer available to the translation protein machinery, thereby reducing levels of the mature protein (reviewed in (Karkare et al. 2004)). They can be introduced *in vitro* to cells in culture, *in vivo* into various target tissues by injection (e.g. intrathecally) and by viral transfection.

There are a number of reports of successful application of siRNA to knockdown connexin levels (e.g. (Nakano et al. 2008; Schock et al. 2008)) although, similarly to the AsODN approach, to date this methodology has not been used *in vivo* to study the effect of depletion of any of the connexin protein family on seizures.

3.5 Other methods for reduction of connexin based cell-to-cell connectivity

Other methods for selective reduction or elimination of cell-to-cell connectivity via gap junctions is via the use of antibodies directed to regions of the connexon extracellular loop. This approach was used by Lin and colleagues (2002) to study the effect of connexin43 blockade on glioma cells. In that study the authors raised an antibody (namely EL1-46) to an epitope (peptide) corresponding to amino acid positions 46-76 in the first external loop (EL1) of the mature protein. The resultant antibodies were shown to produce up to 70% blockade of gap junctions when used at 60mg/mL against cultured astrocytes. In another study, antibodies (EL2-186) raised to an epitope corresponding to amino acids 186-206 in the second extracellular loop of connexin43 were shown to give up to 50% reduction in cell-to-cell coupling in cultured astrocytes (Hofer and Dermietzel 1998).

While antibodies have not been widely used to study seizure by *in vivo* application, the rapid turnover of the connexin family of proteins would likely make them good targets for such an approach.

4. Do gap junctions promote or hinder seizure activity?

Interest in the subject of gap junction involvement in the generation of seizure activity has been driven largely from two complementary ideas: that seizures result from hypersynchronous activation of neuronal populations within the central nervous system; and that direct electrical communication between neurons (via open gap junctions) ought to promote hypersynchronous activity because of the near instantaneous propagation of electrical activity between gap junction-linked cells. The idea that open gap junctions promote seizure activity has been fuelled by a large number of studies showing that gap junction blockade with pharmacological agents is almost universally anticonvulsant (Xiong et al. 2000; Kohling et al. 2001; Bostanci and Bagirici 2007a; Bostanci and Bagirici 2007b; Medina-Ceja et al. 2008; Nassiri-Asl et al. 2008; Nassiri-Asl et al. 2009). However, taking these studies at face value belies the complexity of the nervous system and underestimates the bluntness of many of the tools with which it has been examined.

As we have already proposed, we do not believe it is possible to approach the question of gap junction involvement in seizure mechanisms without considering the distribution of gap junction subtypes within specific cell populations. In the following section we will review the theoretical and experimental basis for pro- and/or anti-convulsant effects of gap junction subtypes on seizures. Because connexin36 and connexin43 subtypes have been most extensively studied, the discussion which follows will focus separately on the role of connexin36-linked neuronal and connexin43-linked astrocytic populations. This does not preclude the possibility that other less well studied gap junction subtypes may also be important.

4.1 Gap junction-linked interneuronal networks

In the mature brain, neuronal gap junction expression is restricted largely to inhibitory interneurons and are almost exclusively of the connexin36 subtype. Connexin36 gap junctions are not expressed uniformly across all interneuron classes. Rather, two main expression patterns predominate: that between same-class parvalbumin-containing multipolar-bursting (MB) cells (Deans et al. 2001; Liu and Jones 2003; Markram et al. 2004; Baude et al. 2007), which synapse onto pyramidal cells in the region of the soma or proximal dendrites (Deans et al. 2001; Liu and Jones 2003; Markram et al. 2004); and that between multipolar calretinin-positive (MCR) and MB interneurons (see Fig 2).

The effect on global brain dynamics of a disruption to gap junction connectivity within these inhibitory networks is not intuitively obvious. Figure 2 is a simplified wiring diagram showing the main synaptic and gap junction connections within the cerebral cortex. According to this schema, blockade of direct electrical communication between inhibitory cells could have *excitatory* effects at the level of pyramidal cell activity via two mechanisms. Firstly, blocking gap junctions between same-class MB interneurons (I_2 in figure 2) will result in a reduction in synchronous firing within this population (Deans et al. 2001) and cause a disruption to inhibitory timing at the pyramidal cell soma. Inhibitory timing is a critical element in maintaining stability in pyramidal cell networks and small inhibitory delays provide a powerful seizurogenic stimulus (Steyn-Ross et al. 2004). Secondly, open gap junctions between MCR and MG cells (I_1 and I_2, respectively in figure 2) provide an "excitation" path between MCR and MB cells, effectively enhancing the inhibitory effect of MB cells at the pyramidal cell soma. Thus, closing these gaps will effectively reduce MB activity and release MB inhibition of the pyramidal cell population.

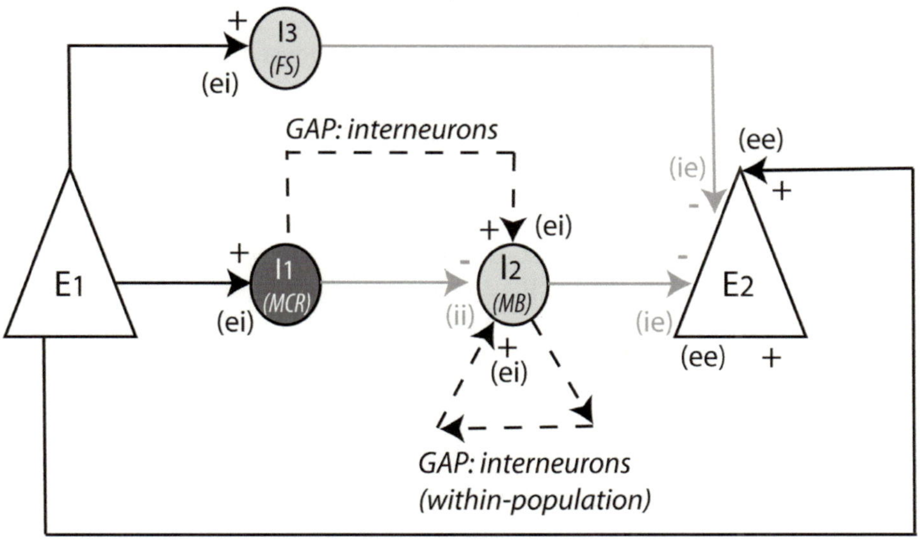

Fig. 2. Schematic showing possible connections involved in seizure spread. Two excitatory (triangles, E_1 and E_2) and two inhibitory (circles, I_1 and I_2) neurons are shown. Chemical synaptic pathways are shown in solid lines and gap-junction mediated pathways are shown in dashed lines. Excitatory pathways are indicated by a "+" and inhibitory pathways by a "-".

The prediction is that connexin36 gap junction blockade will tend to have a pro-seizure effect and there is accumulating experimental evidence to support this hypothesis. Yang and Ling (2007) have shown an increase in excitatory post synaptic potential amplitude following uncoupling of (GABAergic) inhibitory interneurons with carbenoxolone. Carbenoxolone is a broad spectrum gap junction blocker (Gajda et al. 2005; Nilsen et al. 2006) and would have likely blocked all gap junctions in this study. Enhancement of seizure-like event (SLE) frequency has been shown in hippocampal slices following application of carbenoxolone and quinine (Kraglund et al. 2010). The seizure models used in this study (Cs+-induced SLE and low-Ca SLE activity) are non-synaptic in origin, confirming that the excitation effect is not via a synaptic mechanism. Similar excitatory effects have been observed in neocortical slices with mefloquin, which blocks connexin36 gap junctions with greater specificity than carbenoxolone (Voss et al. 2009). This effect is eliminated in connexin36 knockout animals (Voss et al. 2009). Furthermore, connexin36 knockout mice have a greatly enhanced propensity for pentylenetetrazol seizures (Jacobson et al. 2010) and increased hippocampal inter-ictal discharges (Pais et al. 2003) compared to wild-type animals.

Interestingly, connexin32 knockout mice also exhibit neocortical neuronal excitability (Sutor et al. 2000). One of the explanations for this given by the authors is a desynchronisation of inhibitory interneuronal networks; although this is based on the speculation that connexin32 gaps are expressed by interneurons in the cerebral cortex. Currently, there is no evidence that cortical neurons express connexin32 gaps (Dermietzel et al. 1989), although neurons from subcortical nuclei such as the thalamus and basal ganglia show a low level of neuronal expression (Dermietzel et al. 1989).

Contrary to the above findings, hippocampal slices from connexin36 knockout mice show a reduction in ongoing seizure-like activity in response to the convulsant 4-aminopyridine (Maier et al. 2002) and a reduction in fast "ripple" (100-200Hz) oscillations (Maier et al. 2002). Ripples are partly of inhibitory origin (Grenier et al. 2001) and have been implicated in the initiation of seizures (Grenier et al. 2003). The implication is that connexin36 blockade inhibits seizure initiation by disrupting ripple formation.

The discrepancies in experimental findings clearly illustrates that the role of connexin36 gap junctions in seizureogenesis remains to be unequivocally resolved. Many of the studies mentioned above suffer from the limitations already discussed, particularly in terms of non-specificity of pharmacological drug action. In those studies where connexin36 knockout animals have been studied, compensatory effects may also confound the interpretation of results (Voss et al. 2010). Furthermore, the utilisation of different seizure models, analysis methods and choice of tissue between research groups adds further complexity that may account for the apparent contradictions in some results.

4.2 Mathematical models of gap junction effects

A further avenue of investigation that may help to untangle some of this complexity is computer-aided mathematical modelling. Modelling studies have the enviable advantage that selected parameters can be manipulated with absolute specificity. As mentioned in the introduction, no computer model developed to date comes close to representing the brain in all its complexity or functionality; but when aligned with (and refined by) experimental data, computer models can provide an informative adjunct to experimental biology.

Clearly a generalised seizure is the manifestation of a dramatic change in the mode of activity of neuronal populations. It can be most accurately described as a change in the dynamics of a neural mass. The most important conclusion from modelling studies is that the seizure state is principally a transition from a stable steady mode of operation to an oscillatory mode. We would emphasize that the dynamic signature of a seizure is *oscillation*, rather than simple *hyperexcitation* - although often hyperexcitation (manifest clinically as the tonic phase of a generalised seizure) will precipitate a secondary oscillation (manifest clinically as the clonic phase of a generalised seizure). The tendency for this transition to occur depends on both the intrinsic properties of each of the neurons, and also on how they are connected together into networks. The strength and time-course of the interneuronal connections are critical in whether the behaviour of the system will be stable or unstable (oscillatory). The synapses may be chemical or electrical, and are modulated by a variety of glial activities (as mentioned previously). We emphasize that the electrical connections between neurons differ from the chemical synapses in three critical ways:

i. a chemical synapse between inhibitory neurons is inhibitory - i.e. it effectively *reduces* the activity of the downstream neuron, thus allowing downstream excitatory neuronal activation. In contrast an electrical synapse between inhibitory neurons has similar dynamic effects as an *excitatory* glutamatergic synapse - i.e. *increasing* the activity of the second neuron, which in turn dampens the excitatory cells and the system as a whole (see fig 2). Dynamically this is equivalent to an increase in the strength of the basket cells, which tend to control seizure spread.
ii. if the interneuronal gap junctions are open, the inhibitory neurons become a form of *syncitium*, which supports spatial demarcation of areas of high-firing in the neocortex and reduces the tendency of the cortex to become oscillatory.

iii. open gap junctions will reduce input resistance of the neuron, and hence act to *shunt* both excitatory and inhibitory synaptic input, which effectively results in a weakening of chemical synaptic connectivity.

Quantitative modelling of the influences of electrotonic synapses is still at an early stage. There are a number of papers which model the effects of gap junctions on other oscillatory behavior in the brain (gamma rhythms); and quite a few papers that model seizures of various types - but relatively few papers that look at both seizures and gap junctions. Broadly, there are two approaches to quantitative modelling of gap junctions and their modulation of neural dynamics. One is to model, in detail, modest (typically ~ 4 000) numbers of inhibitory and excitatory neurons. We refer to these as "neuron-by-neuron" models. These models try to include the various multicompartmental ion channel conductances within neurons, and chemical and electrotonic synaptic connections between different neuronal subtypes. Whilst these approaches present a seductive verisimilitude with real brain connections, they have significant, and under-appreciated, disadvantages. They are computationally very expensive, and - whilst it is easy to replicate experimentally-derived EEG or ECoG signals in the model output - it is difficult to generalise the results beyond the immediate outputs; and thus achieve some sort of broader analytic understanding of the dynamics of the neuronal populations. The other approach is to use some form of "mean-field" or "neural mass" model. These models quantify the behavior of a 'typical' neuron, and are unable to distinguish individual neurons. Therefore the accurate correspondence of the parameters in the model with neurobiological measurements is more difficult - but the mean-field models are computationally very tractable, and allow a more general understanding of processes that influence the dynamics of the brain. They also allow the full mathematical arsenal of statistical physics to be applied to neurobiology. The seizure state is usually identified as an extreme oscillation in neuronal dynamics. This being the case, the problem of whether the brain will enter a seizure can be rephrased in the language of dynamical systems theory as: "whether the state of the various parameters that control the brain dynamics is such that the brain can enter a region of instability?" If the problem is linearised it simplifies to the question of: "whether the largest real eigenvalue in the system is greater than zero?" We can look at ranges of values for various parameters, that we have deemed to be important in controlling the behaviour of the model system. Certain combinations of parameter ranges will result in a stable neuronal activity (the system will evolve towards a fixed point); and at other ranges the system will be unstable (it will oscillate or undergo irregular chaotic behaviour). The boundary between these two modes of behavior is called a "basin boundary". If the system is close to a basin boundary that encloses an unstable state, minor noise-induced changes in parameter values are more likely to precipitate the neuronal population into a seizure. Typically the choice of parameter values are constrained by experimental estimates from different neuronal populations of such factors as the number of neuronal connections, neuronal membrane potential, and synaptic gain.

4.2.1 Neuron-by-neuron models

Using very detailed neuron-by-neuron models, Traub and co-workers (Traub 2003) have published a number of papers in which they investigate various aspects of the effects of both inhibitory-inhibitory gap junctions and excitatory-excitatory axonal gap junctions. They found that inhibitory-inhibitory gap junctions were not necessary for the presence of gamma oscillations, but that the presence of open gap junctions increased the strength and precision of these oscillations. This has been a recurring theme in almost all experimental and modelling studies of the contribution of gap junctions to neural activity. Namely, that the role of the gap junctions is a secondary one; in which they interact with chemical synaptic function to sculpture and augment existing neuronal rhythms. In these papers this group were primarily interested in testing whether pyramidal cell axo-axonal gap junctions were necessary for the expression of very fast oscillations - which are believed to be important in the process of seizure development (see section 4.3 below). The role of the much more common inhibitory-inhibitory gap junctions was relegated to a few sentences in which they stated "in addition to gamma oscillations, synchronized epileptiform bursts also occur in the connexin36 knockout (but not wild-type) in the presence of kainate (Pais et al. 2003)." (Traub 2005).

The other important attempts at neuron-by-neuron modelling of interneuronal gap junction effects were by van Drongelen (2004) and Di Garbo (2004). Both papers had similar results. They found that inhibitory-inhibitory gap junctions acted to synchronize the inhibitory cell populations, but the actual effects depended strongly on pre-existing activity. If this activity was already strongly synchronous, then whether gaps junctions were open or closed had little influence.

4.2.2 Mean-field models

In mean-field models seizures are usually conceived of as the result of a so-called "Hopf bifurcation" in the dynamics of the brain (Breakspear et al. 2006). There is mathematical precision and complexity behind this statement, but in simple descriptive terms, the dynamics of the brain change from a fixed point to a widespread oscillation between zero firing and high firing states. To date there are no publications of mean field models of the effects of gap junctions in seizure generation, but preliminary communication by Steyn-Ross et al. in general agree with experimental results and the neuron-by-neuron models - i.e. that open inhibitory-inhibitory gap junctions tend to stabilise the brain, whereas excitatory-excitatory gap junctions have the opposite effect. The effects are not very large but may be clinically important. As an example of the sort of output from the mean-field approach, figure 3 shows the regions that are associated with oscillatory behaviour in the presence of open or closed inhibitory-inhibitory gap junctions. The white area is the region of seizure behavior if the gap junctions are open, and the grey area is the *increased area* of oscillation if the gap junctions are closed. It can be seen that closure of these gap junctions increases the size of the basin boundary by about 20%. This means that the range over which combinations of the magnitude of the inhibitory post-synaptic potential and the degree of resting membrane depolarisation result in seizures is modestly greater if the inhibitory-inhibitory gap junctions are closed.

4.3 Gap junction-linked pyramidal axo-axonal networks

A discussion on neuronal gap junctions and seizures would not be complete without considering pyramidal cell axoaxonal junctions. Axoaxonal gap junctions have been demonstrated between pyramidal cells in the hippocampus (Schmitz et al. 2001; Hamzei-Sichani et al. 2007) and are probably of the connexin36 subtype (Hamzei-Sichani et al. 2007). Modeling studies have implicated these junctions in the generation of fast ripple oscillations (Traub et al. 2001) and epileptogenesis (Traub et al. 2002); and blockade is theorised to have an anticonvulsant effect. The finding that neither pharmacological nor genetic connexin36 blockade has an anticonvulsant effect in neocortical slices (Voss et al. 2010) suggest that either these gap junctions are not present in the cortex or are so few as to have minimal impact on seizure processes. If initial findings that axoaxonal gap junctions are composed of connexin36 subunits (Hamzei-Sichani et al. 2007) prove to be correct, this may explain some of the discrepancy in connexin36 gap junction blocking studies. That is, it would provide a rational basis for connexin36 blockade potentially having both pro- or anti-convulsant effects, depending on whether effects on interneuronal or pyramidal cell populations predominated.

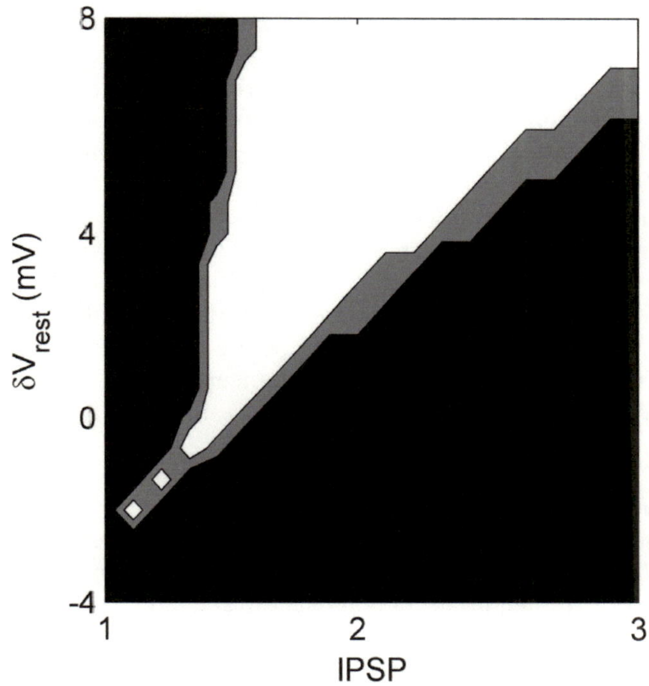

Fig. 3. Size of areas where the model shows seizure-like oscillatory behavior. We have chosen a parameter space with axes of synaptic gain (Inhibitory Postsynaptic Potential (IPSP)) and intrinsic neuronal excitability (change in resting membrane potential (δV_{rest})). The white area is the region of parameter space in which the model cortex is unstable (positive real eigenvalues) when the inhibitory-inhibitory gap junctions are open. The grey area is the region of instability with closed inhibitory-inhibitory gap junctions. The black area is the region of stable cortical dynamics.

4.4 Gap junction-linked astrocytic networks

Increasingly important and diverse roles for glial cells in cortical neurophysiological function and dysfunction are being reported. In particular, the role of astrocytes in epilepsy has been (Penfield 1929) and remains a subject of considerable interest (see Steinhauser and Seifert (2002) for review). Astrocytes are extensively linked by gap junctions (primarily connexin43 and connexin30) and connexin43 is upregulated at epileptic foci in vivo (Fonseca et al. 2002), implicating a role for this gap junction in the seizure process. The nature of this role however is not clearly understood. Two divergent possibilities present themselves from the literature.

Firstly, gap junction-linked astrocytic networks could *contribute* to seizure genesis by facilitating the spread of neuronal activity via propagating calcium waves (Nedergaard 1994) and glutamate release. Astrocytes produce spontaneous slow calcium transients during seizure-like activity in many in vitro models of epilepsy (Tashiro et al. 2002; Stout and Charles 2003; Tian et al. 2005); these events occur independent of neuronal activity (Parri et al. 2001; Wang et al. 2006) and are causally linked to astrocytic release of glutamate (Parpura et al. 1994; Tian et al. 2005) and an increase in neuronal excitability (Fellin et al. 2006) and synchronicity (Fellin et al. 2004). Furthermore, astrocytic release of glutamate can induce epileptiform activity in pyramidal cells independent of synaptic activity (Kang et al. 2005; Tian et al. 2005) and can enhance synaptically driven seizure-like events (Fellin et al. 2006). There is also evidence that gap junction-coupled astrocytes may support epileptiform activity by supplying glucose to neuronal networks (Rouach et al. 2008). Together, these data build a strong case for an important function for gap-junction-linked astrocytes in promoting seizure activity. There is experimental support for this from hippocampal slice studies, where connexin43 gap junction blockade with GAP27 has been shown to attenuate seizure-like activity (Samoilova et al. 2008). An important caveat is that this study may be confounded by effects of the mimetic peptide on pannexin and hemichannels. Indeed, pannexin1 hemichannel blockade with "panx" (100μM, sequence WRQAAFVDSY) has antiepileptic effects in hippocampal slices (Thompson et al. 2008). Pannexin1 hemichannels augment synaptic function by providing an NMDA-linked depolarizing current during intense synaptic activity (Thompson et al. 2008).

Alternatively, gap junction-linked astrocytic networks could *limit* seizure activity by acting as a sink for extracellular potassium ions (Orkand 1986) and/or excitatory neurotransmitters such as glutamate. The effect of an elevation in extracellular potassium is to shift the equilibrium potential for potassium to a more depolarised level; the flow-on effect of which is resting membrane depolarisation and enhanced cell excitability. A similar sequestering role for gap-junction-linked astrocytic networks has been proposed for the excitatory neurotransmitter glutamate (Tanaka et al. 2008). Uncoupling astrocytic connexin43 gap junctions has also been shown to directly reduce the expression of the glutamate transporter GLT-1, resulting in reduced glutamate uptake by astrocytes (Figiel et al. 2007). Astrocytic networks could also limit seizure activity through the coordinated release of ATP (see Halassa and Haydon (2010) for review), the conversion of which to adenosine has an inhibitory effect on neuronal activity. Experimental support for seizure-limiting effects of astrocytic coupling comes from hippocampal slice studies showing that conditional deletion of astrocytic connexin43 and unrestricted deletion of connexin30 results in impaired potassium clearance and reduced seizure threshold (Wallraff et al. 2006). While this study has the advantage of targeted genetic manipulation, one cannot rule out the possibility of confounding compensatory developmental effects in the transgenic animals.

Connexin30 is the other main connexin subtype expressed by astrocytes in the mature CNS. Functional effects of targeted manipulation of connexin30 gap junctions have not been investigated. However, connexin30 has been shown to be up-regulated following kainate-induced seizures in rats (Condorelli et al. 2002). While this implicates connexin30 in the seizure process, an inherent problem with this and similar studies is that changes in connexin or gap junction expression do not necessarily indicate whether these modifications are a cause *or* a consequence of the seizure process. Thus, while there are a growing number of papers documenting alterations in connexin subtype expression (including connexin43 (Fonseca et al. 2002)) during or after seizures (see (Rouach et al. 2002) and tables 2 and 3), studies such as these are generally not helpful in determining the functional role of the subtype in question.

In summary, the role of astrocytic gap junctions in seizureogenesis has not been unequivocally resolved; with theoretical and experimental grounds for both pro- and anticonvulsant effects. It may be that both hypotheses will hold true and that the functional expression of astrocytic gap junction manipulation will be shown to depend upon secondary factors such as the genetic background of the animals (Wiencken-Barger et al. 2007) and/or physiological factors underlying the regulation of astrocytic function.

Gene	*Seizure model*	*Expression change*	*Reference*
Connexin30	Kainate or kindling	No significant changes found	(Sohl et al. 2000)
	Kindling	Upregulated with increased apoptosis	(Condorelli et al. 2002)
Connexin32	In vitro bicuculline (hippocampal slices)	mRNA increased 2-3 fold within 6h and protein increased after 6h	(Li et al. 2001)
	4-aminopyridine	Significantly increased	(Samoilova et al. 2003)
Connexin36	Kainate or kindling	mRNA up 44% reduced by wk4 post application, protein level only slightly reduced (apoptosis linked?)	(Sohl et al. 2000)
	4-aminopyridine	Significantly increased	(Samoilova et al. 2003)
	Kindling	Upregulated during focal seizures then back to basal levels with onset of generalized seizures	(Beheshiti et al. 2010)
	4-aminopyridine	Gradual decrease up to 8h post injection (I.P.)	(Zappala et al. 2006)
Connexin43	4-aminopyridine	Significantly increased	(Samoilova et al. 2003)

Table 1. Connexin expression changes associated with experimentally-induced epilepsy in rodents

Gene	*Epilepsy condition/type*	*Expression change*	*Reference*
Connexin32	Temporal lobe epilepsy	Decreased (hippocampus)	(Collignon et al. 2006)
Connexin36	Temporal lobe epilepsy	Unchanged (hippocampus)	(Collignon et al. 2006)
Connexin43	Intractable seizure disorder	Increased	(Naus et al. 1991)
	Complex partial seizure disorder	No significant change	(Elisevich et al. 1997)
	Temporal lobe epilepsy	Increased (hippocampus)	(Collignon et al. 2006)

Table 2. Connexin expression changes associated with clinical epilepsy

5. Conclusion

In this chapter we have sought to bring together research from a wide range of disciplines encompassing electrophysiology, molecular biology and mathematical modelling, with the aim of addressing the role of gap junctions in the mechanism of seizures. The prevailing notion that open gap junctions promote seizure activity is overly simplistic and does not do justice to a growing body of literature showing that the opposite may be true in certain situations. There is also no evidence to support the idea that gap junctions either cause or ablate seizures *per se;* rather, they perform a modulatory role that is dependent upon the prior activity of the system and upon gap junction subtype. In any discussion it is essential to be precise about the type of experimental manipulation used, and exactly which gap junction subtype is under consideration. Thus, excitatory effects may be expected when pyramidal cell axo-axonal gap junctions are opened, while the opposite is likely with opening of inhibitory interneuronal gap junctions. Electrophysiological and modelling studies support this delineation. However, there is still some way to go before we will fully understand this complex area of neurobiology. The role of astrocytic gap junctions in particular remains an open question. Astrocytes are increasingly being recognised for their complex neuroregulatory functions and gap junctions are well suited for this role. Whether astrocytic gap junctions promote or hinder seizure activity is likely to depend upon prevailing neurophysiological factors governing the state of ongoing neuronal activity. Furthermore, many gap junction subtypes have been poorly studied to date and their possible role in seizure processes is undetermined. Greater understanding of these matters rests upon development and application of experimental techniques and pharmacological tools for targeted modulation of specific gap junction subtypes.

6. Acknowledgement

The authors' research was supported by the Marsden Fund of New Zealand, the Neurological Foundation of New Zealand and the Waikato Medical Research Foundation.

7. References

Amabeoku, G. J. and O. Chikuni (1992). Effects of some GABAergic agents on quinine-induced seizures in mice. *Experientia* Vol. 48, pp. (659-662).

Amabeoku, G. J. and C. C. Farmer (2005). Gamma-aminobutyric acid and mefloquin-induced seizures in mice. *Progress in Neuro-Psychopharmacology and Biological Psychiatry* Vol. 29, pp. (917-921).

Bao, L., S. Locovei, et al. (2004). Pannexin membrane channels are mechanosensitive conduits for ATP. *FEBS Letters* Vol. 572, pp. (65-68).

Baranova, A., D. Ivanov, et al. (2004). The mammalian pannexin family is homologous to the invertebrate innexin gap junction proteins. *Genomics* Vol. 83, pp. (706-716).

Baude, A., C. Bleasdale, et al. (2007). Immunoreactivity for the GABA-A receptor alpha1 subunit, somatostatin and connexin36 distinguishes axoaxonic, basket and bistratified interneurons of the rat hippocampus. *Cerebral Cortex* Vol. 17, pp. (2094-2107).

Beheshiti, S., M. Sayyah, et al. (2010). Changes in hippocampal connexin 36 mRNA and protein levels during epileptogenesis in the kindling model of epilepsy. *Progress in Neuro-Psychopharmacology & Biological Psychiatry* Vol. 34, pp. (510-515).

Belluardo, N., G. Mudo, et al. (2000). Expression of connexin36 in the adult and developing rat brain. *Brain Research* Vol. 865(1), pp. (121-38).

Bostanci, M. O. and F. Bagirici (2007a). Anticonvulsant effects of quinine on penicillin-induced epileptiform activity: an in vivo study. *Seizure* Vol. 16, pp. (166-172).

Bostanci, M. O. and F. Bagirici (2007b). Anticonvulsive effects of carbenoxolone on penicillin-induced epileptiform activity: an in vivo study. *Neuropharmacology* Vol. 52, pp. (362-367).

Breakspear, M., J. A. Roberts, et al. (2006). A unifying explanation of primary generalized seizures through nonlinear brain modeling and bifurcation analysis. *Cerebral Cortex* Vol. 16(9), pp. (1296-1313).

Bruzzone, R., S. G. Hormuzdi, et al. (2003). Pannexins, a family of gap junction proteins expressed in brain. *Proceedings of the National Academy of Sciences of the United States of America* Vol. 100(23), pp. (13644-9).

Buhl, D. L., K. D. Harris, et al. (2003). Selective impairment of hippocampal gamma oscillations in connexin-36 knock-out mouse in vivo. *The Journal of Neuroscience* Vol. 23, pp. (1013-1018).

Collignon, F., N. M. Wetjen, et al. (2006). Altered expression of connexin subtypes in mesial temporal lobe epilepsy in humans. *Journal of neurosurgery* Vol. 105(1), pp. (77-87).

Condorelli, D. F., G. Mudo, et al. (2002). Connexin-30 mRNA Is Up-Regulated in Astrocytes and Expressed in Apoptotic Neuronal Cells of Rat Brain Following Kainate-Induced Seizures. *Molecular and Cellular Neuroscience* Vol. 21, pp. (94-113).

Condorelli, D. F., A. Trovato-Salinaro, et al. (2003). Cellular expression of connexins in the rat brain: neuronal localization, effects of kainate-induced seizures and expression in apoptotic neuronal cells. *European Journal of Neuroscience* Vol. 18, pp. (1807-1827).

Cruikshank, S. J., M. Hopperstad, et al. (2004). Potent block of Cx36 and Cx50 gap junction channels by mefloquine. *Proceedings of the National Academy of Sciences of the United States of America* Vol. 101, pp. (12364-12369).

Dahl, G. (2007). Gap junction-mimetic peptides do work, but in unexpected ways. *Cell Communication and Adhesion* Vol. 14, pp. (259-264).

Deans, M. R., J. R. Gibson, et al. (2001). Synchronous activity of inhibitory networks in neocortex requires electrical synapses containing connexin36. *Neuron* Vol. 31, pp. (477-485).

Dermietzel, R., M. Farooq, et al. (1997). Oligodendrocytes express gap junction proteins connexin32 and connexin45. *GLIA* Vol. 20(2), pp. (101-14).

Dermietzel, R., E. L. Hertzberg, et al. (1991). Gap Junctions between Cultured Astrocytes: Immunocytochemical, Molecular, and Electrophysiological Analysis. *The Journal of Neuroscience* Vol. 11, pp. (1421-1432).

Dermietzel, R., O. Traub, et al. (1989). Differential expression of three gap junction proteins in developing and mature brain tissues. *Proceedings of the National Academy of Sciences of the United States of America* Vol. 86, pp. (10148-10152).

Di Garbo, A., A. Panarese, et al. (2004). Phase locking states between fast-spiking interneurons coupled by electrical and chemical synapses. *Neurocomputing* Vol. 58-60, pp. (159 - 164).

Dow, G. S., T. H. Hudson, et al. (2003). The acute neurotoxicity of mefloquine may be mediated through a disruption of calcium homeostasis and ER function in vitro *Malaria Journal* Vol. 2, pp. (14).

Ebihara, L. (2003). Physiology and biophysics of hemi-gap-junctional channels expressed in Xenopus oocytes. *Acta Physiologica Scandinavica* Vol. 179, pp. (5-8).

Ebihara, L., X. Liu, et al. (2003). Effect of External Magnesium and Calcium on Human Connexin46 Hemichannels. *Biophysical Journal* Vol. 84, pp. (277–286).

Elisevich, K., S. A. Rempel, et al. (1997). Hippocampal connexin 43 expression in human complex partial seizure disorder. *Experimental neurology* Vol. 145(1), pp. (154-64).

Evans, W. H. and S. Boitano (2001). Connexin mimetic peptides: specific inhibitors of gap-junctional intercellular communication. *Biochemical Society Transactions* Vol. 29, pp. (606-612).

Fellin, T., M. Gomez-Gonzalo, et al. (2006). Astrocytic glutamate in not necessary for the generation of epileptiform neuronal activity in hippocampal slices. *The Journal of Neuroscience* Vol. 26, pp. (9312-9322).

Fellin, T., O. Pascual, et al. (2004). Neuronal synchrony mediated by astrocytic glutamate through activation of extrasynaptic NMDA receptors. *Neuron* Vol. 43, pp. (729-743).

Figiel, M., C. Allritz, et al. (2007). Gap junctional control of glial glutamate transporter expression. *Molecular and Cellular Neuroscience* Vol. 35, pp. (130-137).

Fonseca, C. G., C. R. Green, et al. (2002). Upregulation in astrocytic connexin 43 gap junction levels may exacerbate generalized seizures in mesial temporal lobe epilepsy. *Brain Research* Vol. 929, pp. (105-116).

Gajda, Z., Z. Szupera, et al. (2005). Quinine, a blocker of neuronal Cx36 channels, suppresses seizure activity in the rat neocortex in vivo. *Epilepsia* Vol. 56, pp. (1581-1591).

Giaume, C. and M. Theis (2010). Pharmacological and genetic approaches to study connexin-mediated channels in glial cells of the central nervous system. *Brain Research - Brain Research Reviews* Vol. 63, pp. (160-176).

Goodenough, D. A. and D. L. Paul (2003). Beyond the gap: functions of unpaired connexon channels. *Nature Reviews Molecular Cell Biology* Vol. 4, pp. (1-10).

Grenier, F., I. Timofeev, et al. (2001). Focal synchronisation of ripples (80-200Hz) in neocortex and their neuronal correlates. *Journal of Neurophysiology* Vol. 86, pp. (1884-1898).

Grenier, F., I. Timofeev, et al. (2003). Neocortical Very Fast Oscillations (Ripples, 80–200 Hz) During Seizures: Intracellular Correlates. *Journal of Neurophysiology* Vol. 89, pp. (841–852).

Halassa, M. M. and P. G. Haydon (2010). Integrated Brain Circuits: Astrocytic Networks Modulate Neuronal Activity and Behavior. *Annual Review of Physiology* Vol. 72, pp. (335–355).

Hamzei-Sichani, F., N. Kamasawa, et al. (2007). Gap junctions on hippocampal mossy fiber axons demonstrated by thin-section electron microscopy and freeze fracture replica immunogold labeling. *Proceedings of the National Academy of Sciences of the United States of America* Vol. 104(30), pp. (12548-53).

Hauser, W. A. and L. T. Kurland (1975). The epidemiology of epilepsy in Rochester, Minnesota, 1935 through 1967. *Epilepsia* Vol. 16, pp. (1-66).

Herve, J.-C. and S. Dhein (2010). Peptides targeting gap junctional structures. *Current Pharmaceutical Design* Vol. 16, pp. (3056-3070).

Hofer, A. and R. Dermietzel (1998). Visualization and functional blocking of gap junction hemichannels (connexons) with antibodies against external loop domains in astrocytes. *Glia* Vol. 24(1), pp. (141-54).

Hombach, S., U. Janssen-Bienhold, et al. (2004). Functional expression of connexin57 in horizontal cells of the mouse retina. *European Journal of Neuroscience* Vol. 19, pp. (2633-2640).

Jacobson, G. M., L. J. Voss, et al. (2010). Connexin36 knockout mice display increased sensitivity to pentylenetetrazol-induced seizure-like behaviors. *Brain Research* Vol. doi: 10.1016/j.brainres.2010.09.006.

Jiang, J. X. and S. Gu (2005). Gap junction- and hemichannel-independent actions of connexins. *Biochimica et Biophysica Acta* Vol. 1711, pp. (208-214).

Juszczak, G. R. and A. H. Swiergiel (2009). Properties of gap junction blockers and their behavioural, cognitive and electrophysiological effects: animal and human studies. *Progress in Neuro-Psychopharmacology & Biological Psychiatry* Vol. 33, pp. (181-198).

Kang, N., J. Xu, et al. (2005). Astrocytic glutamate release-induced transient depolarisation and epileptiform discharges in hippocampal CA1 pyramidal neurons. *Journal of Neurophysiology* Vol. 94, pp. (4121-4130).

Karkare, S., S. Daniel, et al. (2004). RNA interference silencing the transcriptional message: aspects and applications. *Applied biochemistry and biotechnology* Vol. 119(1), pp. (1-12).

Kohling, R., S. J. Gladwell, et al. (2001). Prolonged epileptiform bursting induced by 0-Mg in rat hippocampal slices depends on gap junctional coupling. *Neuroscience* Vol. 105, pp. (579-587).

Kraglund, N., M. Andreasen, et al. (2010). Differential influence of non-synaptic mechanisms in two in vitro models of epileptic field bursts. *Brain Research* Vol. doi:10.1016/j.brainres.2010.02.015.

Kuhn, R., F. Schwenk, et al. (1995). Inducible gene targeting in mice. *Science* Vol. 269, pp. (1427-1429).

Kuhn, R. and R. M. Torres (2002). Cre/loxP recombination system and gene targeting. *Methods in Molecular Biology* Vol. 180, pp. (175-204).

Kunzelmann, P., W. Schroder, et al. (1999). Late onset and increasing expression of the gap junction protein connexin30 in adult murine brain and long-term cultured astrocytes. *Glia* Vol. 25, pp. (111-119).

Law, L. Y., W. V. Zhang, et al. (2006). In vitro optimization of antisense oligodeoxynucleotide design: an example using the connexin gene family. *Journal of biomolecular techniques* Vol. 17(4), pp. (270-82).

Leybaert, L., K. Braet, et al. (2003). Connexin channels, connexin mimetic peptides and ATP release. *Cell Communication and Adhesion* Vol. 10, pp. (251-257).

Li, J., H. Shen, et al. (2001). Upregulation of gap junction connexin 32 with epileptiform activity in the isolated mouse hippocampus. *Neuroscience* Vol. 105(3), pp. (589-98).

Lin, J. H., T. Takano, et al. (2002). Connexin 43 enhances the adhesivity and mediates the invasion of malignant glioma cells. *The Journal of neuroscience* Vol. 22(11), pp. (4302-11).

Lin, X., S. Chen, et al. Effects of quinine on the excitability and voltage-dependent currents of isolated spiral ganglion neurons in culture. *Journal of Neurophysiology* Vol. 79, pp. (2503-12).

Liu, X. and E. G. Jones (2003). Fine structural localisation of connexin-36 immunoreactivity in mouse cerebral cortex and thalamus. *The Journal of Comparative Neurology* Vol. 466, pp. (457-467).

Locovei, S., L. Bao, et al. (2006). Pannexin 1 in erythrocytes: function without a gap. *Proceedings of the National Academy of Sciences of the United States of America* Vol. 103, pp. (7655-7659).

MacVicar, B. A. and A. J. Thompson (2009). Non-junction functions of pannexin-1 channels. *Trends in Neurosciences* Vol. 33, pp. (93-102).

Maier, N., M. Guldenagel, et al. (2002). Reduction of high-frequency network oscillations (ripples) and pathological network discharges in hippocampal slices from connexin36-deficient mice. *The Journal of Physiology* Vol. 541, pp. (521-528).

Markram, H., M. Toledo-Rodriguez, et al. (2004). Interneurons of the neocortical inhibitory system. *Nature Reviews Neuroscience.* Vol. 5, pp. (793-807).

Maxeiner, S., O. Kruger, et al. (2003). Spatiotemporal transcription of connexin45 during brain development results in neuronal expression in adult mice. *Neuroscience* Vol. 119, pp. (689-700).

Medina-Ceja, L., A. Cordero-Romero, et al. (2008). Antiepileptic effect of carbenoxolone on seizures induced by 4-aminopyridine: a study in the rat hippocampus and entorhinal cortex. *Brain Research* Vol. 1187, pp. (74-81).

Moore, L. K. and J. M. Burt (1994). Selective block of gap junction channel expression with connexin-specific antisense oligodeoxynucleotides. *The American journal of physiology* Vol. 267(5 Pt 1), pp. (C1371-80).

Nakano, Y., M. Oyamada, et al. (2008). Connexin43 knockdown accelerates wound healing but inhibits mesenchymal transition after corneal endothelial injury in vivo. *Investigative ophthalmology & visual science* Vol. 49(1), pp. (93-104).

Nassiri-Asl, M., F. Zamansoltani, et al. (2009). Antiepileptic effects of quinine in the pentylenetetrazole model of seizure. *Seizure* Vol. 18, pp. (129-132).

Nassiri-Asl, M., F. Zamansoltani, et al. (2008). The inhibitory effect of trimethylamine on the anticonvulsant activities of quinine in the pentylenetetrazole model in rats. *Progress in Neuro-Psychopharmacology & Biological Psychiatry* Vol. 32, pp. (1496-1500).

Naus, C. C., J. F. Bechberger, et al. (1991). Gap junction gene expression in human seizure disorder. *Experimental neurology* Vol. 111(2), pp. (198-203).

Nedergaard, M. (1994). Direct signalling from astrocytes to neurons in cultures of mammalian brain cells. *Science* Vol. 263, pp. (1768-1771).

Nilsen, K. E., A. R. Kelso, et al. (2006). Antiepileptic effect of gap-junction blockers in a rat model of refractory focal cortical epilepsy. *Epilepsia* Vol. 47, pp. (1169-1175).

O'Carroll, S. J., M. Alkadhi, et al. (2008). Connexin43 mimetic peptides reduce swelling, astrogliosis, and neuronal cell death after spinal cord injury. *Cell Communication and Adhesion* Vol. 15, pp. (27-42).

Orkand, R. K. (1986). Introductory remarks: glial-interstitial fluid exchange. *Annals of the New York Academy of Sciences* Vol. 481, pp. (269-272).

Pais, I., S. G. Hormuzdi, et al. (2003). Sharp wave-like activity in the hippocampus in vitro in mice lacking the gap junction protein connexin 36. *Journal of Neurophysiology* Vol. 89, pp. (2046-2054).

Parpura, V., T. A. Basarsky, et al. (1994). Glutamate-mediated astrocyte-neuron signalling. *Nature* Vol. 369, pp. (744-747).

Parri, H. R., T. M. Gould, et al. (2001). Spontaneous astrocytic calcium oscillations in situ drive NMDAR-mediated neuronal excitation. *Nature Neuroscience* Vol. 4, pp. (803-812).

Penfield, W. (1929). The Mechanism of cicatricial contraction in the brain. *Brain* Vol. 50, pp. (499-517).

Rouach, N., E. Avignone, et al. (2002). Gap junctions and connexin expression in the normal and pathological central nervous system. *Biology of the Cell* Vol. 94, pp. (457–475).

Rouach, N., A. Koulakoff, et al. (2008). Astroglial metabolic networks sustain hippocampal synaptic transmission. *Science* Vol. 322, pp. (1551-1555).

Samoilova, M., J. Li, et al. (2003). Epileptiform activity in hippocampal slice cultures exposed chronically to bicuculline: increased gap junctional function and expression. *Journal of neurochemistry* Vol. 86(3), pp. (687-99).

Samoilova, M., K. Wentlandt, et al. (2008). Connexin 43 mimetic peptides inhibit spontaneous epileptiform activity in organotypic hippocampal slice cultures. *Experimental Neurology* Vol. 210, pp. (762-775).

Schmitz, D., S. Schuchmann, et al. (2001). Axo-axonal coupling: a novel mechanism for ultrafast neuronal communication. *Neuron* Vol. 31, pp. (831-840).

Schock, S. C., D. Leblanc, et al. (2008). ATP release by way of connexin 36 hemichannels mediates ischemic tolerance in vitro. *Biochemical and biophysical research communications* Vol. 368(1), pp. (138-44).

Singh, S. K., I. D. Clarke, et al. (2003). Identification of a Cancer Stem Cell in Human Brain Tumors. *Cancer Research* Vol. 63, pp. (5821-5828).

Sohl, G., M. Guldenagel, et al. (2000). Expression of connexin genes in hippocampus of kainate-treated and kindled rats under conditions of experimental epilepsy. *Brain research* Vol. 83(1-2), pp. (44-51).

Sohl, G. and K. Willecke (2004). Gap junctions and the connexin protein family. *Cardiovascular Research* Vol. 62, pp. (228– 232).

Song, J. and M. A. Tanouye (2006). Seizure Suppression by shakB2, a Gap Junction Mutation in Drosophila. *Journal of Neurophysiology* Vol. 95, pp. (627–635).

Steinhauser, C. and G. Seifert (2002). Glial membrane channels and receptors in epilepsy: impact for generation and spread of seizure activity. *European Journal of Pharmacology* Vol. 447, pp. (227-237).

Steyn-Ross, M. L., D. A. Steyn-Ross, et al. (2004). Modelling general anaesthesia as a first-order phase transition in the cortex. *Progress in Biophysics and Molecular Biology* Vol. 85, pp. (369-85).

Stout, C. and A. Charles (2003). Modulation of intercellular calcium signalling in astrocytes by extracellular calcium and magnesium. *Glia* Vol. 43, pp. (265-273).

Sutor, B., C. Schmolke, et al. (2000). Myelination defects and neuronal hyperexcitability in the neocortex of connexin 32-deficient mice. *Cerebral Cortex* Vol. 10, pp. (684-697).

Tanaka, M., K. Yamaguchi, et al. (2008). Connexin43 and Bergmann glial gap junctions in cerebellar function. *Frontiers in Neuroscience* Vol. 2, pp. (225-233).

Tashiro, A., J. Goldberg, et al. (2002). Calcium oscillations in neocortical astrocytes under epileptiform conditions. *Journal of Neurobiology* Vol. 50, pp. (45-55).

Thompson, A. J. and S. C. R. Lummis (2008). Antimalarial drugs inhibit human 5-HT3 and GABA-A but not GABA-C receptors. *British Journal of Pharmacology* Vol. 153, pp. (1686-1696).

Thompson, R. J., M. F. Jackson, et al. (2008). Activation of pannexin-1 hemichannels augments aberrant bursting in the hippocampus. *Science* Vol. 322, pp. (1555-1559).

Tian, G.-F., H. Azmi, et al. (2005). An astrocyte basis of epilepsy. *Nature Medicine* Vol. 11, pp. (973-981).

Traub, R. D. (2003). Contrasting roles of axonal (pyramidal cell) and dendritic (interneuron) electrical coupling in the generation of neuronal network oscillations. *Proceedings of the National Academy of Sciences of the United States of America* Vol. 100, pp. (1370-1374).

Traub, R. D. (2005). Transient Depression of Excitatory Synapses on Interneurons Contributes to Epileptiform Bursts During Gamma Oscillations in the Mouse Hippocampal Slice. *Journal of Neurophysiology* Vol. 94, pp. (1225–1235).

Traub, R. D., A. Draguhn, et al. (2002). Axonal gap junctions between principal neurons: a novel source of network oscillations, and perhaps epileptogenesis. *Rev Neurosci* Vol. 13(1), pp. (1-30).

Traub, R. D., M. A. Whittington, et al. (2001). A possible role for gap junctions in generation of very fast EEG oscillations preceding the onset of, and perhaps initiating, seizures. *Epilepsia* Vol. 42, pp. (153-170).

van Drongelen, W., H. C. Lee, et al. (2004). Simulation of neocortical epileptiform activity using parallel computing. *Neurocomputing* Vol. 58-60, pp. (1203 - 1209).

Voss, L. J., G. Jacobson, et al. (2009). Excitatory effects of gap junction blockers on cerebral cortex seizure-like activity in rats and mice. *Epilepsia* Vol. 50, pp. (1971-1978).

Voss, L. J., S. Melin, et al. (2010). GABAergic compensation in connexin36 knock-out mice evident during low-magnesium seizure-like event activity. *Brain Research* Vol. In Press.

Voss, L. J., N. Mutsaerts, et al. (2010). Connexin36 Gap Junction Blockade Is Ineffective at Reducing Seizure-Like Event Activity in Neocortical Mouse Slices. *Epilepsy Research and Treatment* Vol. 2010, pp. (doi:10.1155/2010/310753).

Wallraff, A., R. Kohling, et al. (2006). The impact of astrocytic gap junctional coupling on potassium buffering in the hippocampus. *Journal of Neuroscience* Vol. 26(20), pp. (5438-47).

Wang, J., M. Ma, et al. (2007). Modulation of membrane channel currents by gap junction protein mimetic peptides: size matters. *American Journal of Physiology* Vol. 293, pp. (C1112-C1119).

Wang, T., C. Zhou, et al. (2006). Cellular mechanism for spontaneous calcium oscillations in astrocytes. *Acta Pharmacologica Sinica* Vol. 27, pp. (861-868).

Wellershaus, K., J. Degen, et al. (2008). A new conditional mouse mutant reveals specific expression and functions of connexin36 in neurons and pancreatic beta-cells. *Experimental cell research* Vol. 314(5), pp. (997-1012).

Wiebe, S. (2000). Epidemiology of temporal lobe epilepsy. *Canadian Journal of Neurological Sciences* Vol. 27 (Suppl 1), pp. (S6-S10).

Wiencken-Barger, A. E., B. Djukic, et al. (2007). A role for connexin43 during neurodevelopment. *Glia* Vol. 55, pp. (675-686).

Xiong, Z.-Q., P. Saggau, et al. (2000). Activity-Dependent Intracellular Acidification Correlates with the Duration of Seizure Activity. *The Journal of Neuroscience* Vol. 20, pp. (1290-1296).

Yang, L. and D. S. F. Ling (2007). Carbenoxolone modifies spontaneous inhibitory and excitatory synaptic transmission in rat somatosensory cortex. *Neuroscience Letters* Vol. 416(3), pp. (221-6).

Zappala, A., D. Cicero, et al. (2006). Expression of pannexin1 in the CNS of adult mouse: cellular localization and effect of 4-aminopyridine-induced seizures. *Neuroscience* Vol. 141(1), pp. (167-78).

Part 2

Underlying Mechanisms

6

Recombinant Laforin for Structural Studies

Pedro Castanheira[1], Susana Moreira[2], Margarida Casal[2], Miguel Gama[2] and Carlos Faro[1]
[1]*Biocant – Biotechnology Innovation Centre, Cantanhede*
[2]*Department of Biological Engineering, University of Minho, Braga*
Portugal

1. Introduction

Lafora disease or Lafora progressive myoclonic epilepsy was first described in 1911 by Gonzalo Lafora (Lafora, 1911; Lafora & Glueck, 1911). The disease belongs phenomenologically to the progressive myoclonic epilepsies (Monaghan & Delanty, 2010) and is the most prevalent of such conditions, which include myoclonic epilepsy with ragged-red fibers, action myoclonus-renal failure syndrome, Kuf's disease, infantile neuroaxonal dystrophy, the sialidoses and Unverricht-Lundborg disease (Baltic myoclonus) (Monaghan & Delanty, 2010). These diseases afflict initially healthy children with ever-worsening and soon intractable myoclonus and epilepsy, usually associated with neurodegeneration, eventual dementia and early death (Ramachandran et al., 2009).

The first symptoms of Lafora disease appear between the ages of 8 and 18 years. There is an insidious, near-simultaneous or rapidly successive onset of headaches, difficulties in school work, myoclonic jerks, generalized seizures and in many cases, visual hallucinations of both epileptic and psychotic origin. The myoclonus, seizures and hallucinations gradually worsen and become intractable. For many years, the patient struggles to maintain normal contact and communication, interrupted by extremely frequent myoclonic absence seizures. Gradually, dementia sets in, and by 10 years after onset, the patient is in near continuous myoclonus with absences, frequent generalized seizures, and profound dementia or a vegetative state (Minassian, 2001; Ramachandran et al., 2009; Striano et al., 2008).

A distinctive pathology characterizes Lafora disease. Cells of various types exhibit dense accumulations of malformed and insoluble glycogen molecules, termed polyglucosans, which lack the symmetric branching that allows glycogen to be soluble. These polyglucosan accumulations are called Lafora bodies, and in the central nervous system, they are present profusely in all brain regions and in the majority of neurons, specifically in the cell bodies and dendrites (Minassian, 2001; Ramachandran et al., 2009; Striano et al., 2008).

Genetically, Lafora disease is an autosomal recessive disease caused by mutations in two genes: (1) the EPM2A gene, located on chromosome 6 at 6q24, coding for the protein laforin, a dual-specificity phosphatase (DSP), accounting for the largest group of patients (Minassian et al., 1998) and (2) the EPM2B (NHLRC1) gene, located on chromosome 6 at 6p22, coding for the protein malin, an E3 ubiquitin ligase that interacts with laforin (Chan et al., 2003a; Chan et al., 2003b). About 20% of cases are not explained by abnormalities in genes coding for laforin or malin (Singh & Ganesh, 2009); it is postulated that the mutations involved in these cases involve either an unknown third gene or a regulatory sequence for the EPM2A or EPM2B genes (Monaghan & Delanty, 2010; Singh & Ganesh, 2009).

Laforin is the only human DSP known to have a carbohydrate binding module (CBM) responsible for targeting the phosphatase towards glycogen (Wang et al., 2002). CBMs are typically found in glucosyl hydrolases and glucotransferases in bacterial, fungal or plant genomes (Boraston et al., 2000; Boraston et al., 2004; Gentry & Pace, 2009; Hashimoto, 2006; Shoseyov et al., 2006). The vast majority of enzymes containing CBMs utilize the domain to bind a specific glucan and enzymatically act on the sugar, as in the case of α-amylase (Boraston et al., 2004). Accordingly, it has been demonstrated that laforin and starch excess 4 protein (SEX4), an *Arabidopsis thaliana* protein with laforin-like properties (Gentry et al., 2007), bind and dephosphorylate glucans, such as glycogen and starch (Gentry et al., 2007; Gentry et al., 2005; Tagliabracci et al., 2007; Tagliabracci et al., 2008; Tagliabracci et al., 2011; Worby et al., 2006). While laforin and SEX4 bind similar types of glucans, they utilize distinct CBMs (Boraston et al., 2004). CBMs are classified into 62 evolutionarily distinct families, based on their primary sequence, secondary and tertiary structure predictions, and crystal structures (Boraston et al., 2004; Hashimoto, 2006; Shoseyov et al., 2006). In 2004, laforin was included in the CBM20 family, formerly known as the starch-binding domain of family 4 - SBD4 (CAZy database - http://www.cazy.org/Carbohydrate-Binding-Modules.html) (Coutinho & Henrissat, 1999). At that time, CBM20 family members were only known to be associated with amylases and glucanotransferases in bacteria, fungi and plants (Coutinho & Henrissat, 1999). The degree of homology of laforin and other members of the CBM20 family is very low. Furthermore, the laforin CBM secondary structure does not correlate very well with the other members of the CBM20 family (Girard et al., 2006). Nevertheless, the conservation of three tryptophans is of particular significance. They are invariant both in the few available laforin sequences from other species, as well as in most other CBM20 sequences (Girard et al., 2006).

The phosphatase domain of laforin has been characterized and shown to act as a DSP, based on the differential kinetic parameters of dephosphorylation of the substrates *p*-nitrophenyl phosphate (pNPP) and 3-O-methylfluoresceinyl phosphate (OMFP). For DSPs, the k_{cat}/K_M values are typically more than two orders of magnitude higher with OMFP than with pNPP, whereas they are in the same order of magnitude for protein tyrosine phosphatases (Girard et al., 2006).

The pNPPase activity of laforin has been shown to be inhibited by glycogen and related polysaccharides such as amylopectin and amylose, with inhibition potencies increasing with the decrease in polymer branching (Wang & Roach, 2004). Later, it was observed that laforin can dephosphorylate such polysaccharides (Tagliabracci et al., 2007).

Laforin activity was also shown to be dependent on laforin dimerization via its CBM (Liu et al., 2006) and to interact with proteins involved in glycogen metabolism, such as glycogen synthase (GS) (Worby et al., 2006), and with the glycogen-targeting regulatory subunit R5 of protein phosphatase 1 (PP1) (Fernández-Sánchez et al., 2003). Laforin was also shown to interact with two ubiquitous proteins with unknown functions, EPM2AIP1 (Ianzano, 2003) and HIRIP5, a cytosolic protein predicted to be involved in iron homeostasis (Ganesh et al., 2003). Laforin also interacts with malin, a single subunit E3 ubiquitin ligase containing a RING domain and six NHL domains (Gentry et al., 2005). Malin was shown to interact and to regulate laforin levels by mediating its ubiquitination, and the malin RING domain was necessary and sufficient to mediate laforin polyubiquitination leading to its proteosomal degradation (Gentry et al., 2005). Additionally, laforin was shown to recruit specific substrates to be ubiquitinated by malin (Lohi et al., 2005; Solaz-Fuster et al., 2008). GS and R5 ubiquitination promote the proteasomal degradation of both proteins (Lohi et al., 2005; Solaz-Fuster et al., 2008), and K63-linked ubiquitination of AMP-activated protein kinase (AMPK, a serine/threonine protein kinase that acts as a sensor of the cellular energy status) which extends the protein lifetime (Moreno et al., 2010). Laforin also promotes the dephosphorylation of glycogen synthase kinase 3 (GSK3) at Ser9, activating this enzyme and leading to the GS phosphorylation at multiple sites with subsequent inhibition (Lohi et al., 2005).

Therefore, laforin seems to be involved in glycogen metabolism as a sensor of poorly branched glycogen resulting from GS overactivity relative to glycogen-branching enzyme activity by modulating GS, either via GSK3 dephosphorylation resulting in GS inhibition, or via malin interaction, resulting in GS ubiquitination and subsequent degradation and inhibition of R5-induced glycogen synthesis.

The laforin/malin complex has also been recently implicated in autophagy, acting as a cellular toxicity suppressor by clearing misfolded proteins through the proteasome system (Aguado et al., 2010; Garyali et al., 2009; Knecht et al., 2010). A putative role for laforin in Tau hyperphosphorylation (one of the distinctive hallmarks of Alzheimer's disease) via GSK3 dephosphorylation has also been reported (Puri et al., 2009).

Despite the solid evidence for laforin's involvement in glycogen metabolism and Lafora disease, little is known about the structural mechanism of the glycogen interaction. This is due to the lack of a solid protocol for producing the large amounts of protein needed for structural studies. In this work we report the expression, purification and characterization of both laforin and its CBM, with appropriate yields for future structural and biophysical studies.

2. Heterologous protein expression and purification

In order to produce enough protein to perform structural studies, heterologous systems must be used. *E. coli* is by far the most widely employed host for heterologous protein expression (Rai & Padh, 2001). Its popularity is due to the vast body of knowledge about its genetics, physiology and complete genomic sequence, which greatly facilitates gene cloning and cultivation (Rai & Padh, 2001). High growth rates combined with the ability to express high levels of heterologous proteins, i.e., strains producing up to 30% of their total protein as the expressed gene product, result in high volumetric productivity. Furthermore, *E. coli* can grow rapidly to high densities in simple and inexpensive media (Rai & Padh, 2001).

Laforin cDNA, coding for full-length laforin with a hexahistidine tag at its C-terminus, was cloned into the vector pET21a by Dr. Jack Dixon's laboratory (Gentry et al., 2005). Previously, this tag was associated with problems in laforin purification and stability (Girard et al., 2006; Liu et al., 2006; Wang & Roach, 2004). Therefore, the hexahistidine tag was removed by using site-directed mutagenesis to introduce a stop codon at the end of the full-length laforin coding sequence. This was achieved using the QuickChange Site-Directed Mutagenesis Kit (Stratagene) according to the manufacturer's instructions and using the oligonucleotide primers Laf_ΔHis-for and Laf_ΔHis-rev, whose sequences are presented in Table 1.

The isolated CBM of laforin (Fig. 1, bold sequence) was also produced in order to study the biophysical interaction between the laforin CBM and carbohydrates and for future biotechnology applications. The cDNA sequence of the CBM domain was PCR amplified from the construct provided by Dr. Jack Dixon, using the oligonucleotides Laf_CBM-for and Laf_CBM-rev (Table 1), containing the restriction endonuclease recognition sites for

NcoI and XhoI, respectively, and ligated into NcoI/XhoI linearized pET29a. The Laf_CBM-rev primer introduced a RGD motif followed by a hexahistidine tag at the C-terminus of the CBM. The RGD motif is found in the extracellular matrix and blood proteins, such as fibronectin, vitronectin, osteopontin, collagens, thrombospondin, fibrinogen, and von Willebrand factor and has been described as the major functional group responsible for cellular adhesion (Hwang et al., 2007; Ruoslahti & Pierschbacher, 1987). The inclusion of a RGD motif at the C-terminus of the laforin CBM was intended to be a cell attachment motif in starch-based biomaterial functionalized with the CBM-RGD protein (Moreira et al., 2010).

Primer name	**Primer sequence**
Laf_ΔHis-for	CGTTCTTCTGTGTGTAGCCTGTGAGAGCACCACCACCACCAC
Laf_ΔHis-rev	GTGGTGGTGGTGGTGCTCTCACAGGCTACACACAGAAGAACG
Laf_CBM-for	CATGCCATGGGGATGCGCTTCCGCTTTGGGG
Laf_CBM-rev	CCGCTCGAGATCACCTCTCATGGTTGGTGGCCTGC

Table 1. Oligonucleotide primers used for laforin site-directed mutagenesis and for CBM cloning. The stop codon sequence introduced by site-directed mutagenesis is highlighted in bold. Underlined nucleotides indicate the restriction endonuclease recognition sequences used for cloning.

Full-length Laforin and its CBM were expressed by transforming competent *E. coli* BL21 star strain (Invitrogen; a bacterial strain that is suited for high-level recombinant protein expression, due to improved stability of mRNA and the absence of lon and ompT proteases) with the constructs described above. After transformation, cells were plated onto Luria Broth (LB)-agar plates containing the appropriate antibiotic for positive clone selection, and positive colonies were then grown overnight in liquid LB/antibiotic media. These cultures were used to seed typically 1-2 liters of LB/antibiotic and grown at 37 °C until the bacterial culture reached a cell density corresponding to an OD_{600} of 0.6. At that point, protein expression was induced for 3 h by the addition of isopropyl β-D-1-thiogalactopyranoside (IPTG) to a final concentration of 0.5 mM.

As previously reported, laforin expression in *E. coli* is associated with the appearance of inclusion bodies (Girard et al., 2006), with the CBM behaving in a similar way (Moreira et al., 2010). Our expertise in refolding proteins expressed in the form of inclusion bodies was crucial for the successful production of high amounts of correctly folded protein (Castanheira et al., 2005; Turner et al., 2001; Simões et al., 2007). After cell pellet disruption, the inclusion bodies were washed in 50 mM Tris-HCl, 50 mM NaCl, pH 7.4, followed by a second washing step in 50 mM Tris-HCl, 50 mM NaCl, pH 7.4, 0.1% Triton X-100 (v/v). These washing steps were needed to remove membrane proteins and other contaminants that are released upon cell disruption (Clark, 2001). Purified inclusion bodies were dissolved in 8 M urea buffer (8 M urea, 0.1 M Tris, 1 mM glycine, 1 mM EDTA, pH 10.5) with 100 mM β-mercaptoethanol.

Protein refolding was promoted by rapid dilution (20x) of the dissolved protein into 1 L of 20 mM Tris base, 0.5 mM oxidized/1.25 mM reduced glutathione, 0.5 mM DTT; the pH was then slowly adjusted to pH 8.0 with 6 M HCl solution, and the protein was kept at 4 °C until purification. After 3-7 days in a cold room, the refolded proteins were purified by two

1 atgcgcttccgctttggggtggtggtgccacccgccgtggccggcgcccggccggagctg
M R F R F G V V V P P A V A G A R P E L
61 ctggtggtggggtcgcggcccgagctggggcgttgggagccgcgcggtgccgtccgcctg
L V V G S R P E L G R W E P R G A V R L
121 aggccggccggcaccgcggcgggcgacggggccctggccctgcaggagccgggcctgtgg
R P A G T A A G D G A L A L Q E P G L W
181 ctcggggaggtggagctggcggccgaggaggcggcgcaggacggggcggagccgggccgc
L G E V E L A A E E A A Q D G A E P G R
241 gtggacacgttctggtacaagttcctgaagcgggagccgggaggagagctctcctgggaa
V D T F W Y K F L K R E P G G E L S W E
301 ggcaatggacctcatcatgaccgttgctgtacttacaatgaaaacaacttggtggatggt
G N G P H H D R C C T Y N E N N L V D G
361 gtgtattgtctcccaataggacactggattgaggccactgggcacaccaatgaaatgaag
V Y C L P I G H W I E A T G H T N E M K
421 cacacaacagacttctatttaatattgcaggccaccaagccatgcattattcaagaatt
H T T D F Y F N I A G H Q A M H Y S R I
481 ctaccaaatatctggctgggtagctgccctcgtcaggtggaacatgtaaccatcaaactg
L P N I W L G S C P R Q V E H V T I K L
541 aagcatgaattggggattacagctgtaatgaatttccagactgaatgggatattgtacag
K H E L G I T A V M N F Q T E W D I V Q
601 aattcctcaggctgtaaccgctacccagagcccatgactccagacactatgattaaacta
N S S G C N R Y P E P M T P D T M I K L
661 tatagggaagaaggcttggcctacatctggatgccaacaccagatatgagcaccgaaggc
Y R E E G L A Y I W M P T P D M S T E G
721 cgagtacagatgctgccccaggcggtgtgcctgctgcatgcgctgctggagaagggacac
R V Q M L P Q A V C L L H A L L E K G H
781 atcgtgtacgtgcactgcaacgctggggtgggccgctccaccgcggctgtctgcggctgg
I V Y V H C N A G V G R S T A A V C G W
841 ctccagtatgtgatgggctggaatctgaggaaggtgcagtatttcctcatggccaagagg
L Q Y V M G W N L R K V Q Y F L M A K R
901 ccggctgtctacattgacgaagaggccttggcccgggcacaagaagatttttccagaaa
P A V Y I D E E A L A R A Q E D F F Q K
961 tttgggaaggttcgttcttctgtgtgtagcctgtga
F G K V R S S V C S L -

Fig. 1. Laforin cDNA sequence (lower case letters) and translated protein sequence (upper case letters). The amino acids corresponding to the carbohydrate-binding module (CBM) are in bold.

consecutive chromatographic steps. Each refolded protein was first concentrated to 150 mL by tangential flow ultrafiltration (Sartocon Slice, Sartorius), followed by concentration to 12-15 mL with a N_2-pressurized stirred-cell concentrator (Amicon 8200, Millipore). The protein solution was then clarified by ultracentrifugation (100,000x g, 20 min, 4 °C), and the supernatant was applied to a size-exclusion chromatography column (HiLoad 26/60 Superdex 200 prep grade, GE Healthcare), which was previously equilibrated in 20 mM Tris, 0.4 M urea, pH 8.0, at 2 mL/min in order to separate the aggregated forms from the non-aggregated forms of each protein (Fig. 2A and D). Full-length laforin (Fig. 2A) was shown to elute in two separate peaks. The first peak eluted at the expected column void volume (around 115 mL) and corresponded to soluble protein aggregates, and the second peak eluted at around 188 mL, which according to the column calibration should correspond to a globular protein with a molecular weight of 74 kDa, the expected value for the full-length laforin dimer (2 x 37 kDa). The fractions obtained during size-exclusion purification were analyzed for phosphatase activity in 50 mM Tris/HCl buffer, pH 7.2 at 30 °C using 10 mM pNPP as the substrate by spectrophotometrically following the increase of absorbance at 410 nm induced by the release of *p*-nitrophenol (ε_{410nm} = 18.3 mM^{-1} cm^{-1}) (Girard et al., 2006). The second peak from the size-exclusion was active. The active fractions were combined, and the protein was further purified by anion-exchange chromatography on a Mono Q 5/50 GL (GE Healthcare) (Fig. 2B).

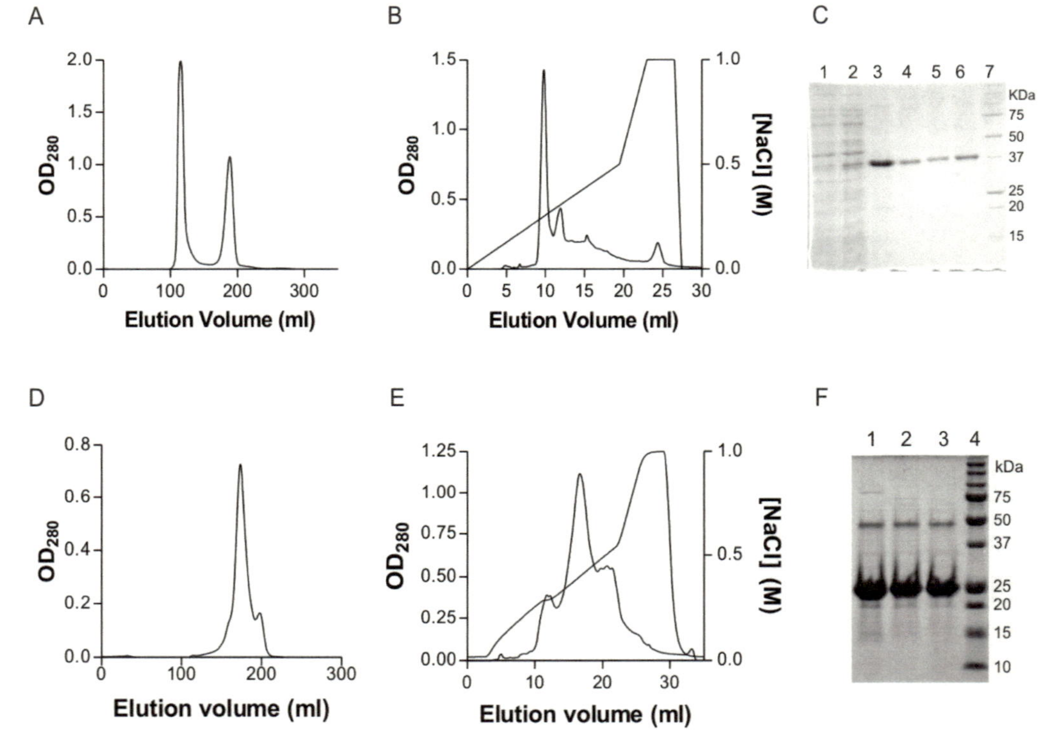

Fig. 2. Protein purification. (A) Full-length laforin size-exclusion chromatogram; (B) Anion-exchange chromatogram of full-length laforin; (C) SDS-PAGE analysis of full-length laforin purification: (1) *E. coli* cells before induction; (2) *E. coli* cells after a 3 h induction, soluble fraction; (3) cells after a 3 h induction, insoluble fraction; (4) concentrated protein applied to a size-exclusion column; (5) second peak from the size exclusion column applied to an anion-exchange column; (6) Anion-exchange major peak; (7) molecular weight standard. The gel was stained with Coomassie brilliant blue. (D) Laforin's CBM size-exclusion chromatogram; (E) Anion-exchange chromatogram of laforin's CBM; (F) SDS-PAGE analysis of laforin's CBM purification: (1) sample applied to a size-exclusion column; (2) second peak (eluted at about 150–200 mL) from the size-exclusion column; (3) highest peak (eluted at about 20 mL) from the anion-exchange column; (4) molecular weight standard. The gel was stained with Coomassie brilliant blue.

Step	Volume (mL)	Total Activity (U)	Total Protein (mg)	Specific Activity (U/mg)	Yield (%)	Purification Factor
Refolded	7	7250	39	186	100	
Superdex	38	5524	22	251	56	1.3
Mono Q	6.5	3400	7	486	47	2.6

Table 2. Full-length laforin purification table. One unit of activity was defined as the activity corresponding to the consumption of 1 µM substrate (pNPP) in one minute at 30 °C.

Most of the protein was eluted in the major peak with a NaCl concentration of approximately 250 mM, which was also the peak where most of the pNPPase activity was found, indicating that most of the protein was correctly folded and relatively homogeneous. At the end of the purification process from several expression batches, we obtained between 5 and 7 mg of purified laforin per liter of expression media. The purification table (Table 2) shows that the starting material after refolding was already relatively pure, as the purification factor was only 2.6, which is again consistent with the lack of contaminant bands in the SDS-PAGE profile of the refolded protein (Fig. 2C, lane 3).

Step	Total Protein (mg)	Estimated amount of total CBM (mg)	Yield (%)	Purity (%)
Cell extract	306	85.7	100	28
Refolded protein	106	72.1	84	68
Applied to size exclusion	43.4	34.7	40	80
Applied to ion exchange	33	29.7	35	90
Mono Q (major peak)	12.8	11.5	13	90

Table 3. Laforin CBM purification table. Purity was determined by analysis of SDS-PAGE band intensities using the Quantity One software, version 4.6 (BioRad).

For the CBM of laforin, a similar procedure was adopted. The first purification step, by size-exclusion chromatography (HiLoad 26/60 Superdex 200 prep grade, GE Healthcare), was run with the same conditions as for the full-length protein and revealed no significant aggregates. Most of the protein eluted at 173 mL, which corresponds to tetrameric laforin CBM, and a minor fraction that eluted at 198 mL corresponds to dimerized protein (Fig. 2D). The fractions corresponding to the major peak were combined and applied to the anion exchange column (Mono Q 5/50 GL, GE Healthcare), with most of the protein eluted at 400 mM NaCl (Fig. 2E). The SDS-PAGE analysis of the purified protein revealed an intense band with a molecular weight close to the expected value (22 kDa), and even under denaturing conditions, a band corresponding to the dimeric form of the protein was observed (Fig. 2F). This result is in agreement with the previously described resistance of laforin to dimer separation, prior to SDS-PAGE (Liu et al., 2006).

The purification table of laforin CBM purification shows a yield of more than 12 mg of purified protein per liter of expression media. This protein expression and purification method is the first successful strategy to obtain the laforin CBM and will thus allow its study and characterization as an independent unit, as well as its use in biotechnology applications (Moreira et al., 2010).

3. Heterologous protein characterization

3.1 Protein oligomerization state

Laforin has been shown to exist in a dimeric state; the CBM is responsible for this dimerization because its deletion completely abolishes the dimerization and phosphatase activity of laforin (Liu et al., 2006). The oligomerization state of both laforin and its CBM were analyzed by two distinct methods: analytical size-exclusion chromatography and dynamic light scattering (DLS) (Fig. 3).

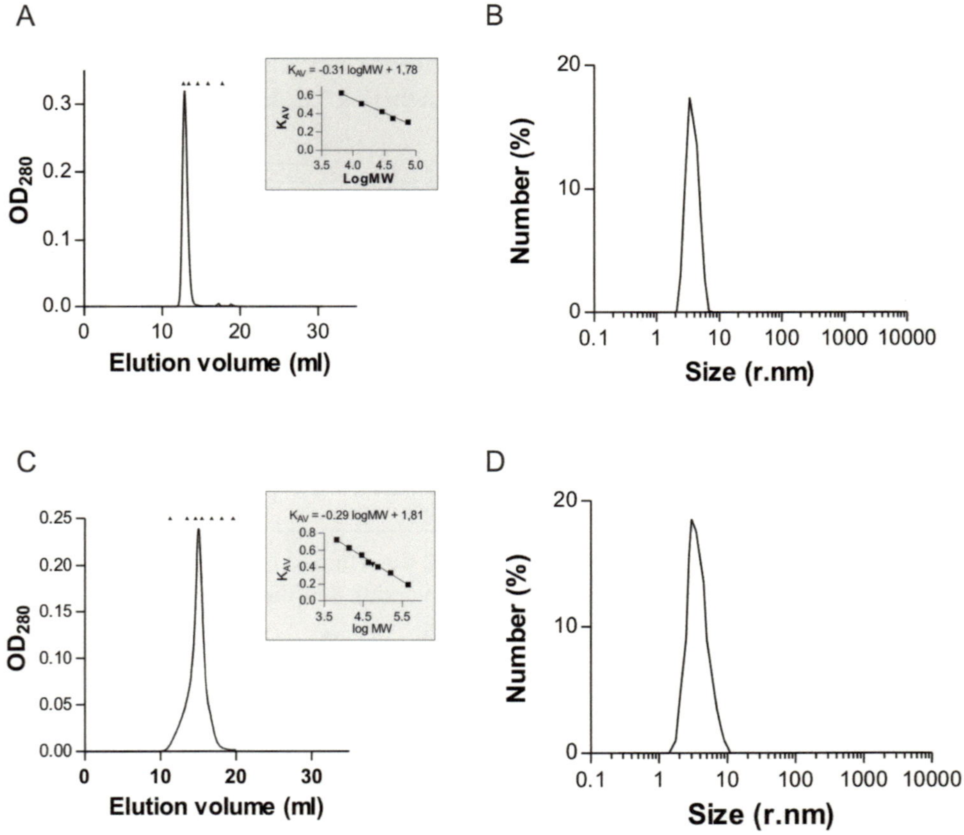

Fig. 3. Protein oligomerization analysis. (A) Analytical size-exclusion chromatography of purified full-length laforin with a Superose 12 10/300 GL column (GE Healthcare); (B) Dynamic Light Scattering analysis of purified full-length laforin; (C) Analytical size-exclusion chromatography of purified laforin CBM with a Superdex 200 10/300 GL column (GE Healthcare); (D) Dynamic Light Scattering analysis of purified laforin CBM.

The analysis of full-length laforin by analytical size-exclusion chromatography on Superose 12 10/300 GL confirmed that laforin is highly homogeneous, eluting with an elution volume corresponding to a globular protein of 64 kDa, based on the column calibration (Fig. 3A, grey box). This result is consistent with the dimer state of full-length laforin (2 x 37 kDa). This result was later confirmed by DLS. The protein was analyzed in both the anion-exchange elution buffer (20 mM Tris, 0.4 M urea, 250 mM NaCl, pH 8.0) and in 50 mM Tris, 50 mM NaCl, pH 7.4, with similar results. The particles detected had a hydrodynamic radius corresponding to a globular protein with a mass of 76 kDa, again consistent with the presence of a dimer.

The analysis of the oligomerization state of the CBM of laforin by analytical size-exclusion chromatography using a Superdex 200 10/300 GL showed that the protein is also in a dimeric state, with a calculated molecular weight of 44 kDa. The differences observed between the preparative size-exclusion chromatography used during protein purification, where the protein eluted as a tetramer, and the analytical size-exclusion chromatography, where the protein eluted as a dimer, are due to the presence of 150 mM NaCl in the analytical size-exclusion chromatography buffer, which was absent from the preparative size exclusion chromatography buffer. The DLS analysis confirmed this result; the protein eluting in the highest peak from the anion-exchange column (Fig. 2E) revealed a hydrodynamic radius corresponding to a 44 kDa protein, thus confirming the dimerization of the isolated protein.

3.2 Protein – carbohydrate interaction assay

The functionality of the CBM, i.e., its ability to bind starch, was evaluated using an adsorption assay, for both the full-length laforin and for the CBM. The purified protein samples were centrifuged (13,000 rpm, 10 min, 4 °C) to remove any precipitated protein, and the protein was then mixed with 50 mg of starch (previously washed with 50 mM Tris-HCl, 150 mM NaCl, pH 7.4 buffer) for 1 h at 4 °C. The mixture was centrifuged (13,000 rpm, 10 min, 4 °C), and the supernatant was analyzed by SDS–PAGE. The starch was washed with buffer (3 x 0.3 mL), and the recombinant protein was eluted from the starch with a 5 mg/mL glycogen solution (0.3 mL, at 4 °C for 1 h). The starch was then treated with buffer containing 2% SDS (0.3 mL, at 95 °C for 5 min) in order to analyze the protein that remained adsorbed after glycogen elution.

The results showed that both full-length laforin and its CBM are able to bind starch and are specifically desorbed from starch when incubated with glycogen. For the full-length laforin, the SDS-PAGE analysis (Fig. 4A) revealed that most of the protein binds to the starch moiety because the protein solution supernatant after starch incubation (Fig. 4A lanes 2) showed a significant decrease in protein levels. This is not due to precipitated protein in the sample because the protein sample was centrifuged prior to the starch incubation. The subsequent washing steps revealed no washed protein (Fig. 4A lanes 3), and after the incubation with glycogen, laforin was effectively eluted from starch (Fig. 4A, lane 4). From the differences in band intensities between the initial protein and the supernatant after incubation, one would expect a stronger band from the glycogen elution, but the relatively faint band resulting from the glycogen elution can be attributed to a stronger binding of laforin to starch rather than glycogen, as previously reported (Chan et al., 2004). The results obtained with the CBM are in line with this assumption because a stronger protein band is observed in the starch pellet after glycogen elution (Fig. 4B, lane 4) than the one resulting from the glycogen elution (Fig. 4B, lane 3).

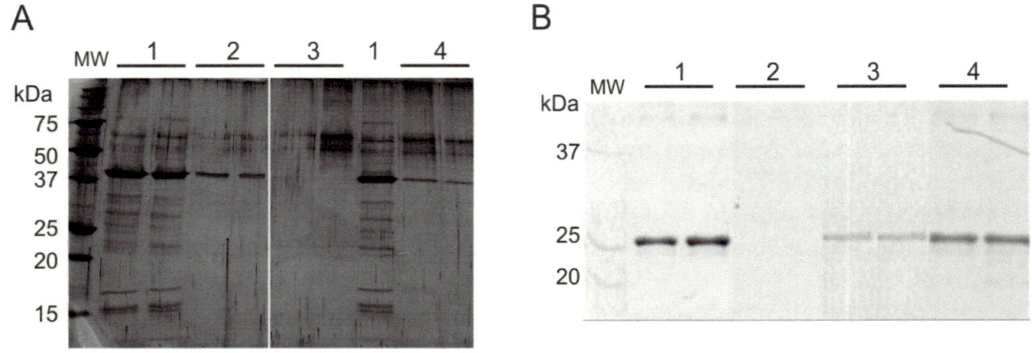

Fig. 4. Protein–starch-binding assay. (A) Full-length laforin starch-binding assay: (1) laforin supernatant before starch incubation; (2) supernatant after starch incubation; (3) starch-washing supernatant; (4) supernatant after glycogen elution. All steps were performed in duplicate. Gel was silver stained. (B) CBM starch-binding assay: (1) CBM supernatant before starch incubation; (2) starch-washing supernatant; (3) supernatant after glycogen elution; (4) starch pellet after glycogen elution. All steps were performed in duplicate. The gel was Coomasie stained.

Together, these results confirmed the starch binding activity of both laforin and its CBM.

3.3 Laforin phosphatase activity characterization

The laforin phosphatase activity was characterized using both pNPP (Montalibet et al., 2005) and OMFP, previously reported to be a better substrate for dual-specificity phosphatases than pNPP (Girard et al., 2006; Gottlin et al., 1996). The kinetic parameters for pNPP as a substrate were measured in a total volume of 1 mL by incubation of the enzyme with various amounts of substrate in 50 mM Tris-HCl buffer, pH 7.2 in a Varian Cary 100 UV/Vis spectrophotometer with the temperature control set to 30 °C by following the absorbance increase at 410 nm induced by the release of *p*-nitrophenol (ε_{410nm} = 18.3 mM^{-1} cm^{-1}) (Girard et al., 2006). For OMFP, the kinetic parameters were obtained by a fluorescence-based assay, using conditions similar to the ones used for pNPP. The assay was performed using a Horiba Jobin Yvon Fluoromax-3 fluorometer by following the fluorescence emission of the product formed with excitation at 485 nm and emission measured at 530 nm. The data were fit to the Michaelis-Menten equation (Eq. 1) using the software Enzyme Kinetics Module v.1.2 - Sigmaplot v 9.01 (Systat Software, Inc.).

$$V = k_{cat}\,[S] \,/\, (K_M + [S]) \qquad (1)$$

The kinetic parameters (Table 4) show that the recombinant laforin produced in this study has similar properties when compared to the previously published kinetic parameters for GST- and His-tagged versions of laforin (Girard et al., 2006), confirming the behavior of laforin as a dual-specificity phosphatase with OMFP better as the substrate than pNPP (Castanheira et al., 2010).

The pH profile of laforin phosphatase activity was also evaluated using OMFP as a substrate. The results presented in Fig. 5A are in agreement with the results published earlier for tagged versions of laforin (Girard et al., 2006; Peters et al., 2003; Wang et al., 2002; Wang & Roach, 2004), with maximal activity at the acidic pH of 6.0. The capability of glycogen to inhibit the phosphatase activity of laforin was also evaluated by including increasing amounts of glycogen in the phosphatase activity assay. The results presented in Fig. 5B show that laforin, in agreement with previously published reports (Girard et al., 2006; Wang & Roach, 2004), is effectively inhibited by glycogen with an AC_{50} of around 50 μg/mL.

Enzyme	pNPP			OMFP		
	k_{cat} (s^{-1})	K_M (mM)	k_{cat}/K_M ($s^{-1}.mM^{-1}$)	k_{cat} (s^{-1})	K_M (mM)	k_{cat}/K_M ($s^{-1}.mM^{-1}$)
Laforin	0.56 ± 0.07	8.4 ± 0.7	0.07 ± 0.01	7.6 ± 1.5	0.21 ± 0.05	36 ± 11
GST-pG laforin	1.1 ± 0.1	11.4 ± 3.0	0.10 ± 0.03	9.5 ± 2.0	0.26 ± 0.04	36 ± 13
His-laforin	1.7 ± 0.2	33 ± 3	0.051 ± 0.004	6.5 ± 1.3	0.75 ± 0.29	8.7 ± 5.1

Table 4. Steady-state kinetic parameters for laforin phosphatase activity. Comparison with published data for tagged versions of laforin, obtained from Girard (2006).

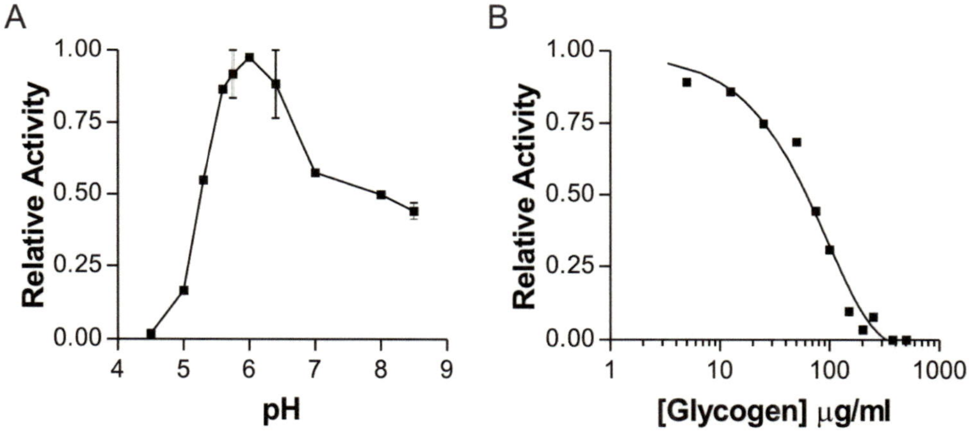

Fig. 5. Laforin phosphatase activity characterization: Optimum pH (A) and inhibition by glycogen (B).

4. Conclusion

In this work, we have shown that both full-length laforin and its CBM can be produced in *E. coli* expression systems in high amounts and purified without the use of fusion tags. The characterization of the purified protein showed that in both cases, the protein is dimerized and has a functional CBM. For full-length laforin, the phosphatase activity was characterized and shown to have similar characteristics to the various forms of laforin previously described. The protein expression methodology used in this study proved to be suited for the production of high amounts of protein. This will enable the structural characterization and determination of the three-dimensional structure of laforin, which will contribute to the understanding of the molecular mechanism of action of laforin. The understanding of both the mechanism of the laforin-laforin or laforin-malin interactions is important for the development of Lafora disease therapies. The protein-protein and protein-carbohydrate interfaces represent targets for the design of new drugs that promote or stabilize laforin's dimerization or its interaction with binding partners (Veselovsky et al., 2002).

5. Future perspectives

The work presented in this chapter paves the way for the structural studies needed to understand the molecular mechanism of protein-carbohydrate interaction. These studies will be performed using techniques such as NMR that will provide site-specific information on the architecture, binding selectivity and plasticity of the carbohydrate-binding sites of laforin. Other biophysical techniques such as Trp fluorescence have been used to address the chemical polarity shifts associated with protein-carbohydrate interactions. Protein-carbohydrate interactions will also be studied by surface plasmon resonance in order to obtain the kinetic parameters of carbohydrate-ligand binding with wild-type and mutant proteins. Finally, X-ray crystallography and solution NMR will be used to obtain the three dimensional structure of laforin and its CBM, respectively.
These studies will most likely provide new insights into the molecular mechanism of protein-carbohydrate binding and into the structural determinants involved in laforin dimerization, which will create new opportunities for the design of Lafora disease therapies and novel biotechnology applications for carbohydrate-binding proteins.

6. Acknowledgements

The authors would like to thank Dr. Jack Dixon (U. Michigan, Ann Arbour, Michigan, USA) for providing the laforin.His-pET29a(+) construct. Susana Moreira was the recipient of a Ph.D. fellowship from Fundação para a Ciência e a Tecnologia (FCT) - Portuguese Government. This work is financed by ERDF funds through Operational Programme - Competitiveness Factors - COMPETE and by Portuguese national funds through FCT - Portuguese Foundation for Science and Technology under the project PTDC/BIA-PRO/111141/2009.

7. References

Aguado, C., Sarkar, S., Korolchuk, V. I., Criado, O., Vernia, S., Boya, P., Sanz, P., Rodriguez de Córdoba, S., Knecht, E. & Rubinsztein, D.C. (2010). Laforin, the most common protein mutated in Lafora disease, regulates autophagy. *Hum. Mol. Genet.*, *19*(14), 2867-76. ISSN: 1460-2083.

Boraston, A. B., Chiu, P., Warren, R. A., & Kilburn, D. G. (2000). Specificity and affinity of substrate binding by a family 17 carbohydrate-binding module from *Clostridium cellulovorans* cellulase 5A. *Biochemistry*, *39*(36), 11129-36. ISSN: 1520-4995.

Boraston, A. B., Bolam, D. N., Gilbert, H. J., & Davies, G. J. (2004). Carbohydrate-binding modules: fine - tuning polysaccharide recognition. *Biochem. J., 382*(Pt 3), 769-81. ISSN: 1470-8728.

Castanheira, P., Samyn, B., Sergeant, K., Clemente, J. C., Dunn, B. M., Pires, E., Van Beeumen, J. & Faro, C. (2005). Activation, proteolytic processing, and peptide specificity of recombinant cardosin A. *J. Biol. Chem., 280*(13), 13047-54. ISSN:1083-351X.

Castanheira, P., Moreira, S., Gama, M., & Faro, C. (2010). *Escherichia coli* expression, refolding and characterization of human laforin. *Protein Expres. Purif., 71*(2), 195-9. ISSN 1046-5928.

Chan, E. M., Bulman, D. E., Paterson, A. D., Turnbull, J., Andermann, E., Andermann, F., Rouleau, G.A., Delgado-Escueta, A.V., Scherer, S.W. & Minassian, B.A. (2003a). Genetic mapping of a new Lafora progressive myoclonus epilepsy locus (EPM2B) on 6p22. *J. Med. Genet., 40*(9), 671-5. ISSN: 0022-2593.

Chan, E. M., Young, E. J., Ianzano, Leonarda, Munteanu, I., Zhao, X., Christopoulos, C. C., Avanzini, G., Elia, M., Ackerley, C.A., Jovic, N.J., Bohlega, S., Andermann, E., Rouleau, G.A., Delgado-Escueta, A.V., Minassian, B.A. & Scherer, S. (2003b). Mutations in NHLRC1 cause progressive myoclonus epilepsy. *Nat. Genet., 35*(2), 125-7. ISSN: 1061-4036.

Chan, E. M., Ackerley, C. a, Lohi, H., Ianzano, Leonarda, Cortez, M. a, Shannon, P., Scherer, S. & Minassian, B.A. (2004). Laforin preferentially binds the neurotoxic starch-like polyglucosans, which form in its absence in progressive myoclonus epilepsy. *Hum. Mol. Genet., 13*(11), 1117-29. ISSN: 1460-2083

Clark, E. D. (2001). Protein refolding for industrial processes. *Curr. Opin. Biotech., 12*(2), 202-7. ISSN: 0958-1669.

Coutinho, P. M., & Henrissat, B. (1999). *Recent Advances in Carbohydrate Bioengineering*. (H.J. Gilbert, G. Davies, B. Henrissat, & B. Svensson, Eds.) (pp. 3-12). Cambridge: The Royal Society of Chemistry. ISBN: 0854047743.

Fernández-Sánchez, M. E., Criado-García, O., Heath, K. E., García-Fojeda, B., Medraño-Fernández, I., Gomez-Garre, P., Sanz, P., Serratosa, J.M. & Rodriguéz de Córdoba, S. (2003). Laforin, the dual-phosphatase responsible for Lafora disease, interacts with R5 (PTG), a regulatory subunit of protein phosphatase-1 that enhances glycogen accumulation. *Hum. Mol. Genet., 12*(23), 3161-71. ISSN: 1460-2083

Ganesh, S., Tsurutani, N., Suzuki, T., Ueda, K., Agarwala, K. L., Osada, H., Delgado-Escueta, A.V. & Yamakawa, K. (2003). The Lafora disease gene product laforin interacts with HIRIP5, a phylogenetically conserved protein containing a NifU-like domain. *Hum. Mol. Genet., 12*(18), 2359-68. ISSN: 1460-2083

Garyali, P., Siwach, P., Singh, P. K., Puri, R., Mittal, S., Sengupta, S., Parihar, R. & Ganesh S. (2009). The malin-laforin complex suppresses the cellular toxicity of misfolded proteins by promoting their degradation through the ubiquitin-proteasome system. *Hum. Mol. Genet., 18*(4), 688-700. ISSN: 1460-2083

Gentry, M.S., Worby, C.A, & Dixon, J.E. (2005). Insights into Lafora disease: malin is an E3 ubiquitin ligase that ubiquitinates and promotes the degradation of laforin. *P. Natl. Acad. Sci. USA, 102*(24), 8501-6. ISSN: 1091-6490.

Gentry, M.S., Dowen, R.H., Worby, C.A., Mattoo, S., Ecker, J.R., & Dixon, J.E. (2007). The phosphatase laforin crosses evolutionary boundaries and links carbohydrate metabolism to neuronal disease. *J. Cell Biol., 178*(3), 477-88. ISSN: 1540-8140.

Gentry, M.S., & Pace, R.M. (2009). Conservation of the glucan phosphatase laforin is linked to rates of molecular evolution and the glucan metabolism of the organism. *BMC Evol. Biol., 9*, 138. ISSN: 1471-2148.

Girard, J.-M., Lê, K. H. & Lederer, F. (2006). Molecular characterization of laforin, a dual-specificity protein phosphatase implicated in Lafora disease. *Biochimie, 88*(12), 1961-71. ISSN: 0300-9084.

Gottlin, E. B., Xu, X., Epstein, D.M., Burke, S.P., Eckstein, J.W., Ballou, D. P. & Dixon, J.E. (1996). Kinetic analysis of the catalytic domain of human cdc25B. *J. Biol. Chem., 271*(44), 27445-9. ISSN:1083-351X.

Hashimoto, H. (2006). Recent structural studies of carbohydrate-binding modules. *Cell. Mol. Life Sci., 63*(24), 2954-67. ISSN: 1420-682X.

Hwang, D.S., Sim, S.B. & Cha, H.J. (2007). Cell adhesion biomaterial based on mussel adhesive protein fused with RGD peptide. *Biomaterials, 28*(28), 4039-46. ISSN: 0142-9612.

Ianzano, L. (2003). Identification of a novel protein interacting with laforin, the epm2a progressive myoclonus epilepsy gene product. *Genomics, 81*(6), 579-587. ISSN: 0888-7543.

Turner III, R.T., Koelsch, G., Hong, L., Castanheira, P., Ghosh, A., & Tang, J. (2001). Subsite Specificity of Memapsin 2 (β-Secretase): Implications for Inhibitor Design. *Biochemistry, 40*(34), 10001-10006. ISSN: 1520-4995.

Knecht, E., Aguado, C., Sarkar, S., Korolchuk, V. I., Criado-García, O., Vernia, S., Boya, P., Sanz, P., Rodríguez de Córdoba, S. & Rubinsztein, D.C. (2010). Impaired autophagy in Lafora disease. *Autophagy, 6*(7), 991-3. ISSN: 1554-8635.

Lafora, G. R. (1911). The presence of amyloid bodies in the protoplasm of the ganglion cells; a contribution to the study of the amyloid substance in the nervous system. *Bull. Gov. Hosp. Insane, 3*, 83-92. ISBN: 1148417796.

Lafora, G. R., & Glueck, B. (1911). Contribution to the histopathology and pathogenesis of myoclonic epilepsy. *Bull. Gov. Hosp. Insane, 3*, 96-111. ISBN: 1148417796.

Liu, Y., Wang, Y., Wu, C., Liu, Yang, & Zheng, P. (2006). Dimerization of Laforin is required for its optimal phosphatase activity, regulation of GSK3beta phosphorylation, and Wnt signaling. *J. Biol. Chem., 281*(46), 34768-74. ISSN:1083-351X.

Lohi, H., Ianzano, L., Zhao, X.-C., Chan, E., Turnbull, J., Scherer, S. W., Ackerley, C.A. and Minassian, B.A. (2005). Novel glycogen synthase kinase 3 and ubiquitination pathways in progressive myoclonus epilepsy. *Hum. Mol. Genet., 14*(18), 2727-36. ISSN: 1460-2083

Minassian, B.A., Lee, J.R., Herbrick, J.A., Huizenga, J., Soder, S., Mungall, A.J., Dunham, I., Gardner, R., Fong, C.-Y., Carpenter, S., Jardim, L., Satishchandra, P., Andermann, E., Snead III, O.C., Lopes-Cendes, I., Tsui, L.C., Delgado-Escueta, A., Rouleau, G. & Scherer, S.W. (1998). Mutations in a gene encoding a novel protein tyrosine phosphatase cause progressive myoclonus epilepsy. *Nat. Genet.*. ISSN: 1061-4036.

Minassian, B. (2001). Lafora's disease: towards a clinical, pathologic, and molecular synthesis. *Pediatric Neurology, 25*(1), 21-29. ISSN: 0887-8994.

Monaghan, T.S., & Delanty, N. (2010). Lafora disease: epidemiology, pathophysiology and management. *CNS drugs, 24*(7), 549-61. ISSN: 1172-7047.

Montalibet, J., Skorey, K.I. & Kennedy, B.P. (2005). Protein tyrosine phosphatase: enzymatic assays. *Methods, 35*(1), 2-8. ISSN: 1046-2023

Moreira, S., Castanheira, P., Casal, M., Faro, C., & Gama, M. (2010). Expression of the functional carbohydrate-binding module (CBM) of human laforin. *Prot. Expres. Purif., 74*(2), 169-74. ISSN 1046-5928.

Moreno, D., Towler, M. C., Hardie, D. G., Knecht, E., & Sanz, P. (2010). The Laforin - Malin Complex , Involved in Lafora Disease , Promotes the Incorporation of K63-linked Ubiquitin Chains into AMP-activated Protein Kinase Subunits. *Mol. Biol. Cell, 21*, 2578 -2588. ISSN 1059-1524.

Peters, G. H., Branner, S., Møller, K. B., Andersen, J. N., & Møller, N. P. H. (2003). Enzyme kinetic characterization of protein tyrosine phosphatases. *Biochimie, 85*(5), 527-34. ISSN: 0300-9084.

Puri, R., Suzuki, T., Yamakawa, K., & Ganesh, S. (2009). Hyperphosphorylation and aggregation of Tau in laforin-deficient mice, an animal model for Lafora disease. *J. Biol. Chem., 284*(34), 22657-63. ISSN:1083-351X.

Rai, M., & Padh, H. (2001). Expression systems for production of heterologous proteins. *Curr. Sci., 80*(9), 1121-1128. ISSN: 0011-3891.

Ramachandran, N., Girard, J.-M., Turnbull, J. & Minassian, B.A. (2009). The autosomal recessively inherited progressive myoclonus epilepsies and their genes. *Epilepsia, 50 Suppl 5*, 29-36. ISSN: 1528-1167.

Ruoslahti, E. & Pierschbacher, M.D. (1987). New perspectives in cell adhesion: RGD and integrins. *Science, 238*(4826), 491-7. ISSN: 1095-9203.

Shoseyov, O., Shani, Z., & Levy, I. (2006). Carbohydrate binding modules: biochemical properties and novel applications. *Microbiol. Mol. Biol. Rev., 70*(2), 283-95. ISSN: 1098-5557.

Simões, I., Faro, R., Bur, D., & Faro, C. (2007). Characterization of recombinant CDR1, an Arabidopsis aspartic proteinase involved in disease resistance. *J. Biol. Chem., 282*(43), 31358-65. ISSN:1083-351X.

Singh, S., & Ganesh, S. (2009). Lafora progressive myoclonus epilepsy: a meta-analysis of reported mutations in the first decade following the discovery of the EPM2A and NHLRC1 genes. *Hum. Mut., 30*(5), 715-23. ISSN: 1098-1004.

Solaz-Fuster, M. C., Gimeno-Alcañiz, J. V., Ros, S., Fernandez-Sanchez, M. E., Garcia-Fojeda, B., Garcia, O.C., Vilchez, D., Dominguez, J., Garcia-Rocha, M., Sanchez-Piris, M., Aguado, C., Knecht, E., Serratosa, J., Guinovart, J.J., Sanz, P. & Rodríguez de Córdoba, S. (2008). Regulation of glycogen synthesis by the laforin-malin complex is modulated by the AMP-activated protein kinase pathway. *Hum. Mol. Genet., 17*(5), 667-78. ISSN: 1460-2083

Striano, P., Zara, F., Turnbull, J., Girard, J.-M., Ackerley, C.A., Cervasio, M., De Rosa, G., De Caro, M.L., Striano, S. & Minassian, B.A. (2008). Typical progression of myoclonic epilepsy of the Lafora type: a case report. *Nat. Clin. Pract. Neurol., 4*(2), 106-11. ISSN: 1759-4758.

Tagliabracci, V.S., Turnbull, J., Wang, W., Girard, J.-M., Zhao, X., Skurat, A.V., Delgado Escueta, A.V., Minassian, B.A., DePaoli-Roach, A.A. & Roach, P.J. (2007). Laforin is a glycogen phosphatase, deficiency of which leads to elevated phosphorylation of glycogen in vivo. *P. Natl. Acad. Sci. USA*, *104*(49), 19262-6. ISSN: 1091-6490.

Tagliabracci, V.S., Girard, J.M., Segvich, D., Meyer, C., Turnbull, Julie, Zhao, X., Minassian, B.A., DePaoli-Roach, A.A. & Roach, P.J. (2008). Abnormal metabolism of glycogen phosphate as a cause for Lafora disease. *J. Biol. Chem.*, *283*(49), 33816-25. ISSN:1083-351X.

Tagliabracci, V. S., Heiss, C., Karthik, C., Contreras, C. J., Glushka, J., Ishihara, M., Azadi, P., Hurley, T.D., DePaoli-Roach, A.A. & Roach, P.J. (2011). Phosphate Incorporation during Glycogen Synthesis and Lafora Disease. *Cell Metab.*, *13*(3), 274-82. ISSN: 1550-4131.

Veselovsky, A.V., Ivanov, Y.D., Ivanov, A.S., Archakov, A.I., Lewi, P. & Janssen, P. (2002). Protein-protein interactions: mechanisms and modifications by drugs. *J. Mol. Recognit.* 15(6):405-422. ISSN:1099-1352.

Wang, J., Stuckey, J.A., Wishart, M.J., & Dixon, J.E. (2002). A unique carbohydrate binding domain targets the lafora disease phosphatase to glycogen. *J. Biol. Chem.*, *277*(4), 2377-80. ISSN:1083-351X.

Wang, W. & Roach, P.J. (2004). Glycogen and related polysaccharides inhibit the laforin dual-specificity protein phosphatase. *Biochem Bioph. Res. Co.*, *325*(3), 726-30. ISSN: 0006-291X.

Worby, C.A., Gentry, M.S., & Dixon, J.E. (2006). Laforin, a dual specificity phosphatase that dephosphorylates complex carbohydrates. *J. Biol. Chem.*, *281*(41), 30412-8. ISSN:1083-351X.

7

Temporal Lobe Epilepsy: Cell Death and Molecular Targets

Maria José da Silva Fernandes[1], Esper Abrão Cavalheiro[1], João Pereira Leite[2] and Daniele Suzete Persike[1]
[1]*Disciplina de Neurologia Experimental, Departamento de Neurologia e Neurocirurgia Universidade Federal de São Paulo, UNIFESP, São Paulo*
[2]*Disciplina de Neurologia, Departamento de Neurociências e Ciências do Comportamento Faculdade de Medicina de Ribeirão Preto, Universidade de São Paulo – USP, São Paulo Brasil*

1. Introduction

According to data from the World Health Organization (WHO), epilepsy is a common chronic brain disorder affecting approximately 50 million people worldwide. The hallmark of epilepsy is the recurrence of seizures, which on a cellular level is characterized by synchronized discharges of large groups of neurons that interrupt normal function. TLE is the most frequent type of human epilepsy (Engel, 2001; Willianson et al., 1993). In about 40% of patients, the seizures are refractory to medical therapy (De Lanerolle & Lee, 2005). The majority of these patients suffer from symptomatic focal epilepsies, which are frequently a consequence of brain trauma, complicated febrile convulsions, prolonged seizures (status epilepticus; SE), ischemic lesions and brain tumors (French et al., 1993; Mathern et al., 1995).
Neuroimaging and cognitive testing of patients with refractory epilepsy also suggest detrimental effects as a result of repeated seizures over time, including volume reduction within the involved brain structures. TLE syndrome is characterized by partial seizures that may or may not be secondarily generalized. The common symptoms include abdominal sensations and fear in patients with mesial temporal sclerosis (Devinski, 2004).
Neuropathological studies indicate that TLE is frequently associated with hippocampal sclerosis that is routinely detected by imaging studies during the presurgical evaluation of patients with an intractable TLE (Mathern et al., 1995). In a review, de Lenarolle and Lee (2005) cited that about 70% of hippocampi removed surgically from patients with TLE showed hippocampal sclerosis, and 30% did not show sclerosis, known as paradoxical TLE. The etiology and the pathogenesis of this type of medial temporal lobe damage are not known. Several studies have shown a correlation between severe childhood illness (infection, febrile convulsions, prolonged seizure and hippocampal atrophy in TLE (Cavanagh & Meyer 1956; Mathern et al., 1995). However, not all TLE patients exhibiting hippocampal damage have a history of an initial insult. Some experimental and human data suggest that recurrent seizures may cause progressive damage to the hippocampus (Sloviter, 1983; Mathern et al., 1995). Until recently, it was unknown whether the damage found in the hippocampus was the cause or the consequence of TLE. However, the surgical

removal of the sclerotic hippocampus results in the best seizure-free outcome (De Lanerolle & Lee, 2005).

2. Neuropathological findings in temporal lobe epilepsy

The hippocampus or Ammon's horn is one of the most vulnerable areas in the temporal lobe to develop cell loss following seizures. The histological pattern of hippocampal sclerosis in TLE patients is characterized by the loss of pyramidal cells in the prosubiculum and the CA1 of the hippocampus (Mathern et al., 1995). These findings also include neuronal loss in the hilus of the dentate gyrus and the adjacent CA3 region of the hippocampus (Mouritzen, 1982; Babb & Lieb 1984). In many cases, the hippocampal damage in TLE was accompanied by aberrant mossy fiber reorganization. Mossy fibers from the dentate granule cells, which normally innervate the hilar mossy cells and the CA3 pyramidal cells and interneurons, reorganize and project into the inner third of the molecular layer of the dentate gyrus (Sutula et al., 1989; Babb et al., 1991; Szabadics & Soltesz, 2009). The term "mesial temporal sclerosis" has been introduced to describe cellular damage in the hippocampus, amygdala and entorhinal cortex (De Lanerolle & Lee, 2005).

3. Epileptogenesis

The development of an epileptic disorder involves a cascade of events that become activated by an initial insult to the brain. Based on studies using animal models (Turski et al., 1983; Leite et al., 1990) or human patients, there is a period so that events triggered by an initial insult (trauma or SE) can generate an active epileptic focus. It is believed that this latency period (weeks in animal models or years in patients) reflects a reaction mechanism resulting from cellular loss and is required for the synaptic reorganization to occur, which leads to an increased excitability and to changes in synchronization that establishes the chronic epileptic disorder. Figure 1 is a schematic diagram showing the events activated at different time points following an insult in human and in animal epilepsy models, which could be involved with the development of spontaneous seizures.

Thus, epilepsy can be considered an active process that results in both ictal phenomena and permanent interictal functional and structural changes in the brain (Mathern et al., 1995). Patients who develop TLE demonstrate a progression in both the number of seizures and in the neurological symptoms related to the seizure, such as cognitive and behavioral disorders (Engel et al., 1991, French et al., 2004). The long latency before the usual complex partial seizures form in TLE offers a potential time window for therapeutic interventions, which may be a good alternative to prevent the appearance of seizures.

4. Experimental animal models of TLE

The experimental animal models provide a useful approach to assess the mechanisms involved in the epileptogenesis. The damage precedes the appearance of spontaneous seizures in several animal models of partial epilepsies. *SE* induced by systemic injection of pilocarpine or kainic acid caused structural brain damage in rats. Cell loss was observed in the hilus and the CA3 region of the hippocampus as well as in the amygdala, entorhinal cortex, thalamus and cerebral cortex (Turski et al., 1983). Moreover, prominent mossy fiber sprouting occurred (Mello et al., 1993). According to Olney et al. (1974), kainic acid and

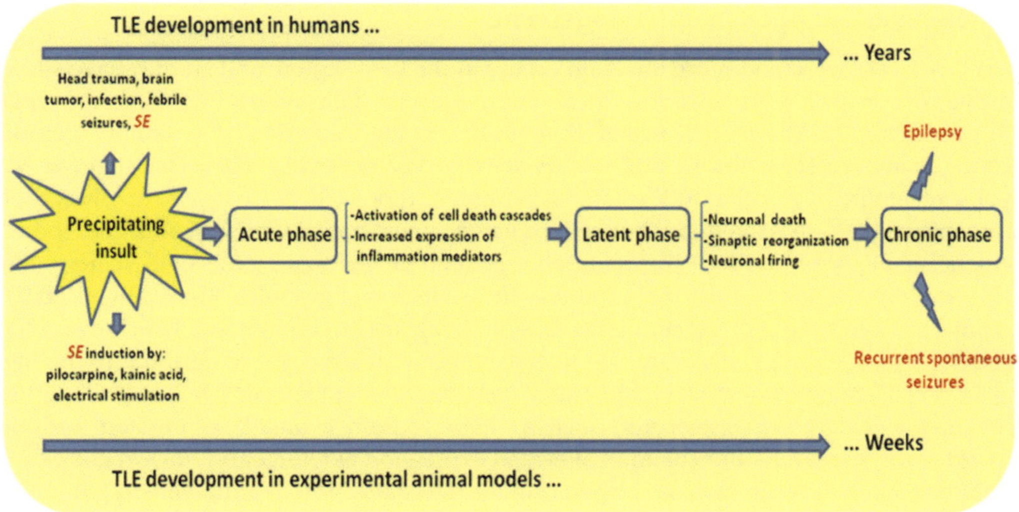

Fig. 1. A schematic diagram of epileptogenesis in patients and an experimental model of TLE. An initial precipitant insult can cause lesioning or functional changes. During a latent period, which can take years (5-10 years) in patients or weeks (2-3 weeks) in animal models, the insult initiates the reorganization of the brain and becomes prone to generate spontaneous motor seizures. Epileptogenesis includes changes that involve cell death, inflammation, neurogenesis, gliosis, sprouting, dendritic plasticity, and blood-brain barrier damage (Pitkanen & Lukasiuk, 2011). The short time frame for the development of the main features of the pathogenesis of TLE in animals encourages use in this study.

other glutamate analogues are toxic because they activate glutamate receptors on neuronal membranes, resulting in prolonged depolarization, neuronal swelling and death. By activating M1 muscarinic receptors, pilocarpine activates phospholipase C, which in turn produces diacylglycerol (DG) and inositol triphosphate (IP3), which results in alterations in calcium and potassium concentrations that lead to enhanced excitability (Raza et al., 2004; Smolders et al., 1997, Smolders et al., 1996).

The increased excitability in the hippocampus resulted in the decreased activity of ATPases that were unable to repolarize the membrane or promote calcium extrusion (Fernandes et al., 1996; Funke et al., 1998). High intracellular calcium can promote glutamate release, which by activating glutamate receptors allows the influx of additional calcium to induce *SE*, excitotoxicity and cell death (Smolders et al., 1997; Fernandes et al., 1996). In these experimental models, the recurrent spontaneous seizures occurred after a latent period, which is reminiscent of the human TLE (Mello et al., 1993). Inflammatory mediators have been described in the hippocampus of rats treated with pilocarpine, and molecules, such as kinins and prostaglandins, and also participate in the pathophysiology of TLE (Naffah-Mazzacoratti et al., 1995; Argañaraz et al., 2003; Perosa et al., 2007).

Kindling is an animal model of TLE where increasingly stronger seizures are induced by electrically stimulating brain areas (Goddard et al., 1969). Repeated seizures induce progressive cellular alterations, not only in the hippocampus, but also in the amygdala and the entorhinal cortex (Cavazos et al., 1994). Furthermore, studies have demonstrated that the neuronal loss is accompanied by aberrant mossy fiber axonal growth of the dentate granule cells in the hippocampus (Cavazos et al., 1991).

5. Molecular changes in epileptogenesis

Significant cell death and reorganization occurs in the CA1 region, and studies have shown an intense synaptic reorganization of calbindin and parvalbumin-positive neurons, which are presumably GABAergic neurons, that results in the inhibition of inhibitory neurons leading to abnormal synchrony and seizure activity (Wittner et al., 2002). This suggests that hyperexcitability is not due to the loss of γ-aminobutyric acid (GABA) but involves other mechanisms that are related to increased excitatory neurotransmission. In addition, there is evidence that mossy cells in the hilus and pyramidal neurons in the CA3 region show increased expression of GluR1 that promotes the excitation of granule cells (Eid et al., 2002).

To date, studies have focused on the increased astrogliosis in this region, which could also contribute to the hyperexcitability. There is evidence that astrocytes contribute to the high levels of glutamate in hippocampal areas where neurons are sparse (De Lanerolle & Lee, 2005). Some changes in astrocytes, such as high sodium channels expression, reduced inward rectifying potassium channels, elevated expression of GluR1 and downregulation of glutamine synthetase, an enzyme responsible for the conversion of glutamate to glutamine, represent potential mechanisms by which astrocytes can release glutamate (O'Connor et al., 1998; Schroder et al., 2000; Eid et al., 2004, van der Hel et al., 2005).

Astrocytes can modulate the inflammatory reactions through the expression of the transcription factor nuclear factor kB (NF-kB) and activation of prostaglandin E2 (PGE2) in response to interleukin-1β (IL-1β) (Dong & Benveniste, 2001). PGE2 increases calcium levels within astrocytes and contributes to glutamate release (Bezzi et al., 1998).

In addition to IL-1β, astrocytes can also produce other immunological agents, such as interleukins (IL-1, IL10 and IL-6), interferon-alpha and beta (IFN-α and β), tumor necrosis factor-alpha (TNF-α) and transforming growth factor-beta (TGF-β) (Dong & Benveniste, 2001; John et al., 2005). Studies have shown that IL-1β is upregulated in the sclerotic hippocampus from patients with TLE and can exacerbate seizures through glutamate release (John et al., 2005). The genes regulated by IL-1β are upregulated in sclerotic hippocampi from TLE patients (John et al., 2005).

Growing evidence indicates that purines are widely involved in the molecular mechanisms underlying the various functions of astrocytes, either by modulating intracellular molecules involved in energy metabolism and nucleic acid synthesis or by activating a variety of membrane receptors (Neary et al., 1996; Abbrachio & Burnstock, 1998). By activating P2 receptors, purines can also modulate calcium influx, and there is substantial evidence that cellular cascades initiated by calcium influx and perturbed intracellular calcium homeostasis are involved in the status epilepticus-induced excitotoxic cell death. Other studies have indicated that large amounts of ATP released from dying cells after the insult might induce reactive astrogliosis, microglia proliferation and act as a powerful chemoattractant at the site of injury (Davalos et al., 2005). Both astrocytes and activated microglia are able to induce the release of cytokines, such as IL-1β, TNF-α, and IL-6, which could influence the neuroinflammatory processes during neurodegeneration (Sanz & Di Virgilio, 2000). The activation of microglial P2X7 receptors by ATP induces TNF-α release, and this effect is regulated by extracellular signal-regulated kinase (ERK) and p38 mitogen-activated protein (MAP) kinase (Suzuki et al., 2004).

It is not known whether microglia protect or damage neurons or whether TNF is beneficial or toxic. However, recent studies have demonstrated that P2X7 receptors were able to modulate the immune response of glial cells, and the expression of P2X7 receptors was increased in the rat hippocampus following pilocarpine-induced SE (Dona et al., 2009; Fernandes et al., 2010). Several authors have reported that the neuroinflammation is an injury-induced glial activation that can contribute to the pathology of epilepsy (Naffah-Mazzacoratti et al., 1995; Rappold et al., 2006; Vezzani & Granata, 2005).

6. Cell death secondary to seizures

The mechanism by which seizures cause neuronal death is understood based on studies that examined glutamatergic neurotransmission. The glutamatergic neurotransmission induced by excitotoxicity leads to the over-activation of glutamate receptors, which causes an excessive influx of Na^+ and Ca^{2+} that induces osmolytic stress, cell swelling/rupturing, free radical production, which damages DNA, and protease activation leading to the proteolysis of cell and organelle membranes. This ultimately culminates with cell necrosis (Fujikawa, 2005, 2006). The glutamate-mediated excitotoxicity and necrosis are primary contributing factors, but seizures also activate programmed cell death pathways, such as apoptosis (Henshall 2007, 2008).

7. Apoptosis

Apoptosis is the physiological process of programmed cell death (Strasser et al., 2000). Apoptotic signals through a highly ordered molecular cascade that is energy-dependent and may involve new gene transcription. Several studies have identified key genes in the nematode worm, *Caenorhabditis elegans*, that promoted (ced-3, ced-4) or inhibited (ced-9) apoptosis (Ellis and Horvitz, 1986; Hengartner et al., 1992). Further, the mammalian homologues of these genes allowed for the characterization of two classes of proteins involved in apoptosis: caspases and Bcl-2 (Hengartner and Horvitz, 1994; Yuan et al., 1993).

8. Caspases and Bcl-2

Caspases are aspartate-specific cysteine proteases present in cells as zymogens. A proteolytic cleavage is required for the enzymes to become active. In mammals, fourteen types of caspases have been identified and were divided into the inflammatory/cytokine-processing caspases that include -1, -4, -5, -11, and -12. The apoptosis-regulatory caspases were divided into initiators of apoptosis that include -8, -9, and -10, and the apoptotic executioners are caspases -3, -6, and -7 (Thornberry and Lazebnik, 1998; Henshall & Simon, 2005). The activation of cell death signaling is initiated by a caspase, which will then activate specific executioner caspases. The executioner caspases will cleave key structural and functional proteins within the cell, such as actin and the inhibitor of caspase-activated DNase (ICAD), as well as providing feedback loops for further processing of caspases (Mashima et al., 1997; Sakahira et al., 1998; Thornberry and Lazebnik, 1998; Henshall and Simon, 2005).

The Bcl-2 gene family is comprised of more than 20 different members that regulate apoptosis positively, pro-apoptotic, or negatively, anti-apoptotic, primarily by affecting the mitochondria (Henshall and Simon, 2005; Kroemer et al., 2007). Many efforts have been made to elucidate the role of Bcl-2 proteins in apoptosis (Henshall & Simon, 2005; Kim et al., 2006). The pro-apoptotic Bcl2 family protein, Bax, becomes active by binding to tBid and can trigger the formation of pores in the mitochondrial membrane, which allows the

release of the apoptogenic factor, cytochrome c. The Bcl-2 pro-apoptotic proteins, Bim and Puma, neutralize the anti-apoptotic protein Bcl2. The proteins Bcl-2 and Bcl-xl confer protection by promoting oligomerization with pro-apoptotic members, by maintaining the integrity of the mitochondria, by mobilizing calcium and by acting as an antioxidant (Henshall & Simon, 2005).
The high level of intracellular calcium (Ca^{2+}) that results from the activation of glutamate can trigger mitochondrial dysfunction directly or activate calcium phosphatases (e.g., PP2B and calcineurin) or regulatory molecules responsible for the release of Bad from the anti-apoptotic protein, 14-3-3 (for details see Henshall & Simon, 2005). The transcription factor, Fox-O, is involved as a second regulatory step, is activated by dephosphorylation and upregulates Bim, whereas p53 upregulates Puma. These BH3-only proteins may promote Bax/Bak by inactivating the anti-apoptotic Bcl-2, Bcl-xl, Bcl-w or by directly activating Bax/Bak. Cytochrome *c* is released from Apaf-1, which then triggers caspase-9 activation, blocks various heat shock protein (HSP) activity and the X-linked inhibitor of apoptosis protein (XIAP). The extrinsic and intrinsic pathways converge on the activation of the executioner caspases, -3 and -7 that can then cleave key substrates (e.g., ICAD).
The endoplasmic reticulum (ER) is an organelle that acts as a key trigger in the induction of the intrinsic pathway of apoptosis (Xu et al., 2005). Protein misfolding that arises from an increased intracellular calcium level can act as a potential ER stressor. Under persistent stress, apoptosis is triggered by a mitochondrial-mediated pathway (Smith & Deshmukh, 2007), and this process requires Bax for the initiation of the pathway and Apaf-1 for cell death execution (Smith & Deshmukh, 2007).

9. Intrinsic and extrinsic pathways of apoptosis

Apoptosis can be initiated by two different routes known as extrinsic death receptor pathway, and intrinsic mitochondrial pathway (see Henshall and Simon, 2005).
In the extrinsic pathway, a cell death-promoting stimulus activates an initiator caspase via a recruitment scaffold. Activation of the cell surface-expressed death receptors, such as the TNF superfamily (TNFR1; TNF receptor 1) or Fas, causes the death effector domains (DED) within the prodomain to bind to homologous regions on the death receptor (DR) adaptor proteins, such as Fas-associated death domain (FADD), which forms an intracellular complex known as the DISC (death-inducing signaling complex), leading to caspase-8 activation (Henshall, 2005, Thornberry and Lazebnik, 1998).
The caspase cascade is initiated by caspase-8 and culminates with the activation of executioner caspases, such as caspase-3, which cleave intracellular structural and survival proteins and activate enzymes responsible for DNA fragmentation (Henshall and Simon, 2005, Thornberry and Lazebnik, 1998).
The intrinsic pathway is triggered following the disruption of intracellular organelle homoeostasis or DNA damage (Verhagen et al., 2000). This pathway is characterized by mitochondrial dysfunction that causes the release of apoptogenic factors, such as cytochrome *c*, which activates Apaf-1 (apoptotic protease-activating factor 1) and caspase-9 and is followed by downstream executioner caspase activation and cell death (Figure 3). Smac/DIABLO is released following mitochondrial damage and blocks active caspase inhibitors (Verhagen et al., 2000).
The cross-talk between the two apoptotic pathways can occur through the cleavage of Bid by activated caspase-8. Cleavage of Bid leads to truncated Bid (tBid) formation, which

translocates into the mitochondria and induces the release of cytochrome c and Smac/DIABLO (Figure 3) (Madesh et al., 2002).

10. Seizures activate apoptosis

Several studies have indicated that seizures can activate the intrinsic and extrinsic apoptotic pathways in the brain (Henshall, 2007). The release of cytochrome *c*, Apaf-1, activated caspase-9 and -3 and subsequent DNA fragmentation in the rat hippocampus after a short *SE* duration indicate activation of the intrinsic pathway (Turski et al., 1983; Leite et al., 1990). Further, the intrinsic pathway can be activated by calcium. Pro-apoptotic Bcl-2 proteins (Bad, Bid and Bim) can be activated via calcium-dependent mechanisms, and each protein was found to be activated by seizures *in vivo* (Weiss et al., 1986; Mello et al., 1993).

The importance of the Bcl-2 family in human epilepsy has been studied extensively. Elevated Bcl-w, reduced Bim and normal levels of Bcl-xl, Bax, Bad and Bid have been reported in the hippocampus obtained from patients with intractable seizures (Murphy et al., 2007; Shinoda et al., 2004, Yamamoto et al., 2006a). Serum analysis has also provided indirect evidence for the modulation of Bcl-2 in patients with epilepsy (El-Hodhod et al., 2006). These Bcl-2 expression patterns may reflect the repertoire of genes that regulate cell death that may lower the vulnerability of the brain to further neuronal loss (El-Hodhod et al., 2006). Indeed, repeated electroshock seizures in rats and mice, a protocol used to evoke a damage-refractory state, adjust the balance of pro- and anti-apoptotic Bim and Bcl-w levels and demonstrate a similar pattern to those observed in patients (Murphy et al., 2007; Shinoda et al., 2004).

The secondary role of the extrinsic pathway in cell death during seizures was demonstrated by the presence of caspase-8 cleavage in the early stages following the seizures (Henshall et al., 2001). The cleavage of a select group of caspases (-3, -7, -8 and -9) was detected in the hippocampus of rats after repeated electroshock seizures, indicating that the progression of apoptosis signaling may occur (Yamamoto et al., 2006b, Schindler et al., 2006, Yamamoto et al., 2006c).

In addition, activated TNFR1 and DISC were detected in a seizure-damaged hippocampus from rats (Henshall et al., 2003; Shinoda et al., 2003), and patients with TLE (Yamamoto et al., 2006).

Currently, it is not known whether TNF is beneficial or toxic to neurons. TNF may enhance injury induced by ischemia and trauma (Barone et al., 1997; Meistrel et al., 1997) as well as provide neuroprotection by inducing the expression of anti-apoptotic and antioxidative proteins (Yang et al., 2002). The dual effect of TNF is mediated by different TNF receptors, with the p55 TNFR1 mediating the neurotoxic effect and p75 TNF receptor 2 (TNFR2) eliciting the neuroprotection (Yang et al., 2002). By blocking protein synthesis, TNFR1 can trigger apoptosis and cause stress to the ER in the hippocampus of a patient during seizures (Yamamoto et al., 2006; Shinoda et al., 2003). These data suggest that glutamate excitotoxicity is not the only mechanism resulting in cell death after seizures. Efforts have been made to determine the temporal order of intrinsic and extrinsic pathway activation to clarify the relevance of these signaling pathways in neuronal death that is secondary to seizures.

In summary, apoptosis signaling pathways contribute to the neurodegenerative mechanism elicited by seizures and may be involved in epileptogenesis. Several apoptotic regulatory proteins have homeostatic functions in the cells involved with seizure or epilepsy susceptibility, such as Bcl-2 members, Bax and Bak, which regulate intracellular calcium at the ER membrane (White et al., 2005). In this vein, altered levels of Bcl-2 proteins in the TLE patient's brain may influence a spectrum of intracellular responses, including excitability. It has been reported that caspases can have other functions in addition to apoptotic signaling. The importance of activated caspases in normal cells during development and signaling has recently been extended to the CNS where these proteases have been shown to contribute to axon guidance, synaptic plasticity and neuroprotection (McLaughlin, 2004; Lamkanfi et al., 2007). Finally, efforts have been made to elucidate the physiological and pathological role of Bcl-2 proteins and caspases in the brain.

11. Caspase activity in temporal lobe epilepsy

Several reports have shown that seizures can occur after the activation of caspase-1 (Eriksson et al., 1999), caspase-3 (Becker et al., 1999; Kondratyev and Gale 2000; Weise et al., 2005), caspase-8 (Tan et al., 2002) or caspases-2 and -9 (Henshall et al., 2001).

Henshall et al. (2001) and Li et al. (2006) reported that caspase-8 and -9 are activated in the hippocampus 40 min after focal SE was induced by kainic acid. The different location of caspase expression after SE suggests different functions in the brain. Weise et al. (2005) reported the expression of activated caspase-3 in hippocampal neurons after pilocarpine-induced SE while other authors (Narkilahti et al., 2003; Ferrer et al., 2000) have detected active caspase-3 primarily in astrocytes and, to a lesser degree, in neurons. These data suggest that caspase-3 could exert an important role in the astrocytic death following SE and may have other unknown functions.

Using biochemical and immunohistochemistry assays, we have demonstrated that inflammatory caspase-1 and the apoptotic executioner caspase-3 are activated in the hippocampus of rats at 90 min after the seizure onset and at 7 days after SE (latent period) (in preparation). Interestingly, the most intense caspase activity was observed in the latent period where the highest amount of neuronal death occurs. The neuronal damage is necessary to generate spontaneous seizures in this model (Turski et al., 1983).

The activation of caspase-1 by SE induced by pilocarpine is involved in inflammatory mediator generation. Fantuzzi et al. (1999) demonstrated that caspase-1 is specifically required for processing pro-IL-1β and pro-IL-18 to their active forms. IL-1β can modulate the hyperexcitability by increasing glutamate release (Kamikawa et al., 1998), inhibiting glutamate reuptake by glial cells (Ye and Sontheimer, 1996) and increasing the calcium influx mediated by NMDAR through activation of Src family kinases (Viviani et al., 2003). There are a growing number of studies showing the role of inflammation in the injury process caused by seizures (Ravizza et al., 2006; Vezzani et al., 1999; 2000). Thus, caspase-1 inhibition may be a promising anticonvulsant and neuroprotective therapy.

12. Caspase inhibition as neuroprotective strategy in temporal lobe epilepsy

Because caspases are differentially activated during epileptogenesis as demonstrated by Gorter et al. (2007) using microarray assays, caspase selective inhibitors are considered potential targets for novel neuroprotective and anticonvulsant agents for epilepsy (Kondratyev and Gale, 2000; Henshall et al., 2001; Ravizza et al., 2006). Inhibition of caspase-1 reduced seizures in rats, whereas the deletion of the caspase-1 gene delayed acute seizure onset (Ravizza et al., 2006). Inhibition of caspase-3 and -9 provides neuroprotection after *SE* was induced by kainate (Henshall et al., 2001), and the inhibition of caspase-8 may attenuate neuronal death by decreasing cleaved Bid, caspase-9, and the release of cytochrome *c* from mitochondria (Li et al., 2006).

The caspase inhibition was also used as a neuroprotective strategy against injury caused by *SE* induced by pilocarpine (Persike et al., 2008).

Several studies determined that tellurium compounds, as the non-toxic AS-101, ammonium trichloro(dioxoethylene-O,O') tellurate, exert anti-apoptotic, anti-inflammatory, and immunomodulatory effects (Okun et al., 2007a; Sredni et al., 2007). These effects are primarily caused by the unique tellurium-thiol chemistry, which enables the interaction between the tellurium compound with the reactive cysteine residues of the inflammatory and apoptotic caspases leading to caspase inhibition (Albeck et al., 1998; Okun et al., 2007b). AS-101 not only interacts with catalytic thiols from cysteine proteases but also interacts with non-catalytic thiols (Okun et al., 2007b). It has been demonstrated that AS-101 can upregulate the anti-apoptotic proteins Bcl-2, p21Ras, PI3 kinase and the glial cell line derived neurotrophic factor (GDNF), and AS-101 can inhibit IL-1β and caspase-1 and -3 (Makarovsky et al., 2003; Okun et al., 2006a,b; Sredni et al., 2007). AS-101 is currently being tested in Phase II clinical trials in cancer patients (Sredni et al., 1995, 1996, Frei et al., 2008) and was recently suggested as a promising agent for treatment of Parkinson's disease (Sredni et al., 2007).

A compound of tellurium(IV), the organotelluroxetane RF-07 (see Figure 2), is an analogue of AS-101 (Persike et al., 2008). The administration of RF-07 prior to pilocarpine significantly blocked the behavioral and electrographic symptoms of SE in rats (Figure 3). To evaluate if this activity could be related to caspase inhibition, RF-07 was used in an "*in vitro*" assay to test recombinant caspases -3 and -8. RF-07 showed a potent inhibitory effect on both caspase -3 and -8 (Persike et al., 2008). The RF-07 was also tested in hippocampal homogenates from rats euthanized 90 min after pilocarpine-induced *SE*. RF-07 was the most potent inhibitor of caspase-like activity compared with commercial caspase inhibitors (Persike et al., 2008). Based on the results of this study, RF-07 inhibits not only caspases but other proteases that were activated during seizures, such as cathepsins, matrix metalloproteinases and plasminogen activators (see Figure 4).

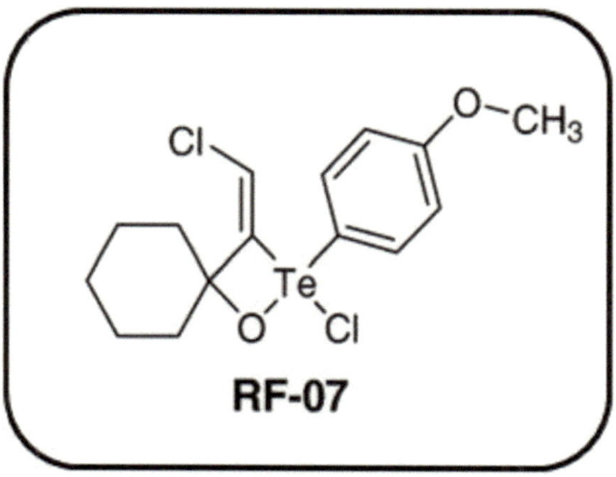

Fig. 2. The molecular structure of the neuroprotector tellurium(IV) compound, (4-{2-Chloro-3-[chloromethylidene]-1-oxa-2l4-telluraspiro[3.5]non-2-yl}phenyl Methyl Ether).

Taken together, these data show that RF-07 represents a promising anti-epileptic and/or agent for epilepsy. Further investigations are ongoing to elucidate the mechanisms by which RF-07 inhibits pilocarpine-induced seizures. Studies using proteomic analysis may help to clarify these mechanisms.

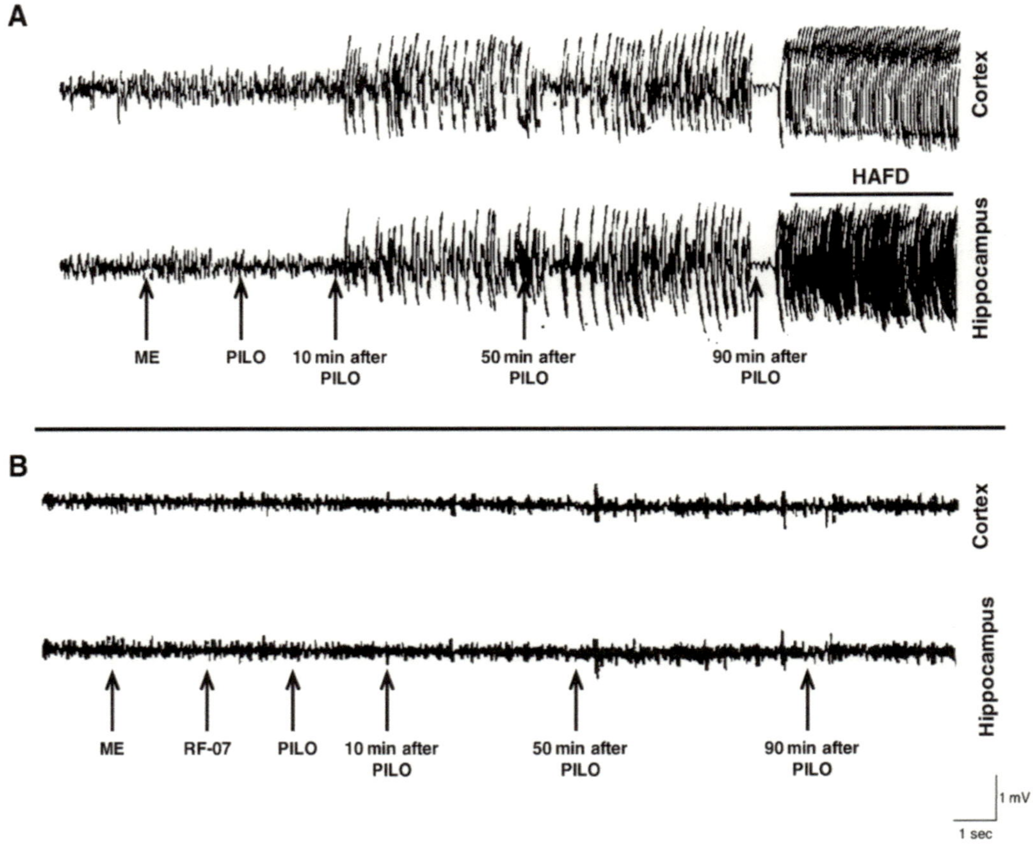

Fig. 3. Electroencephalographic recording showing the blockade of the brain high amplitude and frequency discharges (HAFD) following RF-07 injected prior to pilocarpine in rats. (**A**) N-methyl-scopolamine did not change the control recordings. N-methyl-scopolamine was used to prevent the peripheral effects of pilocarpine. The electrographic seizure started 10 min after pilocarpine administration and was highly synchronized in the hippocampus and cortex. (**B**) The rats were pre-treated systemically with RF-07 15 min prior to pilocarpine. As shown, rats did not develop seizures, which exhibited electrographic activity in the hippocampus and cortex similar to the pre-pilocarpine pattern (Persike et al., 2008).

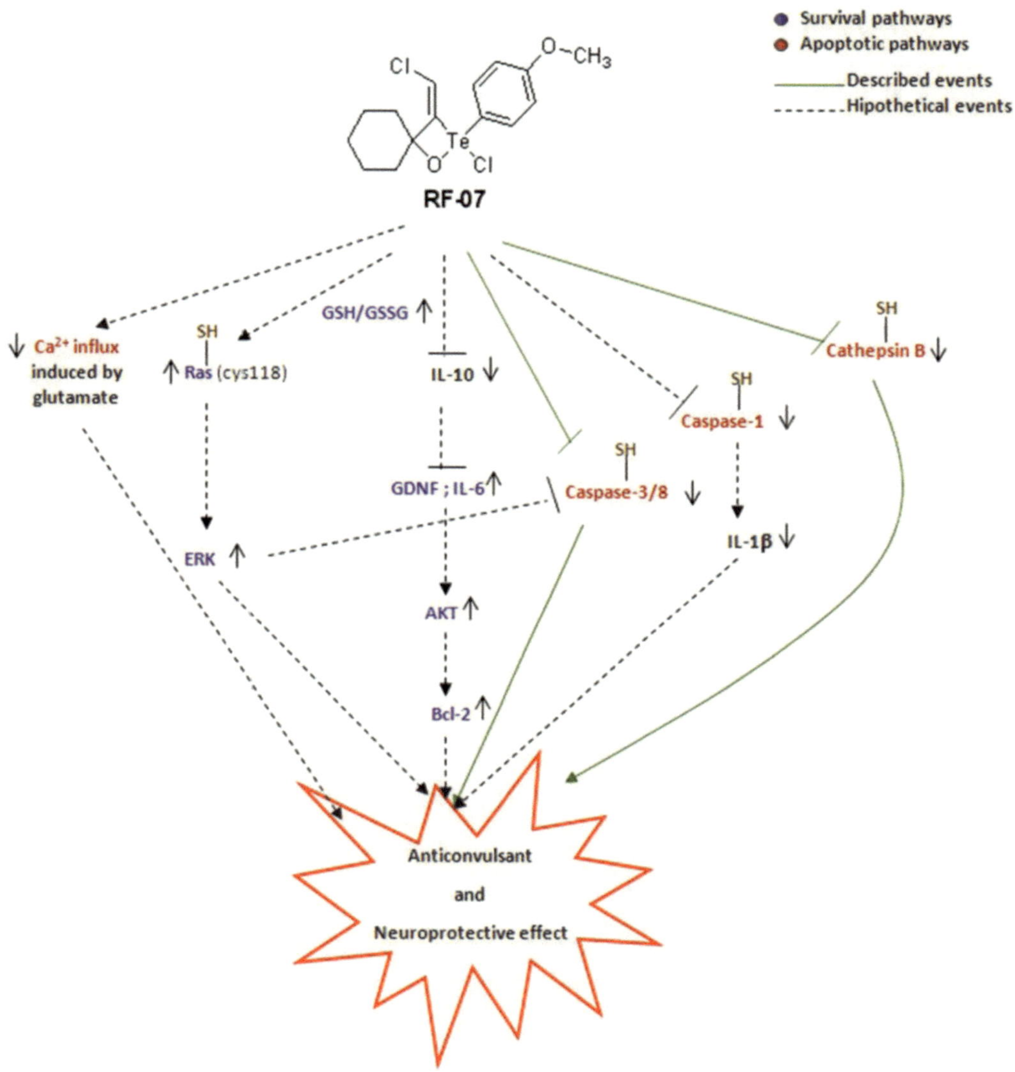

Fig. 4. A hypothetical diagram showing the signaling pathways modulated by RF-07. As previously described for AS-101, the RF-07 can bind to the cysteine residues of several proteins, such as Ras, cathepsins and caspases-1, -3 and -8. By binding to Ras, RF-07 increased the enzymatic activity, but upon binding to caspases, inhibited its activity. Ras activates ERKs, which then induces the expression of Bcl-2 to protect neurons from oxidative stress and mitochondrial disruption. The inhibition of caspases -1, -3 and -8 can prevent apoptosis and reduce the production of the pro-inflammatory cytokine IL-1β. In parallel, RF-07 could inhibit IL-10 production in addition to an increase in the ratio of GSH/GSSG. This inhibition would result in GDNF/IL-6 upregulation. By inhibiting cathepsin, RF-07 reduced the degradation of extracellular matrix components (Based on Sredni et al., 2007; Cunha et al., 2005 and Gorter et al., 2007).

13. Conclusion

Temporal lobe epilepsy is a progressive epileptic syndrome in which most of patients exhibit hippocampal sclerosis characterized by pyramidal cell degeneration, astrogliosis and aberrant mossy fiber sprouting in the inner molecular layer of the dentate gyrus. We have demonstrated that the caspase-mediated inflammatory process has been reported as a possible mechanism involved with the pathogenesis of TLE, and caspase inhibitors could be a promising therapeutic strategy. The knowledge about the physiological role of caspases in the CNS could improve our understanding about the balance between mediators of survival and cell death in the epileptogenesis.

14. Acknowledgements

The authors thank Fapesp-Fapemig, Cinapce-Fapesp, CNPq, Capes and INCT (Fapesp, MCT, CNPq) for financial support.

15. References

Abbrachio M.P. & Burnstock G. 1998 Purinergic signaling pathophysiological roles. Jpn J Pharmacol, 78: 113-45.

Albeck, A., Weitman, H., Sredni, B., Albeck, M., 1998. Tellurium compounds: selective inhibition of cysteine proteases and model reaction with thiols. Inorg. Chem. 37, 1704–1712.

Argañaraz, G.A., Perosa, S.R., Lencioni, E.C., Bader, M., Cavalheiro, E.A., Naffah-Mazzacoratti, M.G., Pesquero, J.B. and Silva, J.A. 2003. Role of kinin B1 and B2 receptors in the development of pilocarpine model of epilepsy. Brain Res. 1013, 30-49.

Babb, T.L., Brown, W.J. 1986. Neuronal, dendritic, and vascular profiles of human temporal lobe epilepsy correlated with cellular physiology in vivo. Adv Neurol. 44:949-66.

Babb, T.L., Kupfer, W.R., Pretorius, J.K., Crandall, P.H., Levesque, M.F. 1991. Synaptic reorganization by mossy fibers in human epileptic fascia dentata. Neuroscience 42: 351-364.

Babb, T.L., Lieb, J.P., Brown, W.J., Pretorius, J., Crandall, P.H. 1984. Distribution of pyramidal cell density and hyperexcitability in the epileptic human hippocampal formation. Epilepsia 25:721-728.

Barone, F.C., Arvin, B., White, R.F., Miller, A., Webb, C.L., Willette, R.N., Lysko, P.G., Fuerstein, G.Z. 1997. Tumor necrosis factor-alpha. A mediator of focal ischemic brain injury. Stroke 28:1233-44.

Becker, A.J., Gillardon, F., Blumcke, I., Langendorfer, D., Beck, H., Wiestler, O.D., 1999. Differential regulation of apoptosis-related genes in resistant and vulnerable subfields of the rat epileptic hippocampus. Brain Res. 67, 172–176.

Bezzi, P., Carmignoto, G., Pasti, L. 1998. Prostaglandins stimulates calcium-dependent glutamate release in astrocytes. Nature 391:281-5.

Cavanagh, J.B., Meyer, A. 1956. Aetiological aspects of Ammon's horn sclerosis associated with temporal lobe epilepsy. BMJ. 2:1403-1407.

Cavazos, J.E., Da, I., Sutula, T.P. 1994. Neuronal loss induced in limbic pathways by kindling: evidence for induction of hippocampal sclerosis by repeated brief seizures. J Neurosci. 14: 3106-3121.

Cavazos, J.E., Golarai, G., Sutula, T.P. 1991. Mossy fiber synaptic reorganization induced by kindling: time course of development , progression, and permanence. J Neurosci. 11: 2795-2803.

Davalos D, Grustzendler J., Yang G., et al. 2005. ATP mediates rapid microglial response to local brain injury in vivo Nat. Neurosci, 8(6): 752-8.

De Lanerolle, N.C., Lee, T.S. 2005. New facets of the neuropathology and molecular profile of human temporal lobe epilepsy. Epilepsy & Behavior 7:190-203.

Devinski, O. 2004. Diagnosis and treatment of temporal lobe epilepsy. Reviews in Neurol Dis. 1(1): 2-9.

Dona, F., Ulrich, H., Persike, D.S., et al. 2009. Alteration of purinergic P2X4 and P2X7 receptor expression in rats with temporal lobe epilepsy induced by pilocarpine. Epilepsy Res., 83:157-67.

Dong, Y., Benveniste, E.N. 2001. Immune function of astrocytes. Glia 36(2):180-90.

Eid, T., Kovacs, I., Spencer, D.D., De Lanerolle, N.C. 2002. Novel expression of AMPA-receptor subunit GluR1 on mossy cells and CA3 pyramidal neurons in the human epileptogenic hippocampus. Eur J Neurosci. 15: 517-27.

Eid, T., Thomas, M., Spencer, D., Rundén-Pran, E., Lai, J., Malthankar, G., Kim, J., Danbolt, N., Ottersen, O., de Lanerolle, N.C. 2004. Loss of glutamine synthetase in the human epileptogenic hippocampus: possible mechanism for raised extracellular glutamate in mesial temporal lobe epilepsy. The Lancet 363(9402): 28-37.

El-Hodhod, M.A., Tomoum, H.Y., Abd, Al-Aziz M.M., Samaan, S.M. 2006. Serum Fas and Bcl-2 in patients with epilepsy. Acta Neurol Scand. 113:315-321.

Ellis, H.M., Horvitz, H.R. 1986. Genetic control of programmed cell death in the nematode C. elegans. Cell 44:817-29.

Engel, J.Jr. 1993. Clinical neurophysiology, neuroimaging, and the surgical treatment of epilepsy. Curr Opin Neurol Neurosurg. 6(2):240-249. Review.

Engel, J. Jr. 2001. Mesial temporal lobe epilepsy: what have we learned? Neuroscientist 7:340-352.

Engel, J. Jr., Bandler, R., Griffith, N.C., Caldecott-Hazard, S. 1991. Neurobiological evidence for epilepsy-induced interictal disturbances. In: Advances in Neurology. Eds. Smith D, Treiman D, Trimble M. Raven Press, New York, 97-111.

Eriksson, C., Van Dam, A.M., Lucassen, P.J., Bol, J.G., Winblad, B., Schultzberg, M., 1999. Immunohistochemical localization of interleukin-1 beta, interleukin-1 receptor antagonist and interleukin-1 beta converting enzyme/caspase-1 in the rat brain after peripheral administration of kainic acid. Neuroscience 93, 915–930.

Fantuzzi, G., Reed, D.A., Dinarello, C.A., 1999. IL-12-induced IFN-gamma is dependent on caspase-1 processing of the IL-18 precursor. J. Clin. Invest. 104 (6), 761–767.

Fernandes, M.J.S., Naffah-Mazzacoratti, M.G., Cavalheiro, E.A. 1996. $Na^{+}K^{+}$ATPase in the rat hippocampus: A study in the pilocarpine model of epilepsy. Neurochem Int. 28:497-500.

Fernandes, M.J.S., Naffah-Mazzacoratti, M.G. Cavalheiro E.A. 2010. Pathophysiological aspects of temporal lobe epilepsy and the role of P2X receptors. The Open Neurosci J. 4: 35-43.

Ferrer, I., Lopez, E., Blanco, R., Rivera, R., Krupinski, J., Marti, E., 2000. Differential c-Fos and caspase expression following kainic acid excitotoxicity. Acta Neuropathol. (Berl) 99 (3), 245–256.

Frei, G.M., Kremer, M., Hanschmann, K.M., Krause, S., Albeck, M., Sredni, B., Schnierle, B.S., 2008. Antitumour effects in mycosis fungoides of the immunomodulatory, tellurium-based compound, AS101. Br. J. Dermatol. 158 (3), 578–586.

French, J.A., Williamson, P.D., Thadani, V.M., Darcey, T.M., Mattson, R.H., Spencer, S.S., Spencer, D.D. 2004. Characteristics of medial temporal lobe epilepsy: I. Results of history and physical examination. Ann Neurol. 34(6): 774-80.

Fujikawa, D.G. 2005: Prolonged seizures and cellular injury: understanding the connection. Epilepsy Behav. 7(Suppl. 3):S3-S11.

Fujikawa, D.G. (2006) in Status Epilepticus: Mechanisms and Management (Wasterlain, C.G. and Treiman, D.M., eds), pp. 463–480, MIT Press, Cambridge.

Funke, M.G., Amado, D., Cavalheiro, E.A., Naffah-Mazzacoratti, M.G. 1998. Tyrosine phosphorylation is increased in the rat hippocampus during the status epilepticus induced by pilocarpine. Brain Res Bul. 47: 87-93.

Goddard, G.V., McIntyre, D.C., Leech, C.K. 1969. A permanent change in brain function resulting from daily electrical stimulation. Exp Neurol. 25: 295-330.

Gorter, J.A., Van Vliet, E.A., Rauwerda, H., Breit, T., Stad, R., Van Schaik, L., Vreugdenhil, E., Redeker, S., Hendriksen, E., Aronica, E., Lopes da Silva, F.H., Wadman, W.J., 2007. Dynamic changes of proteases and protease inhibitors revealed bymicroarray analysis in CA3 and entorhinal cortex during epileptogenesis in the rat. Epilepsia 48 (5), 53–64.

Hengartner, M.O., Ellis, R.E., Horvitz, H.R. 1992. *Caenorhabditis elegans* gene ced-9 protects cells from programmed cell death. Nature 356:494-9.

Hengartner, M.O., Horvitz, H.R. 1994. C. elegans cell survival gene ced-9 encodes a functional homolog of the mammalian proto-oncogene bcl-2. Cell 76:665-76.

Henshall, D.C., Bonislawski, D.P., Skradski, S.L., Lan, J.Q., Meller, R., Simon, R.P. 2001.Cleavage of bid may amplify caspase-8-induced neuronal death following focally evoked limbic seizures. Neurobiol. Dis. 8 (4), 568–580.

Henshall, D.C., Araki, T., Schindler, C.K., Shinoda, S., Lan, J.-Q. and Simon, R.P. 2003. Expression of death-associated protein kinase and recruitment to the tumor necrosis factor signaling pathway following brief seizures. J. Neurochem. 86, 1260–1270.

Henshall, D.C. and Simon, R.P. 2005. Epilepsy and apoptosis pathways. J. Cereb. Blood Flow Metab. 25, 1557–1572.

Henshall, D. C. 2007. Apoptosis signaling pathways in seizure-induced neuronal death and epilepsy. Neurological Disorders: Molecules, Mechanisms and Therapeutics. 421-423.

Henshall, D. C. & Murphy, B. M. Current Opinion in Pharmacology 2008, 8:75–81 Kamikawa, H., Hori, T., Nakane, H., Aou, S., Tashiro, N., 1998. IL-1beta increases norepinephrine level in rat frontal cortex: involvement of prostanoids, NO, and glutamate. Am. J. Physiol. 275 (3 Pt 2), R803–R810.

John, G.R., Lee, S.C., Song, X., Rivieccio, M., Brosnan, C.F. 2005. IL-1-regulated responses in astrocytes: relevance to injury and recovery. Glia 49:161-76.

Kondratyev, A., Gale, K., 2000. Intracerebral injection of caspase-3 inhibitor prevents neuronal apoptosis after kainic acid-evoked status epilepticus. Brain Res. Mol. Brain Res. 75 (2), 216–224.

Kroemer, G., Galluzzi, L., Brenner, C. 2007: Mitochondrial membrane permeabilization in cell death. Physiol Rev. 87:99-163.

Lamkanfi, M., Festjens, N., Declercq, W., Vanden Berghe, T., Vandenabeele, P. 2007. Caspases in cell survival, proliferation and differentiation. Cell Death Differ. 14(1):44-55.

Leite, J.P., Bortolotto, Z.A., Cavalheiro, E.A. 1990. Spontaneous recurrent seizures in rats: an experimental model of partial epilepsy.Neurosci. Biobehav. Rev. 14(4): 511-17.

Leite, J.P., Babb, T.L., Pretorius, J.K., Kulhman, P.A., Yeoman, K.M., Mathern, G.W. 1996. Neuronal loss, mossy fiber sprouting, and interictal spikes after intrahippocampal kainate in developing rats. Epilepsy Res. 26: 219-231.

Li, T., Lu, C., Xia, Z., Xiao, B., Luo, Y. 2006: Inhibition of caspase-8 attenuates neuronal death induced by limbic seizures in a cytochrome c-dependent and Smac/DIABLO-independent way. Brain Res. 1098:204-211.

Liu, X.Q., Sheng, R., Qin, Z.H. 2009. The neuroprotective mechanism of brain ischemic preconditioning. Acta Pharmacol Sin. 30(8):1071-80.

Madesh, M., Antonsson, B., Srinivasula, S.M., Alnemri, E.S., Hajnoczky, G., 2002. Rapid kinetics of tBid-induced cytochrome c and Smac/DIABLO release and mitochondrial depolarization. J. Biol. Chem. 277 (7), 5651–5659.

Makarovsky, D., Kalechman, Y., Sonino, T., Freidkin, I., Teitz, S., Albeck, M., Weil, M., Geffen-Aricha, R., Yadid, G., Sredni, B. 2003. Tellurium compound AS101 induces PC12 differentiation and rescues the neurons from apoptotic death. Ann. N. Y. Acad. Sci. 1010, 659–666.

Mashima, T., Naito, M., Noguchi, K., Miller, D.K., Nicholson, D.W., Tsuruo, T. 1997. Actin cleavage by CPP-32/apopain during the development of apoptosis. Oncogene 14:1007-12.

Mathern, G.W., Babb, T.L., Vickrey, B.G., Melendez, M., Pretorius, J.K. 1995. The clinical-pathogenic mechanisms of hippocampal neuron loss and surgical outcomes in temporal lobe epilepsy. Brain 118: 105-118.

McLaughlin, B. 2004. The kinder side of killer proteases: caspase activation contributes to neuroprotection and CNS remodeling. Apo 9(2):111-21. Review.

Meistrel, III M.E., Botchinka, G.I., Wang, H., Di Santo, E., Cockroft, K.M., Bloom, O., Vishnubhakat, J.M., Ghezzi, P., Tracey, K.J. 1997. Tumor necrosis factor is a brain damaging cytokine in cerebral ischemia. Shock 8:341-48.

Meldrum, B.S. 2002. Implications for neuroprotective treatments. Prog Brain Res. 135:487-495.

Meller, R., Clayton, C., Torrey, D.J., Schindler, C.K., Lan, J.Q., Cameron, J.A., Chu, X.P., Xiong, Z.G., Simon, R.P., Henshall, D.C. 2006. Activation of the caspase 8 pathway mediates seizure induced cell death in cultured hippocampal neurons. Epilepsy Res. 70:3-14.

Mello, L.E.A.M., Cavalheiro, E.A., Tan, A.M., Kupfer, W.R., Pretorius, J.K., Babb, T.L., Finch, D.M. 1993. Circuit mechanisms of seizures in the pilocarpine model of chronic epilepsy: cell loss and mossy fiber sprouting. Epilepsia 34: 985-995.

Mouritzen, Dam. A. 1982. Hippocampal neuron loss in epilepsy and after experimental seizures. Acta Neurol Scand. 66:601-642.

Murphy, B., Dunleavy, M., Shinoda, S., Schindler, C., Meller, R., Bellver-Estelles, C., Hatazaki, S., Dicker, P., Yamamoto, A., Koegel, I., Chu, X. et al. 2007. Bcl-w protects hippocampus during experimental status epilepticus. Am J Pathol. 171: 1258-1268.

Naffah-Mazzacoratti, M.G., Bellissimo, M.I., Cavalheiro, E.A. 1995. Profile of levels in the rat hippocampus in pilocarpine model of epilepsy. Neurochem Int. 27:461-466.

Narkilahti, S., Pirttila, T.J., Lukasiuk, K., Tuunanen, J., Pitkanen, A., 2003. Expression and activation of caspase 3 following status epilepticus in the rat. Eur. J. Neurosci. 18 (6), 1486–1496.

Neary O'Connor, E.R., Sontheimer, H. , Spencer, D.D., de Lanerolle, N.C. 1998. Astrocytes from human hippocampal epileptogenic foci exhibit action potential-like responses. Epilepsia 39(4): 347-54.

Okun, I., Malarchuk, S., Dubrovskaya, E., Khvat, A., Tkachenko, S., Kysil, V., Kravchenko, D., Ivachtchenko, A., 2006a. Screening for caspase-3 inhibitors: effect of a reducing agent on identified hit chemotypes. J. Biomol. Screen. 11 (6), 694–703.

Okun, E., Saida, H., Albeck, M., Sredni, B., Avtalion, R.R., 2006b. Upregulation of carp GDNF mRNA by the immunomodulator AS101. Dev. Comp. Immunol. 30, 441–446.

Okun, E., Arumugam, T.V., Tang, S.C., Gleichmann, M., Albeck, M., Sredni, B., Mattson, M.P., 2007a. The organotellurium compound ammonium trichloro(dioxoethylene-o,o')tellurate enhances neuronal survival and improves functional outcome in an ischemic stroke model in mice. J. Neurochem. 102 (4), 1232–1241.

Okun, E., Dikshtein, Y., Carmely, A., Saida, H., Frei, G., Sela, B.A., Varshavsky, L., Ofir, A., Levy, E., Albeck, M., Sredni, B., 2007b. The organotellurium compound ammonium trichloro(dioxoethylene-o,o')tellurate reacts with homocysteine to form homocystine and decreases homocysteine levels in hyperhomocysteinemic mice. FEBS J. 274 (12), 3159–3170.

Olney, J.W., Rhee, V., Ho, O.L. 1974. Kainic acid: a powerful neurotoxic analogue of glutamate. Brain Res. 77: 507-512.

Perosa, S.R., Argañaraz, G.A., Goto, E.M., Costa, L.G.P., Konno, A.C., Varella, P.P.V., Santiago, J.F.C., Pesquero, J.B., Canzian, M. , Amado, D., Yacubian, E.M., Carrete, H., Centeno, R.S., Cavalheiro, E.A., Silva, Jr. J.Á., Naffah-Mazzacoratti, M.G. 2007. Kinin B1 and B2 receptors are overexpressed in the hippocampus of humans with temporal lobe epilepsy. Hippocampus 17: 26-33.

Persike, D.S., Cunha, R.L.O.R., Juliano, L., Silva, I.R., Rosim, F.E., Vignoli, T., Doná, F., Cavalheiro, E.A., Fernandes, M.J.S. 2008. Protective effect of the organotelluroxetane RF-07 in pilocarpine-induced *status epilepticus*. Neurobiol. Dis. 31:120-126.

Pitkanen &, Lukasiuk, K. 2011. Mechanisms of epileptogenesis and potential treatment targets.The Lancet, 10:173-184

Rappold P.M., Lind-Balta E., Joseph S.A. 2006. P2X7 receptor immunoreactive profile confined to resting and activated microglia in the epileptic brain. Brain Res., 1089(1): 171-8.

Ravizza, T., Lucas, S.M., Balosso, S., Bernardino, L., Ku, G., Noé, F., Malva, J., Randle, J.C., Allan, S., Vezzani, A., 2006. Inactivation of caspase-1 in rodent brain: a novel anticonvulsive strategy. Epilepsia 47 (7), 1160–1168.

Raza, M., Blair, R.E., Sombati, S., Carter, D., Deshpande, L.S., DeLorenzo, R.J. 2004. Evidence that injury-induced changes in hippocampal neuronal calcium dynamics during epileptogenesis cause acquired epilepsy. Proc Natl Acad Sci. 101(50):17522-2.

Sanz J.M. & Di virgilio F. 2000. Kinetics and mechanism of ATp dependente IL-1β release from microglial cells. J. immunol, 164: 4893-8.

Schroder, W., Hinterkeuser, S., Seifert, G. 2000. Functional and molecular properties of human astrocytes in acute hippocampal slices obtained from patients with temporal lobe epilepsy. Epilepsia 41: S181-4.

Schindler, C.K., Pearson, E.G., Bonner, H.P., So, N.K., Simon, R.P., Prehn, J.H., Henshall, D.C. 2006. Caspase-3 cleavage and nuclear localization of caspase-activated DNase in human temporal lobe epilepsy. J Cereb Blood Flow Metab. 26:583-589.

Shinoda, S., Skradski, S.L., Araki, T., Schindler, C.K., Meller, R., Lan, J.-Q., Taki, W., Simon, R.P. and Henshall, D.C. 2003. NF-kappaB at the crossroads of life and death.

Eur. J. Neurosci. 17, 2065–2076.

Shinoda, S., Schindler, C.K., Meller, R., So, N.K., Araki, T., Yamamoto, A., Lan, J.Q., Taki, W., Simon, R.P., Henshall, D.C. 2004. Bim regulation may determine hippocampal vulnerability after injurious seizures and in temporal lobe epilepsy. J Clin Invest. 113:1059-1068.

Sloviter, R.S. 1983. "Epileptic" brain damage in rats induced by sustained electrical stimulation of the perforant path. I. Acute electrophysiological and light microscopic studies. Brain Res Bull. 10:675-697.

Smith, M.I., Deshmukh, M. 2007. Endoplasmic reticulum stress-induced apoptosis requires bax for commitment and Apaf-1 for execution in primary neurons. Cell Death Differ. 14:1011-1019.

Smolders, I., Khan, M., Manil, J., Ebinger, G., Michotte, Y. 1997. NMDA receptor-mediated pilocarpine-induced seizures: characterization in freely moving rats by microdialysis. British Journal of Pharmacology 121(6):1171-79.

Smolders, I., Van Belle, K., Ebinger, G., Michotte, Y. 1996. Hippocampal and cerebellar extracellular amino acids during pilocarpine-induced seizures in freely moving rats. Eur J Pharmacol. 319(1): 21-29.

Sredni, B., Albeck,M., Tichler, T., Shani, A., Shapira, J., Bruderman, I., Catane, R., Kaufman, B., Kalechman, Y., 1995. Bone marrow-sparing and prevention of alopecia by AS101 in non-small-cell lung cancer patients treated with carboplatin and etoposide. J. Clin. Oncol. 13 (9), 2342–2353.

Sredni, B., Geffen-Aricha, R., Duan, W., Albeck, M., Shalit, F., Lander, H.M., Kinor, N., Sagi, O., Albeck, A., Yosef, S., Brodsky,M., Sredni-Kenigsbuch, D., Sonino, T., Longo, D.L., Mattson, M.P., Yadid, G., 2007. Multifunctional tellurium molecule protects and restores dopaminergic neurons in Parkinson's diseasemodels. FASEB J. 21 (8), 1870–1883.

Strasser, A., O'Connor, L., Dixit, V.M. 2000. Apoptosis signaling. Annu Rev Biochem. 69:217-45.

Sutula, T., Cascino, G., Cavazos, J., Parada, I., Ramirez, L. 1989. Mossy fiber synaptic reorganization in the epileptic human temporal lobe. Ann Neurol. 26: 321-330.

Suzuki T., Hide I., Ido K., et al. 2004. Production and release of neuroprotective tumor necrosis fator by P2X7 receptor activated micróglia. J. Neurosci, 24(1): 1-7.

Szabadics, J., Soltesz, I. 2009. Functional Specificity of Mossy Fiber Innervation of GABAergic Cells in the Hippocampus. J Neurosci 29(13): 4239-51.

Tan, Z., Sankar, R., Tu, W., Shin, D., Liu, H., Wasterlain, C.G., Schreiber, S.S., 2002. Immunohistochemical study of p53-associated proteins in rat brain following lithium-pilocarpine status epilepticus. Brain Res. 929 (1), 129–138.

Thornberry, N.A., Lazebnik, Y., 1998. Caspases: enemies within. Science 281 (5381), 1312–1316.

Turski, W.A., Czuczwar, S.J.,Kleinrok, Z., Turski, L. 1983. Cholinomimetics produce seizures and brain damage in rats. Experientia 39:1408-1411.

van der Hel, W.S., Notenboom, R.G.E., Bos, I.W.M., van Rijen, P.C., van Veelen, C.W.M., de Graan, P.N.E. 2005. Reduced glutamine synthetase in hippocampal areas with neuron loss in temporal lobe epilepsy. Neuroogy 64: 326-33.

Verhagen, A.M., Ekert, P.G., Pakusch, M., Silke, J., Connolly, L.M., Reid, G.E., Moritz, R.L., Simpson, R.J., Vaux, D.L., 2000. Identification of DIABLO, a mammalian protein that promotes apoptosis by binding to and antagonizing IAP proteins. Cell 102 (1), 43–53.

Vezzani, A., Conti, M., De Luigi, A., Ravizza, T., Moneta, D., Marchesi, F., De Simoni, M.G., 1999. Interleukin-1beta immunoreactivity and microglia are enhanced in the rat hippocampus by focal kainate application: functional evidence for enhancement of electrographic seizures. J. Neurosci. 19 (12), 5054–5065.

Vezzani A & Granata T. Brain inflammation in epilepsy experimental and clinical evidence. 2005. Epilepsia, 46(11): 1724-43

Vezzani, A., Moneta, D., Conti, M., Richichi, C., Ravizza, T., De Luigi, A., De Simoni, M.G., Sperk, G., Andell-Jonsson, S., Lundkvist, J., Iverfeldt, K., Bartfai, T., 2000. Powerful anticonvulsant action of IL-1 receptor antagonist on intracerebral injection and astrocytic overexpression in mice. Proc. Natl. Acad.Sci. 97 (21), 11534–11539.

Viviani, B., Bartesaghi, S., Gardoni, F., Vezzani, A., Behrens, M.M., Bartfai, T., Binaglia, M., Corsini, E., Di Luca, M., Galli, C.L., Marinovich, M., 2003. Interleukin-1beta enhances NMDA receptor-mediated intracellular calcium increase through activation of the Src family of kinases. J. Neurosci. 23 (25), 8692–8700.

Weise, J., Engelhorn, T., Dorfler, A., Aker, S., Bahr, M., Hufnagel, A., 2005. Expression time course and spatial distribution of activated caspase-3 after experimental status epilepticus: Contribution of delayed neuronal cell death to seizure-induced neuronal injury. Neurobiol. Dis. 18 (3), 582–590.

Weiss, G.H., Salazar, A.M., Vance, S.C., Grafman, J.H., Jabbari, B. 1986. Predicting posttraumatic epilepsy in penetrating head injury. Arch Neurol. 43: 771-773.

White, C., Li, C., Yang, J., Petrenko, N. B., Madesh, M., Thompson, C.B. and Foskett, J.K. 2005. The endoplasmic reticulum gateway to apoptosis by Bcl-X(L) modulation of the InsP3R. Nat. Cell Biol. 7, 1021–1028.

Wittner, L. E., Szabó, S., Tóth, S. Czirják, P. Halász, Freund, T. F., Maglóczky, Z. 2002. Synaptic reorganization of calbindin-positive neurons in the human hippocampal CA1 region in temporal lobe epilepsy. Neuroscience 115(3): 961-78.

Xu, C., Bailly-Maitre, B., Reed, J.C. 2005. Endoplasmic reticulum stress: cell life and death decisions. J Clin Invest. 115:2656-2664.

Yamamoto, A., Schindler, C.K., Murphy, B.M., Bellver-Estelles, C., So, N.K., Taki, W., Meller, R., Simon, R.P. and Henshall, D.C. 2006a. Evidence of tumor necrosis factor receptor 1 signaling in human temporal lobe epilepsy. Exp. Neurol. 202, 410–420.

Yamamoto, A., Murphy, N., Schindler, C.K., So, N.K., Stohr, S., Taki, W., Prehn, J.H., Henshall, D.C. 2006b. Endoplasmic reticulum stress and apoptosis signaling in human temporal lobe epilepsy. J Neuropathol Exp Neurol. 65:217-225.

Yamamoto, A., Schindler, C.K., Murphy, B.M., Bellver-Estelles, C., So, N.K., Taki, W., Meller, R., Simon, R.P., Henshall, D.C. 2006c. Evidence of tumor necrosis factor receptor 1 signaling in human temporal lobe epilepsy. Exp Neurol. 202:410-420.

Yuan, J., Shaham, S., Ledoux, S., Ellis, H.M., Horvitz, H.R. 1993. The C. elegans cell death gene ced-3 encodes a protein similar to mammalian interleukin-1 beta-converting enzyme. Cell 75:641-52.

Yang, L., Lindholm, K., Konishi, Y., Li, R., Shen, Y. 2002. Target depletion of distinct tumor necrosis factor receptor subtypes reveals hippocampal neuronal death and survival through different signal transduction pathaways. J Neurosci. 22:3025-32.

8

The Cross-Talk Between Mitochondria and the Nucleus in the Response to Oxidative Stress Associated with Mitochondrial Dysfunction in Mitochondrial Encephalomyopathies

Yu-Ting Wu[1], Wan-Yu Lee[1], Shi-Bei Wu[1] and Yau-Huei Wei[1,2]
[1]*Department of Biochemistry and Molecular Biology*
School of Life Sciences, National Yang-Ming University
[2]*Department of Medicine, Mackay Medical College*
Taiwan

1. Introduction

Mitochondria are responsible for the supply of the majority of ATP in human cells via respiration and oxidative phosphorylation (OXPHOS). Mitochondria also play a central role in numerous cellular processes including energy production, intracellular Ca^{2+} homeostasis, biosynthesis of pyridine nucleotides and amino acids, and β-oxidation of fatty acids. On the contrary, mitochondria are also involved in the generation of reactive oxygen species (ROS), and initiation and execution of apoptotic cell death. Accumulating evidence show that defects in one or more of these functions may contribute to mitochondrial encephalomyopathies and other neuromuscular diseases. The term "mitochondrial encephalomyopathies" was coined by pediatric neurologists to call the attention of clinicians when the brain disease was first reported in children with mitochondrial alterations in their muscle biopsies (Shapira et al., 1977). Clinically, mitochondrial encephalomyopathies are common disorders that are a result of mutations affecting genes encoding proteins of important mitochondrial function (Leonard & Schapira, 2000a). Most mitochondrial diseases, such as mitochondrial myopathy, lactic acidosis and stroke-like episodes (MELAS), are maternally inherited and frequently manifested as encephalomyopathies (Taylor et al., 2004). Furthermore, typical clinical features of mitochondrial encephalomyopathies include weakness and retardation of the heart, skeletal muscle and brain, where mitochondria are relatively abundant. Common symptoms of mitochondrial encephalomyopathies include loss of cognitive function, sensorineural deafness, optic atrophy, fluctuating encephalopathy, ataxia, seizures, dementia, migraine, stroke-like episodes, spasticity, cardiomyopathy, proximal myopathy and exercise intolerance (Stollberger & Finsterer, 2006).

Epilepsy and seizures are common features of mitochondrial dysfunction associated with mitochondrial encephalomyopathies and have been considered the most common neurological disorders. According to the electroencephalograph (EEG) and seizure procedures, epilepsy is often an important sign in the early progression of mitochondrial encephalomyopathies (Canafoglia et al., 2001). Epilepsy is characterized by spontaneous and recurrent unprovoked seizures that may lead to numerous changes with events of cascades at the cellular level of neurons. Neuronal excitability can be affected by mitochondrial dysfunction including depletion of ATP, generation of ROS, disruption of Ca^{2+} homeostasis, defects in biosynthesis and metabolism of neurotransmitters. However, the mechanism by which mitochondrial dysfunction leads to the onset and progression of epilepsy is still unclear. In this article, we focus on the potential role of mitochondrial function in the pathophysiology of mitochondrial encephalomyopathies. Firstly, we discuss the biochemical consequences of mitochondrial dysfunction-elicited oxidative stress in affected cells of patients with mitochondrial encephalomyopathies. Secondly, we address the possible molecular mechanisms involving in the regulation of communication between defective mitochondria and the nucleus, which is termed "mitochondrial retrograde signaling" in the pathogenesis of mitochondrial encephalomyopathies. Moreover, we also explore the role of mitochondria in the regulation of Ca^{2+} homoeostasis in neuron excitability that influences the normal function of neurons and proceeds towards epileptic seizures. Finally, we discuss the role of stress responsive gene, Sirt1, in the signaling pathway of the cross-talk between mitochondria and the nucleus to be a defense mechanism against neuronal degeneration in the patients with mitochondrial encephalomyopathies. We believe that the above-mentioned information will help us gain a deeper insight into the mechanisms underlying the pathogenesis of epilepsy in patients with mitochondrial disease and guide us to develop novel therapeutic strategies for better treatment of human diseases caused by mitochondrial dysfunction.

2. Oxidative stress and mitochondrial encephalomyopathies

Typical mitochondrial myopathy and encephalomyopathies are caused by mutations in the mtDNA or nuclear DNA that affect the respiratory chain directly (Bertini & D'Amico, 2009). Since mitochondria are responsible for the supply of the majority of ATP in human cells via respiration and OXPHOS, the defective mitochondria in affected tissue cells cause not only inefficient ATP production but also increased production of ROS. The symptoms of mitochondrial encephalomyopathies and neuromuscular disorders caused by mitochondrial dysfunction-elicited oxidative stress have been proven to be similar to those documented in the patients with mitochondrial diseases (Fernández-Checa et al., 2010). Oxidative stress elicited by mitochondrial dysfunction can further increase oxidative damage to various biomolecules in mitochondria. Hence, it has been proposed that the vicious cycle is propagating in mitochondrial diseases and results in the widely observed accumulation of oxidative damage and mutation of mtDNA, which ultimately leads to a progressive decline in the bioenergetic function of mitochondria that affects tissue cells in patients with mitochondrial encephalomyopathies (Fukui & Moraes, 2008). Recently, Katayama and coworkers demonstrated that the occurrence of 8-OHdG-positive neurons was significantly increased in the peri-lesional cortices as compared with the non-lesional and control cortices in the patients with MELAS syndrome (Katayama et al., 2009). Importantly, the spread frequency of stroke-like lesions in MELAS patients was significantly reduced after treatment with the antioxidant edaravone. In addition, a key finding was that failure of adaptive responses to oxidative stress (e.g., DNA repair system) in the brain during epileptogenesis could lead to an increase in the susceptibility of mitochondria to oxidative damage (Jarrett et al., 2008). The mitochondrial base excision repair (BER) pathway involves a highly coordinated process catalyzed by the sequential actions of the DNA repair enzymes 8-oxoguanine glycosylase (OGG1) and DNA polymerase gamma (POLG). It was reported that the RNA and protein expression levels of OGG1 and POLG were decreased during chronic epilepsy in an animal model (Lin et al., 2010). They found that spontaneous seizures coincided with an accumulation of mtDNA damage, increased mitochondrial H_2O_2, and impaired mtDNA repair, which suggest a contribution of mitochondrial defects to epileptogenesis. On the other hand, the regulation of antioxidant enzymes against oxidative stress in the cells with defective mitochondria also plays an important role in the pathophysiology of mitochondrial encephalomyopathies (Wu et al., 2010). Several animal models with the disruption of the antioxidant enzymes such as manganese superoxide dismutase (Mn-SOD) and glutathione peroxidase 1 (GPx-1) genes could lead to neuromuscular disorders that are similar to those documented in the patients with mitochondrial diseases (Li et al., 1995; Esposito et al., 2000). Taken together, the increase of oxidative stress and oxidative damage and the dysregulation of antioxidant enzymes are involved in the deterioration of bioenergetic function of the affected tissues, especially in the brain and skeletal muscle from patients with mitochondrial encephalomyopathies, which depend on mitochondrial function for supply of most of the ATP (Wei & Lee, 2003). Recent studies conducted in our own and other laboratories have provided compelling evidence to support the notion that oxidative stress elicited by impairment of the respiratory chain in the affected tissues of patients plays a role in the pathogenesis and progression of mitochondrial diseases and seizure generation (Waldbaum et al., 2010a; Wu et al., 2010).

3. Biochemical hallmarks in mitochondrial encephalomyopathies

A wide spectrum of the clinical phenotypes in the patients with mitochondrial encephalomyopathies is mostly associated with the defects in the structure or function of mitochondria. The histological and histochemical examinations of affected tissues have provided useful clues to determine the mitochondrial defects in the diagnosis of these diseases (Alhatou et al., 2004). There are well-established dye-staining methods for the assay of enzyme activities of cytochrome *c* oxidase (COX, Complex IV) and succinate dehydrogenase (SDH, Complex II) in affected muscle fibers and brain (DiMauro et al., 2002). Usually, the succinate dehydrogenase (SDH) activity staining clearly shows the subsarcolemmal accumulation of mitochondria (SDH-positive) and the activity assay of COX is particularly useful in the evaluation of mitochondrial myopathies (COX-negative fibers) because Complex IV contains subunits encoded by both the mtDNA and nuclear DNA (Taylor et al., 2004). Recently, Folbergrová et al. (2010) reported that the persistent inhibition of Complex I led to the overproduction of ROS, which could contribute to the neuronal injury in a rat model of seizures and in the patients with epileptogenesis. In a previous study, we observed a significant decrease in the copy number of mtDNA in the leukocytes of patients with mitochondrial encephalomyopathies including MERRF and MELAS syndromes, respectively (Liu et al., 2006). The amplitude of change was related to the proportion of mutant mtDNA, which may serve as a biomarker in the pathogenesis and progression of the mitochondrial diseases. Similarly, a recent study revealed that large amounts of mtDNA with a deletion were observed in hippocampal tissues of patients with epilepsy (Guo et al., 2010). Most importantly, by the establishment of cybrid cells with mitochondrial dysfunction and primary culture of skin fibroblasts from affected tissues, we have been able to intensively study the pathogenesis of mitochondrial encephalomyopathies. Firstly, we found that the glucose metabolism was shifted to enhanced anaerobic glycolysis in the cells from patients with mitochondrial myopathy and encephalopathy. This is consistent with a previous report that glycolysis is up-regulated to compensate for the inefficient ATP production by mitochondrial OXPHOS (Pallotti et al., 2004). Although the increase in glycolysis occurred in affected cells is still equivocal, it revealed cellular adaptation for affected cells to cope with the energy crisis (Qian & van Houten, 2010). Secondly, neuronal mitochondria are important for intracellular Ca^{2+} sequestration, which suggests that mitochondria can modulate neuronal excitability and synaptic transmission which are altered in the patients with epilepsy (Tang & Zucker, 1997). Indeed, loss of Ca^{2+} buffering in hippocampal mitochondria has been demonstrated in kainate-treated chronic epileptic rats (Kunz et al. 1999). Besides, substantial alterations of mitochondrial Ca^{2+} homeostasis were also the predominant feature in cybrids harboring the mtDNA mutation associated with MERRF syndrome (Brini et al., 1999). Finally, since the oxidative damage to proteins was accumulated in the defective mitochondria from the affected tissue cells, an efficient mitochondrial protein quality control system was also essential for the survival of patients with mitochondrial encephalomyopathies (Luce et al., 2010). It has been reported that the mitochondrial Lon protease and heat-shock protein 60 (HSP60) were dysregulated in cultured skin fibroblasts established from patients with MERRF and MELAS syndromes, respectively (Wu et al., 2010). In addition, the decreased expression of mitochondrial HSP60 within the abnormal mitochondria was found in the subsarcolemmal region of muscle from the patients with mitochondrial encephalomyopathies, but HSP60 was over-expressed in the intermyofibrillar mitochondria (Carrier et al., 2000). This finding suggests that the processing and integration of imported precursor proteins are impaired in the subsarcolemmal mitochondrial aggregates of the ragged-red fibers (RRF), whereas the biosynthesis, import and assembly of proteins may still be efficient in the biogenesis of intermyofibrillar mitochondria of these muscle fibers.

4. Mitochondrial dysfunction-induced cell death and mitochondrial encephalomyopathies

Evidence showed that tissue degeneration caused by cell death has been implicated in numerous mitochondrial diseases including mitochondrial encephalomyopathies, neuromuscular disorders and neurodegenerative diseases (Sayre et al., 2008). It is important to unravel the molecular mechanism underlying decreased cell viability in the process of epileptogenesis in the mitochondrial encephalomyopathies. There are at least two mechanisms implicated in neuronal cell death, including activation of the excitotoxic cascades (mitochondrial Ca^{2+} overload; excessive stimulation of glutamate receptors, nitric oxide overproduction; elevated oxidative stress and ROS overproduction), and induction of apoptosis. In this section, we focus on the involvement of programmed cell death (apoptosis) in the mitochondrial encephalomyopathies and provoked epilepsy. Apoptosis is the best understood cell death that can could be manipulated to control the destiny of cells. Indeed, apoptotic pathway has been considered a major physiological process in triggering cell death, which is critical for morphogenesis, tissue homeostasis as well as pathogenesis of diverse diseases (Hetts, 1998). Notably, mitochondria play an important role in the initiation, execution and regulation of apoptosis since mitochondria can release specific proteins and factors to trigger the apoptotic pathway. MtDNA mutation-elicited mitochondrial dysfunction may result in insufficient supply of ATP, excess generation of ROS, elevated oxidative stress, membrane lipids peroxidation, disruption of mitochondrial membrane potential, dysregulation of excitotoxicity, and imbalanced distribution of intracellular Ca^{2+} ions (Kann & Kovacs, 2007). All of these changes can trigger activation of the cascades of caspases and pro-apoptotic proteins, and result in apoptosis.

Clinically, many researchers tried to clarify the correlation between apoptosis-related cell death and pathogenic mechanism involved in the defects in muscle and brain of patients with mitochondrial encephalomyopathies. Many well-documented studies have revealed that apoptosis is involved in the progression of muscle myopathy (Aure et al., 2006; Umaki et al., 2002). Studies showed significant signs of apoptosis in the COX- negative muscle fibers in muscle biopsies from patients who harbored high proportions of specific point mutations in tRNA genes of mtDNA. Distinct expressions of 8-OHdG, 4-HNE, Mn-SOD, cytochrome *c* and DNase I were detected in the COX-negative muscle fibers accompanied by apoptotic markers. These results suggest the importance of apoptosis and the relationship of the oxidative stress with the severity of the muscle myopathy in mitochondrial diseases. Liu and coworkers also showed progressive cortical volume loss in patients with recurrent neocortical epilepsy (Liu et al., 2003). Accumulating evidence substantiated that apoptosis plays a role in seizure-induced neuron death as well as brain damages and also as a cause and consequence for epileptogenesis (Chuang et al., 2009b; Weise et al., 2005). It has been reported that an increase in the expression of caspases molecules was observed in temporal cortex of patients with epilepsy (Henshall et al., 2000). Increased production of ROS, NO and peroxynitrite was also reported to proceed apoptotic cell death in vulnerable brain regions (Chuang et al., 2009a, 2009b). On the other hand, inhibition of pro-apoptotic proteins and caspases activation could reduce seizure-induced neuronal cell death in experimental animal models. It has been reported that inhibition of caspase 3 was efficacious in the protection against neuronal cell loss in several models of brain injury (Liou et al., 2003). Either by short interfering RNA molecules targeting *Bim* in human cells or by knockout of *Bim* in a mouse model could reduce cell death and decrease the degeneration of hippocampal CA3 neurons following seizures (Murphy et al., 2010). In addition, the mice lacking the pro-apoptotic protein, Puma, were found to have a reduced neuronal death by 50% in the hippocampus (Engel et al., 2010). Moreover, a recent study also showed that Bcl-w was an endogenous neuroprotectant in mice and patients with temporal lobe epilepsy (Murphy et al., 2007).

The above-mentioned studies showed the potential neuroprotective effect in epilepsy by targeting apoptosis with caspase inhibitors and genetic manipulation of pro-apoptotic proteins after onset of seizures in animals. Targeting apoptosis signaling pathways to prevent mitochondrial dysfunction-induced neuronal cell death may be a potential strategy for treatment of the patients with mitochondrial encephalomyopathies. However, some researchers showed that reducing cell death by administration of apoptotic inhibitor had no improvement of epilepsy symptoms in experimental animals (Narkilahti et al., 2003). These results revealed the complex cause and consequence of epileptogenesis and epileptic seizures. Therefore, the approach of inhibiting apoptosis to improve epileptic seizures should be evaluated with caution although it is still a potential candidate to collaborate with other antiepileptic drugs.

5. Mechanism of mitochondrial dysfunction caused neuronal excitability

Abnormality of Ca^{2+} homeostasis is thought to be associated with the pathophysiology of neurodegenerative diseases (Mattson, 2007). The disease progression in patients often occurred following epileptic seizures, a cardinal and early symptom of mitochondrial diseases, especially in MERRF and MELAS syndromes (Okumura et al., 2008). Investigators also demonstrated that defects of mitochondrial respiratory chain could evoke seizures by using partial inhibition of ETC enzymes to cause deficiency of cytochrome *c* oxidase (Yamamoto & Tang, 1996). During the episode of epileptic seizures, extreme neuronal cell activity is associated with excessive cytosolic Ca^{2+} influx. It is noteworthy that dysregulation of Ca^{2+} handling in neurons might be a consequence of mtDNA mutation. The energy deficiency and ROS overproduction are the major stressors in human cells harboring disease-associated mtDNA mutations, which play an important role in the induction of the signaling cascades emitted from dysfunctional mitochondria to the nucleus. The abnormality of Ca^{2+} homeostasis induced by insufficiency of cellular ATP and oxidative damage is a potential link between mitochondrial dysfunction and epilepsy-induced hyperexcitability in neurons of patients with mitochondrial encephalomyopathies.

5.1 Redox modulation of Ca^{2+} homeostasis

Mitochondria play an important role in the regulation of Ca^{2+} homoeostasis by effective Ca^{2+} buffering (Tang & Zucker, 1997). Mitochondria can transiently accumulate substantial amounts of Ca^{2+} from the cytosol through the rapid uptake and relatively slow release of the Ca^{2+} ions. Therefore, it is possible that mitochondrial defect could have an impact on Ca^{2+} homoeostasis in cells. Abnormal Ca^{2+} homoeostasis has been reported in various cell types with defects in mitochondrial OXPHOS function (Willems et al., 2008). Many studies also proved that cells with mtDNA mutations could result in the dysregulation of mitochondrial Ca^{2+} buffering and reduction of the Ca^{2+} influx. The increase in the concentration of cytosolic Ca^{2+} was observed in the fibroblasts from patients with mitochondrial encephalomyopathies including MELAS and MERRF. The affected cells have elevated levels of Ca^{2+} ions and cannot normally induce Ca^{2+} influx in response to agonist-stimulated Ca^{2+} uptake by mitochondria (Brini et al., 1999; Moudy et al., 1995). It remains unclear as to how a pathogenic mtDNA mutation affects Ca^{2+} homeostasis. It is thought that mitochondrial Ca^{2+} uptake is dependent on the mitochondrial membrane potential, and thus mitochondrial deficiency-related decline of membrane potential plays an important role in defects of Ca^{2+} homeostasis. It has been proved that diminishment of mitochondrial membrane potential by an uncoupling agent can interfere with the uptake of Ca^{2+} by mitochondria and thus alter the transient cytosolic Ca^{2+} levels in neurons (Werth & Thayer, 1994). Indeed, defect in the mitochondrial Ca^{2+} handling was observed in the skin fibroblasts of patients with the MERRF syndrome. It was reported that cybrids harboring mtDNA mutation derived from a patient with MERRF syndrome exhibited a reduced uptake of the Ca^{2+} ions by mitochondria in response to histamine stimuli (Brini et al., 1999).

Another important factor involving in the dysregulation of cellular Ca^{2+} homeostasis is excessive ROS production induced by mitochondrial dysfunction. More and more studies have supported that ROS and cellular redox state can directly modulate Ca^{2+} signaling through regulation of ion transporters (Hool & Corry, 2007). ROS have been shown to increase the Ca^{2+} channel activity through directly oxidizing the redox-sensing thiols on the Ryanodine receptor channel, and thereby induce the Ca^{2+} uptake from plasma membrane

(Werth & Thayer, 1994), and on IP3 receptor mediating Ca^{2+} release from ER which leads to elevated cytosolic Ca^{2+} (Suzuki & Ford, 1992). On the other hand, alteration of cellular redox states such as the lower GSH/GSSG and NADH/NAD^{+} ratios have been reported to modulate Ca^{2+} homeostasis by elevating the activity of Ca^{2+} channels and inhibiting the Ca^{2+} pump (Kourie, 1998; Zima et al., 2004). In general, Ca^{2+} can be re-uptake by the SR/ER Ca^{2+} ATPase following Ca^{2+} release from SR/ER Ca^{2+} stores or Ca^{2+} influx from PM to maintain the concentration of cytosolic Ca^{2+}. However, the Ca^{2+} ATPase activity is also sensitive to the redox state, but unlike activation of oxidized receptor channels, it is inhibited by oxidative modification and ROS (Kaplan et al., 2003). As described above, mtDNA mutations can elicit over-production of intracellular ROS, which not only damages cellular biomolecules but also change the redox homeostasis of affected cells. Elevated oxidative stress results in a decrease of the GSH/GSSG ratio in the skin fibroblasts and cybrids harboring mtDNA mutation established from patients with mitochondrial diseases. A decrease in the GSH levels and gluthathione reductase activity has been observed in the plasma and brain regions of epileptic patients (Mueller et al., 2001). A large amount of studies have shown that the GSH concentration and the activity of Na^{+}/K^{+} ATPase were decreased and affected the Ca^{2+} pump in the striatum and hippocampus during pilocarpine-induced seizures. It was also demonstrated that restoration of the level of GSH by lipoic acid could abolish the seizure episodes in the rat (de Freitas, 2010). A recent study showed that the tissue levels of GSH, and GSH/GSSG ratio were persistently altered throughout the onset of epileptogenesis in experimental temporal lobe epilepsy (Waldbaum et al., 2010b). The shift of redox state to oxidation would disrupt the Ca^{2+} homeostasis through the stimulation of Ca^{2+} influx and the interference of the Ca^{2+} pump, leading to dysregulation of the cytosolic Ca^{2+} concentration and the perturbation of Ca^{2+} signaling pathways. These findings imply that redox-dependent alterations of Ca^{2+} signaling cascades may contribute to the onset and progression of epileptogenesis.

5.2 Inhibition of Ca^{2+} exchangers by energy deficiency

The defects in the respiration and OXPHOS cause a depletion of ATP, and thus compromise the removal of Ca^{2+} ions by Ca^{2+}-ATPase. Cytoplasmic Ca^{2+} concentration is also maintained by the ATP-dependent Ca^{2+} pump (Leo et al., 2005). Therefore, reduction in ATP synthesis could result in the accumulation of cytosolic Ca^{2+} (Buttgereit & Brand, 1995). A reduction in the capacity of Ca^{2+} clearance might lead to a disruption of Ca^{2+} homeostasis. Besides, lactic acidosis might be associated with an increase of cytosolic Ca^{2+} ions in patients with mitochondrial diseases. An increase in glucose uptake and the rate of glycolysis was observed in the epileptic loci during seizure episodes, which may result in elevated lactate production that is well documented in patients with mitochondrial diseases (Cornord et al., 2002). Intracellular acidification has been shown to inhibit the plasma membrane Na^{+}/H^{+} exchanger (Anderson et al., 2003), which causes an increase in cytosolic Na^{+} concentration and thus interfere with Na^{+}/Ca^{2+} exchange through inhibition of the exchange of cellular Ca^{2+} for extracellular Na^{+}, leading to cellular accumulation of Ca^{2+} ions. These findings suggest that mitochondrial dysfunction-induced insufficient supply of ATP might be another important factor contributing to elevated seizure susceptibility in human epileptic patients through alteration of ion transporters. The scenario described above can explain why an elevation of cytosolic Ca^{2+} ions is often observed in human cells harboring pathogenic mtDNA mutations, especially from MERRF and MELAS patients, respectively.

5.3 Pathological effect of defective Ca^{2+} dyshomeostasis

Proper regulation of the Ca^{2+} influx is critical to neuronal cell function, and to transduce electrochemical signals into molecular signals. Perturbed Ca^{2+} homeostasis would cause excessive amounts of Ca^{2+} within the neurons leading to dysfunction of a variety of cellular processes, followed by degeneration and cell death. When defective mitochondria alter the cellular Ca^{2+} dynamics, it might affect the specificity of Ca^{2+} signals and subsequently result in the induction of improper signaling cascades. Intriguingly, it has been reported that peripheral mitochondria accumulate more Ca^{2+} than do those in perinuclear region (Collins et al., 2002). We have observed that pathogenic mtDNA mutations can alter the distribution and movement of mitochondria, which would affect the regulation of local Ca^{2+} ions (Ma et al., 2005). Thus, the pathogenic deficit of Ca^{2+} signaling might further affect the brain function. Besides, slow elevation of cytosolic Ca^{2+} ions can lead to a corresponding increase in mitochondrial Ca^{2+} concentration. This physiological increase in mitochondrial Ca^{2+} ions could positively regulate mitochondrial metabolism through activation of TCA cycle enzymes, boosting the biosynthesis of reduced respiratory substrates, and stimulation of adenine nucleotide transporter (ANT) and Complex V to promote the production of ATP (Das & Harris, 1990; Mc Cormack & Denton, 1993). However, it has been proposed that the sustained uptake of mitochondrial Ca^{2+} results in the inhibition of Complex I and Complex III activities, which consequently increase the ROS production (Batandier et al., 2004; Jekabsone et al., 2003). When Ca^{2+} ions are overloaded to mitochondria, it temporarily provokes a pathological signal leading to the opening of the permeability transition pore (PTP) to block the intracellular Ca^{2+} homeostasis by Ca^{2+} release, and the subsequent induction of apoptosis through cytochrome *c* release (Crompton, 1999). Therefore, the great amplitude of Ca^{2+} transient in cells harboring a pathogenic mutation of mtDNA may increase the risk of inducing cell death processes. Aforementioned investigations have provided compelling evidence to support the notion that disturbed Ca^{2+} homeostasis elicited by mitochondrial dysfunction in the affected tissues, especially in the neurons of the patients, plays an important role in the epileptogenesis and disease progression of encephalomyopathies.

6. Sirtuin-mediated cellular adaptation in epileptogenesis

There are increasing evidence to reveal that sirtuins play a critical role in regulation of metabolism and the aging process through several pathways (Bordone & Guarente, 2005). Sirt1 is the most extensively studied sirtuin that mediates NAD^+-dependent deacetylation of target proteins and thereby regulates many cellular functions. Overexpression or increase of the activity of Sirt1 has been reported to be neuroprotective in several neurodegenerative diseases. The most important mechanism contributory to Sirt1-induced protective effect is related to the regulation of cell survival (de Oliveira et al., 2010). In addition to alleviating the cell death and inducing the repair system, Sirt1 can modulate cellular response to oxidative stress and promote mitochondrial function (Gerhart-Hines et al., 2007). In human cells with mitochondrial dysfunction, increase of oxidative stress and damage may trigger apoptosis, which is closely related to seizure-induced cell loss. To cope with oxidative stress, the antioxidant defense system has evolved to dispose of excess intracellular ROS. Indeed, an imbalanced expression of antioxidant enzymes has been reported in different brain regions of animals in several studies of experimental status epilepticus. Induction of Mn-SOD and catalase expression was observed in picrotoxin-induced seizures. The catalase levels have been also reported to increase following electrically induced seizures (de Freitas, 2009). Contrary to Mn-SOD and catalase, the GPx showed a tendency to decrease in the animals with status epileptic seizures (Shin et al., 2008). Interestingly, the abnormal expression of antioxidant enzymes was commonly found in the affected tissues of patients with mitochondrial encephalomyopathies caused by pathogenic mtDNA mutations. In previous studies, we observed increased levels of intracellular ROS and imbalanced expression of antioxidant enzymes in skin fibroblasts established from patients with the MERRF syndrome (Wu et al., 2010). Increase in the expression and activity of Mn-SOD rather than other antioxidant enzymes was observed in skin fibroblasts from MERRF and CPEO patients, respectively, which suggests that the expression of antioxidant enzymes was altered and failed to cope with the increase of oxidative stress in tissue cells with mitochondrial defects. Recent studies showed that Sirt1 plays a critical role in the detoxification of ROS since it can deacetylate and activate some of the Foxo family proteins, which in turn increase the transcription of Mn-SOD and catalase genes expressions(Brunet et al., 2004). Several studies have suggested that Sirt1 is a stress responsive gene. In one of our previous studies, we showed that oxidative stress could increase Sirt1 protein expression in human skin fibroblasts upon treatment with 150-300 μM H_2O_2 (Wu et al., 2010). Increased Sirt1 protein expression was also observed in skin fibroblasts from patients with some of the mitochondrial diseases as compared to normal subjects. Therefore, it is possible that increased expression of Sirt1 in affected tissue cells of patients with mitochondrial encephalomyopathies could lead to abnormal expression of antioxidant enzymes in response to mitochondrial dysfunction, which might contribute to epileptic conditions.

On the other hand, Sirt1 may exert the calorie restriction-induced anti-aging effect by modulation of the mitochondrial function. It can promote mitochondrial respiration through deacetylation and activation of the transcription activity of PGC-1α, a master regulator of mitochondrial biogenesis (Nemoto et al., 2005). It is well known that mitochondrial biogenesis is induced in the affected tissue cells of patients with mitochondrial diseases as a compensatory adaptation to compromised bioenergetic function due to defects in OXPHOS, despite the fact that increase in the number of mitochondria might have little contribution to the bioenergetic outcome. In one of our previous studies, we demonstrated that most of the patients with mitochondrial diseases frequently display abnormal mitochondrial proliferation along with an increase in the mitochondrial mass and gene expression of mtTFA (Wu et al., 2010). In addition, we also showed that increased oxidative stress is involved in the aberrant mitochondrial proliferation. Similarly, a change in the number of mitochondria has been reported in some of the patients with seizures or epilepsy. These findings led us to conjecture that compensatory induction of Sirt1 elicited by oxidative stress may be responsible for the unusual cellular status and neurotoxicity in epileptics. This also suggests that Sirt1 may be involved in the signaling pathway of the cross-talk between defective mitochondria and the nucleus to regulate cellular adaptation to mtDNA mutation-elicited oxidative stress.

7. Therapeutic approaches to target mitochondrial bioenergetics and oxidative stress in epilepsy

Therapies for epileptic seizures have largely focused on reducing neuronal excitability and hence alleviating the frequency of occurrence of seizures and epilepsy. Recent therapeutic approaches tend to seek for antiepileptogenic drugs that may inhibit the targets involved in the pathogenesis of epileptogenesis. Mitochondrial dysfunction triggering neuron cell death has been considered as a major contribution to the onset of seizures and is related to the resistance to epileptic therapy. Thus, therapies targeting mitochondrial bioenergetics and oxidative stress pathways could have neuroprotective effect and would be able to improve the seizure activity and attenuate the severity of epilepsy. Administration of creatine is frequently used and has been shown to protect brain injury in animal models of ALS, Huntington's disease and MPTP-induced Parkinsonism (Ferrante et al., 2000; Matthews et al., 1999). Creatine can move through blood to brain and increase the pool of phosphocreatine/creatine by mitochondrial creatine kinase to boost the neuronal energy level. Supplementation of creatine was observed to attenuate hypoxia-induced seizures in both rats and rabbits. Creatine was also found to be neuroprotective in epilepsy induced by pilocarpine (Holtzman et al., 1998). These observations suggest that creatine treatment has the potential neuroprotective effect for patients with epilepsy, although it remains to be proven by clinical trials. Additionally, diet modification by caloric restriction or ketogenic diet has been used to inhibit seizure susceptibility in epileptic EL mice through a reduction of glucose metabolism (Todorova et al., 2000). Accumulating evidence support that chronic use of ketogenic diet can alter mitochondrial function, which includes promotion of mitochondrial biogenesis, decrease of ROS production and induction of GSH biosynthesis that ultimately lead to cellular adaption and restoration of mitochondrial redox state (Jrrett et al., 2008).

On the other hand, to interfere with increased ROS during the onset of epilepsy appears to be another possible strategy for therapy. Natural antioxidant compounds such as vitamin C and E, melatonin and catalase have been shown to decrease oxidative stress and alleviate the seizure-induced brain injury (MacGrego et al., 1996; Tan et al., 1998). It has been reported that clinical trial of vitamin E as a therapy for epilepsy is controversial because it failed to improve seizure activity in pediatric patients. Similarly, although the Mn-SOD knockout mice was shown to exhibit age-dependent spontaneous and handling-induced seizures (Liang & Patel, 2004), and even more susceptible to kainate-induced seizures and neuron cell death, the SOD mimetics only reduced oxidative stress and oxidative damage but not the behavioral seizures (Rong et al., 1999). Hence, the therapeutic effect of antioxidants on epileptogenesis remains to be further investigated.

8. Conclusion

Mitochondrial dysfunction has been identified as a potential cause of epileptic seizures. Specific mtDNA mutations leading to the impairment of mitochondrial respiration and OXPHOS might be associated with epileptic phenotype. Because mitochondria supply the majority of ATP in neurons by OXPHOS and maintain the cellular Ca^{2+} homeostasis, their dysfunction can influence neuronal excitability and synaptic transmission, which may be responsible for epileptogenesis. Mitochondria play critical roles in energy metabolism, apoptosis and Ca^{2+} homeostasis, and respond to intrinsic and external stimuli through a variety of retrograde signaling pathways. Thus, mitochondrial dysfunction may trigger events involved in the cascades of the communication between mitochondria and the nucleus to mediate physiological adaptation of human cells through genetic or metabolic regulation. This may subsequently lead to alterations of the antioxidant defense system, activation of Ca^{2+} signaling, modulation of mitochondrial biogenesis and OXPHOS function.

The energy deficiency and ROS overproduction are the major stressors in human cells harboring disease-associated mtDNA mutations, which may play an important role in the induction of the retrograde signaling cascades sent from dysfunctional mitochondria to the nucleus. These events could interfere with Ca^{2+} homeostasis through decrease of the mitochondrial Ca^{2+} buffering capacity and affecting the Ca^{2+} influx and pump, which lead to the abnormal change of the cytosolic Ca^{2+} concentration and perturbation of Ca^{2+}-related signaling pathways that ultimately trigger the neuronal cell death. Therefore, it is reasonable to consider mitochondria as promising targets of neuroprotective treatment of the patients with epilepsy. In conclusion, a better understanding of the mechanisms underlying epileptics elicited by mitochondrial dysfunction will provide novel information for the design of therapeutic approaches to treat patients with epilepsies or seizures caused by or associated with mitochondrial encephalomyopathies.

9. Acknowledgment

We would like to thank the Nation Science Council of Taiwan for long-term support of the studies on mitochondrial dysfunction and mtDNA mutation in the pathophysiology of mitochondrial diseases. We also would like to express our appreciation to the technical support at National Yang-Ming University in conducting molecular and cellular biology experiments on cultured cells established from patients with various mitochondrial diseases.

10. References

Alhatou, M. I., Sladky, J. T., Bagasra, O. & Glass, J. D. (2004). Mitochondrial abnormalities in dermatomyositis: characteristic pattern of neuropathology, *Journal of Molecular Histology* 35(6): 615-619.

Anderson, S. E., Liu, H., Ho, H. S., Lewis, E. J. & Cala, P. M. (2003). Age-related differences in Na^{+}-dependent Ca^{2+} accumulation in rabbit hearts exposed to hypoxia and acidification, *American Journal of Physiology- Cell Physiology* 284: C1123-1132.

Aure, K., Fayet, G., Leroy, J. P., Lacene, E., Romero, N. B., & Lombes, A. (2006). Apoptosis in mitochondrial myopathies is linked to mitochondrial proliferation, *Brain* 129(Pt 5): 1249-1259.

Batandier, C., Leverve, X. & Fontaine, E. (2004). Opening of the mitochondrial permeability transition pore induces reactive oxygen species production at the level of the respiratory chain complex I, *The Journal of Biological Chemistry* 279(17): 17197-17204.

Bertini, E. & D'Amico, A. (2009). Mitochondrial encephalomyopathies and related syndromes: brief review, *Endocrine Development* 14: 38-52.

Blander, G. & Guarente, L. (2004). The Sir2 family of protein deacetylases, *Annual Review of Biochemistry* 73: 417-435.

Bordone, L. & Guarente, L. (2005). Calorie restriction, SIRT1 and metabolism: understanding longevity, *Nature Reviews Molecular Cell Biology* 6: 298-305.

Brini, M., Pinton, P., King, M. P., Davidson, M., Schon, E. A. & Rizzuto, R. (1999). A calcium signaling defect in the pathogenesis of a mitochondrial DNA inherited oxidative phosphorylation deficiency, *Nature Medicine* 5(8): 951-954.

Brunet, A., Sweeney, L. B., Sturgill, J. F., Chua, K. F., Greer, P. L., Lin, Y., Tran, H., Ross, S. E., Mostoslavsky, R., Cohen, H. Y., Hu, L. S., Cheng, H. L., Jedrychowski, M. P., Gygi, S. P., Sinclair, D. A., Alt, F. W. & Greenberg, M. E. (2004). Stress-dependent regulation of FOXO transcription factors by the SIRT1 deacetylase, *Science* 303: 2011-2015.

Buttgereit, F. & Brand, M. D. (1995). A hierarchy of ATP-consuming processes in mammalian cells, *Biochemical Journal* 312: 163-167.

Canafoglia, L., Franceschetti, S., Antozzi, C., Carrara, F., Farina, L., Granata, T., Lamantea, E., Savoiardo, M., Uziel, G., Villani, F., Zeviani, M. & Avanzini, G. (2001). Epileptic phenotypes associated with mitochondrial disorders, *Neurology* 56(10): 1340-1346.

Carrier, H., Flocard, F., Tagliati, V., Arrigo, A. P. & Godinot, C. (2000). Immunolabelling of mitochondrial superoxide dismutase and of Hsp60 in muscles harbouring a respiratory chain deficiency, *Neuromuscular Disorders* 10(2): 144-149.

Chuang, Y. C., Chen, S. D., Liou, C. W., Lin, T. K., Chang, W. N., Chan, S. H. & Chang, A. Y. (2009a). Contribution of nitric oxide, superoxide anion, and peroxynitrite to activation of mitochondrial apoptotic signaling in hippocampal CA3 subfield following experimental temporal lobe status epilepticus, *Epilepsia* 50(4): 731-746.

Chuang, Y. C., Lin, J. W., Chen, S. D., Lin, T. K., Liou, C. W., Lu, C. H. & Chang, W. N. (2009b). Preservation of mitochondrial integrity and energy metabolism during experimental status epilepticus leads to neuronal apoptotic cell death in the hippocampus of the rat, *Seizure* 18(6): 420-428.

Chuang, Y. C. (2010). Mitochondrial dysfunction and oxidative stress in seizure-induced neuronal cell death, *Acta Neurologica Taiwanica* 19(1): 3-15.

Collins, T. J., Berridge, M. J., Lipp, P. & Bootman, M. D. (2002). Mitochondria are morphologically and functionally heterogeneous within the cells, *The EMBO Journal* 21: 1616-1627.

Cornord, E. M., Shamsa, K., Zeitzer, J. M., Enriquez, C. M. Wilson, C. L., Behnke, E. J., Fried, I. & Engel, J. (2002). Regional analyses of CNS microdialysate glucose and lactate in seizure patients, *Epilepsy* 43: 1360-1371.

Crompton, M. (1999). The mitochondrial permeability transition pore and its role in cell death, *Biochemical Journal* 341(2): 233-239.

Das, A. M. & Harris, D. A. (1990). Control of mitochondrial ATP synthase in heart cells: inactive to active transitions caused by beating or positive inotropic agents, *Cardiovascular Research* 24(5): 411-417.

de Freitas, R. M. (2009). The evaluation of effects of lipoic acid on the lipid peroxidation, nitrite formation and antioxidant enzymes in the hippocampus of rats after pilocarpine induced seizures, *Neuroscience Letters* 455(2): 140-144.

de Freitas, R. M. (2010). Lipoic acid alters delta-aminolevulinic dehydratase, glutathione peroxidase and Na^+,K^+-ATPase activities and glutathione-reduced levels in rat hippocampus after pilocarpine-induced seizures, *Cellular and Molecular Neurobiology* 30(3): 381-387.

de Oliveira, R. M., Pais, T. F. & Outeiro, T. F. (2010). Sirtuin: Common targets in aging and in neurodegeneration, *Current Drug Targets* 11: 1270-1280.

DiMauro, S., Hirano, M., Kaufmann, P., Tanji, K., Sano, M., Shungu, D. C., Bonilla, E. & DeVivo, D. C. (2002). Clinical features and genetics of myoclonic epilepsy with ragged red fibers, *Advanced Neurology* 89: 217-229.

Engel, T., Hatazaki, S., Tanaka, K., Prehn, J. H. & Henshall, D. C. (2010). Deletion of Puma protects hippocampal neurons in a model of severe status epilepticus, *Neuroscience* 168(2): 443-450.

Esposito, L. A., Kokoszka, J. E., Waymire, K. G., Cottrell, B., MacGregor, G. R. & Wallace, D. C. (2000). Mitochondrial oxidative stress in mice lacking the glutathione peroxidase-1 gene, *Free Radical Biology & Medicine* 28(5): 754-766.

Fernández-Checa, J. C., Fernández, A., Morales, A., Marí, M., García-Ruiz, C. & Colell, A. (2010). Oxidative stress and altered mitochondrial function in neurodegenerative diseases: lessons from mouse models, *CNS Neurol Disord Drug Targets* 9(4): 439-454.

Ferrante, R. J., Andreassen, O. A., Jenkins, B.G., Dedeoglu, A., Kuemmerle, S., Kubilus, J. K., Kaddurah-Daouk, R., Hersch, S. M. & Beal, M. F. (2000). Neuroprotective effects of creatine in a transgenic mouse model of Huntington's disease, *The Journal of Neuroscience* 20(12): 4389-4397.

Folbergrová, J., Jesina, P., Haugvicová, R., Lisý, V. & Houstek, J. (2010). Sustained deficiency of mitochondrial complex I activity during long periods of survival after seizures induced in immature rats by homocysteic acid, *Neurochemistry International* 56(3): 394-403.

Fukui, H. & Moraes, C. T. (2008). The mitochondrial impairment, oxidative stress and neurodegeneration connection: reality or just an attractive hypothesis? *Trends in Neurosciences* 31: 251-256.

Gerhart-Hines, Z., Rodgers, J. T., Bare, O., Lerin, C., Kim, S. H., Mostoslavsky, R., Alt, F. W., Wu, Z. & Puigserver, P. (2007). Metabolic control of muscle mitochondrial function and fatty acid oxidation through SIRT1/PGC-1alpha, *The EMBO Journal* 26: 1913-1923.

Guo, X., Popadin, K. Y., Markuzon, N., Orlov, Y. L., Kraytsberg, Y., Krishnan, K. J., Zsurka, G., Turnbull, D. M., Kunz, W. S. & Khrapko K. (2010). Repeats, longevity and the sources of mtDNA deletions: evidence from 'deletional spectra', *Trends in Genetics* 26(8): 340-343.

Henshall, D. C., Clark, R. S., Adelson, P. D., Chen, M., Watkins, S. C. & Simon, R. P. (2000). Alterations in bcl-2 and caspase gene family protein expression in human temporal lobe epilepsy, Neurology 55(2): 250-257.

Hetts, S. W. (1998). To die or not to die: an overview of apoptosis and its role in disease, *the Journal of the American Medical Association* 279(4): 300-307.

Holtzman, D., Togliatti, A., Khait, L. & Jensen, F. (1998). Creatine increases survival and suppresses seizures in the hypoxic immature rat, *Pediatric Research* 44: 410-414.

Hool, L. C. & Corry, B. (2007). Redox control of calcium channels: from mechanisms to therapeutic opportunities, *Antioxidants & Redox Signaling* 9(4):409-435.

Jarrett, S. G., Liang, L. P., Hellier, J. L., Staley, K. J. & Patel, M. (2008). Mitochondrial DNA damage and impaired base excision repair during epileptogenesis, *Neurobiology of Disease* 30(1): 130-138.

Jekabsone, A., Ivanoviene, L., Brown, G. C. & Borutaite, V. (2003). Nitric oxide and calcium together inactivate mitochondrial complex I and induce cytochrome c release, *Journal of Molecular and Cellular Cardiology* 35(7): 803-809.

Jrrett, O., Milder, J. B., Liang, L. P. & Patel, M. (2008). The ketogenic diet increases mitochondrial glutathione, *Journal of Neurochemistry* 106: 1044-1051.

Kann, O. & Kovacs, R. (2007). Mitochondria and neuronal activity, *American Journal of Physiology - Cell Physiology* 292(2): C641-657.

Kaplan, P., Babusikova, E., Lehotsky, J. & Dobrota D. (2003). Free radical-induced protein modification and inhibition of Ca^{2+}-ATPase of cardiac sarcoplasmic reticulum, *Molecular and Cellular Biochemistry* 248(1-2): 41-47.

Katayama, Y., Maeda, K., Iizuka, T., Hayashi, M., Hashizume, Y., Sanada, M., Kawai, H. & Kashiwagi, A. (2009) Accumulation of oxidative stress around the stroke-like lesions of MELAS patients, *Mitochondrion* 9(5): 306-313.

Kourie, J. I. (1998). Interaction of reactive oxygen species with ion transport mechanisms, *American Journal of Physiology* 275(1): C1-24.

Kunz, W. S., Goussakov, I. V., Beck, H. & Elger, C. E. (1999). Altered mitochondrial oxidative phosphorylation in hippocampal slices of kainate-treated rats, *Brain Research* 826(2): 236-242.

Leo, S., Bianchi, K., Brini, M. & Rizzuto, R. (2005). Mitochondrial calcium signaling in cell death, *The FEBS Journal* 272: 4013-4022.

Leonard, J. V. & Schapira, A. H. (2000a). Mitochondrial respiratory chain disorders I: mitochondrial DNA defects, *Lancet* 355(9200): 299-304.

Li, Y., Huang, T. T., Carlson, E. J., Melov, S., Ursell, P. C., Olson, J. L., Noble, L. J., Yoshimura, M. P., Berger, C., Chan, P. H., Wallace, D. C. & Epstein, C. J. (1995). Dilated cardiomyopathy and neonatal lethality in mutant mice lacking manganese superoxide dismutase, *Nature Genetics* 11(4): 376-381.

Liang, L. P. & Patel, M. (2004). Mitochondrial oxidative stress and increased seizure susceptibility in Sod2$^{(-/+)}$ mice, *Free Radical Biology & Medicine* 36(5): 542-554.

Lin, Y., Xu, J., Cao, L., Han, Y., Gao, J., Xie, N., Zhao, X., Jiang, H. & Chi, Z. (2010). Mitochondrial base excision repair pathway failed to respond to status epilepticus induced by pilocarpine, *Neuroscience Letters* 474(1): 22-25.

Liou, A. K., Clark, R. S., Henshall, D. C., Yin, X. M. & Chen, J. (2003). To die or not to die for neurons in ischemia, traumatic brain injury and epilepsy: a review on the stress-activated signaling pathways and apoptotic pathways, *Progress in Neurobiology* 69(2): 103-142.

Liu, C. S., Cheng, W. L., Lee, C. F., Ma, Y. S., Lin, C. Y., Huang, C. C. & Wei, Y. H. (2006). Alteration in the copy number of mitochondrial DNA in leukocytes of patients with mitochondrial encephalomyopathies, *Acta Neurological Scandinavica* 113(5): 334-341.

Liu, R. S., Lemieux, L., Bell, G. S., Hammers, A., Sisodiya, S. M., Bartlett, P. A., Shorvon, S. D., Sander, J. W. & Duncan, J. S. (2003). Progressive neocortical damage in epilepsy, *Annals Neurology* 53(3): 312-324.

Luce, K., Weil, A. C. & Osiewacz, H. D. (2010). Mitochondrial protein quality control systems in aging and disease, *Advances in Experimental Medicine and Biology* 694: 108-125.

Ma, Y. S., Chen, Y. C., Lu, C. Y., Liu, C. Y. & Wei, Y. H. (2005). Upregulation of matrix metalloproteinase 1 and disruption of mitochondrial network in skin fibroblasts of patients with MERRF syndrome, *Annals of the New York Academy of Sciences* 1042: 55-63.

MacGregor, D. G., Higgins, M. J., Jones, P. A., Maxwell, W. L., Watson, M. W., Graham, D. I. & Stone, T. W. (1996). Ascorbate attenuates the systemic kainite-induced neurotoxicity in the rat hippocampus, *Brain Research* 727: 133-144.

Matthews, R. T., Ferrante, R. J., Klivenyi, P., Yang, L., Klein, A. M., Mueller, G., Kaddurah-Daouk, R. & Beal, M. F. (1999). Creatine and cyclocreatine attenuate MPTP neurotoxicity, *Experimental Neurology* 57(1): 142-149.

Mattson, M. P. (2007). Calcium and neurodegeneration, *Aging Cell* 6(3): 337-350.

Mc Cormack, J. G. & Denton, R. M. (1993). Mitochondrial Ca^{2+} transport and the role of intramitochondrial Ca^{2+} in the regulation of energy metabolism, *Developmental Neuroscience* 15(3-5): 165-173.

Moudy, A. M., Handran, S.D., Godberg, M. P., Ruffin, N., Kranz-Eble, P., Darryl, C. DeVivo. & Steven, M. Rothman. (1995). Abnormal calcium homeostasis and mitochondrial polarization in a human encephalomyopathy, *Proceedings of the National Academy of Sciences of the United States of America* 92: 729-733.

Mueller, S. G., Trabesinger, A. H., Boesiger, P. & Wieser, H. G. (2001). Brain glutathione levels in patients with epilepsy measured by in vivo H-MRS, *Neurology* 57:1422-1427.

Murphy, B., Dunleavy, M., Shinoda, S., Schindler, C., Meller, R., Bellver-Estelles, C., Hatazaki, S., Dicker, P., Yamamoto, A., Koegel, I. Chu, X., Wang, W., Xiong, Z., Prehn, J., Simon, R. & Henshall, D. (2007). Bcl-w protects hippocampus during experimental status epilepticus, *American Journal of Pathology* 171(4): 1258-1268.

Murphy, B. M., Engel, T., Paucard, A., Hatazaki, S., Mouri, G., Tanaka, K., Tuffy, L. P., Jimenez-Mateos, E. M., Woods, I., Dunleavy, M. Bonner, H. P., Meller, R., Simon, R. P., Strasser, A., Prehn, J. H. & Henshall D. C. (2010). Contrasting patterns of Bim induction and neuroprotection in Bim-deficient mice between hippocampus and neocortex after status epilepticus, *Cell Death and Differentiation* 17(3): 459-468.

Narkilahti, S., Nissinen, J. & Pitkanen, A. (2003). Administration of caspase 3 inhibitor during and after status epilepticus in rat: effect on neuronal damage and epileptogenesis, *Neuropharmacology* 44(8): 1068-1088.

Nemoto, S., Fergusson, M. M. & Finkel, T. (2005). SIRT1 functionally interacts with the metabolic regulator and transcriptional coactivator PGC-1alpha, *The Journal Biological Chemistry* 280: 16456-16460.

Qian, W. & van Houten, B. (2010). Alterations in bioenergetics due to changes in mitochondrial DNA copy number, *Methods* 51(4): 452-457.

Okumura, A., Kdikoro, H., Itomi, K., Maruyama, K., Kubota, T. & Kondo, Y. Itomi, S., Uemura, N., Natsume, J., Watanabe, K. & Morishima, T. (2008). Subacute encephalopathy: clinical features, laboratory data, neuroimaging, and outcomes, *Pediatric Neurology* 38: 111-117.

Pallotti, F., Baracca, A., Hernandez-Rosa, E., Walker, W. F., Solaini, G., Lenaz, G., Melzi D'Eril, G. V., Dimauro, S., Schon, E. A. & Davidson, M. M. (2004). Biochemical analysis of respiratory function in cybrid cell lines harbouring mitochondrial DNA mutations, *The Biochemical Journal* 384(2): 287-293.

Rong, Y., Doctrow, S. R., Tocco, G. & Baudry, M. (1999). EUK-134, a synthetic superoxide dismutase and catalase mimetic, prevents oxidative stress and attenuates kainate-induced neuropathology, *Proceedings of the National Academy of Sciences of the United States of America* 96(17): 9897-9902.

Sayre, L. M., Perry, G. & Smith, M. A. (2008). Oxidative stress and neurotoxicity, *Chemical Research in Toxicology* 21(1): 172-188.

Shapira, Y., Harel, S. & Russell, A. (1977). Mitochondrial encephalomyopathies: a group of neuromuscular disorders with defects in oxidative metabolism, *Israel Journal of Medical Sciences* 13(2): 161-164.

Shin, E. J., Ko, K. H., Kim, W. K., Chae, J. S., Yen, T. P., Kim, H. J., Wie, M. B. & Kim, H. C. (2008). Role of glutathione peroxidase in the ontogeny of hippocampal oxidative stress and kainate seizure sensitivity in the genetically epilepsy-prone rats, *Neurochemistry International* 52(6): 1134-1147.

Siegwart, R. (2001). Indirect Manipulation of a Sphere on a Flat Disk Using Force Information, *International Journal of Advanced Robotic Systems* 6(4): 12-16.

Stollberger, C. & Finsterer, J. (2006). Autonomic dysfunction in left ventricular hypertrabeculation/noncompaction, *International Journal of Cardiology* 109(2): 286-287.

Suzuki, Y. J. & Ford, G. D. (1992). Superoxide stimulates IP3-induced Ca^{2+} release from vascular smooth muscle sarcoplasmic reticulum, *American Journal of Physiology* 262(1): H114-116.

Tan, D., Manchester, L. P., Reiter, R. J., Qi, W., Kim, S. J. & El-Sokkary, G. H. (1998). Melatonin protects hippocampal neurons in vivo against kainic acid-induced damage in mice, *Journal of Neuroscience Research* 54: 382-389.

Tang, Y. G. & Zucker, R. S. (1997). Mitochondrial involvement in post-tetanic potentiation of synaptic transmission, *Neuron* 18(3): 483-491.

Taylor, R. W., Schaefer, A. M., Barron, M. J., McFarland, R. & Turnbull, D. M. (2004). The diagnosis of mitochondrial muscle disease, *Neuromuscular Disorders* 14: 237-245.

Todorova, M. T., Tandon, P., Madore, R. A., Stafstrom, C. E. & Seyfried, T. N. (2000). The ketogenic diet inhibits epileptogenesis in EL mice: a genetic model for idiopathic epilepsy, *Epilepsia* 41: 933-940.

Umaki, Y., Mitsui, T., Endo, I., Akaike, M. & Matsumoto, T. (2002). Apoptosis-related changes in skeletal muscles of patients with mitochondrial diseases, *Acta Neuropathologica* 103(2): 163-170.

Waldbaum, S. & Patel, M. (2010a). Mitochondria, oxidative stress, and temporal lobe epilepsy, *Epilepsy Research* 88(1): 23-45.

Waldbaum, S., Liang, L. P. & Patel, M. (2010b). Persistent impairment of mitochondrial and tissue redox status during lithium-pilocarpine-induced epileptogenesis, *Journal of Neurochemistry* 115(5):1172-1182.

Wei, Y. H. & Lee, H. C. (2003). Mitochondrial DNA mutations and oxidative stress in mitochondrial diseases, *Advances in Clinical Chemistry* 37: 83-128.

Weise, J., Engelhorn, T., Dorfler, A., Aker, S., Bahr, M. & Hufnagel, A. (2005). Expression time course and spatial distribution of activated caspase-3 after experimental status epilepticus: contribution of delayed neuronal cell death to seizure-induced neuronal injury, *Neurobiology of Disease* 18(3): 582-590.

Werth, J. L. & Thayer, S. A. (1994). Mitochondria buffer physiological calcium loads in cultured rat dorsal root ganglion neurons, *The Journal of Neuroscience* 14(1): 348-356.

Willems, P. H., Valsecchi, F., Distelmaier, F., Verkaart, S., Visch, H. J. & Smeitink, J. A. & Koopman, W. J. (2008). Mitochondrial Ca^{2+} homeostasis in human NADH:ubiqinone oxidoreductase deficiency, *Cell Calcium* 44: 123-133.

Wu, S. B., Ma, Y. S., Wu, Y. T., Chen, Y. C. & Wei, Y. H. (2010). Mitochondrial DNA mutation-elicited oxidative stress, oxidative damage, and altered gene expression in cultured cells of patients with MERRF syndrome, *Molecular Neurobiology* 41(2-3): 256-266.

Wu, Y. T., Wu, S. B., Lee, W. Y. & Wei, Y. H. (2010). Mitochondrial respiratory dysfunction-elicited oxidative stress and posttranslational protein modification in mitochondrial diseases, *Annals of the New York Academy of Sciences* 1201: 147-156.

Yamamoto, H. & Tang, H. W. (1996). Preventive effect of melatonin against cyanide-induced seizures and lipid peroxidation in mice, *Neuroscience Letters* 207: 89-92.

Zima, A. V., Copello, J. A. & Blatter, L. A. (2004). Effects of cytosolic NADH/NAD^+ levels on sarcoplasmic reticulum Ca^{2+} release in permeabilized rat ventricular myocytes, *The Journal of Physiology* 555(3): 727-741.

9

Ghrelin Regulation in Epilepsy

Flavia Prodam, Simonetta Bellone, Roberta Ricotti,
Giulia Genoni, Marina Caputo and Gianni Bona
University of Piemonte Orientale, Amedeo Avogadro, Novara
Italy

1. Introduction

Epilepsy is one of the most common neurological problems worldwide affecting approximately 1% of the population (Browne & Holmes, 2000; Chang & Lowenstein, 2003). It is characterized by recurrent unprovoked behavioural seizures (Beck & Elger, 2008).

In recent decades, the relationship between epilepsy and the neuroendocrine system has gained a great deal of interest and many researchers as neurologists, endocrinologists and basic scientists have investigated it. The main issue is whether hormonal changes in relation to epilepsy are due to seizures activity per se or to consequential effects of antiepileptic drugs. To understand the far-reaching effects of epilepsy and antiepileptic medications on hormonal system and vice versa, several studies have been recently performed. Their results are interesting but still controversial and the neuroendocrine regulation of epilepsy is far to be clearly explained.

However, considering that a role of hormones in epilepsy is known and in part well described, this chapter would firstly review the endocrine regulation mediated by sex hormones, prolactin (PRL), growth hormone (GH), thyrotropin-releasing hormone (TRH), adrenocortical axis and neuropeptide Y (NPY). More recently, also other new hormones have been investigated in this field, bringing to light ghrelin. Ghrelin is a 28 amino acid peptide predominantly produced by the stomach (Kojima et al., 1999). It was discovered as the first natural ligand of the orphan growth hormone segretagogues receptor 1a (GHS-R1a), which exerts, through its activation, a strong GH-releasing activity (Arvat et al., 2001; Howard et al., 1996; Kojima et al., 1999; Kojima & Kangawa, 2005; van der Lely et al., 2004). It also influences glucose and insulin metabolism and controls food and energy intake through many neuroendocrine systems (van der Lely et al., 2004). Furthermore, several evidences suggest that ghrelin not only plays a metabolic role but it is also involved in sleep-wake regulation, affective status, learning and memory processes (Steiger et al., 2011; van der Lely et al., 2004). Besides, the recent discovery of ghrelin has also provided an important insight to the neuroendocrine knowledge in epilepsy. In fact, a relationship between ghrelin and epilepsy has been already shown in animal and human models, although the results are sometimes conflicting. Thus, this chapter would secondly describe the intriguing ghrelin role in relation to seizures activity and discuss open questions and future perspectives.

2. The interplay between epilepsy and the endocrine system

Epilepsy and antiepileptic drugs affect hormones and neuroendocrine system. The relationship between epilepsy and the endocrine system is described, in particular for sex

hormones, GH and NPY system. More recently, the role of new hormones in epilepsy like ghrelin and its modulation on GH and NPY has been investigated (Berilgen et al., 2006; Gallagher et al., 1984; Morrell, 2003; Obay et al., 2007; Quigg, 2002; Stroud et al., 2005).
Overall, endocrine disorders related to epilepsy or antiepileptic drugs are a consequence of the influence of epileptogenic lesions, epilepsy or anticonvulsant medications on the endocrine control centers in the brain. Antiepileptic drugs also impact on peripheral endocrine glands, metabolism of hormones and binding proteins, weight and insulin sensitivity (Opaleke & Helmers, 2007).

2.1 Hypothalamus-pituitary-gonads axis

Sex steroids and hypothalamus-pituitary-gonads axis is the most investigated system in epilepsy. Seizures have consequences, in both sexes, on various aspects of the sexual and reproductive functioning and endocrine dysfunctions are reported during childhood, adolescence and adulthood (Opaleke & Helmers, 2007). Postictal hormonal alterations are not relevant after a single seizure; however, endocrine discharges can follow serial uncontrolled seizures, even unrecognized simple partial seizures (Luef, 2010). This is particularly common in temporal lobe epilepsy and it is probably related to the direct connections between this lobe and the reproductive neuroendocrine axis (Opaleke & Helmers, 2007). For example, menstrual disturbances are more frequent in women with epilepsy as compared with those without epilepsy (Svalheim et al., 2003), both in adulthood and in paediatric age (Herzog et al., 1986). In females with epilepsy the most described reproductive endocrine disorder is the polycystic ovary syndrome (Bilo et al., 1988; Herzog & Schachter, 2001). Other common forms of reproductive dysfunctions in women with epilepsy include: hypothalamic amenorrhea with low gonadotropin and estrogen levels and diminished luteinizing hormone (LH) response to the gonadotropin-releasing hormone (GnRH) (Herzog et al., 1986), poly- or oligo-menorrhea, hirsutism, functional hyperprolactinemia with galactorrhea, sub- or infertility and premature menopause (Bauer & Cooper-Mahkorn, 2008). Decreased libido, abnormal semen analysis with reduced sperm count, abnormal sperm morphology and impaired motility and reduced fertility have also been overrepresented in males with epilepsy (Isojarvi et al., 2004). Antiepileptic drugs, as well as seizures, seem to contribute to these sexual and reproductive dysfunctions. These alterations are likely related to a liver enzyme induction, which leads to an increase of the sex hormone-binding globulin and a reduction of the bioavailability of serum-free sex hormone levels in both genders (Opaleke & Helmers, 2007). In contrast, testosterone and androgens are elevated in association with valproate treatments (Herzog et al., 2006; Isojarvi et al., 2004). Clinical data on gonads dysfunctions led to investigate the role of sex hormones on epilepsy mechanisms.
The ovarian sex steroids act in the central nervous system and alter the frequency and the severity of seizures. In human and animal models, estrogen is a potent proconvulsant and progesterone has anticonvulsant properties (Reddy & Rogawski, 2009). Studies also suggested that these hormones might have complex effects depending on many factors like the endocrine state and their relative concentration and metabolism (Scharfman & MacLusky, 2006). In particular, estrogen can stimulate an increase of excitatory neurotransmitters such as glutamate via the N-methyl-D-aspartate (NMDA) receptor and a decrease of inhibitory neurotransmitters such as dopamine, through non-genomic mechanisms (S.S. Smith, 1989) and gamma-aminobutyric acid (GABA) (Ledoux et al., 2009). Estrogen has also an effect on the synaptic areas of neurons leading to an increase of

dendritic spines and cell-to-cell contacts and promoting the hypersynchronization seen in epilepsy. This can contribute to a lowering of the seizure threshold in both hippocampus and amygdala (S.S. Smith, 1989). In addition, it has been observed that estradiol, in parallel with its proconvulsant action, has a mitigating effect to reduce the seizure severity, related to facilitated and increased release of NPY (Ledoux et al., 2009). Progesterone exerts an inhibitory effect via metabolites such as allopregnanolone, which is a GABA-A receptor-modulating neurosteroid. In fact, progesterone increases the seizure threshold and also has antianxiety and sedating effects (Backstrom et al., 1984; Mayewska et al., 1986; Paul & Purdy, 1992).

Androgen metabolites also have some effect on seizure susceptibility, in animals and humans, through testosterone's conversion, with either anticonvulsant or proconvulsant abilities. In particular, aromatization of testosterone to 17beta-estradiol reduces the seizure threshold, whereas 3alfa-androstanediol, which derives by the testosterone's reduction to 5alfa-dihydrotestosterone, has an anticonvulsant effect through a powerful modulation of GABA-A receptor (Reddy, 2004).

2.2 Prolactin

Acute variations in PRL, as well as in gonadotropin levels, following generalized and partial seizures, support the hypothesis of a relationship between temporolimbic epileptiform discharges and reproductive endocrine disorders. In fact, epileptic activity in the temporal structures may propagate to the hypothalamus, altering the hypothalamic regulation of PRL release via a PRL inhibitory factor or dopamine (Parra et al., 1980). In particular, PRL is elevated during phases of simple partial seizures when consciousness is preserved and also rises during the subsequent seizure evolution (Meierkord et al., 1994). Thus, PRL has an immediate postictal elevation, as well as LH, both thought to have clinical values in the diagnosis of epilepsy (Abbott et al., 1980).

2.3 Noradreline, vasopressin and oxytocin

It has also been described a fast serum increase of noradreline, vasopressin and oxytocin during and after prolonged epileptic temporal seizures. In fact, noradreline, vasopressin and oxytocin levels are low during the aura but rapidly increase during the phase in which the epileptic activity evolves from a simple partial to complex partial and finally to the generalisation. In particular, the peak of oxytocin and noradrenaline characterizes the phase of the generalised attack, whereas vasopressin levels peak in the postictal time and remain constantly high for several hours. These findings suggest that the length or the intensity of seizures is important factors influencing the hormonal concentration of noradrenaline, vasopressin and oxytocin, as well as PRL, during limbic seizures (Meierkord et al., 1994).

2.4 Growth hormone and insulin-like growth factor-1

Although most of the data on the physiology of epilepsy are related to sex-hormones, other neuro-hormones have been investigated.

A role of GH in epilepsy has been shown. Epileptic seizures are a side effect of the rhGH replacement therapy (Clayton & Cowell, 2000). In particular, the Kabi International Growth Study (KIGS), a 10-year wide observational study about the GH therapy, recorded seizures as the seventh side effect of the treatment with a prevalence of about 0.5% (Wilton, 1999). The fact that GH has revealed as an important factor in epileptogenesis also emerged from a study performed by Kato and co-workers, on an amygdala-kindled mice model obtained with electrodes stimulation (Kato et al., 2009). Furthermore, a role of GH for neuronal development, cognitive functions and neuroprotection during hypoxic-ischemic injury, has been reported (Harvey & Hull, 2003; Lyuh et al., 2007; Mahmoud & Grover, 2006; Nyberg, 2000; Ramsey et al., 2004; Scheepens et al., 2001). However, KIGS was the first study that evidenced that GH enhances epileptic seizures progression. This is a consequence of the increase of endogenous GH expression and the signalling of the hormone itself along neuronal circuits, which propagate kindling-stimuli in hippocampus and cortex, but not in the pituitary (Kato et al., 2009). Moreover, the injection of GH into the hippocampus strongly promotes the progression of the kindling, whereas the direct administration of an inhibitor, such as octreotide, elicits a delay in the behavioural development during epileptogenesis (Kato et al., 2009). In particular, GH is involved in a biochemical pathway that seems to affect excitatory postsynaptic potentials on hippocampal synaptic transmission via the modulation of a-amino-3-hydroxy-5-methylisoxazole-4-propionate and NMDA-receptor (Mahmoud & Grover, 2006).

Pathophysiological events, such as ischemia and status epilepticus, increase cell proliferation through insulin-like growth factor-1 (IGF-1). Its expression is up-regulated in the reactive microglia near to the subgranular zone of the dentate gyrus at 2-days after a status epilepticus. It firstly promotes the release of glutamate; secondly, mitogen-activated protein kinase (MAPK) cascade and finally it increases the rate of proliferation of cell's progenitors (Aberg et al., 2000, 2003; Choi et al., 2008; Kurihara et al., 2000). Probably the involvement of GH signalling not regards the GH-receptor (GHR); in fact, an increase of neuronal proliferation in the subgranular zone of the dentate gyrus has been shown in GHR knockout mice (Ransome & Turnley, 2008). The neuronal plasticity related to GH suggests the possibility of therapeutic interventions against neurodegenerative disorders in the older age; however, recent data also indicate that these newly generated neurons are integrated into epileptogenic networks in animal models (Siebzehnrubl & Blumcke, 2008), suggesting that neurogenesis contributes to promote susceptibility to seizures.

2.5 Thyrotropin-releasing hormone

Over the past years, the neuromodulatory role of TRH has been investigated. TRH participates to the regulation of hypothalamic-pituitary-thyroid axis but it is also a neuropeptide and it exerts its functions in the brain, particularly in the hippocampus and in other neural tissues (Gary et al., 2003; Kubek et al., 1977; Nillni & Sevarino, 1999). There are several findings that support an anticonvulsant effect of TRH in the regulation of seizure susceptibility (Jaworska-Feil et al., 1999, 2001; Knoblanch & Kubek, 1997a, 1997b; Kubek et al., 1989; Kubek & Garg, 2002; Wan et al., 1998). Its mechanism of action is poorly understood; however, it seems to be implicated in a protection against neuronal overexcitability. In fact, some authors reported that TRH could inhibit the effects of the glutamate-induced toxicity, in a dose-dependent manner, in cultured fetal rat hippocampal neurons (Pizzi et al., 1999; Veronesi et al., 2007). Furthermore, a paradoxical secretary peak of GH to TRH is more frequent during a status epilepticus. A GH release after an intravenous TRH administration in patients with a status epilepticus suggests an abnormal regulation of GH as a consequence of the long-standing epileptic activity (Lindborn et al., 1999).

2.6 Hypothalamic-pituitary-adrenocortical system

A marked hormonal dysregulation of the hypothalamic-pituitary-adrenocortical system, independent of administered medications, has been found in patients with epilepsy. In fact, in these patients increased circulating levels of cortisol and adrenocorticotropic hormone (ACTH) are measured, relating to a deficient inhibitory feedback system after the suppression by dexamethasone (Zobel et al., 2004). These data have been confirmed by Galimberti and co-workers who reported decreased levels of dehydroepiandrosterone sulphate (DHEAS), in women with frequent seizures; this is not merely due to enzyme-inducing antiepileptic drugs (Galimberti et al., 2005). These findings recognize the involvement of the hippocampus and/or amygdala, which are target regions for the control of hypothalamic-pituitary-adrenocortical system and which contribute to the generation and propagation of seizures (Aliashkevich et al., 2003; Heimer, 2003). Furthermore, repetitive seizures themselves induce a hypothalamic-pituitary-adrenocortical dysfunction, in relation to chronic stressful events, which is independent of the localization of the epileptogenic focus (Checkley, 1996; De Kloet, 1995; Holsboer, 2001; Kudielka et al., 1999).

Increased basal cortisol levels, measured in salivary samples, have been recently described in patients with psychogenic nonepileptic seizures as independent of the acute occurrence of seizures; in addition, a basal hypercortisolism is present in patients with a trauma history, underling an involvement of psychological stress factors (Bakvis et al., 2010). However, further studies about the time of the onset of a blunted inhibitory control of hypothalamic-pituitary-adrenocortical system, are important to understand if this discharge is only a secondary effect of seizures or whether it also determines a susceptibility to epilepsy (Zobel et al., 2004). At this regard, it is known that the hypercortisolism observed in several neuropsychiatric disorders is partially due to reduced neuronal outgrowth and plasticity with a lower hippocampus volume and cognitive deficits (McEwen et al., 1992; Sapolsky, 2000; Sapolsky et al., 1986; Sheline et al., 1996).

In addition, opposite effects on neuron survival have been attributed to cortisol and DHEAS. Cortisol exerts a neurotoxic effect, affecting cerebral glucose metabolism and enhancing calcium influx in hippocampal neurons (McEwen & Magarinos, 1997; Sapolsky et al., 1986). By contrast, DHEAS has a neuroprotective activity, inhibiting GABA-induced chloride transmembrane transport and antagonizing NMDA negative effects on neurons in relation to an increased calcium influx (Baulieu & Robel, 1996; Beyenburg et al., 2001; Kimonides et al., 1998; Mayewska, 1995; Watzka et al., 2000). Thus, these mechanisms are involved in neuron excitability and seizures. However, an intracerebroventricular injection of DHEAS in animals induces seizures (Czlonkowska et al., 2000), so the actual effects in vivo remain further unclear.

Instead it is widely demonstrated that ACTH has a neurotrophic effect, promoting recovery from damages in both the peripheral and central nervous system (Darlington et al., 1996; Kokubo et al., 2002), the ACTH mechanism in epilepsy is not fully understood. It has an anticonvulsant action by itself, enhancing GABA-receptors via deoxycorticosterone synthesis (Rogawski & Reddy, 2002) and downregulating corticothropin releasing hormone (CRH) expression, which is a proconvulsant agent in the immature brain (Baram & Hatalski, 1998). Actually, ACTH is well accepted as an effective therapy for infantile spasms, one of the intractable types of epilepsy that occurs in infancy and early childhood (Mackay et al., 2004).

2.7 Neuropeptide Y

NPY, which is widely distributed throughout the central nervous system, including the hippocampus, is an endogenous anticonvulsant; it is known to prevent seizures in rats (De Quidt & Emson, 1986) by increasing the seizure threshold (Dubè et al., 1999). Although the relationship between NPY and epilepsy has not been completely investigated in humans, the extensively studies in animal models suggest a critical role of NPY in regulating the excessive synaptic excitation associated with an epileptic seizure (Colmers et al., 1987; Haas et al., 1987).

Plasma concentrations of NPY were lower in human patients with atypical febrile convulsions than those with typical ones, suggesting that low NPY levels could increase the risk of long-lasting seizures or recurrent febrile convulsions and make patients more susceptible to epilepsy, independently by gender, both in adults (Lin et al., 2007) and children (Lin et al., 2010).

Recently, ghrelin has been isolated from the stomach and has been recognized as the first endogenous ligand of the GSH-R1a (Korbonits et al., 2004; Weikel et al., 2003). Ghrelin is able to stimulate GH secretion but it also has pleiotropic activities, it influences cardiac and gastrointestinal functions, carbohydrate metabolism, adipose and reproductive tissues, sleep, feeding and energy intake. The control of food and energy intake is mediated by effects on NPY (Korbonits et al., 2004; Tolle et al., 2002; van der Lely et al., 2004; Weikel et al., 2003). Given the relationship between epilepsy and NPY, some authors focused their attention on this new hormone. Actually, the physiologic role of ghrelin in this complex network has not been clearly established and the association between epilepsy and ghrelin is still controversial. However, the recent discovery of ghrelin has provided an important insight to this field and we will focus on these new aspects.

3. Ghrelin regulation and functions

Ghrelin is a 28 amino acid peptide predominantly produced by the stomach, particularly in the A/X-like cells that account for 20-25% of all the endocrine cells in the oxyntic mucosa (Kojima et al., 1999). It was discovered as the first natural ligand of the orphan GHS-R1a, which exerts, through its activation, a strong GH-releasing activity (Howard et al., 1996; Kojima et al., 1999; Kojima & Kangawa, 2005; van der Lely et al., 2004); for its binding to and the activation of the GHS-R1a, the acylation of ghrelin with a medium fatty n-octanoic acid on the Ser3 residue seems to be essential. This mechanism is largely unknown (Kojima et al., 1999; van der Lely et al., 2004). Despite this background, uncylated ghrelin (UAG), which is devoid of the n-octanoil group at Ser3, is the most abundant circulating form and the ratio between UAG and acylated ghrelin (AG) is either 3:1 or 4:1 (Gauna et al., 2004; Kojima et al., 1999; Kojima & Kangawa, 2005; Korbonits et al., 2004). The regulation of AG and UAG circulating levels has not yet been clearly defined. It is thought that UAG could be produced directly from the ghrelin gene, via a different pathway to the acylated form or alternatively it could be derived by the deacylation of ghrelin (Liu et al., 2008; Soares & Leite-Moreira, 2008). Very recently ghrelin O-acyltransferase (GOAT), an enzyme catalyzing the addition of the octanoyl-group, has been identified (Gualillo et al., 2008). It is not known at present whether the GOAT levels regulate changes in ghrelin acylation or, on the contrary, if GOAT itself depends on different metabolic conditions. Originally AG was supposed to be the only biologically active hormonal form (Broglio et al., 2008; Kojima & Kangawa, 2005; van der Lely et al., 2004); however, there is increasing evidence that demonstrates that UAG is also a biologically active molecule, although it is unable to cross the blood brain barrier and to exert a direct action on hypothalamus-pituitary (Broglio et al., 2004a; Gauna et al., 2005; Gil-Campos et al., 2006; Wiedmer et al., 2007). This is consistent with the hypothesis

of the existence of some GHS-R subtypes that are activated independently by the ghrelin's acylation (Kojima et al., 1999; Kojima & Kangawa, 2005; van der Lely et al., 2004).
Ghrelin is predominantly expressed and secreted by the stomach (Kojima et al., 1999), unless during fetal life, when the major site of its production is the endocrine pancreas (Chanoine & Wong, 2004). Ghrelin expression has also been demonstrated in several other tissues, such as adrenal gland, breast, testis, thyroid, myocardium, muscle and colon (Gnanapavan et al., 2002; van der Lely et al., 2004). The ghrelin target, GHS-R1a, is remarkably expressed in the hypothalamus-pituitary unit and, in parallel with ghrelin, it has also been demonstrated in several peripheral endocrine and non-endocrine tissues (van der Lely et al., 2004).
This widespread distribution could mediate the multiple actions of ghrelin. In addition to the GH releasing effect, ghrelin emerged as one of the most powerful orexigenic and adipogenic agents known so far (Arvat et al., 2001; Cummings et al., 2001; Korbonits et al., 2004; Leite-Moreira & Soares, 2007; van der Lely et al., 2004). The NPY and Agouti-related protein (AgRP) co-mediate ghrelin's effects on energy balance in the hypothalamus, in the arcuate nucleus (Chen et al., 2004; Gil-Campos et al., 2006; van der Lely et al., 2004). Furthermore, ghrelin regulation of energy balance also seems to be influenced by efferent and afferent fibers of the vagal nerve and other neuroendocrine factors as orexins, GABA, cocaine-amphetamine regulated transcript (CART) and CRH (Asakawa et al., 2001b; Gil-Campos et al., 2006; Leite-Moreira & Soares, 2007). The adipogenic action of ghrelin consists of an increase in fat mass induced by a reduction of cellular fat oxidation and a promotion of adipogenesis. This action can reflect both its orexigenic action and central modulator effect on energy expenditure (Gil-Campos et al., 2006; Leite-Moreira & Soares, 2007; Thompson et al., 2004; van der Lely et al., 2004; Wiedmer et al., 2007). Furthermore, several studies clearly indicated the existence of direct effects on the adipose tissue (Thompson et al., 2004; van der Lely et al., 2004; W. Zhang et al., 2004); at least in part, this is due to a decrease in fat utilization and an increase in fat tissue content (Leite-Moreira & Soares, 2007; Tschop et al., 2000; van der Lely et al., 2004). Additionally, considering adipose tissue, UAG and AG are active in modulating lipolysis, such both UAG and AG seem to affect in the same way adipocyte function and to determine a lipogenic pattern (Muccioli et al., 2004). In contrast, UAG and AG play opposite effects on food intake, gastric emptying, pancreatic beta-cell secretion and glucose metabolism (Prodam et al., 2008). In fact, if AG may contribute to the worsening of insulin sensitivity, suggesting a diabetogenic function, UAG could exert its metabolic actions counterbalancing those of AG, at least in part at the pancreatic level (Ariyasu et al., 2005; Broglio et al., 2004a; Gauna et al., 2005).
Considering ghrelin regulation, in humans it has a pulsatory secretion, with higher secretion at night-time as it undergoes circadian variations with a decrease following food ingestion that suggests a metabolic control (Cummings, 2006; Cummings et al., 2001; van der Lely et al., 2004). The depth and duration of ghrelin decrease after a meal is related to the total amount of calories ingested and to the type of the macronutrients, such as carbohydrates and proteins in spite of less effective suppression led by lipids (Prodam et al., 2006; Leite-Moreira & Soares, 2007; van der Lely et al., 2004). In particular, meals inhibited secretion of both AG and UAG. Acylation may be regulated independently of secretion by nutrient availability in the gut or by esterases that cleave the acyl-group (Liu et al., 2008). Furthermore, ghrelin secretion is also under cholinergic control (Broglio et al., 2004b) and it is regulated by other factors that are involved in energy balance and metabolism, such as glucan-like peptide 1 (GLP-1), peptide YY (PYY), oxyntomodulin, urocortin, thyroid hormones, glucocorticoids, insulin and gonadal steroids (Baldelli et al., 2006; Gil-Campos et

al., 2006; Korbonits et al., 2004; Leite-Moreira & Soares, 2007; van der Lely et al., 2004; Wiedmer et al., 2007).

As mentioned below, the circulating levels of ghrelin are firstly modulated by energy balance and nutrition status; in particular, ghrelin levels are negatively associated with body mass index, with ghrelin secretion increased in anorexia and cachexia and reduced in obesity, with normalization achieved through the recovery to an ideal body weight (Tschop et al., 2001; Leite-Moreira & Soares, 2007; van der Lely et al., 2004). Furthermore, circadian ghrelin secretion is abnormal in obesity, as there is an absent or an altered ghrelin elevation during fasting (Perreault et al., 2004) and an abolished or a blunted increase during the night or sleep deprivation (Vazquez et al., 2006; Yildiz et al., 2004) and blunted suppression following a meal (English et al., 2002). The most likely explanations could be that low ghrelin levels in essential obesity are related to increased insulin resistance and consequent hyperinsulinemia with weight excess. However, it may also reflect a compensatory mechanism by communicating to central regulatory centres that energy stores are sufficiently filled (Cummings, 2006; van der Lely et al., 2004). Therefore, conditions characterized by insulin resistance, such as polycystic ovarian syndrome (Pagotto et al., 2002), type 2 diabetes and metabolic syndrome (Erdmann et al., 2005; Langenberg et al., 2005), have low ghrelin levels too.

The only clinical exception to this picture is the Prader-Willi syndrome, a complex multi-systemic genetic disease caused by the lack of expression of paternally inherited genes imprinted and located in the chromosome 15q11-q13 region (Goldstone et al., 2008; Nicholls et al., 1989). Although genotype-phenotype correlations have been widely described, it can be summarized that Prader-Willi syndrome is characterized by typical features including neonatal hypotonia, uncontrolled and precocious hyperphagia, severe obesity with typical fat distribution, short stature, hypogonadism and other somatic, endocrine and psychological problems (Goldstone et al., 2004; Goldstone et al., 2008). These many phenotypes may depend on hypothalamus-pituitary and brain signalling derangements (Bellone et al., 2011). Interestingly, it has to be underlined that the Prader-Willi syndrome neuroendocrine and metabolic patterns are partly different to what occurs in simple obesity; in fact, unlike essential obesity, patients with Prader-Willi syndrome show elevated ghrelin levels (DelParigi et al., 2002; Goldstone, 2004; Paik et al., 2004, 2006). Since the exact pathogenetic mechanism leading to the Prader-Willi syndrome phenotype are at present unknown, ghrelin hypersecretion has been obviously hypothesized to participate in the development of at least some symptoms such as hyperphagia and weight excess (DelParigi et al., 2002; Paik et al., 2004). However, growing data suggested that hyperghrelinemia in Prader-Willi syndrome could be more likely a compensatory mechanism to other biochemical and hormonal alterations, in particular neonatal hypoglycaemia and relative hypoinsulinemia, to restore normal glucose levels or glucose sensing (Bellone et al., 2011).

Several studies also suggested that ghrelin is one of the mediators of behaviours linked to food intake and body weight and of those associated with psychological stress, mood and anxiety (Chuang & Zigman, 2010). In fact, ghrelin rises in response to stressful events both in mice (Lutter et al., 2008b) and humans (Rouach et al., 2007). It has been proposed that higher ghrelin levels help in promoting antidepressant-like behavioural adaptations (Lutter et al., 2008b); for example it increases neuronal activity in brain reward centers in humans when images of appealing food are shown (Malik et al., 2008). Studies about the relationship between ghrelin and mood showed that a GSH-R1a polymorphism is related to major depressive disorders (Nakashima et al., 2008). Mechanisms by which ghrelin is able to modulate mood are not completely explained; however, ghrelin's action on mood seems to be due to: 1) direct and indirect feedbacks on the orexin system; 2) interactions with neuronal circuits involved in motivation and rewards; 3) effects on reward-associated memories and the ability to experience pleasure; 4) modulation of hippocampal neurogenesis and brain inflammation (Lutter et al., 2008a, 2008b; Chuang & Zigman, 2010). By contrast, other studies suggested that rising ghrelin would contribute to the development of stress-induced depression and anxiety (Asakawa et al., 2001a; Carlini et al., 2002, 2004; Carvajal et al., 2009).

Furthermore, increasing evidence indicates that ghrelin not only plays a role in anxiety and stress, but it is also involved in promoting learning behaviour and memory processes and in sleep-wake regulation (Steiger et al., 2011). In particular, a sleep-promoting potential of ghrelin has been supported (Steiger et al., 2011). Szentirmai and co-workers reported that ghrelin knock out rodents sleep less than wild type ones (Szentirmai et al., 2007). In according to a sleep-promoting effect of ghrelin, knockout mice for ghrelin had impaired physiologic sleep regulation and thermoregulatory responses too. Thus, in response to fasting at 17 °C, these knockout mice presented hypothermic bousts associated with a reduced sleep (Szentirmai et al., 2009).

Furthermore, also previous studies in humans suggested a sleep-promoting effect of ghrelin, with the evidence of its peaks around the sleep onset (Dzaja et al., 2004). This finding was not supported by Schussler and co-workers, who described in subjects with higher nocturnal ghrelin levels, a lower time spent in the stage 1 of sleep that means shallow sleep suggesting a promotion of sleep by ghrelin (Schussler et al., 2005). Schussler and co-workers also showed increased ghrelin levels during the recovery night after a sleep deprivation period, supporting the idea that an endogenous substance diverse from ghrelin accumulates during the sleep deprivation and it is a candidate to be a promoting factor of sleep. Higher ghrelin levels in sleep deprivation, in association with other hormonal derangements, could be a root cause of the dysregulation of hunger, appetite and metabolism linked to sleep loss or sleep alterations (Van Cauter et al., 2008; Van Cauter & Knutson, 2008). In addition, ghrelin levels are lower in the insomnia patients across the night (Motivala et al., 2009).

In conclusion, the action of ghrelin includes much more than the energetic homeostasis and affects a more complex pathway not yet known.

4. Ghrelin and epilepsy: In vitro and in animal studies

A relationship between ghrelin and epilepsy has been demonstrated in animal and human models, although the results are still controversial (Dag et al., 2010).

Some studies suggested an anticonvulsant effect of ghrelin. In fact, the intraperitoneally injection of ghrelin was able to delay or prevent the development of pentylenetetrazole (PTZ)-induced seizures in rats, supporting the hypothesis of an inhibitory effect on the emergence and the severity of seizures. However, dose-dependent ghrelin administrations reduced but not completely abolished the intensity of PTZ-induced seizures in rats (Obay et al., 2007). The mechanism related to the antiepileptic and the preventive role of ghrelin has been explained, firstly, through the enhancing of NPY and GABA activity in the brain (Cowley et al., 2003). In the arcuate nucleus of the hypothalamus, ghrelin fibers form axo-somatic and axo-dendritic contacts with both proopiomelanocortin (POMC) and NPY/AgRP neurons (Cowley et al., 2003). The direct link between the brain-derived ghrelin and the central melanocortin system has been supported by electrophysiological demonstration: ghrelin increases the firing of arcuate NPY/AgRP neurons, which increase GABA-ergic inhibitory post-synaptic currents into POMC neurons (Cowley et al., 2001). Secondly, ghrelin can be considered as an anticonvulsant agent by stimulating vagal nerve (Macdonalds, 1997). In fact vagal nerve stimulations are associated with a reduction of the seizure frequency more than 50% in about 30% of patients who are refractory to epilepsy treatments (Ben-Menachem et al., 1999; Handforth et al., 1998; Morris & Mueller, 1999).

The oxidative stress in the central nervous system in relation to discharges in the epileptic rat brain has been reported in several rodent models of epilepsy (Bruce & Baudry, 1995; Erakovic et al., 2003; Singh & Pathak, 1990; Veerendra Kumar & Gupta, 2003). At this regard, there is emerging evidence that oxidative stress and mitochondrial dysfunctions result as a consequence and a cause of seizures (Patel, 2002). In fact, free oxygen radicals contribute to the genesis of seizure activity by direct inactivation of glutamine synthase and glutamate decarboxylase, such promoting an abnormal build-up of excitatory (glutamate) and inhibitory GABA neurotransmitters (Atmaca & Fry, 1996; Oliver et al., 1990; Sudha et al., 2001). In addition, seizure itself is associated with an important production of reactive oxygen species (Mueller et al., 2001). It has also been suggested that oxidative stress could occur during anticonvulsant therapies, likely related to detrimental effects on the antioxidant defence system, in particular with a significant decrease in plasma glutathione levels (Ono et al., 2000; Uma Devi et al., 2006). In the light of this knowledge, Obay and co-workers supported the hypothesis that ghrelin might be an antioxidant and an anti-inflammatory agent therefore it exerted protective effects in PTZ-induced epileptic rats (ISeri et al., 2005; Obay et al., 2007). In particular, in PTZ-induced epileptic rats there was an increase in the oxidative stress, with higher lipid peroxidation in erythrocytes, liver and brain tissues, whereas enzymes which have antioxidant activities (superoxide dismutase - SOD, catalase -CAT) and glutathione levels were significantly reduced; all these alterations are prevented by an intraperitoneally ghrelin pretreatment (Obay et al., 2008).

Recently, neuroprotective effects of ghrelin on pilocarpine-induced seizures in rodent models have also been investigated (Xu et al., 2009). Pilocarpine-induced seizures cause a neuronal loss in the hippocampus and ghrelin seems to be able to protect hippocampal neurons against this cell death. According with previous studies reporting that ghrelin activates the phosphoinositide-3-kinase (PI3K)/Akt pathway in hypothamalamic neurons (Chung et al., 2007), a mechanism which plays a central role in intracellular processes such as survival and proliferation (Cuevas et al., 2001; Franke et al., 1997; Henshall et al., 2002), it has been demonstrated that ghrelin strongly up-regulates the seizure-induced decrease in phospho-PI3K and phospho-Akt in the hippocampus, rescuing neuronal cells from death induced by seizures (Xu et al., 2009). Furthermore, anti-apoptotic actions of ghrelin are also confirmed by data of the effects on mithocondrial pathways (Miao et al., 2007; Xu et al., 2009; Y. Zhang et al., 2007). In particular, pilocarpine-induced seizures result in increased Bax and decreased Bcl-2 with consequentially a decreased ratio of Bcl-2 to Bax and an activation of caspase-3 in the hippocampus at 24 h after pilocarpine treatments. The ghrelin pretreatment prevents the decreased ratio of Bcl-2 to Bax induced by seizures and inhibits caspase-3 activation, such protecting by the hippocampal neuronal damage (Xu et al., 2009). However, it is unclear whether the neuroprotective effect of ghrelin is due to the activation of the GHS-R1a or of an unknown receptor in hippocampus (Xu et al., 2009).

Ghrelin also prevents the kainic acid-induced activation of microglia and astrocytes and the expression of pro-inflammatory mediators as well as tumor necrosis factor alpha, interleukin-1bheta and cyclooxygenase-2 with the inhibition of the matrix

metalloproiteinase-3 expression which is related to the damaged of hippocampal neurons (Lee et al., 2010).
A recent study showed not only the effect of ghrelin in the penicillin-induced seizures, confirming its antiepileptic action but also the role of nitric oxide (NO) on the effect of ghrelin (Aslan et al., 2009). In fact, several effects exerted by ghrelin involve NO pathway by stimulating NO synthesis (Korbonits et al., 2004) whom role has also been investigated in neurological diseases such as epilepsy (Bosnak et al., 2007; Gaskin et al., 2003; Korbonits et al., 2004; S. E. Smith et al., 1996). Indeed, the antiepileptiform activity of ghrelin was reversed by a non specific nitric oxide synthase inhibitor (L-NAME), but not by a selective neuronal nitric oxide synthase inhibitor (7-NI). This evidence indicated that ghrelin could need an activation by the endothelial nitric oxide synthase (NOS)/NO route in the brain and suggested NO as an intermediate effector in the functional balance between excitatory and inhibitory neurotransmitter systems related to ghrelin (Aslan et al., 2009).
Some studies have been conduced also in animals focusing on regulation of ghrelin secretion in epilepsy or after seizures. Blood AG levels decreased after the PTZ-induced seizures in rats with a similar but not significant trend for UAG and total blood ghrelin levels (Ataie et al., 2011). These decreases could be modulated by hormones which inhibit the production, acylation or secretion of ghrelin, such as somatostatin and leptin (Ataie et al., 2011). Somatostatin, preferentially released from neurons under conditions of high neuronal activation, for example during seizures (Vezzani & Hoyer, 1999), is able to blunt ghrelin secretion in animals (Shimada et al., 2003; Silva et al., 2005; van der Lely et al., 2004) and humans (Broglio et al., 2002, 2007; van der Lely et al., 2004). In addition, it has been reported that somatostatin decreases the GOAT expression (Gahete et al., 2010; Gualillo et al., 2008). Then, a rapid rebound of UAG levels respect to those of AG, related to this mechanism, may explain the partial reduction of UAG and total ghrelin levels after the PTZ-induced seizure (Ataie et al., 2011). Moreover, some studies described high serum leptin levels in rats after seizures (Bhatt et al., 2005; Hum et al., 2009), which could directly inhibit ghrelin secretion as shown in other animal models (Kamegai et al., 2004). Another possible explanation about lower AG blood levels, is an increased uptake of AG by brain structures influenced by pathophysiological events to modulate epileptic discharges (Ataie et al., 2011; Banks et al., 2002). Furthermore, other mechanisms such as proteolysis of AG and degradation into non-UAG metabolities could occurr during seizures (De Vriese et al., 2004; Ni et al., 2010); both of them may contribute to the reduction of blood ghrelin levels immediately after the epileptic seizures in animals (Ataie et al., 2011).
In conclusion, ghrelin can be considered as a neuroprotective agent, exerting antiepileptic, antioxidant or anti-inflammatory properties at least in vitro and in animal models. However, the anticonvulsant ghrelin mechanism has not been yet completely understood, in particular the regulation of its secretion after seizures.

5. Ghrelin and epilepsy in humans

The attention of researchers has been directed to investigate the role of ghrelin in epilepsy firstly in animals and secondly in humans.
In one of the first studies in epileptic subjects, serum total ghrelin levels were higher in patients than in controls, in contrast to data in animal models (Ataie et al., 2011; Berilgen et al., 2006; Obay et al., 2007). In addition to its effect on weight regulation and glucose and lipid metabolism, ghrelin has also been shown to act on the release of GH, ACTH and PRL

(Arvat et al., 2001; Korbonits et al., 2004, van der Lely et al., 2004). Besides, it is proposed that higher ghrelin levels could facilitate the emergence of seizures by affecting GH and PRL secretion and by disrupting hormonal homeostasis (Berilgen et al., 2006). Furthermore, ghrelin has been described as a factor in sleep regulation able to promote the slow-wave sleep and prolong non rapid eye movements (NREM) sleep during the night (Weikel et al., 2003; Van Cauter et al., 2008; Van Cauter & Knutson, 2008). Therefore, higher serum levels of ghrelin in epileptic patients might be interpreted as a contributing factor to the genesis of seizures, considering that NREM is the stage in which seizures tend to occur (Berilgen et al., 2006). Finally, authors suggested that higher serum ghrelin levels indicate a predisposition toward seizure activity (Berilgen et al., 2006).

Greco and co-workers reported that circulating ghrelin levels in epileptic patients treated with valproic acid were decreased and they were significantly lower than those of patients who did not gain weight; however, this study did not rule out whether lower ghrelin levels were due to weight accrual or puberty (Greco et al., 2005). Taking into account antiepileptic treatments and weight, another study demonstrated that circulating ghrelin levels were decreased in young epileptic prepubertal normal weight children treated with carbamazepine and valproic acid during the first years of therapy, prior to and independent of a consistent drug-induced weight gain (Ness-Abramof & Apovian, 2005; Prodam et al., 2009). The choice to enrol only young prepubertal children was related to avoid the well-known modulation of ghrelin secretion by pubertal stage and age (van der Lely et al., 2004). In fact, the study of Berilgen and co-workers showed controversial results considering all epileptic subjects from childhood to adulthood and their data may be explained by a multitude of factors including the recruitment of an older population with a longer history of antiepileptic therapy and the different auxological stages (Berilgen et al., 2006; Prodam et al., 2009). Moreover, although ghrelin levels were reduced in the entire sample, patients under treatment with valproic acid showed higher ghrelin levels than those under carbamazepine, suggesting an involvement of valproic acid in a positive feedback regulation of ghrelin levels (Berilgen et al., 2006; Prodam et al., 2009).

This study also demonstrated a positive correlation between lower ghrelin levels and the negative variation of the height standard deviation score with respect to the baseline of therapy with carbamazepine in patients who were drug-naïve, hypothesizing that lower ghrelin levels could worsen the variation height standard deviation score (Prodam et al., 2009).

The fact that physical growth seems to be affected in paediatrics patients with epilepsy also emerges in a study recently performed by El-Khayat and co-workers (El-Khayat et al., 2010). Height was lower in patients with epilepsy and they presented significantly lower levels of GH and IGF-1 after provocation with L-dopa compared to the control group (El-Khayat et al., 2010). Actually, the question arises whether the decreased GH release might be related to the direct negative effect on the hypothalamus-pituitary axis due to seizure activity per se or to antiepileptic drugs. Likely, these findings can be explained as a consequence of a hormonal imbalance related to both events (El-Khayat et al., 2010). A possible mechanism is the reduction of GABA concentration and of GABA receptor binding that are both demonstrated in cortical epileptic specimens (Bakay & Harris, 1981). In fact, GABA agonists are able to stimulate GH release (Tamminga et al., 1978). Instead, the possible role of enzyme inducing antiepileptic drugs on promoting GH metabolism wasn't evident in this study (El-Khayat et al., 2010). The reduction of height associated with lower GH and IGF-1 levels in children with epilepsy might be a consequence of lower ghrelin levels or of a blunted ghrelin action on pituitary (van der Lely et al., 2004; Zizzari et al., 2005).

The most recent study was designed to indicate candidate biomarkers for the diagnosis of epilepsy and for the monitoring of the response to anticonvulsant drugs, dosing ghrelin and other hormones with simpler and non-invasive tests (Aydin et al., 2009). Besides, Aydin and co-workers recorded lower ghrelin levels in serum and saliva, in association with higher serum and saliva levels of nesfatin-1 (Aydin et al., 2009). Nesfatin-1 is a satiety hormone recently discovered, expressed in hypothalamic nuclei (Kohno et al., 2008; Oh-I et al., 2006; Pan et al., 2007; T. O. Price et al., 2007) in epileptic patients. These results were more evident before the starting of antiepileptic treatments and they weren't explained yet. However, it has been hypothesized that an excessive release of nesfatin-1 might cause an excitotoxicity, stimulating hyperpolarization and depolarization in paraventricular and arcuate nuclei (T. O. Price et al., 2007; C. J. Price et al., 2008). However, the question whether higher nesfatin-1 and lower ghrelin levels are a root cause of epilepsy or epilepsy modulates them has not been answered yet (Aydin et al., 2009).

Similar results were reported by Dag and co-workers who showed that serum chromogranin A and obestatin were up-regulated whereas serum total ghrelin were down-regulated in epileptic patients previously or currently treated with drugs, with salivary hormone concentrations resembling those in serum (Dag et al., 2010). Chromogranin A is an acidic glycoprotein located in the secretary vesicles of neurons and endocrine cells (Hendy et al., 1995), actually known as a stress indicator (Zheng & Moritani, 2008). Instead, obestatin, a bioactive peptide hormone, derives from the pre-proghrelin sequence and it is also involved in a wide range of physiological functions. It was considered as a ghrelin antagonist but more recent findings not confirm this role (Tang et al., 2008; J. V. Zhang et al., 2005). The exact mechanism of the relationship between ghrelin and obestatin has not been completely explained, in particular in epileptic patients. An important unresolved question is why ghrelin and obestatin levels do not show parallel decrements or increments since they are products of the same gene (Dag et al., 2010). However, also these data supported that ghrelin levels are reduced in epilepsy and that saliva might be a good alternative for measuring these hormones in the diagnosis and follow-up of epilepsy (Dag et al., 2010).

In addition, some authors found reduced high density lipoprotein (HDL)-cholesterol serum levels in epileptic patients (Aydin et al., 2009; Dag et al., 2010); so a parallel decrease both in ghrelin and HDL-cholesterol concentrations may be expected, because ghrelin is a HDL-cholesterol-associated hormone (Beaumont et al., 2003).

Therefore, more studies are needed to clarify the complex pathway system involved in epilepsy and, in particular, the exact role of ghrelin and obestatin.

6. Conclusions

Epilepsy and antiepileptic drugs affect the neuroendocrine system and seizure threshold may be alterated in relation to these hormonal modifications. Actually, the knowledge about neuroendocrine regulation in epilepsy is far to be complete and it is yet elusive. However, current findings suggest a complex network in which hormones play a crucial role as both as a cause and as a consequence of the epileptic activity. Thus, further studies are needed, in particular to fully define the role of new identified hormones, as ghrelin. Since the current knowledge, the effects of ghrelin include much more than those on pituitary and energy homeostasis. Increasing evidence indicates that ghrelin plays a role in anxiety and stress, in promoting learning behaviour, memory processes and sleep-wake regulation. Considering ghrelin pleiotropic functions, it has a relationship with epilepsy and seizures. Actually, the results of the studies in vitro and in vivo are still controversial. However, it could be assured that ghrelin has anticonvulsant properties. In fact, focusing on regulation of ghrelin secretion in epilepsy or after seizure activity, blood ghrelin levels are shown decreased both in experimental epileptic rodents and in humans. Therefore ghrelin results as a neuroprotective agent, exerting antiepileptic, antioxidant and anti-inflammatory effects on neuronal brain cells. A better understanding of ghrelin's activities may help to develop new therapeutic approaches to epilepsy, the most common neurological problem worldwide and, in particular, to refractory seizure forms.

7. Acknowledgements

This study was supported by Regione Piemonte and University of Piemonte Orientale Amedeo Avogadro. The Authors wish to thank Gillian Walker, Valentina Agarla and Caterina Balossini for their technical assistance.

8. References

Aberg, MA., Aberg, ND., Hedbäcker, H., Oscarsson, J. & Eriksson, PS. (2000). Peripheral infusion of IGF-1 selectively induces neurogenesis in the adult rat hippocampus. *The Journal of Neuroscience,* Vol.20, No.8, pp. 2896-2903, ISNN 0270-6474

Aberg, MA., Aberg, ND., Palmer, TD., Alborn, AM., Carlsson-Skwirut, C., Bang, P., Rosengren, LE., Olsson, T., Gage, FH. & Eriksson, PS. (2003). IGF-1 has a direct proliferative effect in adult hippocampal progenitor cells. *Molecular and Cellular Neuroscience,* Vol.24, No.1, pp. 23-40

Abbott, RJ., Browning, MC. & Davidson, DL. (1980). Serum prolactin and cortisol concentrations after grand mal seizures. *Journal of Neurolology, Neurosurgery and Psychiatry,* Vol.43, No.2, pp. 163-167, ISNN 1468-330X

Aliashkevich, AF., Yilmazer-Hanke, D., Van Roost, D., Mundhenk, B., Schramm, J. & Blümcke, I. (2003). Cellular pathology of amygdala neurons in human temporal lobe epilepsy. *Acta Neuropathologica,* Vol.106, No.2, pp. 99-106

Ariyasu, H., Takaya, K., Iwakura, H., Hosoda, H., Akamizu, T., Arai, Y., Kangawa, K. & Nakao, K. (2005). Transgenic mice overexpressing des-acyl ghrelin show small phenotype. *Endocrinology,* Vol.146, No.1, pp. 355-364

Arvat, E., Maccario, M., Di Vito, L., Broglio, F., Benso, A., Gottero, C., Papotti, M., Muccioli, G., Dieguez, C., Casanueva, FF., Deghenghi, R., Camanni, F. & Ghigo, E. (2001). Endocrine activities of ghrelin, a natural growth hormone secretagogue (GHS), in humans: comparison and interactions with hexarelin, a non-natural peptidyl GHS, and GH-releasing hormone. *The Journal of Clinical Endocrinology & Metabolism,* Vol.86, No.3, pp. 1169-1174

Asakawa, A., Inui, A., Kaga, T., Yuzuriha, H., Nagata, T., Fujimiya, M., Katsuura, G., Makino, S., Fujino, MA. & Kasuga, M. (2001a). A role of ghrelin in neuroendocrine and behavioral responses to stress in mice. *Neuroendocrinology,* Vol.74, No.3, pp. 143-147

Asakawa, A., Inui, A., Kaga, T., Yuzuriha, H., Nagata, T., Ueno, N., Makino, S., Fujimiya, M., Niijima, A., Fujino, MA. & Kasuga, M. (2001b). Ghrelin is an appetite-stimulatory signal from stomach with structural resemblance to motilin. *Gastroenterology*, Vol.120, No.2, pp. 337-345

Aslan, A., Yildirim, M., Ayyildiz, M., Güven, A. & Agar, E. (2009). The role of nitric oxide in the inhibitory effect of ghrelin against penicillin-induced epileptiform activity in rat. *Neuropeptides*, Vol.43, No.4, pp. 295-302

Ataie, Z., Golzar, MG., Babri, S., Ebrahimi, H. & Mohaddes, G. (2011). Does ghrelin level change after epileptic seizure in rats? *Seizure*, [Epub ahead of print], doi:10.1016/j.seizure.2011.01.001

Atmaca, M. & Fry, JR. (1996). Adenosine-mediated inhibition of glutathione synthesis in rat isolated hepatocytes. *Biochemical Pharmacology*,Vol.52, No.9, pp. 1423-1428

Aydin, S., Dag, E., Ozkan, Y., Erman, F., Dagli, AF., Kilic, N., Sahin, I., Karatas, F., Yoldas, T., Barim, AO. & Kendir, Y. (2009). Nesfatin-1 and ghrelin levels in serum and saliva of epileptic patients: hormonal changes can have a major effect on seizure disorders. *Molecular and Cellular Biochemistry*, Vol.328, No.1-2, pp. 49-56

Bäckström, T., Zetterlund, B., Blom, S. & Romano, M. (1984). Effects of intravenous progesterone infusions on the epileptic discharge frequency in women with partial epilepsy. *Acta Neurologica Scandinavica*, Vol.69, No.4, pp. 240-248

Bakay, RA. & Harris, AB. (1981). Neurotransmitter, receptor and biochemical changes in monkey cortical epileptic foci. *Brain Research*, Vol.206, No.2, pp. 387-404

Bakvis, P., Spinhoven, P., Giltay, EJ., Kuyk, J., Edelbroek, PM., Zitman, FG. & Roelofs, K. (2010). Basal hypercortisolism and trauma in patients with psychogenic nonepileptic seizures. *Epilepsia*, Vol.51, No.5, pp. 752-759

Baldelli, R., Bellone, S., Castellino, N., Petri, A., Rapa, A., Vivenza, D., Bellone, J., Broglio, F., Ghigo, E. & Bona, G. (2006). Oral glucose load inhibits circulating ghrelin levels to the same extent in normal and obese children. *Clinical Endocrinology* (Oxf), Vol.64, No.3, pp. 255-259

Banks, WA., Tschöp, M., Robinson, SM. & Heiman, ML. (2002). Extent and direction of ghrelin transport across the blood-brain barrier is determined by its unique primary structure. *The Journal of Pharmacology and Experimental Therapetics*, Vol.302, No.2, pp. 822-827, ISSN 0022-3565

Baram, TZ. & Hatalski, CG. (1998). Neuropeptide-mediated excitability: a key triggering mechanism for seizure generation in the developing brain. *Trends in Neurosciences*, Vol.21, No.11, pp. 471-476

Bauer, J. & Cooper-Mahkorn, D. (2008). Reproductive dysfunction in women with epilepsy: menstrual cycle abnormalities, fertility, and polycystic ovary syndrome. *International Reviews of Neurobiology*, Vol.83, pp. 135-155

Baulieu, EE. & Robel, P. (1996). Dehydroepiandrosterone and dehydroepiandrosterone sulfate as neuroactive neurosteroids. *Journal of Endocrinology*, Vol.50, pp. S221-239

Beaumont, NJ., Skinner, VO., Tan, TM., Ramesh, BS., Byrne, DJ., MacColl, GS., Keen, JN., Bouloux, PM., Mikhailidis, DP., Bruckdorfer, KR., Vanderpump, MP. & Srai, KS. (2003). Ghrelin can bind to a species of high density lipoprotein associated with paraoxonase. *The Journal of Biological Chemistry,* Vol.278, No.11, pp. 8877-8880, ISSN 0021-9258

Beck, H. & Elger, CE. (2008). Epilepsy research: a window onto function to and dysfunction of the human brain. *Dialogues in Clinical Neuroscience,* Vol.10, No.1, pp. 7-15

Bellone, S., Busti, A., Belcastro, S., Aimaretti, G., Bona, G. & Prodam, F. (2011). Children obesity, glucose tolerance, ghrelin and Prader-Willi syndrome, In: *Global perspective on childhood obesity,* Debasis Bagchi, pp. 191-200, Elsevier, ISBN 978-0-12-374985-6

Ben-Menachem, E., Hellström, K., Waldton, C. & Augustinsson, LE. (1999). Evaluation of refractory epilepsy treated with vagus nevre stimulation for up to 5 years. *Neurology,* Vol.52, No.6, pp. 265-267

Berilgen, MS., Mungen, B., Ustundag, B. & Demir, C. (2006). Serum ghrelin levels are enhanced in patients with epileptic patients. *Seizure,* Vol.15, No.2, pp. 106-111

Beyenburg, S., Stoffel-Wagner, B., Bauer, J., Watzka, M., Blümcke, I., Bidlingmaier, F. & Elger, CE. (2001). Neuroactive steroids and seizure susceptibility. *Epilepsy Research,* Vol.44, No.2-3, pp. 141-153

Bhatt, R., Bhatt, S., Rameshwar, P. & Siegel, A. (2005). Long-term kindled seizures induce alterations in hematopoietic functions: role of serum leptin. *Epilepsy Research,* Vol.65, pp. 169-178

Bilo, L., Meo, R., Nappi, C., Annunziato, L., Striano, S., Colao, AM., Merola, B. & Buscaino, GA. (1988). Reproductive endocrine disorders in women with primary generalized epilepsy. *Epilepsia,* Vol.29, No.5, pp. 612-619

Bosnak, M., Ayyildiz, M., Yildirim, M. & Agar, E. (2007). The role of nitric oxide in the anticonvulsant effects of pyridoxine on penicillin-induced epileptiform activity in rats. *Epilepsy Research,* Vol.76, No.1, pp. 49-59

Broglio, F., Koetsveld, Pv P., Benso, A., Gottero, C., Prodam, F., Papotti, M., Muccioli, G., Gauna, C., Hofland, L., Deghenghi, R., Arvat, E., van der Lely, AJ. & Ghigo, E. (2002). Ghrelin secretion is inibited by either somatostatin or cortistatin in humans. *The Journal of Clinical Endocrinology and Metabolism,* Vol.87, No.10, pp. 4829-4832

Broglio, F., Gottero, C., Prodam, F., Gauna, C., Muccioli, G., Papotti, M., Abribat, T., van der Lely, AJ. & Ghigo, E. (2004a). Non-acylated ghrelin counteracts the metabolic but not the neuroendocrine response to acylated ghrelin in humans. *The Journal of Clinical Endocrinology and Metabolism,* Vol.89, No.6, pp. 3062-3065

Broglio, F., Gottero, C., Van Koetsveld, P., Prodam, F., Destefanis, S., Benso, A., Gauna, C., Hofland, L., Arvat, E., van der Lely, AJ. & Ghigo, E. (2004b). Acetylcholine regulates ghrelin secretion in humans. *The Journal of Clinical Endocrinology and Metabolism,* Vol. 89, No.5, pp. 2429-2433

Broglio, F., Papotti, M., Muccioli, G. & Ghigo, E. (2007). Brain-gut communication: cortistatin, somatostatin and ghrelin. *Trends in Endocrinology & Metabolism,* Vol.18, No.6, pp. 246-251

Broglio, F., Prodam, F., Riganti, F., Gottero, C., Destefanis, S., Granata, R., Muccioli, G., Abribat, T., van der Lely, AJ. & Ghigo, E. (2008). The continuous infusion of acylated ghrelin enhances GH secretion and worsen glucose metabolism in humans. *Journal Endocrinological Investigation,* Vol.31, No.9, pp. 788-794

Browne, TR. & Holmes, GL. (2000). *Handbook of Epilepsy* (2nd Edition), Lippicott Williams & Wilkins, ISBN-13 978-0-7817-7397-3, Philadelphia

Bruce, AJ. & Baudry, M. (1995). Oxygen free radicals in rat limbic structures after kainite-induces seizures. *Free Radical Biology and Medicine,* Vol.18, pp. 993-1002

Carlini, VP., Monzón, ME., Varas, MM., Cragnolini, AB., Schiöth, HB., Scimonelli, TN. & de Barioglio, SR. (2002). Ghrelin increases anxiety-like behavior and memory retentions in rats. *Biochemical and Biophysical Research Communications,* Vol.299, No.5, pp. 739-743

Carlini, VP., Varas, MM., Cragnolini, AB., Schiöth, HB., Scimonelli, TN. & de Barioglio, SR. (2004). Differential role of the hippocampus, amygdala, and dorsal raphe nucleus in regulating feeding, memory, and anxiety-like behavioral responses to ghrelin. *Biochemical and Biophysical Research Communications,* Vol.313, No.3, pp. 635-641

Carvajal, P., Carlini, VP., Schiöth, HB., de Barioglio, SR. & Salvatierra, NA. (2009). Central ghrelin increases anxiety in the Open Field test and impairs retention memory in a passive avoidance task in neonatal chicks. *Neurobiology of Learning and Memory,* Vol.91, No.4, pp. 402-407

Chang, BS. & Lowenstein, DH. (2003). Epilepsy. *The New England Journal of Medicine,* Vol.349, No.13, pp. 1257-1266

Chanoine, JP. & Wong, AC. (2004). Ghrelin gene expression is markedly higher in fetal pancreas compared with fetal stomach: effect of maternal fasting. *Endocrinology,* Vol.145, No.8, pp. 3813-3820

Checkley, S. (1996). The neuroendocrinology of depression and chronic stress. *British Medical Bullettin,* Vol.52, No.3, pp. 597-617

Chen, HY., Trumbauer, ME., Chen, AS., Weingarth, DT., Adams, JR., Frazier, EG., Shen, Z., Marsh, DJ., Feighner, SD., Guan, XM., Ye, Z., Nargund, RP., Smith, RG., Van der Ploeg, LH., Howard, AD., MacNeil, DJ. & Qian, S. (2004). Orexogenic functions of peripheral ghrelin is mediated by neuropeptide Y and Agouti-related protein. *Endocrinology,* Vol.145, No.6, pp. 2607-2612

Choi, YS., Cho, HY., Hoyt, KR., Naegele, JR. & Obrietan, K. (2008). IGF-1 Receptor-mediated ERK/MAPK signaling couples status epilepticus to progenitor cell proliferation in the subgranular layer of the dentate gyrus. *Glia,* Vol.56, No.7, pp. 791-800

Chuang, JC. & Zigman, JM. (2010). Ghrelin's roles in stress, mood, and anxiety regulation. *International Journal of Peptides,* ID 460549, doi: 10.1155/2010/460549

Chung, H., Kim, E., Lee, DH., Seo, S., Ju, S., Lee, D., Kim, H. & Park, S. (2007) Ghrelin inhibits apoptosis in hypothalamic neuronal cells during oxygen-glucose deprivation. *Endocrinology,* Vol.148, No.1, pp. 148-159

Clayton, PE. & Cowell, CT. (2000). Safety issues in children and adolescents during growth hormone therapy: a review. *Growth Hormone & IGF Research,* Vol.10, No.6, pp. 306-317

Cowley, MA., Smart, JL., Rubinstein, M., Cerdán, MG., Diano, S., Horvath, TL., Cone, RD. & Low, MJ. (2001). Leptin activates anorexigenic POMC neurons through a neutral network in the arcuate nucleus. *Nature,* Vol.411, No.6836, pp. 480-484

Cowley, MA., Smith, RG., Diano, S., Tschöp, M., Pronchuk, N., Grove, KL., Strasburger, CJ., Bidlingmaier, M., Esterman, M., Heiman, ML., Garcia-Segura, LM., Nillni, EA., Mendez, P., Low, MJ., Sotonyi, P., Friedman, JM., Liu, H., Pinto, S., Colmers, WF., Cone, RD. & Horvath, TL. (2003). The distribution and mechanism of action of ghrelin in the CNS demonstrated a novel hypothalamic circuit regulating energy homeostasis. *Neuron,* Vol.37, No.4, pp. 649-661

Colmers, WF., Lukowiak K. & Pittman, QJ. (1987). Presynaptic action of neuropeptide Y in area CA1 of the rat hippocampal slice. *The Journal of Physiology,* Vol.41, pp. 737-44

Cuevas, BD., Lu, Y., Mao, M., Zhang, J., LaPushin, R., Siminovitch, K. & Mills, GB. (2001). Tyrosine phosphorylation of p85 relieves its inhibitory activity on phosphatidylinositol-3-kinase. *The Journal of Biological Chemistry,* Vol.276, No.29, pp. 27455-27461, ISSN 0021-9258

Cummings, DE. (2006). Ghrelin and the short- and long-term regulation of appetite and body weight. *Physiology & Behavior,* Vol.89, No.1, pp. 71-84

Cummings, DE., Purnell, JQ., Frayo, RS., Schmidova, K., Wisse, BE. & Weigle, DS. (2001). A preprandial rise in plasma ghrelin levels suggests a role in meal initiation in humans. *Diabetes,* Vol.50, No.8, pp. 1714-1719, ISSN 0012-1797

Czlonkowska, AI., Krzaścik, P., Sienkiewicz-Jarosz, H., Siemiatkowski, M., Szyndler, J., Bidziński, A. & Płaźnik, A. (2000). The effects of neurosteroids on picrotoxin-, bicuculline- and NMDA-induced seizures, and a hypnotic effect of ethanol. *Pharmacology, Biochemistry & Behavior,* Vol. 67, No.2, pp. 345-353

Dag, E., Aydin, S., Ozkan, Y., Erman, F., Dagli, AF. & Gurger, M. (2010). Alteration in chromogranin A, obestatin and total ghrelin levels of saliva and serum in epilepsy cases. *Peptides,* Vol.31, No.5, pp. 932-937

Darlington, CL., Gilchrist, DP. & Smith, PF. (1996). Melanocortics and lesion-induced plasticity in the CNS: a review. *Brain Research Reviews,* Vol.22, No.3, pp. 245-257

De Kloet, ER. (1995). Steroids, stability and stress. *Frontiers in Neuroendocrinology,* Vol.16, No.4, pp. 416-425

DelParigi, A., Tschöp, M., Heiman, ML., Salbe, AD., Vozarova, B., Sell, SM., Bunt, JC. & Tataranni, PA. (2002). High circulating ghrelin: a potential cause for hyperphagia and obesity in Prader-Willi syndrome. *The Journal of Clinical Endocrinology and Metabolism,* Vol.87, No.12, pp. 5461-5464

De Quidt, ME. & Emson, PC. (1986). Distribution of neuropeptide Y-like immunoreactivity in the rat central nervous system: II. Immunohistochemical analysis. *Neuroscience,* Vol.18, No.3, pp. 545-618

De Vriese, C., Gregoire, F., Lema-Kisoka, R., Waelbroeck, M., Robberecht, P. & Delporte, C. (2004). Ghrelin degradation by serum and tissue homogenates: identification of the cleavage sites. *Endocrinology,* Vol.145 , No.11, pp. 4997-5005

Dubè, C., Brunson, KL., Eghbal-Ahmadi, M., Gonzalez-Vega, R. & Baram, TZ. (1999) Endogenous neuropeptide Y prevents recurrence of experimental febrile seizure by increasing seizure threshold. *Journal of Molecular Neuroscience*, Vol.25, No.3, pp. 275-284

Dzaja, A., Dalal, MA., Himmerich, H., Uhr, M., Pollmächer, T. & Schuld, A. (2004). Sleep enhances nocturnal plasma ghrelin levels in healthy subjects. *American Journal of Physiology Endocrinology and Metabolism*, Vol.286, No.6, pp. E963-E967, ISSN 0193-1849

El-Khayat, HA., Aly, GS., Tomoum, HY., Mamdouh, RM., Al-Badani, AK. & Mohamed, EI. (2010). Growth hormone levels in children and adolescents with epilepsy. *European Journal Paediatric Neurology*, Vol.14, No.6, pp. 508-512

English, PJ., Ghatei, MA., Malik, IA., Bloom, SR. & Wilding, JP. (2002). Food fails to suppress ghrelin levels in obese humans. *The Journal of Clinical Endocrinology & Metabolism*, Vol.87, No.6, pp. 2984-2987

Erdmann, J., Lippl, F., Wagenpfeil, S. & Schusdziarra, V. (2005). Differential association of basal and postprandial plasma ghrelin with leptin, insulin, and type 2 diabetes. *Diabetes*, Vol.54, No.5, pp. 1371-1378, ISSN 0012-1797

Erakovic, V., Zupan, G., Varljen, J. & Simonić, A. (2003). Pentylenetetrazole-induced seizures and kindling: changes in free fatty acids, superoxide dismutase, and glutathione peroxidase activity. *Neurochemistry International*, Vol.42, No.2, pp. 173-178

Franke, TF., Kaplan, DR. & Cantley, LC. (1997). PI3K: downstream AKTion blocks apoptosis. *Cell*, Vol.88, No.4, pp. 435.437

Gahete, MD., Córdoba-Chacón, J., Salvatori, R., Castaño, JP., Kineman, RD. & Luque, RM. (2010). Metabolic regulation of ghrelin O-acytransferase (GOAT) expression in the mouse hypothalamus, pituitary, and stomach. *Molecular and Cellular Endocrinology*, Vol.317, No.1-2, pp. 154-160

Galimberti, CA., Magri, F., Copello, F., Arbasino, C., Cravello, L., Casu, M., Patrone, V. & Murialdo, G. (2005). Seizure frequency and cortisol and dehydroepiandrosterone sulfate (DHEAS) levels in women with epilepsy receiving antiepileptic drug treatment. *Epilepsia*, Vol.46, No.4, pp. 517-523

Gallagher, BB., Murvin, A., Flanigin, HF., King, DW. & Luney D. (1984). Pituitary and adrenal function in epileptic patients. *Epilepsia*, Vol.25, No.6, pp. 683-689

Gary, KA., Sevarino, KA., Yarbrough, GG., Prange, AJ Jr. & Winokur, A. (2003). The thyrotropin-releasing hormone (TRH) hypothesis of homeostatic regulation: implications for TRH-based therapeutics. *The Journal of Pharmacology and Experimental Therapeutics*, Vol.305, No.2, pp. 410-416, ISSN 0022-3565

Gaskin, FS., Farr, SA., Banks, WA., Kumar, VB. & Morley, JE. (2003). Ghrelin-induced feeding is dependent on nitric oxide. *Peptides*, Vol.24, No.6, pp. 913-918

Gauna, C., Meyler, FM., Janssen, JA., Delhanty, PJ., Abribat, T., Van Koetsveld, P., Hofland, LJ., Broglio, F., Ghigo, E. & van der Lely, AJ. (2004). Administration of acylated ghrelin reduces insulin sensitivity, whereas the combination of acylated plus unacylated ghrelin strongly improves insulin sensitivity. *The Journal of Clinical Endocrinology & Metabolism*, Vol.89, No.10, pp. 5035-5042

Gauna, C., Delhanty, PJ., Hofland, LJ., Janssen, JA., Broglio, F., Ross, RJ., Ghigo, E. & van der Lely AJ. (2005). Ghrelin stimulates, while des-octanoyl ghrelin inhibits, glucose output by primary hepatocytes. *The Journal of Clinical Endocrinology & Metabolism*, Vol.90, No.2, pp. 1055-1060

Gil-Campos, M., Aguilera, CM., Cañete, R. & Gil, A. (2006). Ghrelin: a hormone regulating food intake and energy homeostasis. *British Journal of Nutrition*, Vol.96, No2, pp. 201-226

Gnanapavan, S., Kola, B., Bustin, SA., Morris, DG., McGee, P., Fairclough, P., Bhattacharya, S., Carpenter, R., Grossman, AB. & Korbonits, M. (2002). The tissue distribution of mRNA of ghrelin and subtypes of its receptor, GHS-R, in humans. *The Journal of Clinical Endocrinology & Metabolism*, Vol.87, No.6, pp. 2988-2991

Goldstone, AP. (2004). Prader-Willi syndrome: advances in genetics, pathophysiology and treatment. *Trends in Endocrinology & Metabolism*, Vol.15, No.1, pp. 12-20

Goldstone, AP., Thomas, EL., Brynes, AE., Castroman, G., Edwards, R., Ghatei, MA., Frost, G., Holland, AJ., Grossman, AB., Korbonits, M., Bloom, SR. & Bell, JD. (2004). Elevated fasting plasma ghrelin in Prader-Willi syndrome adults is not solely explained by their reduced visceral adiposity and insulin resistance. *The Journal of Clinical Endocrinology & Metabolism*, Vol.89, No.4, pp. 1718-1726

Goldstone, AP., Holland, AJ., Hauffa, BP., Hokken-Koelega, AC. & Tauber, M. (2008). Recommendations for diagnosis and management of Prader-Willi syndrome. *The Journal of Clinical Endocrinology & Metabolism*, Vol.93, No.11, pp. 4183-4197

Greco, R., Latini, G., Chiarelli, F., Iannetti, P., Verrotti, A. (2005). Leptin, ghrelin, and adiponectin in epileptic patients treated with valproic acid. *Neurology*, Vol.65, No.11, pp. 1808-1809

Gualillo, O., Lago, F. & Dieguez, C. (2008). Introducing GOAT: a target for obesity and anti-diabetic drugs? *Trends Pharmacological Science*, Vol.29, No.8, pp. 398-401

Haas, HL., Hermann, A., Greene, RW. & Chan-Palay, V. (1987). Actions and location of neuropeptide tyrosine (Y) on hyppocampal neurons of the rat in slice preparations. *Journal of Comparative Neurology*, Vol.257, No.2, pp. 208-15

Handforth, A., DeGiorgio, CM., Schachter, SC., Uthman, BM., Naritoku, DK., Tecoma, ES., Henry, TR., Collins, SD., Vaughn, BV., Gilmartin, RC., Labar, DR., Morris, GL 3rd., Salinsky, MC., Osorio, I., Ristanovic, RK., Labiner, DM., Jones, JC., Murphy, JV., Ney, GC. & Wheless, JW. (1998). Vagus nerve stimulation therapy for partial onset seizures. A randomized active-control trial. *Neurology*, Vol.51, No.1, pp. 48-55

Harvey, S. & Hull, K. (2003). Neural growth hormone: an update. *Journal of Molecular Neuroscience*, Vol.20, No.1, pp. 1-13

Heimer, TR. (2003). A new anatomical framework for neuropsychiatric disorders and drug abuse. *The American Journal of Psychiatry*, Vol.160, No.10, pp. 1726-1739

Hendy, GN., Bevan, S., Mattei, MG. & Mouland, AJ. (1995). Chromogranin A. *Clinical and Investigative Medicine*, Vol.18, No.1, pp. 47-65

Henshall, DC., Araki, T., Schindler, CK., Lan, JQ., Tiekoter, KL., Taki, W. & Simon, RP. (2002). Activation of Bcl-2-associated death protein and counter-response of Akt within cell populations during seizure-induced neuronal death. *The Journal of Neuroscience*, Vol.22, No.19, pp. 8458.8465, ISSN 0270-6474

Herzog, AG., Seibel, MM., Schomer, DL., Vaitukaitis, JL. & Geschwind, N. (1986). Reproductive endocrine disorders in women with partial seizures of temporal lobe origin. *Archivies of Neurology*, Vol.43, No.4, pp. 341-346

Herzog, AG. & Schachter, SC. (2001). Valproate and the polycystc ovarian syndrome. *Epilepsia*, Vol.42, No.3, pp. 311-315

Herzog, AG., Drislane, FW., Schomer, DL., Pennell, PB., Bromfield, EB., Dworetzky, BA., Farina, EL. & Frye, CA. (2006). Differential effects of antiepileptic drugs on neuroactive steroids in men with epilepsy. *Epilepsia*, Vol.47, No.11, pp. 1945-1948

Holsboer, F. (2001). Stress, hypercortisolism and corticosteroid receptors in depression: implications for therapy. *Journal of Affective Disorders*, Vol.62, No.1-2, pp. 77-91

Howard, AD., Feighner, SD., Cully, DF., Arena, JP., Liberator, PA., Rosenblum, CI., Hamelin, M., Hreniuk, DL., Palyha, OC., Anderson, J., Paress, PS., Diaz, C., Chou, M., Liu, KK., McKee, KK., Pong, SS., Chaung, LY., Elbrecht, A., Dashkevicz, M., Heavens, R., Rigby, M., Sirinathsinghji, DJ., Dean, DC., Melillo, DG., Patchett, AA., Nargund, R., Griffin, PR., DeMartino, JA., Gupta, SK., Schaeffer, JM., Smith, RG. & Van der Ploeg, LH. (1996). A receptor in pituitary and hypothalamus that functions in growth hormone release. *Science*, Vol.273, No.5277, pp. 974-977

Hum, KM., Megna, S. & Burnham, WM. (2009). Lack of laterality in the effects of right and left amygdale kindling on weight gain in female rats. *Epilepsy Research*, Vol.87, No.1, pp. 40-46

Işeri, SO., Sener, G., Yüksel, M., Contuk, G., Cetinel, S., Gedik, N. & Yegen, BC. (2005). Ghrelin against alendronate-induced gastric damage in rats. *Journal of Endocrinology*, Vol.187, No.3, pp. 399-406

Isojarvi, JI., Löfgren, E., Juntunen, KS., Pakarinen, AJ., Päivänsalo, M., Rautakorpi, I. & Tuomivaara, L. (2004). Effect of epilepsy and antiepileptic drugs on male reproductive health, *Neurology*, Vol.62, No.2, pp. 247-253

Jaworska-Feil, L., Turchan, J., Przewłocka, B., Budziszewska, B., Leśkiewicz, M. & Lasoń, W. (1999). Effects of pilocarpine- and kainite-induced seizures of thyrotropin-releasing hormone biosynthesis and receptors in the rat brain. *Journal of Neural Transmission*, Vol.106, No.5-6, pp. 395-407

Jaworska-Feil, L., Kajta, M., Budziszewska, B., Leśkiewicz, M. & Lasoń, W. (2001). Protective effects of TRH and its stable analogue, RGH-2202, on kainite-induced seizures and neurotoxicity in rodents. *Epilepsy Research*, Vol.43, No.1, pp. 67-73

Kamegai, J., Tamura, H., Shimizu, T., Ishii, S., Sugihara, H. & Oikawa, S. (2004). Effects of insulin, leptin, and glucagon on ghrelin secretion from isolated perfused rat stomach. *Regulatory Peptide*, Vol.119, No.1-2, pp. 77-81

Kato, K., Suzuki, M., Kanno, H., Sekino, S., Kusakabe, K., Okada, T., Mori, T., Yoshida, K. & Hirabayashi, Y. (2009). Distinct role of growth hormone on epilepsy progression in a model of temporal lobe epilepsy. *Journal of Neurochemistry*, Vol.110, No.2, pp. 509-519

Kimonides, VG., Khatibi, NH., Svendsen, CN., Sofroniew, MV. & Herbert, J. (1998). Dehydroepiandrosterone (DHEA) and DHEA-sulfate (DHEAS) protect hippocampal neurons against excitatory amino acid-induced neurotoxicity.

Proceedings of the National Academy of Sciences of the National States of America, Vol.95, No.4, pp. 1852-1857

Knoblanch, SM. & Kubek, MJ. (1997a). Changes in thyrotropin-releasing hormone levels in hippocampal subregions induced by a model of human temporal lobe epilepsy: effect of partial and complete kindling. *Neuroscience*, Vol.76, No.1, pp. 97-104

Knoblanch, SM. & Kubek, MJ. (1997b). Increases in thyrotropin-releasing hormone messenger RNA expression induced by a model of human temporal lobe epilepsy: effect of partial and complete kindling. *Neuroscience*, Vol.76, No.1, pp. 85-89

Kohno, D., Nakata, M., Maejima, Y., Shimizu, H., Sedbazar, U., Yoshida, N., Dezaki, K., Onaka, T., Mori, M. & Yada, T. (2008). Nesfatin-1 neurons in paraventricular and supraotic nuclei of the rat hypothalamus coexpress oxytocin and vasopressin and are activated by refeeding. *Endocrinology*, Vol.149, No.3, pp. 1295-1301

Kojima, M., Hosoda, H., Date, Y., Nakazato, M., Matsuo, H. & Kangawa, K. (1999). Ghrelin is a growth-hormone-releasing acylated peptide from stomach. *Nature*, Vol.402, No.6762, pp. 656-660

Kojima, M. & Kangawa, K. (2005). Ghrelin: structure and function. *Physiological Reviews*, Vol.85, No.2, pp. 495-522

Kokubo, M., Asai, K., Yamamoto, N., Aoyama, M., Morikawa, M., Togari, H., Wada, Y. & Kato, T. (2002). ACTH1-24 downregulates expression of ciliary neurotrophic factor mRNA in cultured rat astrocyte. *Pediatric Research*, Vol.52, No.6, pp. 950-957

Korbonits, M., Goldstone, AP., Gueorguiev, M. & Grossman, AB. (2004). Ghrelin - a hormone with multiple functions. *Frontiers in Neuroendocrinology*, Vol.25, No.1, pp. 27-68

Kubek, MJ., Lorincz, MA. & Wilber, JF. (1977). The identification of thyrotropin releasing hormone (TRH) in hypothalamic and extrahypothalamic loci of the human nervous system. *Brain Res*earch, Vol.126, No.1, pp. 196-200

Kubek, MJ., Low, WC., Sattin, A., Morzorati, SL., Meyerhoff, JL. & Larsen, SH. (1989). Role of TRH in seizure modulation. *Annals of New York Academy of Sciences*, Vol.553, pp. 286-303

Kubek, MJ. & Garg, BP. (2002). Thyrotropin-releasing hormone in the treatment of intractable epilepsy. *Pediatric Neurology*, Vol.26, No.1, pp. 9-17

Kudielka, BM., Schmidt-Reinwald, AK., Hellhammer, DH. & Kirschbaum, C. (1999). Psychological and endocrine responses to psychosocial stress and dexamethasone/corticotrophin-releasing hormone in healthy postmenopausal women and young controls: The impact of age and a two-week estradiol-treatment. *Neuroendocrinology*, Vol.70, No.6, pp. 422-430

Kurihara, S., Hakuno, F. & Takahashi, SI. (2000). Insulin-like growth factor-I-dependent signal transduction pathways leading to the induction of cell growth and differentiation of human neuroblastoma cell line SH-SY5Y: the roles of MAP kinase pathway and PI 3-kinase pathway. *Endocrine Journal*, Vol.47, No.6, pp. 739-751, ISSN: 0918-8959

Langenberg, C., Bergstrom, J., Laughlin, GA. & Barrett-Connor, E. (2005). Ghrelin and the metabolic syndrome in older adults. *The Journal of Clinical Endocrinology & Metabolism*, Vol.90, No.12, pp. 6448-6453

Ledoux, VA., Smejkalova, T., May, RM., Cooke, BM. & Woolley, CS. (2009). Estradiol facilitates the release of neuropeptide Y to suppress hippocampus-dependent seizures. *The Journal of Neuroscience*, Vol.29, No.5, pp. 1457-1468

Lee, J., Lim, E., Kim, Y., Li, E. & Park, S. (2010). Ghrelin attenuates kainic acid-induced neuronal cell death in mouse hippocampus. *Journal of Endocrinology*, Vol.205, No. 3, pp. 263-270

Leite-Moreira, AF. & Soares, JB. (2007). Physiological, pathological and potential therapeutic roles of ghrelin. *Drug Discovery Today*, Vol.12, No.7-8, pp. 276-288

Lin, LC., Lin, HS. & Yang, RC. (2007). Neuropeptide Y gene polymorphism and plasma neuropeptide Y level in febrile seizure patients in Taiwan. *Kaohsiung Journal of Medical Sciences*, Vol.23, No.11, pp. 560-565

Lin, LC., Lee, WT., Chen, IJ. & Yang, RC. (2010). Lower plasma neuropeptide Y level in patients with atypical febrile convulsions. *Kaohsiung Journal of Medical Sciences*, Vol.26, No.1, pp. 8-12

Lindborn, U., Hulting, AL. & Tomson, T. (1999). Paradoxical GH response to TRH during status epilepticus in man. *European Journal of Endocrinology*, Vol.140, No.4, pp. 307-314

Liu, J., Prudom, CE., Nass, R., Pezzoli, SS., Oliveri, MC., Johnson, ML., Veldhuis, P., Gordon, DA., Howard, AD., Witcher, DR., Geysen, HM., Gaylinn, BD. & Thorner, MO. (2008). Novel ghrelin assays provide evidence for independent regulation of ghrelin acylation and secretion in healthy young men. *The Journal of Clinical Endocrinology & Metabolism*, Vol.93, No.5, pp. 1980-1987

Luef, G. (2010). Hormonal alterations following seizures. *Epilepsy & Behavior*, Vol.19, No.2, pp. 131-133

Lutter, M., Lutter, M., Krishnan, V., Russo, SJ., Jung, S., McClung, CA. & Nestler, EJ. (2008a). Orexin signalling mediates the antidepressant-like effect of calorie restriction. *Journal of Neuroscience*, Vol.28, No.12, pp. 3071-3075

Lutter, M., Sakata, I., Osborne-Lawrence, S., Rovinsky, SA., Anderson, JG., Jung, S., Birnbaum, S., Yanagisawa, M., Elmquist, JK., Nestler, EJ. & Zigman, JM. (2008b). The orexogenic hormone ghrelin defends against depressive symptoms of chronic stress. *Nature Neuroscience*, Vol.11, No.7, pp. 752-753, ISSN 1097-6256

Lyuh, E., Kim, HJ., Kim, M., Lee, JK., Park, KS., Yoo, KY., Lee, KW. & Ahn, YO. (2007). Dose-specific or dose dependent effect of growth hormone treatment on the proliferation and differentiation of cultured neuronal cells. *Growth Hormon & IGF Research*, Vol.17, No.4, pp. 315-322

Macdonalds, RL. (1997) Cellular effects of antiepileptic drugs, In: Epilepsy. A comprehensive textbook, Engel Jr., Pedley TA., pp. 1383-1391, Lippincott-Raven, New York

Mackay, MT., Weiss, SK., Adams-Webber, T., Ashwal, S., Stephens, D., Ballaban-Gill, K., Baram, TZ., Duchowny, M., Hirtz, D., Pellock, JM., Shields, WD., Shinnar, S., Wyllie, E., Snead, OC. 3rd & American Academy of Neurology; Child Neurology Society. (2004). American Academy of Neurology: Child Neurology Society. Practice parameter: medical treatment of infantile spasms: report of the American

Academy of Neurology and the Child Neurology Society. *Neurology*, Vol.62, No.10, pp. 668-81

Mahmoud, GS. & Grover, LM. (2006). Growth hormone enhances excitatory synaptic transmission in area CA1 of rat hippocampus. *Journal of Neurophysiology*, Vol.95, No.5, pp. 2962-2974, ISSN 0022-3077

Malik, S., McGlone, F., Bedrossian, D. & Dagher, A. (2008). Ghrelin modulates brain activity in areas that control appetitive behaviour. *Cell Metabolism*, Vol.7, No.5, pp. 400-409

Mayewska, MD., Harrison, NL., Schwartz, RD., Barker, JL. & Paul, SM. (1986). Steroid hormones metabolites are barbiturate-like modulators of the GABA receptor. *Science*, Vol.232, No.4753, pp. 1004-1007

Mayewska, MD. (1995). Neuronal actions of dehydroepiandrosterone: possible roles in brain development, aging, memory and affect. *Annals of New York Academy of Sciences*, Vol.774, pp. 111-120

McEwen, BS., Gould, EA. & Sakai, RR. (1992). The vulnerability of the hippocampus to protective and destructive effects of glucocorticoids in relation to stress. *British Journal of Psychiatry (Suppl)*, Vol.160, No.15, pp. 18-24

McEwen, BS. & Magarinos, AM. (1997). Stress effects on morphology and function of the hippocampus. *Annals of New York Academy of Sciences*, Vol.821, pp. 271-284

Meierkord, H., Shorvon, S. & Lightman, SL. (1994). Plasma concentrations of prolactin, noradrenaline, vasopressin and oxcytocin during and after a prolonged epileptic seizure. *Acta Neurologica Scandinavica*, Vol.90, No.2, pp. 73-77

Miao, YY., Xia, Q., Hou, Z., Zheng, Y., Pan, H. & Zhu, S. (2007). Ghrelin protects cortical neuron against focal ischemia/reperfusion in rats. *Biochemical and Biophysical Research Communications*, Vol.359, No.3, pp. 780-795

Morrell, MJ. (2003). Reproductive and metabolic disorders in women with epilepsy. *Epilepsia*, Vol.44, Suppl.4, pp. 11-20

Morris, GL. 3rd. & Mueller, WM. (1999). Long-term treatment with vagus nevre stimulation in patients refractory epilepsy. The Vagus Nevre Stimulation Study Group E01-E05. *Neurology*, Vol.53, No.8, pp. 1731-1735

Motivala, SJ., Tomiyama, AJ., Ziegler, M., Khandrika, S. & Irwin, MR. (2009). Nocturnal levels ghrelin and leptin and sleep in chronic insomnia. *Psychoneuroendocrinology*, Vol.34, No.4, pp. 540-545

Muccioli, G., Pons, N., Ghè, C., Catapano, F., Granata, R. & Ghigo, E. (2004). Ghrelin and des-acyl ghrelin both inhibit isoproterenol-induced lipolysis in rat adipocytes via a non-type 1a growth hormone segretagogue receptor. *European Journal of Pharmacology*, Vol.498, No.1-3, pp. 27-35

Mueller, SG., Trabesinger, AH., Boesiger, P. & Wieser, HG. (2001). Brain glutathione levels in patients with epilepsy measured by in vivo (1) H-MRS. *Neurology*, Vol.57, No.8, pp. 1422-1427, ISSN 0028-3878

Nakashima, K., Akiyoshi, J., Hatano, K., Hanada, H., Tanaka, Y., Tsuru, J., Matsushita, H., Kodama, K. & Isogawa, K. (2008). Ghrelin gene polymorphism is associated with depression, but not panic disorder. *Psychistric Genetics*, Vol.18, No.5, pp. 257, ISSN 0955-8829

Ness-Abramof, R. & Apovian CM. (2005). Drug-induced weight gain. *Timely Topics in Medicine Cardiovascular Disease,* Vol.28, No.9, pp. E31, ISSN 1699-3993

Ni, H., Walia, P. & Chanoine, JP. (2010). Ontogeny of acylated ghrelin degradation in the rat. *Peptides,* Vol.31, No.2, pp. 301-306

Nicholls, RD., Knoll, JH., Butler, MG., Karam, S. & Lalande, M. (1989). Genetic imprinting suggested by maternal heterodisomy in non-deletion Prader-Willi syndrome. *Nature,* Vol. 342, No.6247, pp. 281-285

Nillni, EA. & Sevarino, KA. (1999). The biology of pro-thyrotropin-releasing hormone-derived peptides. *Endocrine Reviews,* Vol.20, No.5, pp. 599-648

Nyberg, F. (2000). Growth hormone in the brain: characteristics of specific brain targets for the hormone and their functional significance. *Frontiers in Neuroendocrinology,* Vol.21, No.4, pp. 330-348

Obay, BD., Tasdemir, E., Tümer, C., Bilgin, HM. & Sermet, A. (2007). Antiepileptic effects of ghrelin on pentylenetetrazole-induced seizures in rats. *Peptides,* Vol.28, No.6, pp. 1214-1219

Obay, BD., Taşdemir, E., Tümer, C., Bilgin, HM. & Atmaca, M. (2008). Dose dependent effects of ghrelin on pentylenetetrazole-induced oxidative stress in a rat seizure model. *Peptides,* Vol.29, No.3, pp. 448-455

Oh-I, S., Shimizu, H., Satoh, T., Okada, S., Adachi, S., Inoue, K., Eguchi, H., Yamamoto, M., Imaki, T., Hashimoto, K., Tsuchiya, T., Monden, T., Horiguchi, K., Yamada, M. & Mori M. (2006). Identification of nefastin-1 as a satiety molecule in the hypothalamus. *Nature,*Vol.443, No.7112, pp. 709-712

Oliver, CN., Starke-Reed, PE., Stadtman, ER., Liu, GJ., Carney, JM. & Floyd, RA. (1990). Oxidative damage to brain proteins, loss of glutamine synthetase activity and production of free radicals during ischemia/reperfusion induced injury to gerbil brain. *Proceedings of the National Academy of Sciences of the National states of America,* Vol.87, No.13, pp. 5144-5147

Ono, H., Sakamoto, A. & Sakura, N. (2000). Plasma total glutathione concentrations in epileptic patients taking anticonvulsants. *Clinica Chimica Acta,* Vol.298, No.1-2, pp. 135-143

Opaleke, A. & Helmers, SL. (2007). Hormonal consequences of epilepsy. *Seminars in Pediatric Neurology,* Vol.14, No.4, pp. 189-195

Pagotto, U., Gambineri, A., Vicennati, V., Heiman, ML., Tschöp, M. & Pasquali, R. (2002). Plasma ghrelin, obesity, and the polycystic ovary syndrome: correlation with insulin resistance and androgen levels. *The Journal of Clinical Endocrinology & Metabolism,* Vol.87, No.12, pp. 5625-5629

Paik, KH., Song, SY., Lee, JE., Ko, SH., Song, SM., Kim, JS., Oh, YJ., Kim, SW., Lee, SH., Kim, SH., Kwon, EK. & Choe, YH. (2004). Correlation between fasting plasma ghrelin levels and age, body mass index (BMI), BMI percentiles, and 24-hour plasma ghrelin profiles in Prader-Willi syndrome. *The Journal of Clinical Endocrinology & Metabolism,* Vol.89, No.8, pp. 3885-3889

Paik, KH., Choe, YH., Park, WH., Oh, YJ., Kim, AH., Chu, SH., Kim, SW., Kwon, EK., Han, SJ., Shon, WY. & Jin, DK. (2006). Suppression of acylated ghrelin during oral glucose tolerance test is correlated with whole body insulin sensitivity in children with Prader-Willi syndrome. *The Journal of Clinical Endocrinology & Metabolism,* Vol.91, No.5, pp. 1876-1881

Pan, W., Hsuchou, H. & Kastin, AJ. (2007). Nesfatin-1 crosses the blood-brain barrier without saturation. *Peptides,* Vol.28, No.11, pp. 2223-2228

Paul, SM. & Purdy, RH. (1992). Neuroactive steroids. *The FASEB Journal,* Vol.6, No.6, pp. 2311-2322

Parra, A., Velasco, M., Cervantes, C., Muñoz, H., Cerbón, MA. & Velasco, F. (1980). Plasma prolactin increase following electrical stimulation of the amygdala in humans. *Neuroendocrinology,* Vol.31, No.1, pp. 60-65

Patel, MN. (2002). Oxidative stress, mythocondrial dysfunction, and epilepsy. *Free Radical Research,* Vol.36, No.11, pp. 1139-1146

Perreault, M., Istrate, N., Wang, L., Nichols, AJ., Tozzo, E. & Stricker-Krongrad, A. (2004). Resistance to the orexigenic effect of ghrelin in dietary-induced obesity in mice: reversal upon weight loss. *International Journal of Obesity and Related Metabolic Disorders,* Vol.28, No.7, pp. 879-885

Pizzi, M., Boroni, F., Benarese, M., Moraitis, C., Memo, M. & Spano, P. (1999). Neuroprotective effect of thyrotropin-releasing hormone against excitatory amino acid-induced cell death in hippocampal slices. *European Journal of Pharmacology,* Vol.370, No.2, pp. 133-137

Price, TO., Samson, WK., Niehoff, ML. & Banks, WA. (2007). Permeability of the blood-brain barrier to a novel satiety molecule nesfatin-1. *Peptides,* Vol.28, No.12, pp. 2372-2381

Price, CJ., Samson, WK. & Ferguson, AV. (2008). Nesfatin-1 inhibits NPY neurons in the arcuate nucleus. *Brain Research,* Vol.1230, pp. 99-106

Prodam, F., Me, E., Riganti, F., Gramaglia, E., Bellone, S., Baldelli, R., Rapa, A., van der Lely, AJ., Bona, G., Ghigo, E. & Broglio, F. (2006). The nutritional control of ghrelin secretion in humans: The effects of enteral vs. parenteral nutrition. *European Journal of Nutrition,* Vol. 45, No.7, pp. 399-405

Prodam, F., Bellone, S., Corneli, G., Golisano, G. & Bona, G. (2008). Ghrelin: a molecular target for weight regulation, glucose and lipid metabolism. *Recent Patents on Endocrine, Metabolic & Immune Drug Discovery,* Vol.2, No.3, pp. 1-16

Prodam, F., Bellone, S., Casara, G., De Rienzo, F., Grassino, EC., Bonsignori, I., Demarchi, I., Rapa, A., Radetti, G. & Bona, G. (2009). Ghrelin levels are reduced in prepubertal epileptic children under treatment with carbamazepine or valproic acid. *Epilepsia,* Vol.51, No.2, pp. 1-4

Quigg M. (2002). Seizures and circadian rhythms, In: *Sleep and epilepsy: the clinical spectrum,* Bazil CW., Malow BA., Sammaritano MR., pp 31, The Netherlands: Elsevier B.V.

Ramsey, MM., Weiner, JL., Moore, TP., Carter, CS. & Sonntag, WE. (2004). Growth hormone treatment attenuates age-related changes in hippocampal short-term plasticity and spatial learning. *Neuroscience,* Vol.129, No.1, pp. 119-127

Ransome, MI. & Turnley, AM. (2008). Growth hormone signaling and hippocampal neurogenesis: insights from genetic models. *Hippocampus,* Vol.18, No.10, pp. 1034-1050

Reddy, DS. (2004). Anticonvulsant activity of the testosterone-derived neurosteroid 3alfa-androstanediol. *Neuroreport,* Vol.15, No.3, pp. 515-518

Reddy, DS. & Rogawski, MA. (2009). Neurosteroid replacement therapy for catamenial epilepsy. *Neurotherapeutics,* Vol.6, No.2, pp. 392-401

Rogawski, MA. & Reddy, DS. (2002). Neurosteroids and infantile spasms; the deoxycorticosterone hypothesis. *International Review of Neurobiology,* Vol.49, pp. 199-219

Rouach, V., Bloch, M., Rosenberg, N., Gilad, S., Limor, R., Stern, N. & Greenman, Y. (2007). The acute ghrelin response to a psychological stress challenge does not predict the post-stress urge to eat. *Psychoneuroendocrinology,* Vol.32, No.6, pp. 693-702

Sapolsky, RM. (2000). Glucocorticoids and hippocampal atrophy in neuropsychiatric disorders. *Archivies of General Psychiatry,* Vol.57, No.10, pp. 925-935

Sapolsky, RM., Krey, LC. & McEwen, BS. (1986). The neuroendocrinology of stress and aging: the glucocorticoid cascade hypothesis. *Endocrine Reviews,* Vol.7, No.3, pp. 284-301

Scharfman, HE. & MacLusky, NJ. (2006). The influence of gonadal hormones on neuronal excitability, seizures, and epilepsy in the female. *Epilepsia,* Vol.47, No.9, pp. 1423-1440

Scheepens, A., Sirimanne, ES., Breier, BH., Clark, RG., Gluckman, PD. & Williams, CE. (2001). Growth hormone as a neuronal rescue factor during recovery from CNS injury. *Neuroscience,* Vol.104, No.3, pp. 677-687

Sheline, YI., Wang, PW., Gado, MH., Csernansky, JG. & Vannier, MW. (1996). Hippocampal atrophy in recurrent major depression. *Proceedings of the National Academy of Sciences of the National states of America,* Vol.93, No.9, pp. 3908-3913

Shimada, M., Date, Y., Mondal, MS., Toshinai, K., Shimbara, T., Fukunaga, K., Murakami, N., Miyazato, M., Kangawa, K., Yoshimatsu, H., Matsuo, H. & Nakazato, M. (2003). Somatostatin suppressed ghrelin secretion from the rat stomach. *Biochemical and Biophsycal Research Communication,* Vol.302, No.3, pp. 520-525

Schussler, P., Uhr, M., Ising, M., Schmid, D., Weikel, J. & Steiger, A. (2005). Nocturnal ghrelin levels -relationship to sleep EEG, the levels of growth hormone, ACTH and cortisol - and gender differences. *Journal of Sleep Research,* Vol.14, No.4, pp. 329-336

Siebzehnrubl, FA. & Blumcke, I. (2008). Neurogenesis in the human hippocampus and its relevance to temporal lobe epilepsies. *Epilepsia,* Vol.49, Suppl.5, pp. 55-65

Silva, AP., Bethmann, K., Raulf, F. & Schmid, HA. (2005). Regulation of ghrelin secretion by somatostatin analogs in rats. *European Journal of Endocrinology,* Vol.152, No.6, pp. 887-894

Singh, R. & Pathak, DN. (1990). Lipid peroxidation and glutathione peroxidase, glutathione reductase, superoxide dismutase, catalase, and glucose-6-phosphate dehydrogenase activities in FeCl3-induced epileptogenic foci in the rat brain. *Epilepsia,* Vol.31, No.1, pp. 15-26

Smith, SE., Man, CM., Yip, PK., Tang, E., Chapman, AG. & Meldrum, BS. (1996). Anticonvulsant effects of 7-nitroindazole in rodents with reflex epilepsy may result from L-arginine accumulation or a reduction in nitric oxide or L-citrulline formation. *British Journal of Pharmacology,* Vol.119, No.1, pp. 165-173

Smith, SS. (1989). Estrogen administration increases neuronal responses to excitatory amino acids as a long term effect. *Brain Research,* Vol.503, No.2, pp. 354-357

Soares, JB. & Leite-Moreira, AF. (2008). Ghrelin, des-acyl ghrelin and obeostatin: three pieces of the same puzzle. *Peptides,* Vol.29, No.7, pp. 1255-1270

Steiger, A., Dresler, M., Schüssler, P. & Kluge, M. (2011). Ghrelin in mental health, sleep, memory. *Molecular and Cellular Endocrinology,* [Epub ahead of print], doi:10.1016/j.mce.2011.02.013

Stroud, LM., O'Brien, TJ., Jupp, B., Wallengren, C & Morris, MJ. (2005). Neuropeptide Y suppresses absence seizures in a genetic rat model. *Brain Research,* Vol.1033, No.2, pp. 151-156

Sudha, K., Rao, AV. & Rao, A. (2001). Oxidative stress and antioxidants in epilepsy. *Clinica Chimica Acta,* Vol.303, No.1-2, pp. 19-24

Svalheim, S., Taubøll, E., Bjørnenak, T., Røste, LS., Mørland, T., Saetre, ER. & Gjerstad, L. (2003). Do women with epilepsy have increased frequency of menstrual disturbances? *Seizure,* Vol.12, No.8, pp. 529-533

Szentirmai, E., Kapás, L. & Krueger, JM. (2007). Ghrelin microinjection into forebrain sites induces wakefulness and feeding in rats. *American Journal of Physiology Regulatory, Integratory and Comparative Physiology,* Vol.292, No.1, pp. R575-R585

Szentirmai, E., Kapás, L., Sun, Y., Smith, RG. & Krueger, JM. (2009). The preproghrelin gene is required for the normal integration of thermoregulation and sleep in mice. *Proceedings of the National Academy of Sciences of the National states of America,* Vol.106, No.33, pp. 14069-14074

Tamminga, CA., Neophytides, A., Chase, TN. & Frohman, LA. (1978). Stimulation of prolactin and growth hormone secretion by muscimol, a gamma-aminobutyric acid agonist. *The Journal of Clinical Endocrinology & Metabolism,* Vol.47, No.6, pp. 1348-1351

Tang, SQ., Jiang, QY., Zhang, YL., Zhu, XT., Shu, G., Gao, P., Feng, DY., Wang, XQ. & Dong, XY. (2008). Obestatin: its physicochemical characteristics and physiological functions. *Peptides,* Vol.29, No.4, pp. 639-645

Thompson, NM., Gill, DA., Davies, R., Loveridge, N., Houston, PA., Robinson, IC. & Wells, T. (2004). Ghrelin and des-octanoyl ghrelin promote adipogenesis directly in vivo by a mechanism independent of the type 1a growth hormone segretagogue receptor. *Endocrinology,* Vol.145, No.1, pp. 234-242

Tolle, V., Bassant, MH., Zizzari, P., Poindessous-Jazat, F., Tomasetto, C., Epelbaum, J. & Bluet-Pajot, MT. (2002). Ultradian rhythmicity of ghrelin secretion in relation with GH, feeding behavior, and sleep-wake patterns in rats. *Endocrinology,* Vol.143, No.4, pp. 1353-1361

Tschop, M., Smiley, DL. & Heiman, ML. (2000). Ghrelin induces adiposity in rodents. *Nature,* Vol.407, No.6806, pp. 908-913

Tschop, M., Weyer, C., Tataranni, PA., Devanarayan, V., Ravussin, E. & Heiman, ML. (2001). Circulating ghrelin levels are decreased in human obesity. *Diabetes,* Vol.50, No.4, pp. 707-709

Uma Devi, P., Pillai, KK. & Vohora, D. (2006). Modulation of penthylenetetrazole-induced seizures and oxidative stress parameters by sodium valproate in the absence and the presence of N-acetylcysteine. *Fundamental and Clinical Pharmacology,* Vol.20, No.3, pp. 247-253

Van Cauter, E. & Knutson, KL. (2008). Sleep and the epidemic of obesity in children and adults. *European Journal of Endocrinology,* Vol.159, Suppl.1, pp. S59-S66, ISSN 0804-4643

Van Cauter, E., Spiegel, K., Tasali, E. & Leproult, R. (2008). Metabolic consequences of sleep and sleep loss. *Sleep Medicine,* Vol.9, Suppl. 1, pp. S23-S28

van der Lely, AJ., Tschöp, M., Heiman, ML. & Ghigo, E. (2004). Biological, physiological, pathophysiological, and pharmacological aspects of gherlin. *Endocrine Reviews,* Vol.25, No.3, pp. 426-657

Vazquez, RMI., Camilleri, M., Stephens, DA., Jensen, MD., Burton, DD., Baxter, KL. & Zinsmeister, AR. (2006). Gastric sensorimotor functions and hormone profile in normal weight, overweight, and obese people. *Gastroenterology,* Vol.131, No.6, pp. 1717-1724

Veerendra Kumar, MH. & Gupta, YK. (2003). Effect of centella asiatica of pentylenetetrazol induced kindling, cognition and oxidative stress in rats. *Pharmacology, Biochemistry & Behavior,* Vol.74, No.5-6, pp. 579-585

Veronesi, MC., Yard, M., Jackson, J., Lahiri, DK. & Kubek, MJ. (2007). An analog of thyrotropin-releasing hormone (TRH) is neuroprotective against glutamate-induced toxicity in fetal rat hippocampal neurons in vitro. *Brain Research,* Vol.1128, No.1, pp. 79-85

Vezzani, A. & Hoyer, D. (1999). Brain somatostatin: a candidate inhibitory role in seizures and epileptogenesis. *European Journal of Neuroscience,* Vol.11, No.11, pp. 3767-3776

Wan, RQ., Noguera, EC. & Weiss, SR. (1998). Anticonvulsant effects of intra-hippocampal injection of TRH in amygdala kindled rats. *Neuroreport,* Vol.9, No.4, pp. 677-682

Watzka, M., Beyenburg, S., Blümcke, I., Elger, CE., Bidlingmaier, F. & Stoffel-Wagner, B. (2000). Expression of mineralcorticoid and glucocorticoid receptor mRNA in the human hippocampus. *Neuroscience Letters,* Vol.290, No.2, pp. 121-124

Wilton P. (1999). Adverse events during GH treatment: 10 years experience in KIGS, a pharmaco-epidemiological survey, In: *Progress in growth hormone therapy-10 years of KIGS,* Ranke MB., Wilton P., pp. 349-364, Ja Barh Verlag

Weikel, JC., Wichniak, A., Ising, M., Brunner, H., Friess, E., Held, K., Mathias, S., Schmid, DA., Uhr, M. & Steiger, A. (2003). Ghrelin promotes slow-wave sleep in humans. *American Journal of Physiology Endocrinology and Metabolism,* Vol.284, No.2, pp. E407-415

Wiedmer, P., Nogueiras, R., Broglio, F., D'Alessio, D. & Tschöp, MH. (2007). Ghrelin, obesity and diabetes. *Natural Clinical Practice Endocrinology & Metabolism,* Vol.3, No.10, pp. 705-712, ISNN 1759-5037

Xu, J., Wang, S., Lin, Y., Cao, L., Wang, R. & Chi, Z. (2009). Ghrelin protects against cell death of hippocampal neurons in pilocarpine-induced seizures in rats. *Neuroscience Letters,* Vol.453, No.1, pp. 58-61

Yildiz, BO., Suchard, MA., Wong, ML., McCann, SM. & Licinio, J. (2004). Alterations in the dynamics of circulating ghrelin, adiponectin, and leptin in human obesity.

Proceedings of the National Academy of Sciences of the National states of America, Vol.101, No.28, pp. 10434-10439

Zhang, JV., Ren, PG., Avsian-Kretchmer, O., Luo, CW., Rauch, R., Klein, C. & Hsueh, AJ. (2005). Obestatin, a peptide encoded by the ghrelin gene, opposes ghrelin's effects on food intake. *Science*, Vol.310, No.5750, pp. 996-999

Zhang, W., Zhao, L., Lin, TR., Chai, B., Fan, Y., Gantz, I. & Mulholland, MW. (2004). Inhibition of adipogenesis by ghrelin. *Molecular Biology of the Cell*, Vol.15, No.5, pp. 2484-2491

Zhang, Y., Ying, B., Shi, L., Fan, H., Yang, D., Xu, D., Wei, Y., Hu, X., Zhang, Y., Zhang, X., Wang, T., Liu, D., Dou, L., Chen, G., Jiang, F. & Wen, F. (2007). Ghrelin inhibit cell apoptosis in pancreatic beta cell line HIT-T15 via mitogen-activated protein kinase/phosphoinositide3-kinase pathways. *Toxicology*, Vol.237, No.1-3, pp. 194-202

Zheng, A. & Moritani, T. (2008). Effect of the combination of ginseng, oriental bezoar and glycyrrhiza on autonomic nervous activity and immune system under mental arithmetic stress. *Journal of Nutritional Science and Vitaminology (Tokjo)*, Vol.54, No.3, pp. 244-249

Zizzari, P., Halem, H., Taylor, J., Dong, JZ., Datta, R., Culler, MD., Epelbaum, J. & Bluet-Pajot, MT. (2005). Endogenous ghrelin regulates episodic growth hormone (GH) secretion by amplifying GH pulse amplitude: evidence from antagonism of the GH segretagogue R1a-receptor. *Endocrinology*, Vol.146, No.9, pp. 3836-3842

Zobel, A., Wellmer, J., Schulze-Rauschenbach, S., Pfeiffer, U., Schnell, S., Elger, C. & Maier, W. (2004). Impairment of inhibitory control of the hypothalamic pituitary adrenocortical system in epilepsy. *European Archivies of Psychiatry and Clinical Neuroscience*, Vol.254, No.5, pp. 303-311

10

Regulation of GluR6-PSD95-MLK3 Signaling in KA-Induced Epilepsy

Chong Li and Guang-Yi Zhang
Xuzhou Medical College
P. R. China

1. Introduction

Glutamate receptors are classified into two groups: metabotropic glutamate receptors (mGluRs) and ionotropic glutamate receptors (iGluRs). The ionotropic glutamate receptors are superfamily of ligand-gated cation channels that encompass three receptor families identified by the agonists that selectively activate them: *N*-methyl-D-aspartate (NMDA), α-amino-3-hydroxy-5-methyl-4-isoxazole propionate (AMPA), and kainic acid (KA) receptors (Dingledine *et al.* 1999, Mayer & Armstrong 2004, Kew & Kemp 2005). KA is a potent exogenous agonist of KA receptors and AMPA receptors, and systemic administration of KA produces epilepsy in rats and mice accompanied by neuronal damage mainly in limbic structures. In particular, hippocampal pyramidal neurons are highly vulnerable to the excitotoxicity of KA (Sperk *et al.* 1983). KA-induced seizures in rodents have been widely used as a model of human temporal lobe epilepsy on the basis of both behavioral and pathological similarities (Ben-Ari 1985).

KA receptors are comprised of five different subunits: KA1, KA2, GluR5, GluR6 and GluR7 (Lilliu *et al.* 2002, Porter *et al.* 1997). It is reported that GluR6 subunit-deficient and *Jnk3* gene knock-out mice resistance to KA-induced seizures and neuronal toxicity (Yang *et al.* 1997, Mulle *et al.* 1998). And the Glur6 midiated JNK3 (c-Jun N-terminal kinase 3) signaling pathway has been pay more attention in the study of neuron damage during epilepsia. C terminus of GluR6 can bind to the PDZ1 domain of the postsynaptic density protein PSD95/SAP90 through specific interaction (Garcia *et al.* 1998, Mehta *et al.* 2001). Previous studies have also shown that MLK3 (mixed lineage kinase-3), an upstream kinase of JNK (Tibbles *et al.* 1996), can interact with the SH3 (Src homology) domain of PSD95 (Savinainen *et al.* 2001). The triple complex GluR6-PSD95-MLK3 may exist and facilitate JNK activation.

In our previous studies on brain ischemia, it has demonstrated that KA enhanced the assembly of GluR6-PSD95-MLK3 module, increased the autophosphorylation of MLK3 and the phosphorylation of MKK7 (mitogen-activated protein kinase kinase 7), JNK3, c-Jun and Bcl-2 (B-cell lymphoma 2), raised the expression of Fas-Ligand (FasL) and caused the release of Bax (Bcl-2 associated x protein) from Bcl-2/Bax dimmers and the release of cytochrome c from mitochondria (Pei *et al.* 2006). Consequently, the activation of Caspase 3 led to delayed neuronal death in the hippocampal CA1/CA3 subfield (Tian *et al.* 2005, Pei *et al.* 2005, Pan *et al.* 2005). The activation of mitochondrion-linked apoptotic signaling pathways after seizures, including activation of caspase-9, -3, and -8, has also been reported (Henshall *et al.* 2000). And we further found that KA-induced neuronal death is mediated by the GluR6-

PSD95-MLK3 signaling module via FasL/Fas and cytochrome c pathways in KA-induced seizures and interference of the interaction between GluR6 and PSD95 with a peptide can protect neurons from KA-induced death (Liu *et al.* 2006).

Regulation of GluR6 mediated apoptotic pathway has emerged as a possible approach to protect neuron damage against seizure. One idea is down-regulating excitatory GluR6-containing KA receptors by activation of inhibitory GABA receptors. GABA plays a key role in modulating neuronal activity via distinct receptor systems, the ionotropic $GABA_A$ and metabotropic $GABA_B$ receptors. It has been proposed that coactivation of $GABA_A$ and $GABA_B$ receptors induced by muscimol and baclofen respectively can result in neuroprotection during *in vitro* ischemia (Costa *et al.* 2004), and coapplication of the two agonists is more effective than when solely used (Zhang *et al.* 2007). Data acquired from our lab demonstrated that coapplication of muscimol with baclofen has neuroprotective effects in rat hippocampal CA1 and CA3 regions and inhibits the assembly of the GluR6-PSD95-MLK3 signaling module and subsequently activates JNK downstream signaling pathways (Li et al.).

2. Neuroprotective effects of peptide Tat-GluR6-9c and GABA receptors activation against neuronal death induced by KA in rat hippocampus

Based on our previous study, activation of GluR6-PSD95-MLK3 signaling is an important reason for neuron death in rat KA-induced epilepsy model. Interference of this signaling might have protective effects against neuron death, so we designed two different strategies to carry out the goal. First, we constructed a peptide comprising the conserved nine COOH-terminal residues of GluR6 (Arg-Leu-Pro-Gly-Lys-Glu-Thr-Met-Ala, named GluR6-9c), which was fused to Tat protein (cell-membrane transduction domain of the human immunodeficiency virus-type 1, Tyr-Gly-Arg-Lys-Lys-Arg-Arg-Gln-Arg-Arg-Arg). The Tat-GluR6-9c peptide can be delivered into hippocampal neurons and destroy the interaction between GluR6 and PSD95, and further suppress the GluR6-PSD95-MLK3 signaling. Second, elevating the inhibition of GABA receptors can significantly decrease KAR-mediated excitation in KA-induced epilepsy. The major finding is that Muscimol and/or Baclofen can suppress the assembly of the GluR6-PSD95-MLK3 signaling. One possible explanation is that the activation of $GABA_A$ receptor by muscimol can induce the hyperpolarization of postsynaptic nrurons via activating ligand-gated Cl- channels, which decrease the depolarization of the neurons (Attwell *et al.* 1993), and activation of G protein-coupled $GABA_B$ receptor by baclofen can attenuate glutamate release from presynaptic neurons (Moldavan *et al.* 2006). The mechanism and roles of these two strategies are described below.

2.1 Assembly of the GluR6-PSD95-MLK3 signaling module during seizure induced by KA in hippocampal CA1 and CA3/DG regions

Immunoprecipitation and immunoblotting were performed to examine the interactions of GluR6 and MLK3 with PSD95 at various times of KA injection. The interactions of GluR6 and MLK3 with PSD95 increased rapidly after KA injection, reached peak levels at 6 h, and then gradually decreased to control levels at 3 days in both CA1 and CA3/DG regions.

2.2 Tat-GluR6-9c peptide suppresses the increased assembly of the GluR6-PSD95-MLK3 signaling module induced by KA in hippocampal CA1 and CA3/DG regions

Tat-GluR6-9c, a GluR6 C terminus-containing peptide conjugated to the cell membrane transduction sequence of the human immunodeficiency virus Tat protein, can be delivered into hippocampal neurons *in vitro* and *in vivo*. Reciprocal immunoprecipitation experiments demonstrated that the peptide perturbed the GluR6-PSD95-MLK3 signaling module. Administration of Tat-GluR6-9c 40 min prior to KA injection diminished the increased interactions of GluR6 and MLK3 with PSD95 at 6 h after kainate treatment in CA1 and CA3/DG subregions, whereas the protein levels of GluR6, PSD95, and MLK3 were not altered.

2.3 Tat-GluR6-9c inhibits the activation of MLK3, MKK7, and JNK induced by KA in hippocampal CA1 and CA3/DG regions

KA treatment resulted in a remarkable increase in the phosphorylation of MLK3 in CA1and CA3/DG regions. Pretreatment with Tat-GluR6-9c significantly diminished the increase in the phosphorylation of MLK3. And, the activation of MKK7 and JNK at 6 h after KA injection was significantly suppressed by application of the Tat-GluR6-9c peptide in CA1 and CA3/DG regions.

2.4 Tat-GluR6-9c inhibits the phosphorylation of c-Jun and the expression of FasL induced by KA in hippocampal CA1 and CA3/DG regions

The phosphorylation and expression of transcription factor c-Jun was significantly increased at 6 and 12 h in both CA1 and CA3/DG regions after KA injection. Prior administration of Tat-GluR6-9c significantly diminished the increase in phospho-c-Jun at 6 h after KA treatment. The protein levels of c-Jun were not affected. The increased phosphorylation of c-Jun leads to increased expression of FasL. The expression of FasL increased rapidly at 6 h and returned to the basal level at 3 days in CA1 and CA3/DG regions. Prior application of Tat-GluR6-9c diminished the increased expression of FasL.

2.5 Tat-GluR6-9c decreases Bax expression and increases Bcl-2 expression induced by KA in hippocampal CA1 and CA3/DG regions

It is known that Bcl-2 is an anti-apoptotic protein, whereas Bax is an pro-apoptotic protein. The expression of Bax increased dramatically at 6 h after KA injection and lasted 3 days, whereas the level of Bcl-2 decreased sharply at 6 h after KA injection and reached the lowest at 3 days in the CA1 region. Prior application of Tat-GluR6-9c resulted in the decreased expression of Bax at 6 h after KA treatment in both CA1 and CA3/DG regions, whereas the level of Bcl-2 was obviously increased at 6 h after KA injection.

2.6 Tat-GluR6-9c attenuates Bax translocation and the release of cytochrome c induced by KA in Hippocampal CA1 and CA3/DG regions

A previous study reported mitochondrial Bax accumulation after seizure (Henshall *et al.* 2002). Tat-GluR6-9c can inhibit Bax translocation in the mitochondrial fraction in both CA1 and CA3/DG regions. Moreover, Tat-GluR6-9c inhibited the release of cytochrome c from mitochondria to the cytosol in CA1 and CA3/DG fields.

2.7 Tat-GluR6-9c inhibits the activation of caspase-3 and neuronal apoptosis induced by KA in hippocampal CA1 and CA3/DG regions

Tat-GluR6-9c pretreatment diminished the activation of caspase-3 at 6 h after KA injection. TUNEL (Terminal Transferase dUTP Nick End Labeling) staining was used to examine the apoptosis of CA1 and CA3 neuronal cells in the hippocampus. Administration of Tat-GluR6-

9c 40 min before KA injection significantly decreased TUNEL-positive cells. Tat-GluR6-9c significantly decreased neuronal degeneration (Fig. 1).

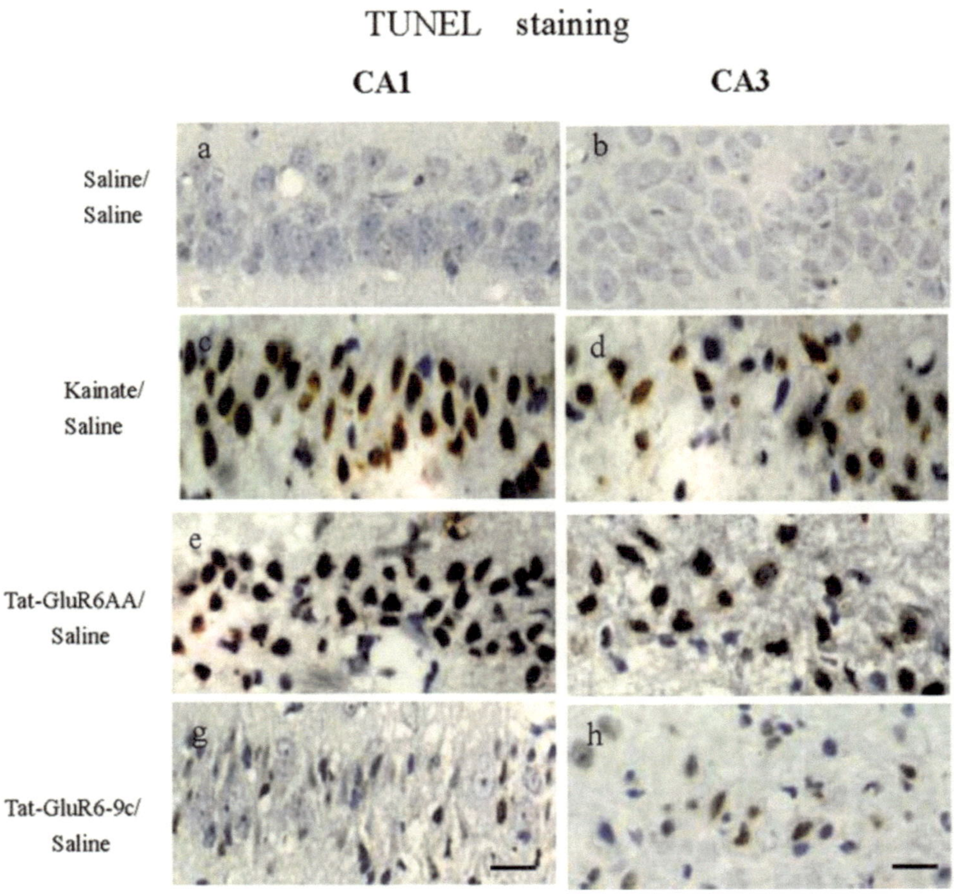

Fig. 1. Neuroprotection of peptide Tat-GluR6-9c in hippocampal CA1 and CA3 subfields.

2.8 Muscimol and baclofen suppress the increased assembly of the GluR6-PSD95-MLK3 signaling module induced by KA in hippocampal CA1 and CA3/DG regions

The GABA receptors can be activated by two GABA agonists: muscimol, a $GABA_A$ agonist, and baclofen, a $GABA_B$ agonist. Reciprocal immunoprecipitation experiments suggested that the administration of two agonists resulted in the disassembly of GluR6-PSD95-MLK3 signaling module. Co-administration of muscimol and baclofen 40 min prior to KA injection diminished the increased interactions of GluR6 and MLK3 with PSD95 at 6 h after KA treatment in CA1 and CA3/DG subregions, whereas the protein levels of GluR6, PSD95 and MLK3 were not altered.

2.9 Muscimol and baclofen inhibit the activation of MLK3, MKK7 and JNK3 induced by KA in hippocampal CA1 and CA3/DG regions

Pretreatment with muscimol and baclofen significantly diminished the increase of the MLK3 phosphorylation. Meanwhile, the activation of MKK7 at 6 h after KA injection was significantly suppressed by co-application of muscimol and baclofen in CA1 and CA3/DG regions. Furthermore, similar results were obtained with JNK3.

2.10 Muscimol and baclofen inhibit the phosphorylation of c-Jun and the expression of FasL induced by KA in hippocampal CA1 and CA3/DG regions

Prior administration of muscimol and baclofen significantly diminished the increase of phospho-c-Jun at 6 h after KA treatment. Prior application of musimol and baclofen attenuated the increased expression of FasL at 6 h induced by KA in hippocampal CA1 and CA3/DG regions.

2.11 Muscimol and baclofen decrease Bax expression and increase Bcl-2 expression induced by KA in hippocampal CA1 and CA3/DG regions

Prior application of muscimol and baclofen resulted in the decreased expression of Bax at 6 h after KA treatment in both CA1 and CA3/DG regions, whereas the level of Bcl-2 was obviously increased at 6 h after KA injection.

2.12 Muscimol and baclofen attenuate Bax translocation and the release of cytochrome c induced by KA in hippocampal CA1 and CA3/DG regions

Muscimol and baclofen inhibited Bax translocation in the mitochondrial fraction at 6 h after KA administration compared with the saline control in both CA1 and CA3/DG regions. In the cytosolic fraction, cytochrome c immunoreactivity was evident as a single band at 6 h of KA injection. However, it was weakly detected in the saline group. A significant amount of mitochondrial cytochrome c was detected in the saline group, and it decreased at 6 h after KA injection corresponding to a marked increase in the cytosolic fraction. Moreover, muscimol and baclofen inhibited the release of cytochrome c from mitochondria to the cytosol in CA1 and CA3/DG fields.

2.13 Muscimol and baclofen inhibit the activation of caspase-3 and neuronal apoptosis induced by KA in hippocampal CA1 and CA3/DG regions

Muscimol and baclofen pretreatment diminished the activation of caspase-3 at 6 h after KA injection. Furthermore, significant numbers of TUNEL-positive cells were observed in the KA-treated group after 7 days, but administration of muscimol and baclofen 40 min before KA injection significantly decreased TUNEL-positive cells.

3. Conclusion

KA induced the assembly of the GluR6-PSD95-MLK3 signaling module and subsequently activated JNK downstream signaling pathways, ultimately resulting in neuronal cell death. Application of Tat-GluR6-9c, a GluR6 C terminus-containing peptide, suppressed the clustering of GluR6 in the postsynaptic regions by competitively binding to the PDZ1 domain of PSD95 and subsequently inhibited the assembly of the GluR6-PSD95-MLK3 signaling module. As a result, the peptide attenuated the activation of MLK3 and JNK. Furthermore, Tat-GluR6-9c inhibited the activation of the nuclear and non-nuclear pathways of JNK induced by KA. Notably, the peptide had neuroprotective effects against rat epileptic brain damage. In conclusion, the kainate receptor subunit GluR6 plays an important role in brain damage induced by KA, and Tat-GluR6-9c provides a new approach for epileptic seizure therapy.

Co-application of muscimol ($GABA_A$ receptor agonist) and baclofen ($GABA_B$ receptor agonist) inhibited the assembly of the GluR6-PSD95-MLK3 signaling module. The two agonists attenuated the activation of MLK3 and JNK. Furthermore, muscimol and baclofen inhibited the activation of the nuclear and non-nuclear pathways of JNK induced by KA. Notably, the coapplication the two agonists had neuroprotective effects against rat epileptic brain damage. This highlighted that the balance between neuronal excitation and inhibition is critical for maintaining normal function.

4. Acknowledgment

This work was supported by Grant from the Key Project of the National Natural Science Foundation of China (30330190), grants from the National Natural Science Foundation of China (No. 90608015; No. 30870543; No. 31000360), the Natural Science Funds of Jiangsu Province (No. BK2010176), the Education Departmental Nature Science Funds of Jiangsu Province (09KJB310015) and the Science and Technology Development Funds (XF10C077). Dr. Chong Li was supported by "Six Talent Peaks Program" of Jiangsu Province of China in 2009.

5. References

Attwell, D., Barbour, B. and Szatkowski, M. (1993) Nonvesicular release of neurotransmitter. *Neuron,* 11, 401-407.

Ben-Ari, Y. (1985) Limbic seizure and brain damage produced by kainic acid: mechanisms and relevance to human temporal lobe epilepsy. *Neuroscience,* 14, 375-403.

Costa, C., Leone, G., Saulle, E., Pisani, F., Bernardi, G. and Calabresi, P. (2004) Coactivation of GABA(A) and GABA(B) receptor results in neuroprotection during in vitro ischemia. *Stroke,* 35, 596-600.

Dingledine, R., Borges, K., Bowie, D. and Traynelis, S. F. (1999) The glutamate receptor ion channels. *Pharmacological reviews,* 51, 7-61.

Garcia, E. P., Mehta, S., Blair, L. A., Wells, D. G., Shang, J., Fukushima, T., Fallon, J. R., Garner, C. C. and Marshall, J. (1998) SAP90 binds and clusters kainate receptors causing incomplete desensitization. *Neuron,* 21, 727-739.

Henshall, D. C., Araki, T., Schindler, C. K., Lan, J. Q., Tiekoter, K. L., Taki, W. and Simon, R. P. (2002) Activation of Bcl-2-associated death protein and counter-response of Akt within cell populations during seizure-induced neuronal death. *J Neurosci,* 22, 8458-8465.

Henshall, D. C., Chen, J. and Simon, R. P. (2000) Involvement of caspase-3-like protease in the mechanism of cell death following focally evoked limbic seizures. *J Neurochem,* 74, 1215-1223.

Kew, J. N. and Kemp, J. A. (2005) Ionotropic and metabotropic glutamate receptor structure and pharmacology. *Psychopharmacology,* 179, 4-29.

Li, C., Xu, B., Wang, W. W., Yu, X. J., Zhu, J., Yu, H. M., Han, D., Pei, D. S. and Zhang, G. Y. (2010) Coactivation of GABA receptors inhibits the JNK3 apoptotic pathway via disassembly of GluR6-PSD-95-MLK3 signaling module in KA-induced seizure. *Epilepsia,* 51, 391-403.

Lilliu, V., Perrone-Capano, C., Pernas-Alonso, R., Diaz Trelles, R., Luca Colucci d'Amato, G., Zuddas, A. and di Porzio, U. (2002) Ontogeny of kainate receptor gene expression in the developing rat midbrain and striatum. *Brain research,* 104, 1-10.

Liu, X. M., Pei, D. S., Guan, Q. H., Sun, Y. F., Wang, X. T., Zhang, Q. X. and Zhang, G. Y. (2006) Neuroprotection of Tat-GluR6-9c against neuronal death induced by kainate in rat hippocampus via nuclear and non-nuclear pathways. *J Biol Chem,* 281, 17432-17445.

Mayer, M. L. and Armstrong, N. (2004) Structure and function of glutamate receptor ion channels. *Annual review of physiology,* 66, 161-181.

Mehta, S., Wu, H., Garner, C. C. and Marshall, J. (2001) Molecular mechanisms regulating the differential association of kainate receptor subunits with SAP90/PSD-95 and SAP97. *J Biol Chem,* 276, 16092-16099.

Moldavan, M. G., Irwin, R. P. and Allen, C. N. (2006) Presynaptic GABA(B) receptors regulate retinohypothalamic tract synaptic transmission by inhibiting voltage-gated Ca2+ channels. *Journal of neurophysiology,* 95, 3727-3741.

Mulle, C., Sailer, A., Perez-Otano, I. et al. (1998) Altered synaptic physiology and reduced susceptibility to kainate-induced seizures in GluR6-deficient mice. *Nature,* 392, 601-605.

Pan, J., Zhang, Q. G. and Zhang, G. Y. (2005) The neuroprotective effects of K252a through inhibiting MLK3/MKK7/JNK3 signaling pathway on ischemic brain injury in rat hippocampal CA1 region. *Neuroscience,* 131, 147-159.

Pei, D. S., Guan, Q. H., Sun, Y. F., Zhang, Q. X., Xu, T. L. and Zhang, G. Y. (2005) Neuroprotective effects of GluR6 antisense oligodeoxynucleotides on transient brain ischemia/reperfusion-induced neuronal death in rat hippocampal CA1 region. *Journal of neuroscience research,* 82, 642-649.

Pei, D. S., Wang, X. T., Liu, Y. et al. (2006) Neuroprotection against ischaemic brain injury by a GluR6-9c peptide containing the TAT protein transduction sequence. *Brain,* 129, 465-479.

Porter, R. H., Eastwood, S. L. and Harrison, P. J. (1997) Distribution of kainate receptor subunit mRNAs in human hippocampus, neocortex and cerebellum, and bilateral reduction of hippocampal GluR6 and KA2 transcripts in schizophrenia. *Brain Res,* 751, 217-231.

Savinainen, A., Garcia, E. P., Dorow, D., Marshall, J. and Liu, Y. F. (2001) Kainate receptor activation induces mixed lineage kinase-mediated cellular signaling cascades via post-synaptic density protein 95. *J Biol Chem,* 276, 11382-11386.

Sperk, G., Lassmann, H., Baran, H., Kish, S. J., Seitelberger, F. and Hornykiewicz, O. (1983) Kainic acid induced seizures: neurochemical and histopathological changes. *Neuroscience,* 10, 1301-1315.

Tian, H., Zhang, Q. G., Zhu, G. X., Pei, D. S., Guan, Q. H. and Zhang, G. Y. (2005) Activation of c-Jun NH2-terminal kinase 3 is mediated by the GluR6.PSD-95.MLK3 signaling module following cerebral ischemia in rat hippocampus. *Brain Res,* 1061, 57-66.

Tibbles, L. A., Ing, Y. L., Kiefer, F., Chan, J., Iscove, N., Woodgett, J. R. and Lassam, N. J. (1996) MLK-3 activates the SAPK/JNK and p38/RK pathways via SEK1 and MKK3/6. *EMBO J*, 15, 7026-7035.

Yang, D. D., Kuan, C. Y., Whitmarsh, A. J., Rincon, M., Zheng, T. S., Davis, R. J., Rakic, P. and Flavell, R. A. (1997) Absence of excitotoxicity-induced apoptosis in the hippocampus of mice lacking the Jnk3 gene. *Nature*, 389, 865-870.

Zhang, F., Li, C., Wang, R., Han, D., Zhang, Q. G., Zhou, C., Yu, H. M. and Zhang, G. Y. (2007) Activation of GABA receptors attenuates neuronal apoptosis through inhibiting the tyrosine phosphorylation of NR2A by Src after cerebral ischemia and reperfusion. *Neuroscience*, 150, 938-949.

11

Biophysical Aspects of the Nonsynaptic Epileptiform Activity

Antônio-Carlos G. Almeida[1], Antônio M. Rodrigues[1], Mário A. Duarte[1], Gilcélio da Silveira[1], Fulvio A. Scorza[2], Ricardo M. Arida[2], Jaderson C. Costa[3] and Esper A. Cavalheiro[2]
[1]Universidade Federal de São João del-Rei
[2]Universidade Federal de São Paulo
[3]Pontifícia Universidade Católica do Rio Grande do Sul
Brazil

1. Introduction

Since the demonstration that the hippocampus slice exposed to low calcium external solution is able to sustain nonsynaptic epileptiform activity, it has been accepted that nonsynaptic interactions may be sufficient, in some conditions, for generating seizure like activity in cortical network. Recently, evidences have suggested that the reductions in calcium are not essential for nonsynaptic mechanisms to contribute to epileptic activity. Therefore, evidences allow demonstrating that the conjoint actuation of nonsynaptic mechanisms and nonsynaptic connections are able to induce and sustain seizures. The nonsynaptic mechanisms considered in this context are all mechanisms which are not directly involved with synaptic transmission, but comprehending important action on the homeostasis equilibrium and, consequently, on the neuronal excitability.

The non-synaptic connections are all types of neuronal coupling that are not mediated by synaptic transmission. The concomitant actuation of nonsynaptic mechanisms and connections seems to be a relevant process for the seizure intensity modulation. Therefore, it may be conjectured that the nonsynaptic mechanisms and connections could be considered a natural target for investigations aiming to control refractory seizures. Within this perspective, the scope of the present chapter will cover the following topics:

- nonsynaptic events: experimental induction and electrophysiological characteristics;
- nonsynaptic mechanisms;
- nonsynaptic connections;
- biophysical aspects of the nonsynaptic epileptiform activities;
- possible targets for controlling refractory seizures.

2. Nonsynaptic epileptiform events

In *in vivo* experiments, chemically induced focal cortical seizures were observed to be sometimes preceded by small reductions in $[Ca^{2+}]_o$ and to become intense during the paroxysms (Heinemann et al., 1977; Krnjevic et al., 1980). Those findings lead to suspect that the calcium reduction may influence the course to the paroxysms. As the description by Jefferys & Haas (1982) and Taylor & Dudek (1982) show, it is well known that the hippocampus slice exposed to low calcium external solution is able to sustain nonsynaptic epileptiform activity. Based on the fact that low Ca^{2+} seizures occur in conditions of suppressed excitatory synaptic transmission, experimental findings demonstrate that nonsynaptic interactions may be sufficient, in some situations, for generating seizurelike activity in cortical network (Konnerth et al., 1986). More recently, evidences have suggested that the reductions in calcium are not essential for nonsynaptic mechanisms to contribute to epileptic activity (Bikson et al., 2002). Therefore, the nonsynaptic connections may have wider relevance than it could be initially suspected.

The nonsynaptic epileptiform activity was first observed in CA1 region of hippocampus slice involving the use of solutions with low $[Ca^{2+}]$. Later, observations of the occurrence of prolonged field bursts in the dentate gyrus (DG) have been reported (Schweitzer et al., 1992). These authors pointed out the effect of deletion of Ca^{2+} from the bath solution on burst firing in CA3, CA1, and DG. When a calcium-free 5 mM $[K^+]_o$ solution was used, spontaneous bursts could still be observed in CA3 and CA1, but not in DG. However, at 9 mM $[K^+]_o$, although absent in CA3 and CA1, in DG spontaneous bursts characterized by an abrupt prolonged negative shift in the extracellular field potential could be observed followed by the appearance of large paroxysmal population spikes. The DG spontaneous bursts exhibited similarity to the "maximal dentate activation" (MDA), observed in vivo in the same region (Somjen et al., 1985; Stringer et al., 1989, 1991; Stringer & Lothman, 1991). Therefore, the ability of each region to generate or sustain nonsynaptic epileptiform activity depends on the circumstances, more specifically on the level of calcium reduction and potassium increase.

In the hippocampus, especially in the DG, the tight packing of the cell bodies of neurons and glial cells constitutes an adequate substrate for the nonsynaptic connections. In high-potassium and zero-Ca^{2+} conditions the granule cells have some endogenous bursting capabilities able to sustain synchronization and, consequently, spontaneous epileptiform activity (Pan & Stringer, 1996). As these observations have been made in the absence of synaptic transmission, because Ca^{2+} has been deleted from the bath solution, synchronization mechanisms must have nonsynaptic origin (Schweitzer et al., 1992; Pan & Stringer, 1996) and could be mediated by gap-junctions, ionic fluctuations, or field effect.

It is known that the electrical signaling in neurons and glial cells is based on the activities of the ion pumps and carriers that establish transmembrane ionic gradients, and on the operation of ionic channels that generate current and voltage response based on electrodiffusion. Therefore, the cellular mechanisms described in the present study and investigated in the context of the epilepsy, by means of a computational simulation, are: membrane ionic currents, Na^+/K^+-ATPase, cotransporters, and exchangers. The cell activity of the network was nonsynaptically connected using extracellular electrodiffusion calculation, as well as the electric field effect and the gap-junctional coupling.

2.1 Experimental induction and electrophysiological characteristics

2.1.1 Inducing non-synaptic epileptiform activity and experimental apparatus

Hippocampal slices from Wistar rats were prepared (4-6 weeks old, male). After eutanized in a CO_2 chamber, the brains were removed. Transverse slices (400 μm) through the hippocampus were cut with a tissue chopper. After cutting, slices were stored in an oxygenated holding chamber for ≥ 1 h before recording. All recordings were acquired in an interface-chamber and continuously perfused with artificial cerebrospinal fluid (ACSF) at 32°C under a stream of humidified 95% O_2/5% CO_2. Composition of the ACSF was (in mM): NaCl 127, KCl 2, $MgSO_4$ 1.5, KH_2PO_4 1.1, $NaHCO_3$ 26, $CaCl_2$ 2 and glucose 10. All solutions were bubbled constantly with 95% O2/5% CO2. Slices were allowed to equilibrate for 1 h in normal ACSF. Recording electrodes were made of microfilament capillary thin-walled glass (0.9 mm ID, 1.2 mm OD) pulled on a micropipette puller (DMZ Universal Puller - Zeitz-Instruments). Electrodes were filled with 2 M NaCl and had impedances between 5 and 10 MΩ. Recording electrodes were placed in the cell body layer of the region of interest. Nonsynaptic epileptiform activity was induced in the hippocampus by changing to ACSF containing 0-added calcium and high potassium. The potassium was raised to 6 mM to induce epileptiform activity in the CA1 region and was raised to 8 mM to induce epileptiform activity in the dentate gyrus. The non-synaptic epileptiform activity can take more than an hour to appear, but once it appears, the interval between field bursts and the burst duration remain stable for many hours (Bikson et al., 1999; Pan & Stringer, 1996).

In our laboratory, the interface-chamber is a variant of those used in several studies aimed at studying with in vitro slices (Pan & Stringer, 1996; Schwartzkroin, 1975). The chamber consists of two coupled modules: the perfusion module and the heating module. The slice perfusion module (top view of the chamber, Fig. 1) consists of two cylinders and an acrylic base, which attaches superiorly to the heating module (see side view of the chamber, Fig. 1). The central cylinder is where a Millipore membrane (0.4 μm Millicell culture plate inserts; Milleppori, Bedford, MA, USA) is inserted. The slices are deposited on the membrane. The region in between the membrane and the acrylic base has approximately 0.34 ml, allowing the solution in contact with the slices, through the membrane, to be constantly renewed. The acrylic base has small holes through which carbogen, after crossing the water bath of the heating module, can humidify and oxygenate the slices. A disc-shaped lid covers the perfusion module ensuring homogeneity of the environment surrounding the slice. The lid has a central hole that allows insertion of the recording electrode and the carbogen release.

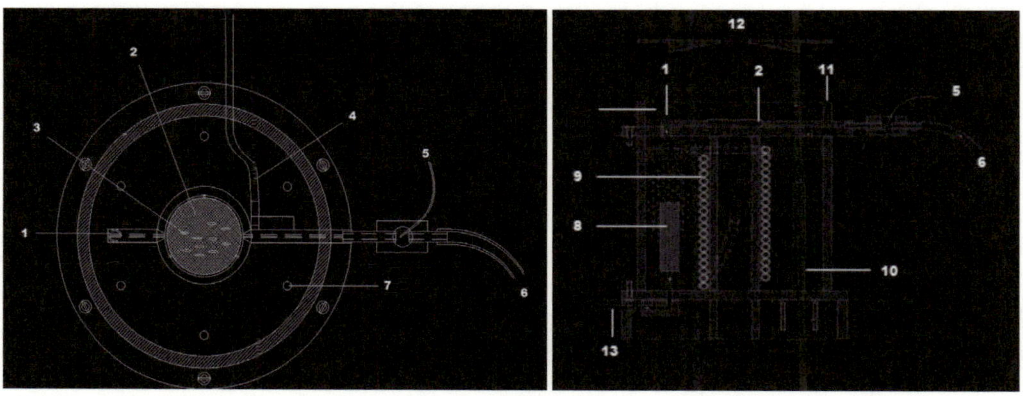

Fig. 1. Interface chamber. Schematic diagram of the interface chamber. (left) superior view - (right) lateral view. (1) perfusion solution entry; (2) Millipore membrane; (3) brain slices; (4) thermometer; (5) ground wire; (6) solution output; (7) holes for conduct the warm and moisturized carbogen into the chamber; (8) carbogen bubbler; (9) heating the perfusion solution; (10) heater; (11) chamber external cylinder; (12) carbogen release; (13) carbogen input.

The heating module is composed of four heating points and two bubblers that disperse carbogen in the water. The equipment, computer controlled, is capable of maintaining the temperature around 34 ° C. The water in the bath warms the perfusion solution when it flows through the tube, around the central cylinder.
To monitor regions of the slices where the activities spontaneously emerge and to guide the electrode positioning and also to evaluate the extension of the recruitment, the slices were transilluminated from below using a halogen lamp from the illuminating system of the upright binocular microscope (model SMZ 1500 - Nikon, Japan). The slices were viewed from above through a 3× or 4× objective, depending on the size of the region studied. The video images were captured using a CCD camera (Cool SNAP-Pro cf 1.4 megapixel cooled, USA). The images were processed on-line for composing the STF images. For this purpose the frames were digitalized by means of a frame-grabber board (DC10 Plus, Pinnacle, USA), controlled by an acquisition software developed in MatLab platform. All the images were captured at a rate of 30 frames per second. Optionally, the images can be processed offline. In this case, all captured frames were stored on a DVD disc. The electrographic signal was used to control the range of frames to be captured.
To obtain images of the light transmittance changes (LTC), the calculation was carried out similarly to the method described by Andrew et al. (1996). Briefly, the averages of the corresponding pixels of the first 50 frames, before the wave propagation, formed the control image (T_{cont}), which was subtracted, pixel by pixel, from each subsequent experimental image (T_{exp}). The resultant image of this subtraction was divided, pixel by pixel, by the T_{cont}. Specifically

$$LTC = \frac{(T_{\exp} - T_{cont})}{T_{cont}} \qquad (1)$$

Using a gray intensity scale, the series of LTC images revealed areas of the slice where the light transmittance changes with time. To condense on a single image the spatiotemporal features (STF) of paroxysmal activity, the contour of the layer involved in the activity is resembled by a polygonal, drawn manually, by setting pixel positions that are then linked forming the polygonal (Figure 2.A).
The STF images were built column by column. For each LTC image, the average intensity of the pixels of a square region (21×21 pixels) centered in each pixel of the polygonal was calculated. These values are the intensities of each pixel of the column obtained rectifying the polygonal over a vertical line. The STF image is composed disposing these columns, from left to right, following the temporal sequence (Figure 2.B and 2.C).

2.1.2 Electrophysiological and spatial characteristics

Electrographically, the non-synaptic epileptiform activity, recorded in the extracellular space of the granular layer of the dentate gyrus, is characterized by ictogenic period with intense population spikes bursts with amplitudes around 10 mV, duration between 30 - 60s and interevent interval around 50s (Fig. 3). These bursts are always accompanied by a negative DC-shift (5-10 mV). Concurrently to the electrographic manifestations, the optical images show that the spatial recruitment engages a portion of the granular layer, preferably the infra-piramidal portion. Although it is possible to estimate with two electrodes the velocity of propagation of the events in the order of mm/s, it is not unusual to observe the

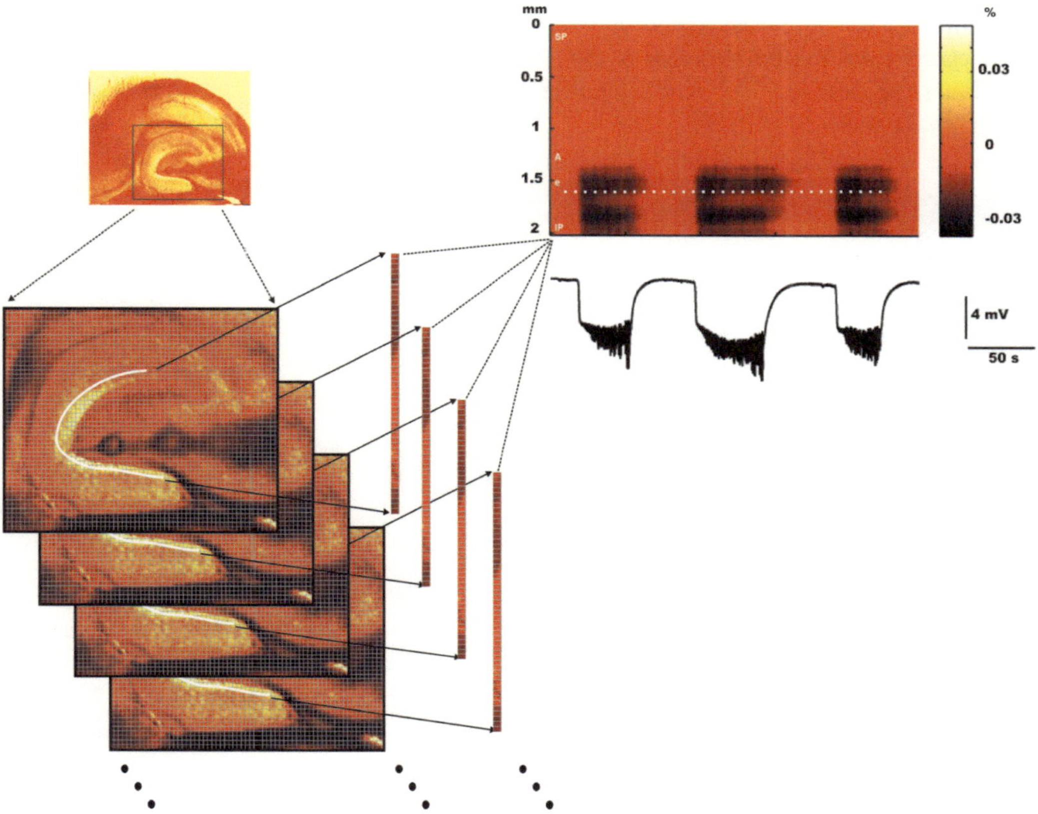

Fig. 2. Schematic representation of the procedure for composing the STF images. (A) The brain slice and the polygonal representing the contour of the layer of interest. (B) Temporal sequence of frames showing the rectified polygonal extracted from each of them. (C) Disposing each polygonal rectified and side by side, the STF images are composed and the pixels are calculated according to the equation 1. The scale indicates the percentage of the light transmittance change according to equation (1).

simultaneous build up of the whole neuronal region recruited, identified by no delays between the signals, suggesting a synergistic excitation of the neuronal tissue involved (Fig 2) The paroxysmal activity sustains stable for up to 3-4h after Ca^{2+} washout has begun. In our experiments, spreading depression usually appears spontaneously after this period. This occurrence of a few episodes of spreading depression normally precedes the irreversible deterioration of the preparation (Fig. 3).

In a substantial portion of the slices investigated in our laboratory, the increase of the DC shift can be associated with a decrease of the population spikes amplitude. This observation, when correlated with the optical signal, shows that it is not always valid to inspect synchrony by means of evaluating the population spikes amplitudes. In fact, as exemplified in Fig. 4, the eugenol effect, a blocker of sodium voltage-sensitive channel, is the reduction of the neuronal population recruited, accompanied by increase of the population spike amplitudes and decrease of the DC shift amplitude. Correlating this observation with the biophysical mechanisms of the bursts generation, analyzed in session 5.2, it can be proposed that the population spike amplitude can also be modulated by the transmembrane ionic gradients. These gradients, when involving a large neuronal population, may change significantly resulting the decrease of the action potentials amplitude and, therefore, of the population spikes. In these circumstances, the association with synchronism decrease doesn't make sense.

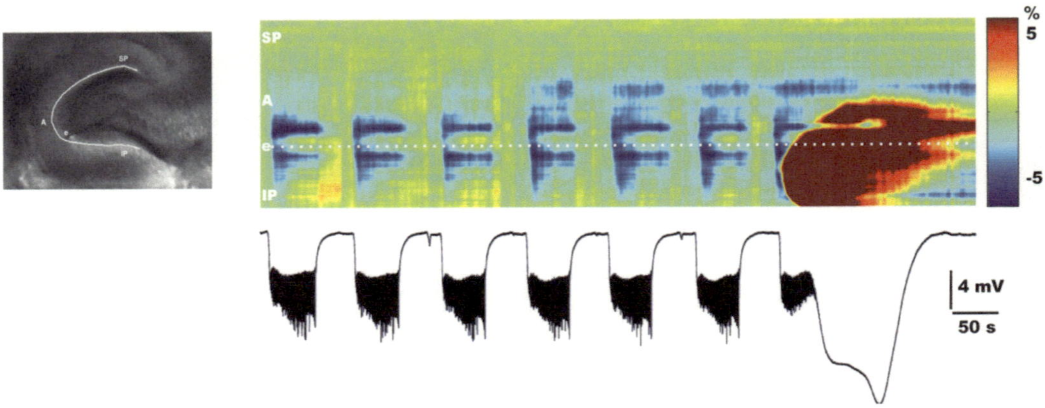

Fig. 3. STF image of a sequential nonsynaptic bursts and the transition to spreading depression. Simultaneous extracellular potential is shown in the bottom. The scale indicates the percentage of the light transmittance change according to equation (1).

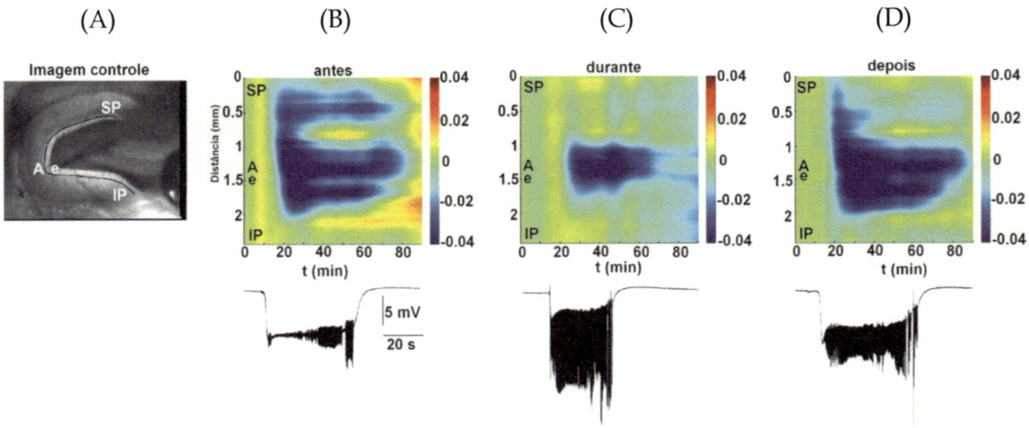

Fig. 4. Optical image and extracellular potential measured simulataneously. (A) Hippocampus slice magnified to show details of the dentate gyrus (A: apex; SP: suprapiramidal; IP: infrapiramidal). Along of the granular layer, the poligonal line used to extract the STF images shown in (B – before eugenol), (C – during eugenol) and (D - after eugenol).

3. Nonsynaptic mechanisms

The processes of neuronal depolarization and hyperpolarization can not be described simply by Na^+ channels and voltage-sensitive K^+ or by the movement of Na^+, K^+, Cl^- associated with the activation of neurotransmitter receptors. In fact, for processes that involve the activation of populations of neurons and glial cells synchronously, such as epileptiform activity, in particular those of origin not only synaptic, ionic balance is also determined by the activity of a large number of pumps, exchangers and cotransporters. The net effect of the performance of these mechanisms is therefore critical to cellular excitability. It is important to observe that ion flux associated with transporter molecules is electrically neutral and is mediated by ionic gradients established primarily by Na/K pump. Therefore, as pointed out by Schwartzkroin at al. (1998), the identification of the nonsynaptic mechanisms participating on this dynamic process and their location (e.g. neuron versus glia) is critical to our understanding of excitability controls. In this item, we will describe the nonsynaptic mechanisms whose actions on the epileptiform activity will be considered in our investigation.

3.1 Na/K pump

The pumping process mediated by the Na/K pump is an ionic transport mechanism responsible for maintaining the Na^+ and K^+ transmembrane concentration gradients, essentials for several cellular functions. The Na/K pump promotes the coupled Na^+ efflux and K^+ influx, in a 3:2 rate and using the energy liberated by the ATP hydrolyses (Glitsch, 2001). Nowadays, the functioning of the Na/K pump in terms of the Albers-Post alternating gate model (Scheiner-Bobis, 2002; Horisberger, 2004) is very well accepted. The Na/K pump is conceived as ionic channel with two gates, one external and other internal. The opening and closing of these gates are coupled and controlled by phosphorylation and dephosphorylation of the Na/K-ATPase, occurring alternately and promoting the transport of Na^+ to the extra- and K^+ to the intracellular space.

3.2 Cation-chloride co-transporter and exchanger mechanisms

Investigations from hippocampal slices in vitro show that cation chloride cotransporter antagonists block epileptiform activity in a variety of seizure models, regardless of the synaptic mechanisms involved. For example, furosemide blocked epileptiform activity in the zero-calcium model in which all chemical synaptic activities are absent, and in which epileptiform discharges must be fully mediated by mechanisms other than chemical synapses. Other in vitro studies showed that furosemide decreases the cellular swelling during conditions of increased $[K^+]_o$ and blocks ECS decreases in hippocampal slices during stimulation-evoked discharges and epileptiform activity. These results show that the cation-chloride antagonists affect some mechanisms common to all seizure models tested, including those that are not dependent on chemical synaptic interactions, and therefore, are required for maintenance of epileptiform activity.

At the start of investigations into the cotransporter it was difficult to differentiate one type of cation-chloride cotransporter (CCC) from the other. However, it is currently known that the CCC family in mammals consists of nine members encoded by the genes Slc12a1-9. Two members are Na-K-2Cl cotransporters (NKCCs; isoforms NKCC1 and KCC2), one is an Na-Cl cotransporter (NCC), and four are K-Cl cotransporters (KCCs; isoforms KCC1-4). The physiological roles of the remaining two CCCs (CIP1 or Slc12a8, and CCC9 or Slc12a9) are yet unknown. With the exception of NKCC2 and NCC, which are predominantly found in kidney, all CCCs are expressed in neurons or glial cells—or both—at least at some stage of CNS development. For all CCCs members, the Na-K ATPase generates plasmalemmal K^+ and Na^+ gradients that provide the main source of energy for their function. The transport

stoichiometry of CCCs renders them electrically silent, thus they do not directly influence the neuronal membrane potential (Blaesse et al., 2009).
The NKCC has the following characteristics (Russell, 2000): 1) displacement of ions through the NKCC requires that all three ionic species (Na^+, K^+ and Cl^-) are simultaneously present in a same face of the membrane, 2) furosemide and congeners bind to proteins co-carrier and inhibit the transport of the three ions; 3) under normal ionic conditions, it functions with the influx of ions and the process has a stoichiometry of 1 (Na^+): 1 (K^+): 2 (Cl^-) for the majority of cells. However, during epileptiform events, which occur in large influxes of Na^+ and Cl^-, the direction of flow can reverse NKCC, therefore carrying the ions to the extracellular environment. The magnitude and direction of ion flux mediated by the NKCC, described by Geck and Pfieffer (1985), are functionally proportional to the difference between the products of concentrations.
Similar to NKCC, the KCC is characterized by a cotransporter protein that mediates the movement of ions, obligatorily coupled in the same direction (in this case, K^+ and Cl^-). The direction of flow depends on the concentration gradients of the two ions across the membrane. Thus, under normal conditions, the KCC promotes the efflux of ions K^+ and Cl^-. The KCC is also blocked by the diuretic furosemide and its congeners, but with less efficiency. In most cells where the KCC has been found, their main function seems to be the regulation of cell volume by removal of K^+ ions and the Cl^- intracellularly. As with the NKCC, the KCC flow is functionally proportional to the difference between the products of ions concentrations (Hochman et al., 1999).
Another type of ion transporter similar to the cotransporter mechanisms is the exchangers. These transporters activity constitutes an electroneutral transport based on the simultaneous exchange of a pair of anions or cations. These mechanisms are present in the hippocampus and their functions are associated with transmembrane ionic gradient recovery, cell volume regulation, and pH (Chesler, 2003). The exchangers under investigation in our group are Na^+/H^+ and HCO_3^-/Cl^-. The last exchanger is considered to have, in each side, sites whose affinities are exclusive to the ions involved. However, for the Na^+/H^+ exchanger, there are evidences of different behaviour; the enzyme is known to have also affinity to K^+ (Sychrova, 2004).

3.3 Osmotic regulation and cell volume changes

Investigating the effect of osmolarity on synchronized neuronal activities supported by non-synaptic mechanisms, Dudek et al. (1990) found that decreasing the extracellular osmolarity, which reduces extracellular volume, the epileptiform bursts become more intense. Additionally, the increase in osmolality with solutes which do not permeate the cell membranes, causing an increase in extracellular volume, ends up blocking or lowering epileptiform discharges. Therefore, reductions in extracellular volume can enhance the synchronization between hippocampal CA1 neurons mediated by non-synaptic communications. Indeed, while changes in the volume of the extracellular space (ECS) are small during normal physiological activity, during synchronized excitatory activity, such as bursts of epileptiform discharges, such variations can be considerable. Specifically in the case of non-synaptic epileptiform activity, the consequence of these changes in ECS can be: (i) effect of extracellular ion accumulation would be magnified due to the reduced level of dilution (ii) ephaptic interactions, mediated by current flow through ECS, would increase due to the high resistance of the ECS.

3.4 Membrane ionic currents

The main ionic species involved in the nonsynaptic paroxysms are sodium, potassium and chloride. These ions flow through the neuronal and glial membranes. During the excitation process of the nonsynaptic bursts their actuations, therefore, are not related with the neurotransmission through the synaptic cleft. The permeability changes of each ionic specie through the corresponding channels are responsible for the changes in the intracellular potential. The ionic channel types considered in the present investigation were: sodium and potassium voltage dependent channels, persistent sodium channels, A-type potassium channel, chloride channel (with constant permeability), chloride channel voltage channel, sodium, potassium and chloride fluxes through gap junctions, sodium, potassium and chloride channels with constant permeability (Fig. 5)

4. Nonsynaptic connections

The types of nonsynaptic interactions that may be involved in the synchronization include: electrotonic interactions mediated by gap-junctions (Naus et al., 1991; Perez-Velazques et al., 1994), changes in extracellular space (Roper et al., 1992), field effects (Jefferys & Haas, 1982; Taylor & Dudek, 1982; Dudek et al., 1986), and extracellular ionic fluctuations (Taylor & Dudek, 1984). In the hippocampus, especially in the DG, the tight packing of the cell bodies of neurons and glial cells constitutes an adequate substrate for the nonsynaptic connections. In high-potassium and zero-Ca^{2+} conditions the granule cells have some endogenous bursting capabilities able to sustain synchronization and, consequently, spontaneous epileptiform activity (Pan & Stringer, 1996). As these observations have been made in the absence of synaptic transmission, because Ca^{2+} has been deleted from the bath solution, synchronization mechanisms must have nonsynaptic origin (Schweitzer et al., 1992; Pan & Stringer, 1996) and could be mediated, as already mentioned, by gap-junctions, ionic fluctuations, or field effect (Fig. 6)

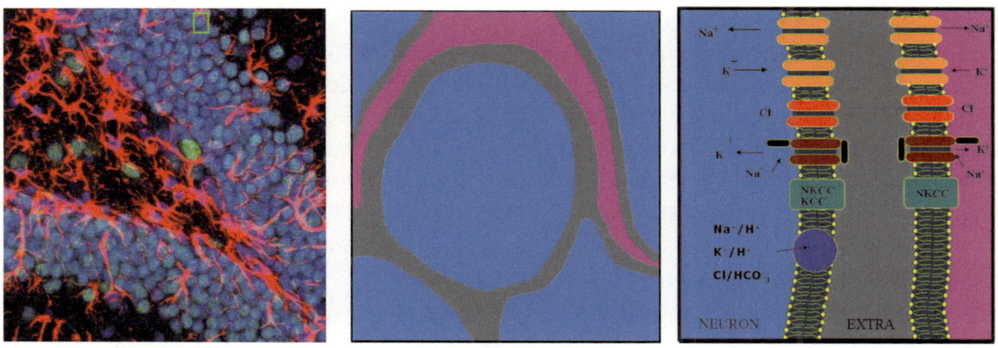

(A) (B) (C)

Fig. 5. Diagramatic conception of the tissue and its cell membranes component representation. (A) DG granullar layer - neurons (blue/green) in the dendate gyrus surrounded by astrocytic processes (red) (extracted from J. Breunig, Rakic Lab.) allows to extract the basic constituents. From the squared region in (A) and magnified in (B), it can be defined the functional unit of the tissue. From this functional unit an additional magnification (C) allow to define the main components of the neuronal and glial membranes. Na^+ (orange), K^+ (orange) and Cl^- (red) channels, Na/K pumps (brown), cotransporters (green) and exchangers (blue).

5. Biophysical aspects of the nonsynaptic epileptiform activities

The complexity of the mechanisms involved in the nonsynaptic epileptiform activities comprehend a puzzle where the collection of experimental data is not enough to unravel the biophysical aspects of the initiation, the build up, and the termination of these activities. In other words, the main mechanisms responsible for the transition from the interictal to the ictal state must be explored by means of a methodology able to translate all experimental observations in a single systemic representation of the neuronal tissue that is the source of the activity. In this section, we show the mathematical description of subcellular mechanisms suspected to have significant involvement in the non-synaptic epileptiform activity. Next, neurons and glial cells are represented by the composition of these mechanisms. Finally, with population of neurons and glial cells, nonsynaptically connected, the neuronal tissue is represented and the epileptiform activities can be computationally simulated. With the simulations, the mechanisms are manipulated allowing investigating their contributions.

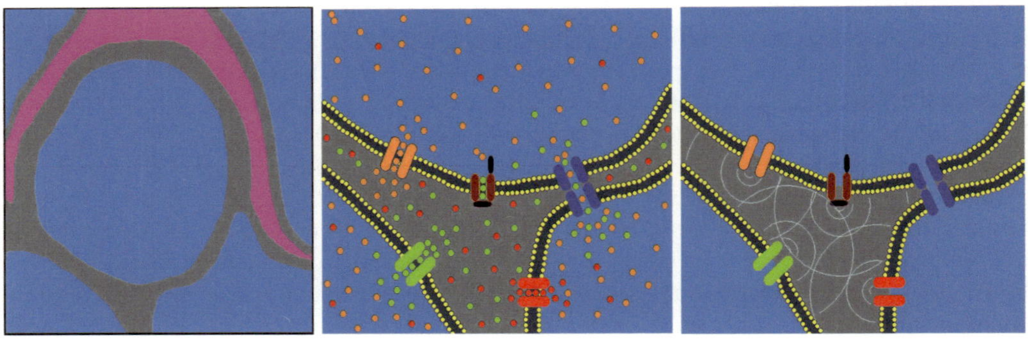

(A) (B) (C)

Fig. 6. Nonsynaptic connections can be seen magnifing the squared region of the functional unit represented in (A). In (B), the ionic flow through ionic channels (green, red and blue), pumps (brown), cotransporters and exchangers (not shown) results extracellular ionic concentration changes which consists a nonsynaptic connection. The gap-junctions are the second type of nonsynaptc connections which also is responsible for the mutual coumpling between neurons. In (C), the third type of nonsynaptic connectons, the eletric field effect. The electric field generated by the ionic currents trough a given cell membrane is able to interfere with the intracellular potential of the immediate vicinity cells.

5.1 Modelling the dentate gyrus

5.1.1 Geometric representation of the cell body layer

The cell body layer of the DG, characterized by a packing of neurons and glial processes, was represented by a network of functional units. Each functional unit was composed by the cell body of a neuron and a segment of a glial process, as depicted in Fig. 7 (left). The specific geometry of each cell population was not characterized, only the threedimensional (3D) distribution of the functional units, representing the cell body layer, was incorporated. To simulate the experimental maneuver for inducing the nonsynaptic epileptiform activity in the hippocampal slice maintained in an interface chamber, the bathing fluid was represented by two shells of compartments covering the inferior and lateral sides of the cell body layer. The internal shell was composed by compartments with inactive membranes allowing the electrodiffusion of ions through the extracellular space. The most external shell was composed by compartments with constant ionic concentrations, representing the relative infinite volume of the bathing fluid in respect to the extracellular volume of each functional unit. The superior face of the cell body layer was not covered and depicted the slice in the liquid/gas interface. As there is no fluidic perfusion at this face, the ionic gradient was null in the orthogonal direction. In Fig. 7 (right), a schematic representation of the interfaces neuron/extracellular/glial cells, with the corresponding mechanisms simulated, is shown.

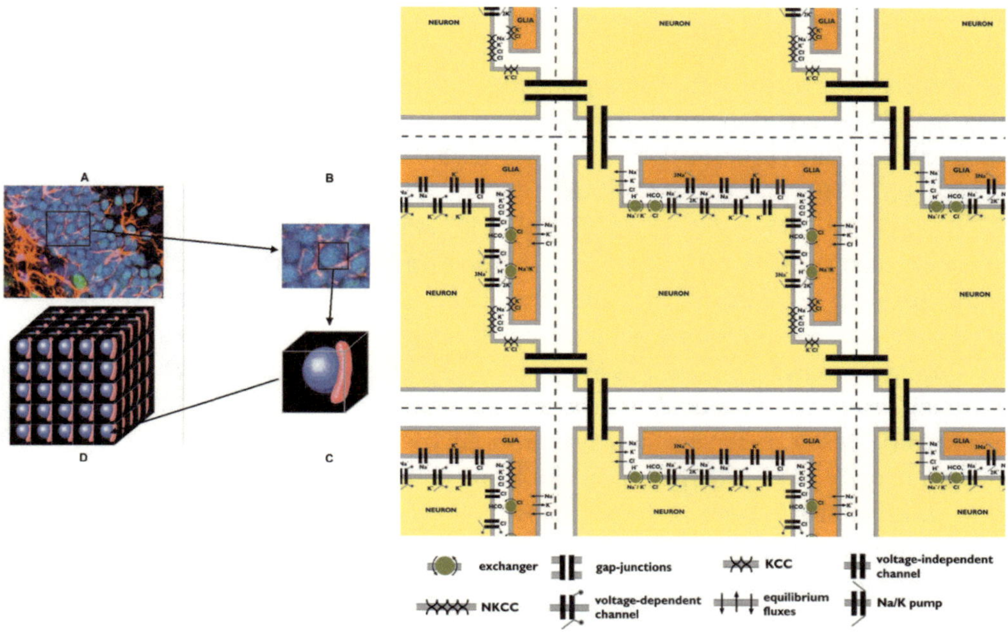

Fig. 7. Left: (A) DG granullar layer—the picture of the neurons (blue/green) in the dentate gyrus surrounded by astrocytic processes (red) (extracted from J. Breunig, Rakic Lab) allows to extract the basic constituents (B) of the functional unit (C), which will form the nodes of the tridimensional computational network used to simulate the DG (D). Right: Schematic representation of the interfaces neuron/extracellular/glial cells with the corresponding mechanisms embedded in the simulated membranes. Each neuron is connected to the neurons of the functional units of the immediate vicinity. The glial cells connection with the vicinity is mediated exclusively by the extracellular space. Modified from Almeida et al (2008).

5.1.2 Mathematical description

The fluxes through the ionic channels, gap-junctions, or Na/K pumps were described by GHK current equation (Hille, 1992):

$$\Phi_{c,\,type}^{CELL} = P_{c,\,type} z_c F \frac{V_k}{RT} \frac{[C]_i \, e^{\frac{Z_c F V_k}{RT}} - [C]_o}{e^{\frac{Z_c F V_k}{RT}} - 1}, \qquad (2)$$

where $\phi_{c,\,type}$ is the flux of the ion C associated to the *type* (channel, pump, gap junction) of mechanism described, $P_{c,type}$ is the permeability, V_k is the transmembrane potential in the case of the ionic channels and the electrogenic current pump. When referring to gap-junctions, V_k is the potential difference between the neighboring cells connected by the connexins, $[C]_i$ and $[C]_o$ are the intracellular and extracellular concentration, respectively. When calculating the gap-junction current, $[C]_o$ is replaced by the intracellular ionic concentration of the cell connected, z_c is the valence of the ion C, F (96.487 C/mmol) the Faraday constant, R (8.314 mV.C/K.mmol) the gas constant and T (210.16 K) the temperature.

The permeabilities of the sodium and potassium voltage dependent channels were simulated using the Hodgkin-Huxley formalism (Supplemental Material – Almeida et al., 2008). The ionic permeability parameters $\overline{P}_{Na,fast}^{neuron}$ (7.78×10-4 cm/s), $\overline{P}_{K}^{neuron}$ (1.80×10-4 cm/s), $\overline{P}_{Na,persistent}^{neuron}$ (7.20×10^{-8} cm/s), $\overline{P}_{K,A}^{neuron}$ (3.60 × 10^{-4} cm/s), $P_{Cl,const}^{neuron}$ (3.60 × 10^{-6} cm/s), $\overline{P}_{Cl,volt-depend}^{neuron}$ (1.08 × 10^{-5} cm/s) and P_{A}^{neuron} (2.04 × 10^{-3} cm/s) are the quantitative representation of the population of each mechanism (in this case, channels or pumps) involved. Since these parameters were adjusted to reproduce the activity inductions, they were considered as *investigation parameters*. This means that these parameters were adjusted heuristically aiming at reproducing the activities, as well as investigating the preponderance of each mechanism for generating the events and their characteristics, always respecting the experimental observations. These experimental observations were collected from experiments carried out in our laboratory or from published data, like Xiong and Stringer (2000) and Pan and Stringer (1996). Based on this inspection, the associations observed between each parameters and their influences on the activities are, basically: i) $\overline{P}_{Na,fast}^{neuron}$ - depolarizing phase of the action potential; ii) $\overline{P}_{K}^{neuron}$ - polarizing phase of the action potential, neuronal excitability and extracellular potassium accumulation; iii) $\overline{P}_{Na,persistent}^{neuron}$ – initial cell depolarization (preceding the action potential firing), neuronal excitability and action potential frequency; iv) $\overline{P}_{K,A}^{neuron}$ – action potential frequency; v) $P_{Cl,const}^{neuron}$ and $\overline{P}_{Cl,volt-depend}^{neuron}$ – neuronal resting potential and extracellular chloride concentration; vi) P_{A}^{neuron} – Na/K pump activity.

The parameters $P_{gj,Na}$ (6.73 × 10^{-8} cm/s), $P_{gj,K}$ (9.92 × 10^{-8} cm/s) and $P_{gj,Cl}$ (1.84 × 10^{-8} cm/s) represent the intercellular permeability through the gap-junctions. The adjustment of these parameter was guided by the experiments from MacVicar and Dudek (1982). The permeability parameters for the glial cells, P_{Na}^{glia} (1.00 × 10^{-8} cm/s), P_{K}^{glia} (1.08 × 10^{-7} cm/s) and P_{Cl}^{glia} (2.50 × 10^{-8} cm/s), were adjusted aiming at reproducing the resting potential typical for these cells (Pan & Stringer, 1996). The Na/K pump parameter, P_{A}^{glia} (2.04 × 10^{-2} cm/s), was tuned to control the $[Na^+]_i$ of the glial cells and also to contribute to controlling the $[K^+]_o$ during the epileptiform events. The activation and inactivation factors values (m_{fast} = 0.03, h_{fast} = 0.78, n = 0.1, w_{pers} = 0.0003, a_A = 0.1, b_A = 0.8) of the voltage dependent channels correspond to the resting state defined before the activities induction.

The sodium potassium ATPase function was modeled considering the main reactions involved, always following the Albers–Post model (Heyse et al., 1994; Rodrigues et al., 2008). From the reactions describing the Albers–Post cycles, two reactions were derived, one for the forward cycle, 3NaiEi + 2KoEo + ATPEi ↔ Ai, and other for the reverse cycle, 3NaoEo + 2KiEi + ADPEi + PEi ↔ Ao.

The reactions predict the formation of a fictitious ion A+, product of each exchange of 3 Na+ by 2 K+, in the intra- or extracellular space, depending on the cycle direction. The reactions from the Albers–Post model were used to predict the substates formation and to deduce equations for the intra- and extracellular concentrations of the ion A+ :

$$[A^+]_i = K_A^i C_{E_{Na,K}}^{m,total} \left(\frac{[ATP]_i}{[ATP]_i + K_{ATP}^i \left(1 + \frac{[ADP]_i C_P^i}{K_{ADP,P}^i}\right)} \right) \left(\frac{[Na^+]_i}{[Na^+]_i + K_{Na,pump}^i \left(1 + \frac{[K^+]_i}{K_{K,pump}^i}\right)} \right)^3 \left(\frac{[K^+]_o}{[K^+]_o + K_{K,pump}^o \left(1 + \frac{[Na^+]_o}{K_{Na,pump}^o}\right)} \right)^2 \quad (3)$$

$$[A^+]_o = K_A^o C_{E_{Na,K}}^{m,total} \left(\frac{[ADP]_i [P]_i}{[ADP]_i [P]_i + K_{ADP,P}^i \left(1 + \frac{[ATP]_i}{K_{ATP}^i}\right)} \right) \left(\frac{[Na^+]_o}{[Na^+]_o + K_{Na,pump}^o \left(1 + \frac{[K^+]_o}{K_{K,pump}^o}\right)} \right)^3 \left(\frac{[K^+]_i}{[K^+]_i + K_{K,pump}^i \left(1 + \frac{[Na^+]_i}{K_{Na,pump}^i}\right)} \right)^2 \quad (4)$$

The investigations carried on by Nakao and Gadsby (1989) about the Na/K pump activity dependence on the extracellular concentrations of Na^+ and K^+ allowed to guide the pump parameters adjustment. During the experiments, [ADP] was kept constant and equal to 0 mM and a Na^+-free solution was used as extracellular medium. Therefore, normalizing the current in terms of the current for $[K^+]_o = 5.4$ mM, from equation 2, the following equation could be derived:

$$\Phi_{A^P,pump}^{norm} = \left(\frac{[K^+]_o}{[K^+]_o + K_K^o} \right)^2 \Big/ \left(\frac{5,4}{5,4 + K_K^o} \right)^2 , \quad (5)$$

where $\Phi_{Ap,pump}^{norm}$ is the normalized pump current. Using this equation to fit a curve to the experimental data, K_K^o was estimated ($K_K^o = 0.094$ mM). Once this constant was determined, considering the experimental conditions described by the authors, $[Na^+]_o = 150$ mM and $V_m = 0$ mV, and with the previous value determined for K_K^o, K_{Na}^o could be calculated finding the best curve fitting to the data, using the following equation, which gave $K_{Na}^o = 34,7$ mM.

$$\Phi_{A^P,pump}^{norm} = \left(\frac{[K^+]_o}{[K^+]_o + K_K^o \left(1 + \frac{150}{K_{Na}^o}\right)} \right)^2 \Big/ \left(\frac{5,4}{5,4 + K_K^o \left(1 + \frac{150}{K_{Na}^o}\right)} \right)^2 , \quad (6)$$

The intracellular sodium dissociation constant, K_{Na}^i, was adjusted using the data from Barmashenko *et al.* (1999). These authors measured the Na/K pump current in relation to the intracellular Na^+. The cells used in the investigation were kept in K^+-free solution and the transmembrane potential was clamped in 0 mV. The normalized current (normalization with respect to $[Na^+]_i = 50$ mM) could then be described using the next equation. By a curve fitting to the experimental data, K_{Na}^i was estimated equal to 0.856 mM.

$$\Phi^{norm}_{A^+,pump} = \left(\frac{[Na^+]_i}{[Na^+]_i + K^i_{Na}}\right)^3 \bigg/ \left(\frac{50}{50 + K^i_{Na}}\right)^3 \tag{7}$$

Hansen *et al.* (2002) measured the Na/K pump activation with respect to intracellular Na^+ in the presence of intracellular K^+ (80 mM). The experiments were conducted with intra and extracellular ADP-free and Na^+-free solutions. These conditions gave the following equation for the normalized current:

$$\Phi^{norm}_{A^+,pump} = \left(\frac{[Na^+]_i}{[Na^+]_i + K^i_{Na}\left(1 + \frac{80}{K^i_K}\right)}\right)^3 \Bigg/ \left(\frac{79{,}8}{79{,}8 + K^i_{Na}\left(1 + \frac{80}{K^i_K}\right)}\right)^3 \tag{8}$$

Using this equation for the curve fitting to the experimental data, $K_K{}^i$ was estimated equal to 4.831 mM.

Friedrich *et al.* (1996) studied the Na/K pump dependence on intracellular ATP. The experiments were conducted with ADP-free intracellular medium and the transmembrane potential was clamped in 0 mV. The Equation (6), describing the normalized current with respect to current for [ATP] = 0.204 mM, could then be deduced. Using this equation for calculating the best curve fitting to experimental data, the ATP dissociation constant, K_{ATP}, was estimated equal to 0.155 mM.

$$\Phi^{norm}_{A^+,pump} = \left(\frac{[ATP]^i}{[ATP]^i + K^i_{ATP}}\right) \bigg/ \left(\frac{0{,}204}{0{,}204 + K^i_{ATP}}\right) \tag{9}$$

The lacking of information about the Na/K pump activity with respect to the intracellular ADP and P, the intracellular dissociation constant of ADP and P, $K_{ADP,P}{}^i$, was estimated assuming that the formation and consuming rate of ATP are equal. Additionally, this constant must be high enough to reduce the pump rate in the reverse direction, when Na^+ is transported to the intracellular medium and K^+ to the extra. To provide these conditions $K_{ADP,P}$ was assumed equal to 5 mM.

The ratio between the equilibrium constants $K_A{}^i$ and $K_A{}^o$, of the Na/K pump reactions, could be calculated by means of the reverse potential of the Na/K pump. Therefore, the condition of null Na/K current gives:

$$V^{rev}_A = \frac{RT}{F} \ln \frac{[A^+]_o}{[A^+]_i} \tag{10}$$

Glistsch (2001) estimated the Na/K pump reverse potential equal to –232 mV. Substituting in Equation (10), and taking into account the normal intra and extracellular $[Na^+]$ and $[K^+]$, and the corresponding dissociation constants, the ratio $[A^+]_o/[A^+]_i$ can be described in terms of $K_A{}^o/K_A{}^i$. The convenient substitutions allowed estimating $K_A{}^o/K_A{}^i$ equal to 0.012. Since each parameter of this ratio could not be estimated, it was necessary to concentrate parameters:

$$P_A^{cell} = \bar{P}_A^{cell} C_{E_{Na,K}}^{m,total} K_A^i \tag{11}$$

where P_A^{cell} is a parameter related to the density of the Na/K pumps and was considered an *investigative parameter* and its value was attributed directly simulating the epileptiform activity.

The equations (12) and (13) were derived from reactions describing the KCC enzyme interaction with its ligands. The neuronal and glial KCC co-transporters proportionality constants convey the expression intensity of these enzymes in the cellular membranes. In this case, the constant Q_{KCC}^{neur} (4.21 × 10^{-3} µmol/s.cm^2) was assumed as an *investigative parameter*. Therefore, its value was adjusted along the investigation about the Cl^- and K^+ levels control, during the nonsynaptic epileptiform activities induction. On the other hand, the Q_{KCC}^{glia} (5.35×10^{-4} µmol/s.cm^2) was estimated aiming at controlling the $[Cl^-]_i$ in the steady state.

$$\Phi_{KCC} = Q_{KCC} \frac{[K^+]_i[Cl^-]_i}{\left([K^+]_i + K^i_{K,KCC}(1+\frac{[K^+]_o}{K^o_{K,KCC}})\right)\left([Cl^-]_i + K^i_{Cl,KCC}(1+\frac{[Cl^-]_o}{K^o_{Cl,KCC}})\right)} - \frac{[K^+]_o[Cl^-]_o}{\left([K^+]_o + K^o_{K,KCC}(1+\frac{[K^+]_i}{K^i_{K,KCC}})\right)\left([Cl^-]_o + K^o_{Cl,KCC}(1+\frac{[Cl^-]_i}{K^i_{Cl,KCC}})\right)} \tag{12}$$

$$\Phi_{NKCC} = Q_{NKCC} \frac{[Na^+]_i[K^+]_i[Cl^-]_i^2 - [Na^+]_o[K^+]_o[Cl^-]_o^2}{\left(K_{Na,NKCC} + [Na^+]_i + [Na^+]_o\right)\left(K_{K,NKCC} + [K^+]_i + [K^+]_o\right)\left(K_{Cl} + [Cl^-]_i + [Cl^-]_o\right)^2} \tag{13}$$

Payne (1997) measured the Rb^+ influx by the KCC cotransporters in dependence on the $[Rb^+]_o$ and $[Cl^-]_o$. For each variation of Rb^+ or Cl^-, the initial rate of the Rb^+ influx was measured. Since for the cation-chloride cotransporters the Rb^+ and K^+ affinities were undistinguishable, the K^+ effects on the cotrasnporters could be inferred using Rb^+ in the investigations. The experiments carried out by Payne (1997), were used to adjust the dissociation constants for K^+ ($K_{K,KCC}^{o,neur}$ = 7.34 mM) and Cl^- ($K_{Cl,KCC}^{o,neur}$ = 92.02 mM). Considering the corresponding conditions, the following equations were deduced and used to simulate the experimental data from Payne (1997). The first one was obtained considering the $[Rb^+]_o$ changing and keeping the $[Cl^-]_o$ constant. The second equation for $[Cl^-]_o$ changing, keeping $[Rb^-]_o$ constant.

$$\Phi_{KCC}^{norm} = \frac{[Rb]_o}{\left(K_{Rb} + [Rb]_o\right)} \Big/ \frac{25}{\left(K_{Rb} + 25\right)} \tag{14}$$

$$\Phi_{KCC}^{norm} = \frac{[Cl]_o}{\left(K_{Cl,KCC}^{o,neur} + [Cl]_o\right)} \Big/ \frac{144,2}{\left(K_{Cl,KCC}^{o,neur} + 144,2\right)} \tag{15}$$

For the neurons, the intracellular dissociation constants for K^+ and Cl^-, in the membrane internal face, respectively $K_{K,KCC}^{i,neur}$ and $K_{Cl,KCC}^{i,neur}$ were assumed equal to that at the external face. This simplification assumes that the KCC cotransporters are mainly influenced by the K^+ and Cl^- transmembrane gradients and less by the enzyme affinities.
In the case of K^+ and Cl^- dissociation constants for the glial KCC cotransporters, $K_{K,KCC}^{i,glia}$ (2.3 mM), $K_{Cl,KCC}^{i,glia}$ (0.1 mM), $K_{K,KCC}^{o,glia}$ (200 mM) and $K_{Cl,KCC}^{o,glia}$ (500 mM), the parameters were adjusted to maintain the steady state of the intracellular concentrations of the glial cells.
The neuronal and glial proportionality constants of the NKCC cotransporters, Q_{NKCC}^{neur} (4.72×10^{-3} μmol/s.cm²) and Q_{NKCC}^{glia} (2.80×10^{-2} μmol/s.cm²), were used to represent the expression intensity of the cotransporter enzymes in the cells membrane. Supposing that this expression intensity guides the contribution of the mechanisms to the activities studied, these parameters were considered as *investigative parameters*. In this sense, they were adjusted aiming at contributing for the intra and extracellular ionic concentrations of Na^+, K^+ and Cl^-.
Concerning the NKCC dissociation constants, the values were estimated simulating experimental data. Tas *et al.* (1987) measured, in rat brain astrocytes, the Rb^+ influx, promoted by these cotransporters in dependence on the extracellular concentrations of Na^+, K^+ and Cl^-. The measurements were carried out for cells incubated in Na^+-free solution (A), in $[K^+]$ = 1 mM (B) and in Cl^--free solution (C). To adjust the parameters, like as with the KCC cotransporters, the Na^+, K^+ and Cl^- intracellular concentrations were admitted null, respectively, in (A), (B) and (C) conditions. The following corresponding equations (16, 17 and 18) were used to simulate the Rb^+influx, Φ_{NKCC}^{norm}, in dependence on the Na^+, K^+ and Cl^- concentrations.

$$\Phi_{NKCC}^{norm} = \frac{[Na^+]_o}{\left(K_{Na,NKCC} + [Na^+]_o\right)} \Bigg/ \frac{150,4}{\left(K_{Na,NKCC} + 150,4\right)} \tag{16}$$

$$\Phi_{NKCC}^{norm} = \frac{[K^+]_o}{\left(K_{K,NKCC} + [K^+]_o\right)} \Bigg/ \frac{39,9}{\left(K_{K,NKCC} + 39,9\right)} \tag{17}$$

$$\Phi_{NKCC}^{norm} = \left(\frac{[Cl^-]_o}{\left(K_{Cl,NKCC} + [Cl^-]_o\right)}\right)^2 \Bigg/ \left(\frac{153,4}{\left(K_{Cl,NKCC} + 153,4\right)}\right)^2 \tag{18}$$

Analogously to KCC, the extracellular dissociation constants for Na^+, K^+ and Cl^-, in the membrane internal face, $K_{Na,NKCC}^{neur}$ (70.0 mM), $K_{K,NKCC}^{neur}$ (2.33 mM), $K_{Cl,NKCC}^{neur}$ (25.0 mM), $K_{Na,NKCC}^{glia}$ (70.0 mM), $K_{K,NKCC}^{glia}$ (2.33 mM) and $K_{Cl,NKCC}^{glia}$ (25.0 mM), were assumed equal to their values at the internal face. Therefore, the direction of net movement of Na^+, K^+ and Cl^- through the cotransporter will be very sensitive Na^+, K^+ and Cl^- transmembrane gradients.
The chloride exchangers were implemented in the model aiming at obtaining the internal ionic equilibrium of the cells during the steady state (Equation 19). Therefore the parameters $Q_{HCO_3^-,Cl}^{neur}$ (9.81×10^{-5} μmol/s.cm²), $Q_{HCO_3^-,Cl}^{glia}$ (3.38×10^{-4} μmol/s.cm²), $K_{Cl,exch}^{neur}$ (6.00 mM) and $K_{Cl,exch}^{glia}$ (0.10 mM) were considered as *equilibrium parameters* and were adjusted for the steady state.

$$\phi_{Cl} = Q_{HCO3/CL} \frac{\left[Cl^-\right]_i}{\left[Cl^-\right]_i + K_{Cl-exch}} \tag{19}$$

Similarly to the chloride exchangers, the sodium exchangers were also included to obtain the internal ionic equilibrium of the cells during the steady state (Equation 20). For the same reasons, the *equilibrium parameters* $Q^{neur}_{Na,exch}$ (1.09 × 10^{-4} μmol/s.cm^2), $Q^{glia}_{Na,exch}$ (7.94 × 10^{-4} μmol/s.cm^2), $K^{neur}_{Na,exch}$ (10.0 mM) and $K^{glia}_{Na,exch}$ (13.0 mM) were adjusted for the steady state. According to Sychrová (2004), K^+ may also be transported by the sodium exchangers. In the model this function helped to control the level of K^+ accumulation (Equation 21). Therefore, the parameters $K^{neur}_{K,exch}$ (800 mM) and $K^{glia}_{K,exch}$ (300 mM) were assumed as *investigative parameters* and adjusted along the simulation of the activities.

$$\phi_{Na} = Q_{Na/H} \frac{\left[Na^+\right]_i}{\left[Na^+\right]_i + K_{Na-exch}\left(1 + \frac{\left[K^+\right]_i}{K_{K-exch}}\right)} \tag{20}$$

$$\phi_{K} = Q_{Na/H} \frac{\left[K^+\right]_i}{\left[K^+\right]_i + K_{K-exch}\left(1 + \frac{\left[Na^+\right]_i}{K_{Na-exch}}\right)} \tag{21}$$

The electric field effect on the extracellular space at the immediate vicinity of the sources was estimated by:

$$V_{extra,fast} = \tau F \sum_{n=1}^{N} \frac{(\Phi^{NEURON}_{Na,fast} + \Phi^{NEURON}_{K,fast})_n}{d_n}, \tag{22}$$

where d_n means the distance between the current source 'n' and the neuron, and τ a constant that translates the resistivity of the medium at the vicinity of the neuron.
The τ changing in dependence on the intracellular volume change was described by:

$$\tau = \overline{\tau}\left[\left(\frac{-1}{e^{-\frac{Vol_{extra} - 2{,}97\times10^{-13}}{6\times10^{-16}}} + 1} + 1\right)\times 15 + 1\right] \tag{23}$$

This equation was deduced to translate a sigmoidal dependence of τ on the Vol_{extra}, where Vol_{extra}, representing the extracellular volume, was calculated by means of the equation 42. The parameter $\overline{\tau}$ (6.25 × 10^{-3} mV.s/mM) controls the population spikes amplitude and was adjusted to reproduce the typical amplitudes observed experimentally in our laboratory in the same conditions of the simulation. Therefore, this parameter was assumed as *experimental parameter*.

The electric field effect on the membranes on the immediate vicinity of the sources was estimated by:

$$I_{elect-effect} = \varepsilon V_{extra,fast} , \tag{24}$$

where ε (7.30 × 10-6 mA/ mV.m2) was used to tune the field effect in the simulations. This *experimental parameter* was adjusted to reproduce the findings from Snow and Dudek (1986). It was tuned to obtain an electrical field effect to induce an intracellular depolarization around 50% of the population spikes.
Hence,

$$\frac{\partial[C]_i^{NEURON}}{\partial t} = -\Phi_{C(INTRA \to EXTRA)}^{NEURON} - \Phi_{C,Gap-Junction}^{NEURON} , \tag{25}$$

$$\frac{\partial[C]_i^{GLIA}}{\partial t} = -\Phi_{C(INTRA \to EXTRA)}^{GLIA} \tag{26}$$

and

$$\frac{\partial[C]_o}{\partial t} = \Phi_{C(INTRA \to EXTRA)}^{NEURON} + \left(\frac{\partial[C]}{\partial t}\right)_{Electrodiffusion} + \Phi_{C(INTRA \to EXTRA)}^{GLIA} \tag{27}$$

where

$$\begin{aligned}\Phi_{Na(INTRA \to EXTRA)}^{NEURON} &= \Phi_{Na,fast}^{NEURON} + \Phi_{Na,presist}^{NEURON} + \Phi_{NKCC}^{NEURON} + \\ &3.\Phi_{PUMP}^{NEURON} + \Phi_{Na,exchanger}^{NEURON} + \Phi_{Na,leak}^{NEURON}\end{aligned} , \tag{28}$$

$$\begin{aligned}\Phi_{K(INTRA \to EXTRA)}^{NEURON} &= \Phi_{K,fast}^{NEURON} + \Phi_{K,TypeA}^{NEURON} + \Phi_{NKCC}^{NEURON} + \Phi_{KCC}^{NEURON} - \\ &-2.\Phi_{PUMP}^{NEURON} + \Phi_{K,exchanger}^{NEURON} + \Phi_{K,leak}^{NEURON}\end{aligned} , \tag{29}$$

$$\begin{aligned}\Phi_{Cl(INTRA \to EXTRA)}^{NEURON} &= \Phi_{Cl}^{NEURON} + \Phi_{Cl,voltage}^{NEURON} + 2.\Phi_{NKCC}^{NEURON} + \\ &\Phi_{KCC}^{NEURON} + \Phi_{Cl,exchanger}^{NEURON} + \Phi_{Cl,leak}^{NEURON}\end{aligned} \tag{30}$$

and

$$\Phi_{Na(INTRA \to EXTRA)}^{GLIA} = \Phi_{Na}^{GLIA} + \Phi_{NKCC}^{GLIA} + 3.\Phi_{PUMP}^{GLIA} + \Phi_{Na,leak}^{GLIA} + \Phi_{Na,exchanger}^{GLIA} , \tag{31}$$

$$\Phi_{K(INTRA \to EXTRA)}^{GLIA} = \Phi_{K}^{GLIA} + \Phi_{K,Inw-Ret}^{GLIA} + \Phi_{NKCC}^{GLIA} - 2.\Phi_{PUMP}^{GLIA} + \Phi_{K,leak}^{GLIA} + \Phi_{K,exchanger}^{GLIA} + \Phi_{KCC}^{GLIA} , \tag{32}$$

$$\Phi_{Cl(INTRA \to EXTRA)}^{GLIA} = \Phi_{Cl}^{GLIA} + 2.\Phi_{NKCC}^{GLIA} + \Phi_{Cl,leak}^{GLIA} + \Phi_{Cl,exchanger}^{GLIA} + \Phi_{KCC}^{GLIA} . \tag{33}$$

The equilibrium fluxes $\Phi_{Na,leak}^{neuron}$ (-1.73 × 10-8 mmol/s.cm2), $\Phi_{K,leak}^{neuron}$ (-3.95 × 10-8 mmol/s.cm2), $\Phi_{Cl,leak}^{neuron}$ (-3.00 × 10-8 mmol/s.cm2), $\Phi_{Na,leak}^{glia}$ (-1.39 × 10-7 mmol/s.cm2), $\Phi_{K,leak}^{glia}$ (−2.43 × 10−7 mmol/s.cm2) and $\Phi_{Cl,leak}^{glia}$ (-2.23 × 10-7 mmol/s.cm2) are related to the steady state in normal conditions, therefore, before perfusion with high K^+ solution. In this sense, they were assumed as *steady state parameters* and adjusted to keep the resting conditions stable.

The equation used to calculate the extracellular electrodiffusion effect on the ionic concentration changes was:

$$\left(\frac{\partial[C]_o}{\partial t}\right)_{Electrodiffusion} = \frac{D_c}{\lambda^2}\cdot\nabla^2[C]_o + \frac{z\cdot F\cdot D_c}{R\cdot T\cdot\lambda^2}\cdot\vec{\nabla}[C]_o\cdot\vec{\nabla}V + \frac{z\cdot F\cdot D_c}{R\cdot T\cdot\lambda^2}\cdot[C]_o\cdot\nabla^2 V\,. \quad (34)$$

The extracellular electrical field, $\vec{\nabla}V$, was estimated by the following equation:

$$\vec{\nabla}V = -\frac{RT}{F}\frac{z_{Na}D_{Na}\vec{\nabla}[Na^+]_o + z_K D_K\vec{\nabla}[K^+]_o + z_{Cl}D_{Cl}\vec{\nabla}[Cl^-]_o}{z_{Na}{}^2 D_{Na}[Na^+]_o + z_K{}^2 D_K[K^+]_o + z_{Cl}{}^2 D_{Cl}[Cl^-]_o} + \vec{\nabla}V_{extra,\,fast}\,, \quad (35)$$

and $\nabla^2 V$ was estimated in terms of the $\vec{\nabla}V$. The first term of (35) was deduced assuming the continuity of the ionic currents along the extracellular space. The value of the parameters D_{Na} (1.33×10^{-5} cm²/s), D_K (1.96×10^{-5} cm²/s), and D_{Cl} (2.03×10^{-5} cm²/s), as constants, were obtained from the literature (Hille, 1992). The tortuosity ($\lambda = 1.6$) is an *experimental parameter* and along the granular layer was extracted from (Nicholson, 2001). In the case of the lateral shell of the network simulating this layer, the tortuosity was increased ($\lambda = 4.0$) aiming at representing the layers in between the solution and the granular layer. With this simplification, the computation could be reduced.

The functional unity dimensions, Δx, Δy e Δz, were admitted equal to 20 µm, assuming that the diameters of the neuronal and glial cells can be considered around 10 µm. The iteration interval, Δt, adopted was 0.1 ms. This value was defined considering the compromise between the computational time of the simulations and the maximal numerical error acceptable.

The transmembrane potential was estimated by the following equation:

$$V_m = \frac{RT}{F}\ln\left(\frac{P_{Na}[Na^+]_o + P_K[K^+]_o + P_{Cl}[Cl^-]_o + P_A[A^+]_o + f_{gj} + f_{ef} + \gamma}{P_{Na}[Na^+]_i + P_K[K^+]_i + P_{Cl}[Cl^-]_i + P_A[A^+]_i + 2 + \xi}\right), \quad (36)$$

where

$$f_{gj} = -\frac{I_{gj}A_{gj}}{A_m}\cdot\left(e^{\frac{FV_m}{RT}} - 1\right)\cdot\frac{RT}{F^2 V_m} + e^{\frac{FV_m}{RT}}\,, \quad (37)$$

with I_{gj} representing the resultant current induced by all gap-junctions with the neighboring neurons, calculated by

$$I_{gj} = \sum_{\substack{NEURON= \\ NEIGHBORING}}\ \sum_{C=Na,K,Cl} z_C F\Phi^{NEURON}_{C,Gap-Junction} \quad (38)$$

and

$$f_{ef} = -I_{elect\text{-}effect}\cdot\left(e^{\frac{FV_m}{RT}} - 1\right)\cdot\frac{RT}{F^2 V_m} + e^{\frac{FV_m}{RT}}\,, \quad (39)$$

where $I_{elect\text{-}effect}$ is the current referred to the electric field effect, and γ and ζ representing the ionic leakage through the membrane. The parameters γ^{neur} (8 mMcm/s), ξ^{neur} (72 mMcm/s), γ^{glia} (1 mMcm/s) and ξ^{glia} (70 mMcm/s) were adjusted aiming at establishing transmembrane potentials, for neurons and glial cells, in the same range observed experimentally (Pan & Stringer, 1996) and, therefore, were assumed as *steady state parameters*. The superficial area of the neuronal membrane, A_m, was estimated assuming a spherical cellular body for the granular cells and with diameter equal to 20 μm. This allowed to estimate $A_m = 1.26 \times 10^{-5}$ cm². The parameter A_{gj}, which represents the area of each gap-junction pore, is equal to 1.77×10^{-14} cm² (Jeffery, 1995).

The extracellular field potential sensed by a microelectrode was calculated in terms of the extracellular electric field, as the following equation describes:

$$V_{ext} = -\int_{\lambda} \vec{\nabla} V \bullet d\vec{l} \,, \tag{40}$$

where λ represented a trajectory linking the electrode tip position to a remote point in the bath solution.

The following equation describes the volume change of the cells and the extracellular space:

$$\frac{dVol_{\text{int}-neur}}{dt} = \upsilon\left(\sum_{C=Na,K,Cl} [C]_o + [S]_i - \sum_{C=Na,K,Cl} [C]_i + [S]_o \right), \tag{41}$$

where

$$Vol_{extra} = Vol_{total,constant} - Vol_{\text{int}-neur}\,, \tag{42}$$

$[S]^i = n_s^i / Vol^{\text{intra},neur}$, $[S]^o = n_s^o / Vol^{\text{intra},neur}$, n_s^i (9.01×10^{-10} mmol) and n_s^o (3.15×10^{-11} mmol) represent the quantity of the impermeant solutes S, $Vol^{\text{intra}-neur}$ (4.19×10^{-12} dm³) the neuronal intracellular volume, Vol_{extra} (3.15×10^{-13} dm³) the extracellular volume of the functional unit and $Vol_{total,constant}$ (4.19×10^{-12} dm³) the total volume of the functional unit. The parameters ν (4.50×10^{-17} cm²/s) and n_s^o (3.15 × 10-11 mmol), assumed as *investigative parameters*, act on the cell volume variation along of the neuronal discharges. The parameter n_s^i (9.01 × 10-10 mmol) is a *steady state parameter* and was adjusted to keep the volume constant when the system is in steady state conditions.

The neuronal and glial initial volumes were determined considering spherical cellular bodies with diameter equal to 20 μm. The extracellular volume was calculated according to the extracellular volume fraction, assumed equal to 0.07, considering that the bursts inductions were obtained placing the slices in an interface chamber.

Some parameters were involved in almost all equations described above. This is the case of the initial ionic concentrations of the extracellular medium ($[Na]_o$ = 131 mM, $[K]_o$ = 4 mM, $[Cl]_o$ = 130 mM). These values were admitted equal to the values commonly used in the experimental investigations. The intracellular concentrations ($[Na]_{i,neur}$ = 10 mM, $[K]_{i,neur}$ = 130 mM, $[Cl]_{i,neur}$ = 9 mM, $[Na]_{i,glia}$ = 10 mM, $[K]_{i,glia}$ = 130 mM, $[Cl]_{i,glia}$ = 9 mM) were adjusted in the ranges normally assumed experimentally (Kager et al., 2002; Xiong & Stringer, 2000; Almeida et al, 2004). The neuronal transmembrane potential at the steady state was considered equal to -69 mV. This value was assumed reasonable because

experimentally the Ca^{2+}-free solution induces a desinhibition that leads to a depolarization around the same level (Pan & Stringer, 1996). For glial cells, the initial transmembrane potential was set around -79 mV and this value is in the range of the experimental observations (Orkand, 1991). Normally, it is assumed that the glial intracellular potential is more negative because of the elevated K^+ permeability of the membrane of these cells.
The equations of the model were solved numerically by means of the finite difference method and the maximum error tolerance was 10^{-4}. The computational language used was FORTRAN 90. To run the simulations, a computer cluster was necessary. The main configuration used for the simulations presented: (1) One front end Athlon 64 3000+ Dual Core, 2 GB RAM, 300 GB HD; (2) 10 Slaves Athlon 64 3000+ Dual Core, 2 GB RAM, 80 GB HD; (3) One switch with 16 ports; (4) Operational System Rocks Cluster 4.1 (Linux), and (5) FORTRAN 90 and MPI (message passing interface).

5.2 Investigating the biophysics of the nonsynaptic epileptiform activity

Comparing the measured and simulated extracellular potential, as shown in Fig. 8, it can be observed that all main features of the extracellular potential were captured by the simulations. The simulation corresponds to the experimental maneuver for inducing the nonsynaptic epileptiform activities. The $[K^+]_o$ of the compartments representing the bath solution was increased from 4 to 8 mM. The cells of the network were coupled exclusively with nonsynaptic connections, as described in item 5.1, aiming at representing the deletion of Ca^{2+} in the bath solution. The great advantage offered by the computational simulation is that once the experimental data are reproduced, then it is possible to analyze all mechanisms and variables involved and infer about the biophysics.
The model allows predicting the concomitant concentration changes along the period preceding the paroxysm induction and also along the paroxysm, when the interictal and ictal states transitions occur, as it is seen in Fig. 8. The DC-shift components of the nonsynaptic events simulated were in agreement with the experimental data and were calculated (see equations 35 and 36) based on the hypothesis of being generated by a Goldman-Hodgkin-Katz potential established along the extracellular space, therefore, the same mechanism proposed for the DC-shift during spreading depression (Almeida et al., 2004).
As described in our previous work (Almeida et al. 2008), the simulations show that Cl^- concentration changes, in response to the $[K^+]_o$ increase, are able to promote the Cl^- Nernst potential overcoming the transmembrane potential (Fig. 8). These changes are the main responsible cause of the excitation sustained along of the paroxysm. Therefore, it should be treated as a target for the paroxysms reduction. This means that the mechanisms involved must be investigated. The first step is to analyze the ion flux of each mechanism, shown in Fig. 8. It can be observed that the cotransporters, in particular the NKCC, exhibited valuable contributions for the changes, differently from the exchangers, which were almost insensitive to the $[K^+]_o$ increase. Before induction, the Cl^- efflux by KCC was greater than its influx by NKCC and this situation changed in the course of the induction. This can also be associated with situations in which the excitability of a brain region increases and the recruited neuronal depolarization is enough to increase the $[K^+]_o$. From the simulation we can propose that brain regions under these circumstances are able to induce nonsynaptic epileptiform activity. The biophysical process captured by the simulation can then be described. In normal conditions, the KCC cotransporter is responsible for the Cl^- extrusion, counteracted by the NKCC cotransporter, which is in charge of the Cl^- influx. The $[K^+]_o$

elevation increases the driving force for NKCC influx. This influx increase provides more Cl^- to the intracellular space, increasing, by its turn, the driving force for KCC extrusion. However, the dynamic equilibrium occurs for Cl^- accumulated in the intracellular space. This accumulation is sufficient to make the Cl^- Nernst potential overcoming the transmembrane potential. In these circumstances, the inward Cl^- current through the channels become outward, inducing the neuronal depolarization.

The simulations showing the concomitant ionic concentration changes and fluxes allow analyzing the mechanisms acting along the transitions between itcal and interictal states. AS shown in Fig. 8, in the extracellular space, the $[Na^+]$ and $[Cl^-]$ decreased quickly at the transition of the states, reached a trough, followed by a slow increase until the end of the ictal state (transition to the interictal state), from which the concentrations returned quickly to the baseline. Almost the same behavior was exhibited by the $[K^+]_o$, however in an inverted manner. In the neuronal intracellular space, the simulations showed, during the ictal state, the $[Na^+]$ and $[Cl^-]$ increasing slowly and monotonically and $[K^+]$ decreasing also monotonically. The recovery of the concentrations along the interictal state did not have the same time course. Different from the extracellular, where the concentrations return quickly to the baseline, in the intracellular the $[K^+]$ increase covers almost the entire interictal state, as well as the $[Na^+]$ and $[Cl^-]$ reduction. Of course, these changes have a definitive influence on the Nernst potential of each ionic specie and, therefore, on the excitability.

During the ictal period, the direction of the transmembrane passive ionic fluxes simulated, as illustrated in Fig. 8, in almost all the cases, were guided by the transmembrane concentration gradient. The Na^+ flux through the ionic channels was directed to the intracellular space and the K^+ to the extracellular. The Cl^- flux direction was in some situations against its transmembrane concentration gradient, sustained by the transmembrane electric field originated from the Nernst potential of this ion overcoming the transmembrane potential. According to the simulations, these were observed during the interictal state and during the interval between subsequent action potentials along the ictal period (Almeida et.al, 2008).

Through the Na/K pump, the Na^+ and K^+ fluxes were, as expected, against their gradients. Sensitive to intracellular Na^+, the pump increased its activity during the ictal period, when Na^+ accumulated in the intracellular space. Only about the end of the period, the pump started to decrease the Na^+ efflux. This decrease happened simultaneously with the Na^+ influx decrease through the voltage dependent channels. The Na^+ influx by the cotransporter NKCC as well as its efflux by the Na^+/H^+ exchanger had minor changes on their intensities along the neuronal activity transition from the interictal to the ictal state. However, their baselines showed significant magnitude, sustaining the ionic equilibrium during the interictal state (Fig. 8). The K^+ influx through the pump, in comparison with its efflux through the channels, behaves similarly to Na^+, however, with inverted flow direction. The K^+ fluxes through the NKCC cotransporter and the Na^+/H^+ exchanger also had the same behavior as described for Na^+ and its H^+ exchanger. On the other hand, the neuronal KCC cotransporter not only had a significant baseline, but the changes on the transitions from the interictal to ictal states were also prominent. The Cl^- fluxes simulated suggest that the cotransporter mechanisms were the ones mainly responsible for the intra- and extracellular concentration changes of this ion. The Cl^- accumulation in the intracellular space during the ictal state was mediated by the NKCC cotransporter, which happened with almost the same flux along of the ictal state. The Cl^- efflux was dominated by the KCC cotransporter and during the ictal state it was always smaller than the Cl^- NKCC influx.

Only at the transition between the ictal/interictal states, the KCC efflux overcame the NKCC influx and was responsible for the intracellular Cl^- concentration decrease.

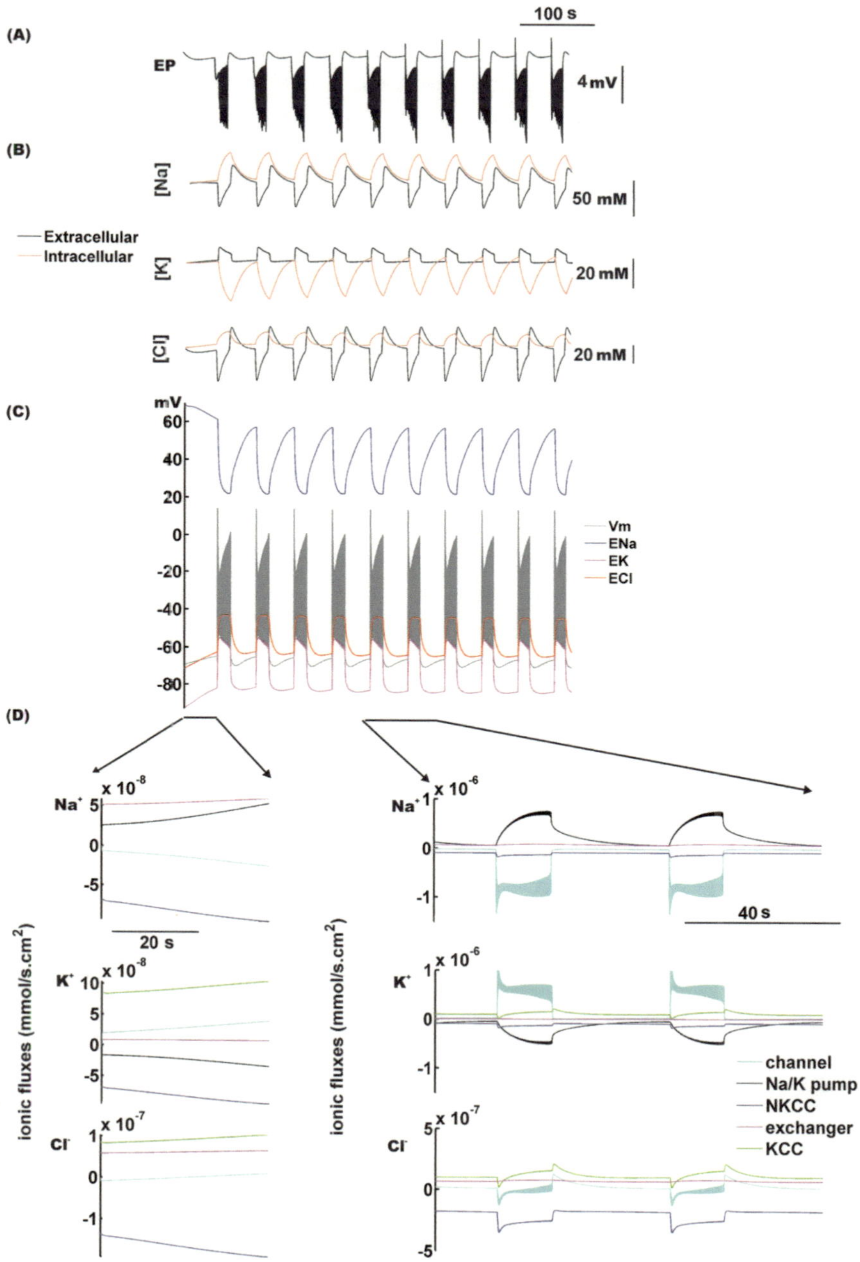

Fig. 8. Nonsynaptic epileptiforme activity simulated. (A) Extracellular potential; Concomitantly, (B) intra- and extra-cellular ionic concentrations and (C) Nernst potential for Na^+, K^+ and Cl^-, and the transmembrane potential. Detailed in (D) the fluxes associated with each nonsynaptic mechanism considered in the model.

Observations on the effect of the antiepileptic furosemide (Geck& Pfeiffer, 1985; Alvarez-Leefman, 1990) are in accordance with the hypothetical Cl- current sustaining the nonsynaptic epileptiform activities. It has been observed that furosemide, a blocker of the NKCC and KCC cotransporters, blocks spontaneous epileptiform activities induced in a variety of experimental maneuvers and models. The blockage can be explained considering the blockage of the net effect of both cotransporters, therefore the Cl- influx. This suggests that the preferential blockage or depression of the NKCC activities would be more efficient and that it would be a possible target for an antiepileptic drug. The simulation of this hypothesis, shown in Fig. 9, confirms the assumption and experimental observations also corroborate this finding (Haglund & Hochman, 2005).

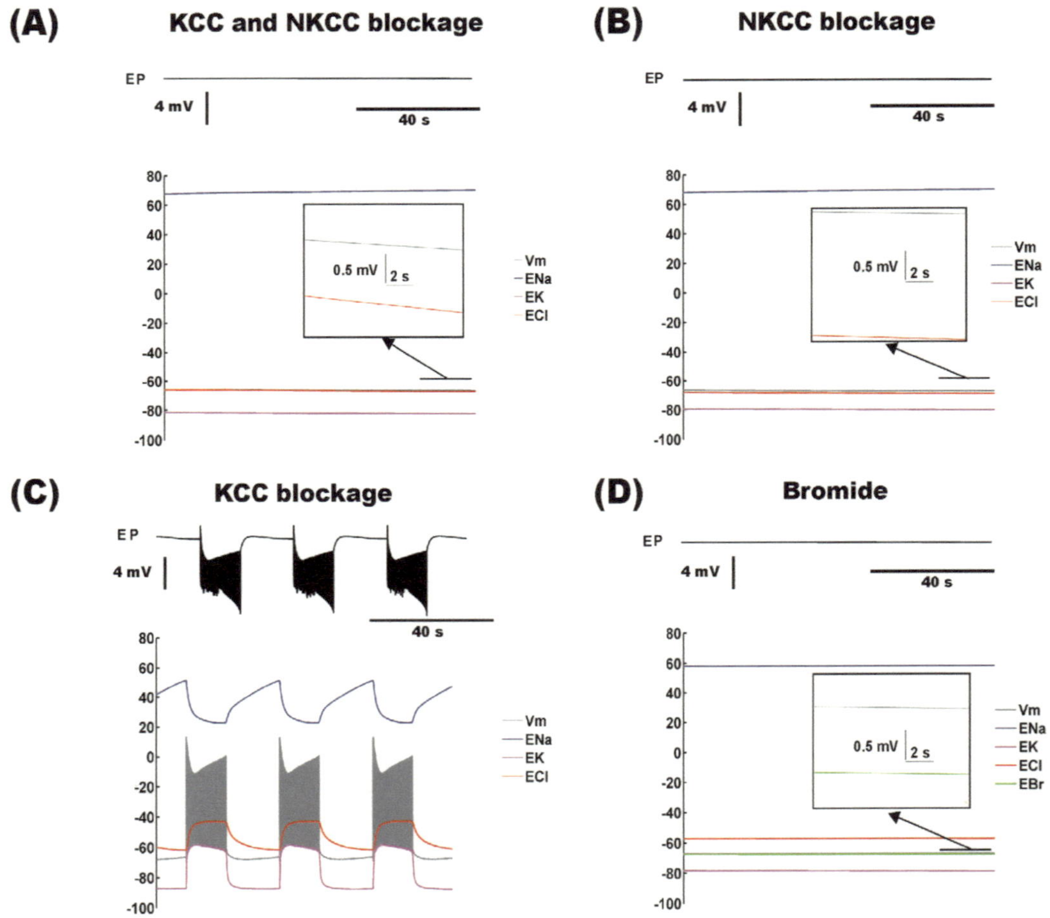

Fig. 9. Simulated experimental maneuver. (A) simultaneous blockage of NKCC and KCC, inducing a Cl- Nernst potential negative in respect to the transmembrane potential. (B) NKCC blockage, when the polarization is even more effective than in (B). (C) KCC blockage, promoting excitability increase. (D) Inhibition by means of the negativity of the Br- Nernst potential in respect to the membrane potential.

Focusing the same target, another possible strategy for the seizure control would be to counteract the Cl^- Nernst potential depolarization. An anion capable of permeating the Cl^- channels and, at the same time, having low affinity to KCC and NKCC enzymes - thus able to sustain a more negative Nernst potential - would be a good candidate. In fact, this seems to be the bromide effect, whose mechanisms are being investigated in our group. A simulation of the resultant effect of such kind of anion is shown in Fig. 9.

Analyzing the excitatory and inhibitory contributions of each mechanism involved (Almeida et al. 2008) it was possible to demonstrate that the Na^+ current was the most intense during the ictal state and that it was counteracted along the whole ictal state by the Na/K pump electrogenic current. The simulations shown in Fig. 10 suggest that it was exactly when the electrogenic current pump overcame the Na^+ current through the channels that the ictal states finalized, therefore, the ictal/interictal transition took place. In contrast, along the interictal state, the Cl^- current was the most prominent. This current decreased

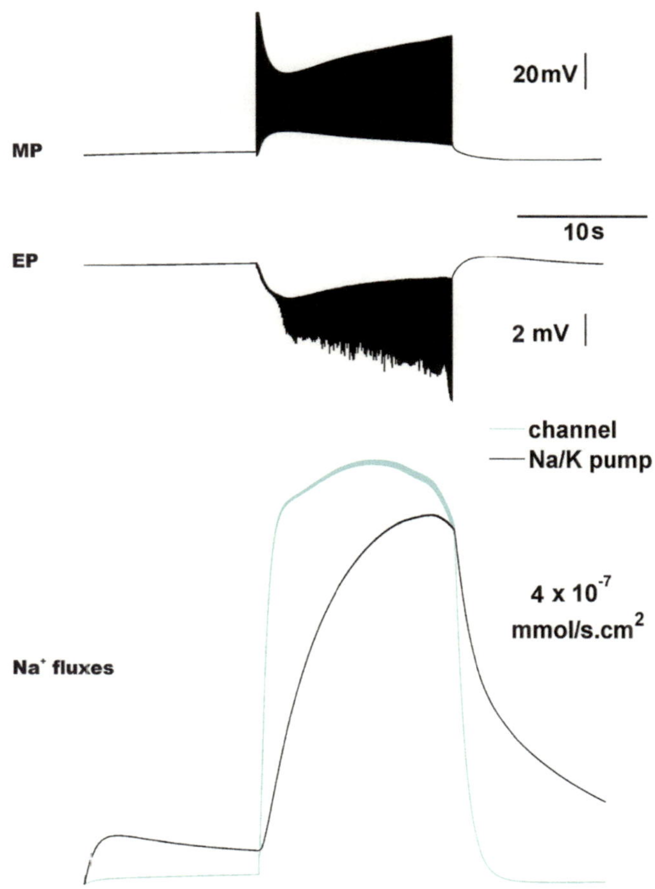

Fig. 10. Nonsynaptic burst simulation. (MP) membrane potential; (EP) extracellular potential. Na^+ fluxes shown on the bottom traces: (blue) voltage dependent channels. (black) Na/K pump. When the efflux trough the Na/K pump overcame the influx trough the voltage dependent channels, the event terminates.

during the state and, at the same time, Na^+ current increased in almost the same rate. The crossing point of the currents occurred about the end of the state and was immediately followed by the transition point between the interictal/ictal states. The most important contributors for this transition were again Na^+ current and the pump electrogenic current. The abrupt increase of the Na^+ current allowed the excitatory current overcoming the inhibitory pump current due to the electrogenic effect. These observations emphasize the importance to target the Cl^- mechanisms responsible for its intracellular accumulation and also to counteract is Nernst potential. Additionally, the Na^+ influx is also revealed as another possible target, placing in perspective strategies to antagonize ionic currents through Na^+ persistent channels.

6. Possible targets for controlling refractory seizures

From the biophysical mechanisms suggested by the simulations, the therapeutic use of bumetanide and bromide may be proposed combined for the treatment of patients with refractory epilepsy (Almeida et al., 2011). Bumetanide would reduce intracellular chloride concentration and bromide would reinforce E_{GABA} negativity, as seen in Fig. 9, where the systemic effects of bumetanide and bromide are depicted. Although acting through different mechanisms, both drugs reduce neuronal excitability. Once the effects are complementary, the doses of bumetanide and bromide could be reduced and, consequently, their side effects

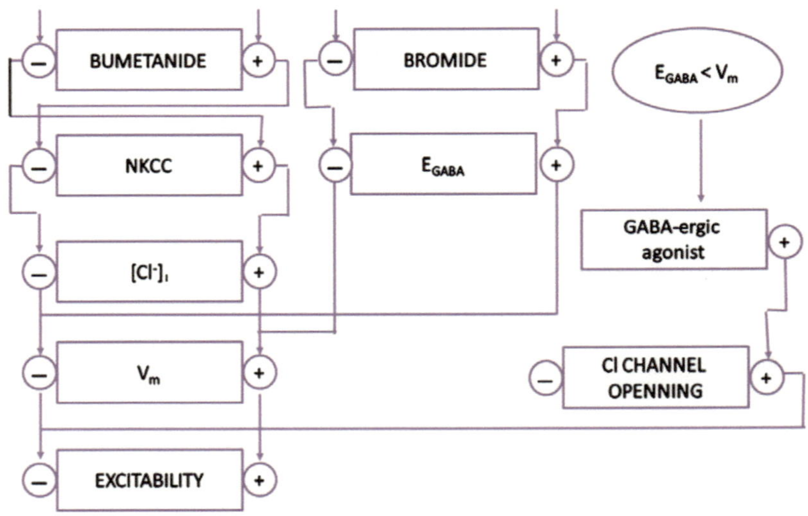

Fig. 11. Block diagram indicating the systemic action of the conjoint effect of bumetanide, bromide, and $GABA_A$ agonist. Bromide acts by blocking NKCC activity. This co-transporter is responsible for Cl- influx, which induces the accumulation of this ion in the intracellular space, inducing an increase in excitability. An NKCC antagonist is, therefore, able to counteract the chloride accumulation, decreasing excitability. Bromide acts directly on E_{GABA}, improving its negativity and also decreasing excitability. The conjoint effects of an NKCC antagonist and bromide are therefore complementary. The clinical observation of seizure reduction could be indicative of induced E_{GABA} negativity with respect to Vm (intracellular potential), when the use of GABAergic drugs can be useful. NKCC=Na^+, K^+, 2Cl- co-transporter; E_{GABA}=GABA reverse potential. Extracted from Almeida et al. 2011.

would be minimized as well. In fact, in a recent case reported on the use of bumetanide for treatment of autism, the authors did not observe, at the dosage investigated, any side effect (Franciolini & Nonner, 1987). To overcome the severe side effects of bromide described (Meierkord et al., 2000), it is paramount that bromide be administered with care, that follow-up testing be carried out, and that serum bromide levels be monitored periodically. We also propose that effort should be directed to find anions or anionic compounds that can replace bromide with the aim of avoiding its side effects. These proposals reflect a new perspective on the use of bromide: valuing its clinical efficacy associated with a reduction of its side effects. Furthermore, we also hypothesize that clinical observation of seizure reduction would be indicative of E_{GABA} negativity (Fig. 11). Under such clinical conditions, after the effect of bumetanide and bromide has already been established, shifting GABA from excitation to inhibition, the administration of GABA agonists should be considered in the treatment of uncontrollable seizures. With the action of these agonists, it is assumed that the doses of bumetanide and bromide could be further reduced.

7. Conclusion

The investigation of the biophysical aspects of the nonsynaptic epileptiform activities may guide the design of experimental investigations aiming at unraveling the intricate interdependence of the several process that are not only responsible for the neuronal activities but also for the ionic homeostasis of the whole network. The development of antiepileptic medications targeted to the conditions that sustain seizures would be facilitated if the basic mechanisms, in terms of their complex interdependence during normal or epileptiform activities, were taken into consideration. Such kind of approach would offer the necessary information for designing pharmacological agents able to antagonize the interplay of the mechanisms responsible for maintaining the homeostasis that favour the conditions for the abnormal functions.

8. Acknowledgment

This work was supported by *Fundação de Amparo à Pesquisa do Estado de Minas Gerais* (**FAPEMIG**), *Conselho Nacional de Desenvolvimento Científico e Tecnológico* (**CNPq**), PROCAD/*Coordenação de Aperfeiçoamento de Pessoal de Nível Superior* (**CAPES**), *Pandurata Ltda,* FAPESP, CInAPCe-FAPESP *and* FAPESP/CNPq/MCT- *Instituto Nacional de Neurociência Translacional.*

9. References

Almeida, A.; Texeira, H.; Duarte, M. & Infantosi, A. (2004). Modeling extracellular space electrodiffusion during Leão's spreading depression, *IEEE Trans Biomed Eng,* Vol. 51, No. 3, (March), pp. 450-458, ISSN 0018-9294

Almeida, A.; Rodrigues, A.; Scorza, F.; Cavalheiro. E.; Teixeira HZ, Duarte MA, Silveira G. & Arruda, E. (2008). Mechanistic hypotheses for nonsynaptic epileptiform activity induction and its transition from the interictal to ictal state--computational simulation, *Epilepsia,* Vol. 49, No. 11, (November), pp. 1908-1924, ISSN 1528-1167

Almeida, A.; Scorza, F.; Rodrigues, A.; Arida, R.; Carlesso, F.; Batista, A.; Duarte, M. & DaCosta, J. (2011). Combined effect of bumetanide, bromide, and GABAergic agonists: an alternative treatment for intractable seizures, *Epilepsy Behav*, Vol. 20, No. 1, (January), pp. 147-149, ISSN 1525-5050

Alverez-Leefman F. (1990). Intracellular Cl− regulation and synaptic inhibition in vertebrate and invertebrate neurons. In: *Chloride channels and carriers in nerve, muscle, and glial cells*, Alvarez-Leefmans FJ, Russell JM, pp. 109–158. Plenum, ISBN-10: 0306434261 New York

Andrew, R.; Adams, J. & Polischuk, T. (1996). Imaging NMDA- and kainate-induced intrinsic optical signals from the hippocampal slice, *J Neurophysiol*. Vol. 76, No. 4, (October), pp. 2707-2717, ISSN 0022-3077

Barmashenko, G.; Kockskamper, J. & Glitsch, H. (1999). Depolarization increases the apparent affinity of the Na+-K+ pump to cytoplasmic Na+ in isolated guinea-pig ventricular myocytes, *J Physiol* Vol. 517, No. 15, (Jun), pp. 691-698, 0022-3751

Bikson, M.; Ghai, R.; Baraban, S. & Durand DM. (1999). Modulation of burst frequency, durantion, and amplitude in the zero-Ca(2+) model of epileptiform activity, *J Neurophysiol*, Vol. 82, No.: 5, (November), pp. 2262–2270, ISSN 0022-3077

Bikson, M.; Baraban, S. & Durand, D. (2002) Conditions sufficient for nonsynaptic epileptogenesis in the CA1 region of hippocampal slices, *J Neurophysiol*, Vol. 87, No. 1, (January), pp. 62–71, ISSN 0022-3077

Blaesse, P.; Airaksinen, M.; Rivera, C. & Kaila, K. (2009). Cation-Chloride Cotransporters and Neuronal Function, *Neuron*, Vol.61, No. 6, pp. 820-838, ISSN 0896-6273

Chesler, M. (2003). Regulation and modulation of pH in the brain, *Physiol Rev*, Vol. 83, No. 4, (October), pp.1183–1221, ISSN 0031-9333

Dudek, F.; Snow, R. & Taylor, C. (1986). Role of electrical interactions in synchronization of epileptiform bursts, *Adv Neurol*, Vol. 44, pp. 593–617, ISSN 0091-3952

Dudek, F.; Obenaus, A. & Tasker, J. (1990). Osmolality-induced changes in extracellular volume alter epileptiform bursts independent of chemical synapses in the rat: importance of non-synaptic mechanisms in hippocampal epileptogenesis. *Neurosci Lett*, Vol. 11, No. 2, (December), pp. 267-270, ISSN 0304-3940

Franciolini, F. & Nonner, W. (1987). Anion and cation permeability of a chloride channel in rat hippocampal neurons. *J Gen Physiol*, Vol. 90, No. 4, (October), pp. 453–478, ISSN 0022-1295

Friedrich, T.; Bamberg, E. & Nagel, G. (1996). Na+,K+-ATPase pump currents in giant excised patches activated by an ATP concentration jump. *Biophys. J.*, Vol. 71, No. 5, (Nov), pp. 2486-2500, ISSN 0006-3495

Geck, P. & Pfeiffer, B. (1985). Na++ K++ 2Cl−cotransport in animal cells—its role in volume regulation. *Ann N Y Acad Sci*, Vol. 456, pp. 166–182, ISSN 0077-8923

Glitsch, H. (2001). Electrophysiology of the sodium-potassium-ATPase in cardiac cells. *Physiol. Rev*, Vol. 81, No. 4, (October), pp 1791-1826, ISSN 0031-9333

Hansen, P.; Buhagiar, K.; Kong, B. (2002). Dependence of Na^+-K^+ pump current-voltage relationship on intracellular Na^+, K^+ and Cs^+ in rabbit cardiac myocytes. *Am J Physiol Cell Physiol*, Vol. 283, (Dec), pp. C1511-1521, ISSN 0363-6143

Heinemann, U.; Lux, H. & Gutnick, M. (1977). Extracellular free calcium and potassium during paroxysmal activity in cerebral cortex of the cat. *Exp Brain Res*, Vol. 27, No. 3-4, (March), pp. 237–243, ISSN 0014-4819

Heyse. S.; Wuddel, I.; Apell, H. & Sturmer, W. (1994). Partial reactions of the Na, K-ATPase: determination of rate constants. *J Gen Physiol*, Vol. 104, No. 2, (August), pp.197–240, ISSN 0022-1295

Hille, B. (1992). *Ionic channels of excitable membranes* (2nd ed.), Sinauer Associates, Inc., ISBN 0878933239, Sunderland, MA.

Hochman, D.; D'Ambrosio, R.; Janigro, D. & Schwartzkroin, P. (1999). Extracellular chloride and the maintenance of spontaneous epileptiform activity in rat hippocampal slices. *J Neurophysiol*, Vol. 81, No. 1, (January), pp. 49-59, ISSN 0022-3077

Haglund, M. & Hochman, D. (2005). Furosemide and mannitol suppression of epileptic activity in the human brain. *J Neurophysiol*, Vol. 94, No. 2, (August),, pp. 907-918, ISSN 0022-3077

Horisberger, J. (2004). Recent insights into the structure and mechanism of the sodium pump. *Physiology*, Vol. 19, (December), pp. 377-387, ISSN: 1548-9213

Jefferys, J. (1995). Nonsynaptic modulation of neuronal activity in the brain: electric currents and extracellular ions. *Physiol Rev*, Vol. 75, No. 4, (October), pp. 689–723, ISSN 0031-9333

Jefferys, J. & Haas, H. (1982). Synchronized burstings of CA1 pyramidal cells in the absence of synaptic transmission. *Nature*, Vol. 300, No. 5891, (December), pp. 448–450, ISSN 0028-0836

Kager, H.; Wadman, W. & Somjen G. (2007). Seizure-like afterdischargers simulated in a model neuron. *J Comput Neurosci*, Vol. 22, No. 2, (April), pp. 105–128, ISSN 0929-5313

Konnerth, A.; Heinemann, U. & Yaari, Y. (1986). Nonsynaptic epileptogenesis in the mammalian hippocampus in vitro. I. Development of seizurelike activity in low extracellular calcium. *J Neurophysiol*, Vol. 56, No. 2, (August), pp. 409–423, ISSN 0022-3077

Krnjevic, K.; Morris, M. & Reiffenstein, R. (1980). Changes in extracellular Ca^{2+} and K^{+} activity accompanying hippocampal discharges. *Can J Physiol Pharmacol*, Vol. 58, No. 5, (May), pp. 570–583, ISSN 0008-4212

MacVicar, B. & Dudek, F. (1982). Electrotonic coupling between granule cells of rat dentate gyrus: physiological and anatomical evidence. *J Neurophysiol*, Vol. 47, No. 4, (April), pp. 579-592, ISSN 0022-3077

Meierkord, H.; Grünig, F. ; Gutschmidt U, et al. (2000). Sodium bromide: effects on different patterns of epileptiform activity, extracellular pH changes and GABAergic inhibition. *Naunyn Schmiedebergs Arch Pharmacol*, Vol. 361, No. 1, (January), pp. 25–32, ISSN: 0028-1298

Nakao, M. & Gadsby, D. (1989). [Na] and [K] Dependence of the Na/K Pump Current-Voltage Relationship in Guinea Pig Ventricular Myocytes. *J. Gen. Physiol.* Vol. 94, No. 3, (September), pp. 539-565, ISSN 0022-1295

Naus, C.; Bechberger, J.; Caveney, S; & Wilson, J. (1991). Expression of gap junction genes in astrocytes and C6 glioma cells. *Neurosci Lett*. Vol. 126, No. 1, (May), pp. 33-36

Nicholson, C. (2001). Diffusion and related transport mechanisms in brain tissue. *Rep. Prog. Phys*, Vol. 64, No. 7, (July), 815-884, ISSN 0034-4885

Orkand, R. (1991). Glial Electrophysiology and Transport. *Annals of the New York Academy of Sciences*. Vol. 633, (December), pp. 245–247, ISSN 0077-8923

Pan, E. & Stringer, J. (1996). Burst Characteristics of dentate gyrus granule cells: evidence for endogenous and nonsynaptic properties. *J Neurophysiol*, Vol. 75, No. 1, (January), pp. 124–132, ISSN 0022-3077

Payne, J. (1997). Functional characterization of the neuronal-specific K-Cl cotransporter: implications for $[K^{+}]_{o}$. *Am J Physiol*, Vol. 273, Vol. 5, (November), pp. C1516-C1525, ISSN 0363-6143

Perez-Velazques JL, Valiant TA, Carlen PL. (1994). Modulation of gap junction mechanisms during calcium-free induced field activity: a possible role for electrotonic coupling in epileptogenesis. *J Neurophysiol*, Vol.14, No. 7, (July), pp. 4308–4317, ISSN 0022-3077

Rodrigues, A.; Almeida, A. & Infantosi, A. (2008). Effect of palytoxin on the sodium-potassium pump: model and simulation. *Phys Biol*, Vol. 5, No. 3, (July), pp. 036005 1-11, ISSN 1478-3967

Roper, S.; Obenaus, A. and Dudek, F. (1992). Osmolality and nonsynptic epileptiform bursts in rat CA1 and dentate gyrus. *Ann Neurol*, Vol. 31, No. 1, (January), pp. 81–85, ISSN 0364-5134

Russell, J. (2000). Sodium-potassium-chloride cotransport. *Physiol Rev*, Vol. 80, No.1, (January), pp. 211–276, ISSN 0031-9333

Scheiner-Bobis, G. (2002). The sodium pump. Its molecular properties and mechanics of ion transport. *Eur. J. Biochem*, Vol. 269, No. 10, (May), pp. 2424-2433, ISSN 0014-2956

Schwartzkroin, P. (1975). Characteristics of CA1 Neurons Recorded Intracellularly in the Hippocampal in Vitro Slice Preparation, *Brain Res*, v. 85, No. 3, (March), p. 423-436, ISSN 0006-8993

Schwartzkroin, P.; Baraban, S. & Hochman, D. (1998). Osmolarity, ionic flux, and changes in brain excitability. *Epilepsy Res*, Vol. 32, No. 1-2, (September), pp. 275–285, ISSN 0920-1211

Schweitzer, J.; Patrylo, P. & Dudek, F. (1992). Prolonged field bursts in the dentate gyrus: dependence on low calcium, high potassium, and nonsynaptic mechanisms. *J Neurophysiol*, Vol. 68, No. 6, pp. 2016–2025, ISSN 0022-3077

Snow, R. & Dudek, F. (1986). Evidence for neuronal interactions by electrical field effects in the CA3 and dentate regions of rat hippocampal slices. *Brain Res*, Vol. 367, No. 1-2, (March), pp. 292–295, ISSN 0006-8993

Somjen, G.; Aitken, P.; Giacchino, J. & McNamara, J. (1985). Sustained potential shifts and paroxysmal discharges in hippocampal formation. *J Neurophysiol*, Vol. 53, No. 4, (April), pp.1079–1097, ISSN 0022-3077

Stringer, J.; Williamson, J. & Lothman, E. (1989). Induction of paroxysmal discharges in the dentate gyrus: frequency dependence and relationship to afterdischarge production. *J Neurophysiol*, Vol. 62, No. 1, (July), pp. 126–135, ISSN 0022-3077

Stringer, J. & Lothman, E. (1991). Cholinergic and adrenergic agents modify the initiation and termination of epileptic discharges in the dentate gyrus. *Neuropharmacology* Vol. 30, No.1, (January), pp. 59–65, ISSN 0028-3908

Sychrová, H. (2004). Yeast as a model organism to study transport and homeostasis of alkali metal cations. *Physiol Res*, Vol. 53, No. Suppl 1, pp. S91–S98, ISSN 0862 - 8408

Tas, P.; Massa, P.; Kress, H. & Koschel, K. (1987). Characterization of an $Na^+/K^+/Cl^-$ co-transport in primary cultures of rat astrocytes. *Biochim Biophys Acta*, Vol. 903, No. 3, (October), pp. 411–416, ISSN 0006-3002

Taylor, C. & Dudek, F. (1982). Synchonous neural afterdischarges in rat hippocampal slices without active chemical synapses. *Science*, Vol. 218, No. 4574, (November), pp. 810–812, ISSN 0036-8075

Taylor, C. & Dudek, F. (1984). Synchronization without active chemical synapses during hippocampal afterdischarges. *J Neurophysiol*, Vol. 52, No. 1, (July), pp. 143–155, ISSN 0022-3077

Xiong, Z. & Stringer, J. (2000). Sodium Pump Activity, not Glial Spatial Buffering, clears Potassium after Epileptiform Activity Induced in The Dentate Gyrus. *J. Neurophysiol*, Vol. 83, No. :1443-1451, ISSN 0022-3077

12

A Tale of Two Epiphenomena: The Complex Interplay of Epigenetics and Epilepsy

Stacey Beth Foti and A. Jane Roskams
Department of Zoology, Life Science Institute, Brain Research Centre
Canada

1. Introduction

Epilepsy is a disorder primarily characterized by the spontaneous recurrence of unprovoked seizures. Seizures can be triggered by multiple factors including genetic mutations, head injury, toxins, a fever, high or low blood sugar, a tumor, electrolyte imbalance, drug withdrawal; and are also a core component of developmental and degenerative disorders (Loscher and Brandt 2010). However, not all patients that have seizures go on to develop epilepsy, and the mechanisms of epileptogenesis are still poorly understood. Only a small number of genetic mutations identified in ion channels or proteins associated with these channels have been directly linked to causing epilepsy (Greenberg and Pal 2007). In fact, complex epidemiological studies indicate that the interplay of environmental factors with relatively minor genetic alterations may contribute to the difference between the susceptibility to suffer seizures, and the development of epilepsy (Ottman et al. 1996). Evidence is emerging that epileptogenesis involves changes in the expression patterns of several classes of functionally or genomically-grouped genes that coordinate neural development, homeostasis and stress responses, and neural network formation (Lukasiuk et al. 2006 and references therein). This has led to speculation that minor and modifiable changes outside the open reading frames of affected genes could alter the course of epilepsy. How entire groups of genes may be co-regulated with precision during different stages of neural development and function could be the result of epigenetic changes in histone and chromatin structure and DNA methylation that accompany shifts in neural "state."

Chromatin structure and function can be altered to silence gene expression by DNA methylation leading to the recruitment of methyl-DNA binding proteins and histone deacetylation. Histones can also be modified at their N-terminus by phosphorylation, acetylation, methylation, ubiquitination, ADP ribosylation, carbonylation, SUMOylation, glycosylation and biotinylation. Here we will focus on DNA methylation and histone acetylation, and discuss how these epigenetic modifications could regulate developmental alterations that may contribute to the process of epileptogenesis. We will summarize how epigenetic changes may both regulate and be regulated by activity-dependent synaptic plasticity, and how involvement of common mechanisms underlying glial-neuronal interactions could lead to epileptogenesis. Finally, we will discuss how intervening in epilepsy by treating with widely-used drugs that themselves can alter chromatin state (like Valproic Acid) may further affect ongoing epileptogenesis, and discuss which specific epigenetic modifications may be novel therapeutic targets for the treatment of epilepsy.

2. Epigenetics and development

With limited exceptions, all cells in the human body have an identical genotype, and yet development produces a wide range of differentiated cell types with distinct functions that form highly specialized tissues and organs. This is especially true in the immensely complex and highly structured central nervous system (CNS). Cells differentiate from a stem cell to become increasingly specialized through a process of state-dependent (stage- and lineage-specific) gene activation and gene silencing, as many genomic regions become folded into heterochromatin, and are excluded from transcription (silenced) (MacDonald and Roskams 2009). Thus, progressive cell differentiation results, in part, from the epigenetic regulation of gene expression, which has been operationally defined as the study of heritable changes in gene function that are independent of changes in the underlying DNA sequence (Berger et al. 2009).

2.1 Chromatin and histone modifications

Both DNA and its associated histone proteins are subject to epigenetic modifications that change the overall structure of chromatin and the physical appearance of DNA within the nucleus (Goldberg, Allis and Bernstein 2007) (Figure 1). The fundamental unit of eukaryotic chromatin is the nucleosome, and it is composed of 147 base pairs of DNA wrapped around an octamer of four core histone proteins (H3, H4, H2A and H2B). The core histones are predominantly globular with flexible tails located at the N-terminus (Luger et al. 1997, Strahl and Allis 2000, Wade 2001). These tails vary in length and are composed of amino acids that allow for at least nine distinct types of modifications: phosphorylation, acetylation, methylation, ubiquitination, ADP ribosylation, carbonylation, SUMOylation, glycosylation and biotinylation (reviewed in Kouzarides 2007). Histone modifications correlate with gene activation or repression (Jenuwein and Allis 2001), and recently, histone domains containing both activating and repressive modifications have been identified (Azuara et al. 2006, Bernstein et al. 2005, Bernstein et al. 2006). These modifications can be context-dependent allowing gene transcription or silencing depending on the localization in the coding region versus the regulatory regions flanking the promoter (Kouzarides 2007, Vakoc et al. 2005). In addition to distinct histone modifications, DNA methylation can also silence gene transcription; and there is evidence of significant cross-talk between these processes to dynamically modify chromatin structure in response to external stimuli (Bernstein, Meissner and Lander 2007, Fuks 2005, Goldberg et al. 2007, Kouzarides 2007).
Both DNA and histone proteins are subject to epigenetic modifications like DNA methylation and histone acetylation that change the overall structure of chromatin, and alter the extent to which DNA is wrapped around histones and therefore the availability of genes to be activated.

2.1.1 DNA methylation

DNA methylation takes place post-synthesis, and is a chief determinant of the stability of gene expression states (Jaenisch and Bird 2003). In vertebrates, and in humans specifically, DNA methylation happens almost exclusively within cytosine-phosphate-guanine (CpG) dinucleotides, and 70-80% of all CpG dinucleotides are methylated (Ehrlich et al. 1982); (reviewed in Bird 2002, Goll and Bestor 2005). DNA methylation is catalyzed by DNA methyltransferases, or DNMTs, which covalently bind a methyl group to position C5 of cytosine residues (Bird 1992). DNA methylation represses transcription directly by

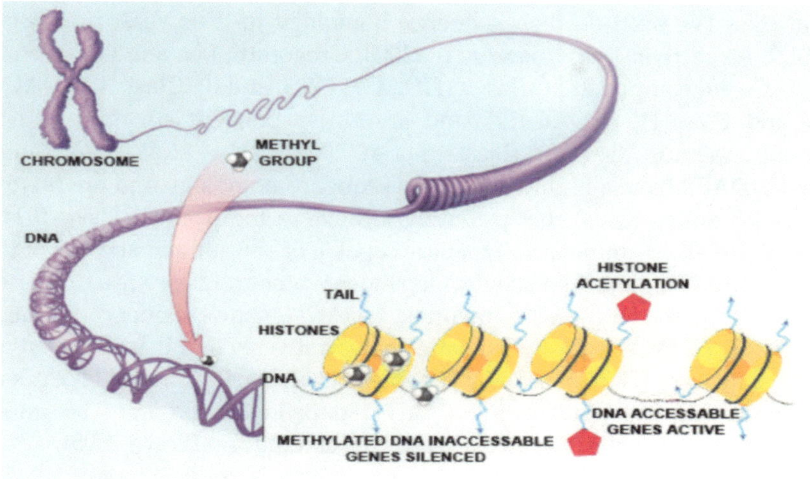

Fig. 1. Epigenetic regulation in the nucleosome (modified from the NIH http://nihroadmap.nih.gov/EPIGENOMICS/images/epigeneticmechanisms.jpg) Both DNA and histone proteins are subject to epigenetic modifications like DNA methylation and histone acetylation that change the overall structure of chromatin, and alter the extent to which DNA is wrapped around histones and therefore the availability of genes to be activated.

inhibiting the binding of specific transcription factors, and indirectly, by recruiting methyl-CpG-binding (MBD) proteins and their associated repressive chromatin remodeling activities (Robertson 2005). DNMT1 is the predominant enzyme in mammals, and is responsible for maintenance methylation (post-replicative restoration of hemi-methylated sites to full methylation), whereas DNMT3A and DNMT3B are thought to be involved primarily in *de novo* methylation (Laird 2003). Methylation is necessary for mammalian development, and mice with DNMT knocked out die during development (Li, Bestor and Jaenisch 1992, Okano et al. 1999). This absolute requirement for DNA methylation in development likely reflects the diverse range of cellular functions and pathologies to which it contributes, including silencing of repetitive and centromeric sequences, tissue-specific gene expression, genomic imprinting, maintenance of X chromosome inactivation, carcinogenesis and aging (Bird 2002, Jaenisch and Bird 2003, Jones and Baylin 2002, Paulsen and Ferguson-Smith 2001).

2.1.2 Histone deacetylation

Histone deacetylases (HDACs) regulate gene expression by removing the acetyl groups of specific lysine residues from histone protein tails, thereby increasing their positive charge, and enhancing their interaction with the negatively charged phosphate groups in the DNA backbone. The functional consequence of deacetylation is to stabilize compacted forms of chromatin, which can restrict binding of transcription factors to promoter regions of genes. This is a reversible reaction, and histone acetyl transferases (HATs) can add acetyl groups to lysine residues, removing the positive charge and loosening the chromatin from the histone core. In general, increased histone acetylation (hyperacetylation) is associated with increased transcriptional activity, whereas decreased acetylation (deacetylation or hypoacetylation) is associated with repression of gene expression (Strahl and Allis 2000, Wade 2001). There are four main classes of HDACs which are grouped into class I, class II, class III and class IV based on their sequence homology to their yeast orthologues Rpd3, HdaI and Sir2, respectively (de Ruijter et al. 2003, Gregoretti, Lee and Goodson 2004). The classical HDACs are comprised of Class I (HDACs 1, 2, 3, and 8), Class II (HDACs 4, 5, 6, 7, 9, and 10), and Class IV (HDAC 11), and are zinc-dependent enzymes with divergent patterns of expression in the brain (Bjerling et al. 2002, Fischle et al. 2002, Yang and Seto 2008). Class I HDACs have a highly conserved sequence homology and are relatively small proteins (377–488 amino acids) that primarily localize in the nucleus. Class II HDACs are larger proteins (669–1215 amino acids) that are capable of shuttling in and out of the nucleus in response to cellular signals like activity-dependent calcium release (de Ruijter et al. 2003, Yang and Seto 2008). The lone class IV member, HDAC11, shows sequence similarity to both class I and class II HDACs, but phylogenetic analysis reveals that it is divergent enough to warrant a separate class (Gao et al. 2002, Gregoretti et al. 2004). Class III HDACs or sirtuins are nicotinamide adenine dinucleotide (NAD+) dependent and may be important for linking metabolic state in cells to gene expression (Guarente and Picard 2005).

3. Epigenetically regulated developmental changes in the brain can lead to epilepsy

As many cell types throughout the brain differentiate, there is a concurrent shift in expression of DNMTs, HATs and HDACs that subsequently alter the compaction of chromatin. Developmental changes in epigenetic state thus underlie distinct shifts in gene expression that ultimately allow for structural and functional organization of the brain through control of neuro- and gliogenesis, and activity-dependent synaptic plasticity. Each stage of neural development carries a signature gene expression pattern, with a progressive restriction in the expression of developmentally regulated genes as maturation proceeds (Schuurmans and Guillemot 2002, Tietjen et al. 2003, Abramova et al. 2005, Lim et al. 2006). How repression or silencing as a result of epigenetic changes in chromatin contributes to these shifts in gene expression is slowly becoming better understood. Perhaps more importantly, improper regulation of each of these steps can lead to a variety of pathologies - apoptosis, alterations in neuro- and gliogenesis, aberrant neuronal migration, ectopic integration of neurons and glia causing structural malformations, and the formation of hyperexcitable circuits, all of which may contribute to seizure activity. Moreover, seizure activity itself can exacerbate many of these pathologies, and further perturb epigenetic factors, resulting in epileptogenesis and cognitive impairment.

3.1 Methylation state modulates neuro- and gliogenesis

In general, the known developmental effects of DNA methylation on gene expression involve long-term silencing of gene expression such as the establishment of parental-specific imprints during meiosis and X-chromosome inactivation (Jaenisch and Bird 2003), but recently much attention has been paid to its role in regulating gene expression during neuro- and gliogenesis. DNMTs are directly involved in neuronal maturation and survival (Fan et al. 2001, MacDonald, Gin and Roskams 2005, Feng et al. 2005). In a study by Fan and colleagues, conditional knock out of DNMT1 in nestin-positive cells is prenatal lethal, but mosaic mice with 30% of their neural cells missing DNMT1 survive into adulthood (Fan et al. 2001). In these animals, DNMT1-deficient neural precursor cells give rise to hypo-methylated progeny cells, including postmitotic neurons. However, within three weeks postnatal, all DNMT1-negative cells are eliminated, suggesting that these neurons were not stable enough to functionally mature (Fan et al. 2001). The *de novo* DNMTs (DNMT3a and DNMT3b) are sequentially expressed during neurogenesis, and are critical for regulating genes directly implicated in neurogenesis and neural function (Jin et al. 2008, Feng et al. 2005). Dnmt3b may be important for the early phase of neurogenesis, while Dnmt3a regulates prenatal progenitors as well as the maturation of post-mitotic neurons (Feng et al. 2005).

DNMT1 is also a critical cell-intrinsic determinant of astrocyte differentiation. For example, the promoter of glial fibrillary acid protein (GFAP) is methylated in progenitor cells during the neurogenic stages of embryonic development, but at later stages during gliogenesis, the promoter becomes demethylated (Teter et al. 1996). Methylation of the STAT binding element within the GFAP promoter inhibits association of activated STATs with the glial promoter (Takizawa et al. 2001), thereby repressing transcription of GFAP and preventing cells from proceeding down an astroglial lineage during the neurogenic stages of brain development (reviewed in MacDonald and Roskams 2009). However, if DNMT1 is knocked out, precocious astroglial differentiation occurs, presumably through hypomethylation of the GFAP promoter and other genes encoding the core components of the gliogenic JAK-STAT pathway (Fan et al. 2005). Since neurons rely on radial glial cells in order to migrate to the appropriate position during development, one consequence of precocious astrocyte formation could be the loss of radial glial "guide wires" and subsequent structural malformations caused by aberrant neuronal migration. These structural malformations are increasingly being discovered in epileptic patients as brain imaging technology advances (Scaravilli 1998).

MBD proteins are also regulators of neurogenesis, particularly in adult neurogenic niches like the subventricular zone. While MBD1 knockout mice are viable and appear relatively normal, they do have decreased neuronal differentiation of adult stem cells and diminished hippocampal neurogenesis (Zhao et al. 2003). MeCP2 is perhaps the best characterized MBD protein, because mutations within its coding region cause Rett syndrome (Amir et al. 1999, Bienvenu and Chelly 2006). Analysis of MeCP2 knockout mice revealed aberrant regulation of factors responsible for neurotransmitter biosynthesis and for promoting the differentiation and maturation of various neural cell types (Urdinguio et al. 2008), suggesting that MeCP2 regulates genes that are known to be involved in epileptogenesis. Furthermore, because seizures occur in many Rett patients (Glaze, Schultz and Frost 1998), there is strong evidence for a direct relationship between dysregulated MBD proteins and epilepsy.

3.2 Acetylation state modulates neuro- and gliogenesis

HDAC1 and HDAC2 are expressed at distinct stages of neuronal commitment and differentiation during CNS development (MacDonald and Roskams 2008), allowing them to modulate gene expression across neurodevelopmental stages. HDAC1 is enriched in progenitors clustered in neurogenic zones throughout the CNS (MacDonald and Roskams 2008). Neural progenitors that maintain the expression of HDAC1 largely differentiate into glial cells, while those that lose HDAC1 expression and begin to upregulate HDAC2 differentiate into neurons (MacDonald and Roskams 2008). In fact, HDAC1 is also highly expressed in the corpus callosum during oligodendrocyte differentiation, and when HDACs are inhibited, oligodendrocytes fail to differentiate and cause hypomyelination in the corpus callosum of postnatal rats (Shen, Li and Casaccia-Bonnefil 2005). Further to this, an elegant body of work has placed Class 1 HDACs, and HDAC1 in particular, as a critical regulator of the production and differentiation of oligodendrocyte precursor cells (Shen and Casaccia-Bonnefil 2008). HDAC1 can also directly regulate stem cell proliferation, as HDAC1 null animals display a significant reduction in cell proliferation (Lagger et al. 2002). HDAC2, on the other hand, is necessary to inhibit astrocyte differentiation, while HDAC1 is not (Humphrey et al. 2008). Taken together, HDAC2 may be involved in silencing glial gene expression, while HDAC1 likely silences neuronal genes.

HDAC1 and HDAC2 have been proposed to work in concert through large multi-protein complexes like REST nuclear protein (RE-1 silencing transcription factor, also called NRSF) and Co-REST. Through these complexes, HDAC-mediated acetylation can enable the transcriptional repression of genes containing a repressor element-1 (RE1/NRSE) in their promoter (Huang, Myers and Dingledine 1999). Because many neuron-specific genes that encode ion channels, synaptic vesicle proteins and neurotransmitter receptors contain an RE-1 motif, it has been proposed that REST silences these genes in all other cell types and acts as a master regulator of neurogenesis and neuronal differentiation (Ooi and Wood 2007, Ballas and Mandel 2005, Hsieh and Gage 2005). Intriguingly, REST is responsible for regulating the expression of several genes implicated in epileptogenesis, including growth factors, ion channels, neurotransmitter receptors, gap junctions, and neurosecretory vesicles, as well as those involved in seminal neural developmental processes and adult neurogenesis (reviewed in Qureshi and Mehler 2009, Qureshi and Mehler 2010)

In summary, abnormal activity of epigenetic mediators including DNMTs, MBDs, HDACs and repressor complexes could result in altered neuro- and gliogenesis, aberrant migration of newly born cells, and improper integration of these cells into circuits, thereby causing hyper-excitable circuits and seizures (Figure 2).

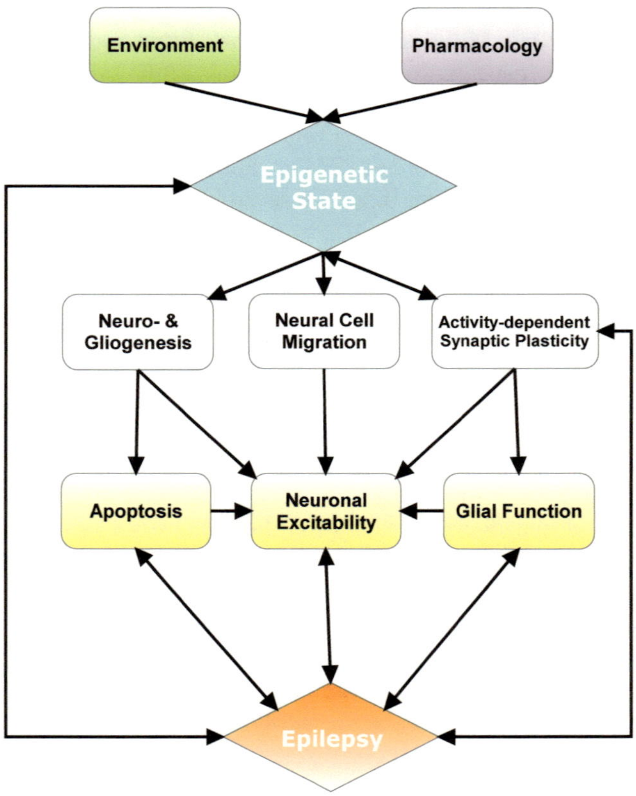

Fig. 2. Epigenetic gene regulation can dynamically impact numerous physiological processes in the nervous system.

Epigenetic state can be altered by extrinsic factors such as environmental stimulation and pharmacological manipulation, and internal factors that regulate neuronal activity. Since epigenetic factors such as DNMTs, MBDs, HDACs and repressor complexes modulate processes that include neuro- and gliogenesis, neural cell migration, and activity-dependent synaptic plasticity; dysregulation of these epigenetic factors can lead to apoptosis, neuronal hyperexcitability, impaired glial function, and ultimately can contribute to seizure activity, epileptogenesis, and epilepsy. Conversely, the hyperexcitability associated with epilepsy can also impact the expression of genes that regulate epigenetic state.

4. Epilepsy modulates epigenetic state and affects brain morphology

Clearly a dysregulation of epigenetic factors during development causes changes in neuro- and gliogenesis that may increase the likelihood of developing seizures, but the reversed scenario can also occur. It is now clear that seizures themselves can regulate epigenetic factors that then affect neurogenesis, neuronal migration, synapse formation, and neural activity.

It is well established that seizures cause alterations in neurogenesis in animal models and humans, but there is an age-dependent paradoxical effect in how seizures alter cell genesis in the CNS. For example, there is a postictal decrease in dentate granule cell birth in one week old rats subjected multiple brief seizures (Houser 1990, McCabe et al. 2001, Liu et al. 2003). This postictal decrease is age-related because a similar seizure paradigm performed in adult rats causes an increase in dentate granule cell birth (Houser 1990, McCabe et al. 2001, Liu et al. 2003). Furthermore, these effects depend on the frequency and severity of the seizures. Acute seizure activity causes a proliferative surge in neural stem cells of the subgranular zone of the hippocampus leading to increased production of new neurons during the first few weeks after the seizure episode, while chronic epilepsy is associated with declined hippocampal neurogenesis (Houser 1990, Parent et al. 1997, Scharfman, Goodman and Sollas 2000, McCabe et al. 2001, Porter 2008, Kuruba, Hattiangady and Shetty 2009). Surgically resected hippocampi from children with extra-hippocampal seizures also reveal a significant decrease in hippocampal neurons (Mathern et al. 1994), suggesting that the rate of cell death is exceeding the rate of neurogenesis and potential cell replacement.

Other pathologies associated with epilepsy-induced dysregulation of epigenetic factors include altered neuronal migration and increased mossy fiber (MF) sprouting. Examination of surgically resected hippocampal tissue from patients with temporal lobe epilepsy (TLE) confirms aberrant supragranular inner molecular layer MF sprouting, and a pathology known as granule cell dispersion (GCD), which has been linked to decreased expression of the glycoprotein Reelin (Haas et al. 2002, Haas and Frotscher 2010, Mathern et al. 1994). Reelin is critical for mediating neuronal migration throughout the CNS, and hippocampal patterning during brain development (Stanfield and Cowan 1979, Forster, Zhao and Frotscher 2006), and its expression is regulated directly by promoter methylation (Levenson, Qiu and Weeber 2008, Kobow et al. 2009). Recently, hippocampal tissue samples from TLE patients revealed increased promoter methylation in TLE specimens compared to controls, and this was significantly correlated with GCD (Kobow et al. 2009), implying that chronic epilepsy can cause epigenetic changes that may exacerbate disease pathology. In fact, seizure activity can perturb the migration of newly born neurons postnatally, resulting in their ectopic location in the hilus (and even as far as CA3), aberrant synapse formation, and consequently enhanced excitability (Scharfman et al. 2000).

Seizures can induce histone modifications for a number of genes involved in neuronal plasticity and synapse formation, including the neurotrophin brain-derived neurotrophic factor (BDNF) and the glutamate receptor GluR2 (Tsankova, Kumar and Nestler 2004, Huang, Doherty and Dingledine 2002). Seizure activity induces acetylation of the BDNF promoter, thereby up-regulating BDNF (Tsankova et al. 2004). BDNF upregulation following seizure activity is thought to contribute to epileptogenesis, and BDNF infusion in epileptic animals can trigger seizure-like events (Scharfman, Goodman and Sollas 1999). In addition, transgenic mice that overexpress BDNF display heightened seizure susceptibility, spontaneous seizures and hyperexcitability of the hippocampus (Croll et al. 1999). Furthermore, BDNF has been shown to attenuate γ-aminobutyric acid (GABA)ergic inhibitory neurotransmission (Tanaka, Saito and Matsuki 1997), which can lead to an imbalance in neuronal excitatory transmission. At the same time, seizure activity leads to deacetylation of histones at the GluR2 promoter, and reduced expression of the receptor, resulting in enhanced AMPA receptor-mediated epileptogenesis (Sanchez et al. 2001). Thus, seizure activity can induce epigenetic changes that contribute to epileptogenesis, but why does this occur? It is highly likely that seizure activity harnesses much of the same molecular machinery involved in activity-dependent synapse formation and learning and memory.

5. Epigenetic factors can both regulate, and be regulated by, synaptic plasticity

Repeated patterns of synaptic transmission lead to diverse forms of synaptic plasticity at excitatory and inhibitory synapses, including long-term potentiation (LTP) and long-term depression (LTD), whereby the strength of synaptic transmission is increased or decreased respectively (reviewed in Malenka and Bear 2004). Certain forms of LTP and LTD are long lived and are dependent on lasting changes in gene expression (Borrelli et al. 2008). Based on the critical role that epigenetics plays in mediating lasting alterations in gene expression, DNA and histone modifiers are poised to provide a mechanism that both encodes and stabilizes these changes in synaptic strength. This is already the case in mice who over-express HDAC2 in neurons, and exhibit decreased dendritic spine density, synapse number, synaptic plasticity and memory formation (Guan et al. 2009). These results suggest that deacetylation may cause transcriptional repression of the neuronal genes involved in forming and maintaining functional synapses. Since seizures result in synchronized neuronal firing, it is possible that they trigger the same types of epigenetic responses as LTP, and that aberrant stabilization of hyper-excitable circuits could lead to progressive epileptogenesis. Theoretically, specific treatment of the area of seizure-genesis with targeted HDAC2 inhibition could thus interrupt this cycle, and may be a promising therapeutic strategy.

DNA methylation can also be dynamically regulated by synaptic activity. For example, neuronal activity and learning can produce DNA methylation of distinct genomic sites in the human brain (Siegmund et al. 2007), and this methylation signature varies by brain region (Ladd-Acosta et al. 2007). These observations are consistent with the recent findings that DNA methylation can occur rapidly and reversibly in the nervous system (Levenson et al. 2006) in contrast to the previous dogma that methylation state is permanent. BDNF exemplifies this principle, and is demethylated upon neuronal activity. It is proposed that neural activity via increases in cellular Ca^{2+} levels and activation of Ca^{2+}/calmodulin kinases leads to the phosphorylation of MeCP2, and its release from the CoREST complexes on the BDNF promoter (Ballas et al. 2005), resulting in increased BDNF expression (reviewed in Borrelli et al. 2008). Increased BDNF expression is associated with alterations in GABA receptor subunit composition which can lead to reduced neuronal inhibition (Lagrange, Botzolakis and Macdonald 2007), and increased excitatory neurotransmission by enhancing presynaptic glutamate release and phosphorylating NMDA receptors (Takei et al. 1997, Lin et al. 1998). Thus, DNA methylation is regulated by neuronal activity, and in turn can also influence neural plasticity through the regulation of activity-dependent neuronal genes. Collectively, this neuronal excitability can play a modulatory role in learning and memory, but in the context of disease, it can feed-forward into the cycle of epileptogenesis.

6. Environmental and nutritional factors that influence epigenetic state and vulnerability to epilepsy

In mammalian development, the prenatal and postnatal periods are characterized by dynamic structural and functional re-organization of the brain, as its pathways become shaped by stimulation and experience. During this highly plastic period, environmental experiences influence neural structure, synaptic strength, and consequently our behavior. There is increasing evidence that epigenetic factors are at the interface of environment and gene regulation, and that changes in epigenetic state are stable enough to be heritable, but not static, thereby allowing future experience to modify them. A particularly good example of this is maternal diet, which can cause heritable changes in epigenetic state that then alter gene expression and behavior in offspring. Mechanistically, protein-restricted diets can inhibit DNMTs and cause hypomethylation of specific gene promoters in the offspring (Lillycrop et al. 2007). In addition, folate and vitamin B12 are essential cofactors for the methylation cycle, thus deficiencies in these vitamins also inhibit DNMTs and DNA methylation, which can cause oxidative stress and neuronal cell death (Kruman et al. 2002, Duan et al. 2002, Seshadri et al. 2002, Shea, Lyons-Weiler and Rogers 2002). Another B-vitamin, biotin, modulates chromatin regulation through histone biotinylation (Hassan and Zempleni 2006). Moreover, biotin deficiency can cause epilepsy as well as other clinical features including hypotonia, ataxia, mental retardation, and fetal malformations (Zempleni et al. 2008). These studies suggest that eating a diet with plenty of protein and foods rich in B vitamins may help lower seizure vulnerability through epigenetic regulation of gene expression. In fact, a ketogenic diet (high fat, adequate protein, low carbohydrate) has been used for decades to control refractory seizures in children (Lefevre and Aronson 2000, Stafstrom 2004), and a recent study by Garriga-Canut et al. provides a potential epigenetic mechanism for the antiepileptic properties of the ketogenic diet and of a potentially new treatment for epilepsy, 2-deoxy-D-glucose (2DG) (Garriga-Canut et al. 2006). Metabolic intermediates including NADH can modulate co-activators and co-repressors, thereby linking energy availability to chromatin structure and transcriptional output (Guarente and Picard 2005). Since 2DG is a glycolytic inhibitor, it may act as a small molecule regulator of the NAD+ HDAC III sirtuins, thereby repressing transcription of genes that contribute to epileptogenesis. In fact, Garriga-Canut and colleagues (2006) show that 2DG can reduce the progression of epileptogenesis in kindled rats by raising the after-discharge threshold, reinforcing that diet can induce changes in epigenetic state that impact the development of epilepsy.

Prenatal and postnatal stress can also influence epigenetic state and neurodevelopment, subsequently changing our behavior patterns. Early-life stress can cause epigenetic changes in the methylation status of certain promoters including the glucocorticoid receptor (GR).

Stress can increase levels of DNA methylation in the NGFI-A binding site of the GR 17 promoter and decrease histone H3-K9 acetylation (a marker of transcriptional activation), the functional consequence of which is a heightened stress response (Weaver et al. 2004, Weaver et al. 2007). Severe early-life stress can increase excitotoxic cell death of hippocampal neurons (Brunson et al. 2003), whereas prenatal stress contributes to the susceptibility for febrile convulsions, afebrile seizures, and cerebral palsy (Greenwood et al. 1998, Weinstock 2001). Perhaps the most striking finding is that maternal stress in the latter half of pregnancy lowers the seizure threshold, potentially increasing seizure susceptibility in the unborn offspring (Edwards et al. 2002). Thus the nervous system is particularly sensitive to alterations in epigenetic regulation, probably because of the fine balance needed to maintain heritable cellular memory while still being capable of adapting to changing environmental conditions.

7. DNA methylation inhibitors and HDAC inhibitors are potential epigenetic targets for epilepsy treatment

Since epigenetic factors play such an important role in regulating gene expression during neuro- and gliogenesis and key phases of synaptic plasticity and learning, pharmacological manipulation of these factors in targeted time windows in the etiology of disease holds enormous therapeutic potential. This is particularly important for a complex disease like epilepsy which involves multiple genes and downstream effectors. Recent evidence has emerged that modifying chromatin structure can indeed alter the disease course of epilepsy, and serves as a fertile ground for exploring targeted remodeling of chromatin as a potential therapeutic strategy in epilepsy (summarized in Table 1).

7.1 DNA methylation inhibitors and treatment of epilepsy

In humans, a variety of mental retardation syndromes with an epileptic phenotype including Rett syndrome, Fragile-X, Rubinstein–Taybi, Prader-Willi and Angelman syndromes, have all been linked to mutations or disruptions in methylation factors (Egger et al. 2004), suggesting that methylation inhibitors may be a novel therapeutic target for epilepsy. Current generation DNMT inhibitors are methylcytosine analogues that reduce DNA methylation through covalent sequestering of DNMTs as opposed to the direct removal of methyl groups from DNA (Juttermann, Li and Jaenisch 1994). These inhibitors are widely used clinically for their anti-cancer efficacy (reviewed in Das and Singal 2004), but have not been systematically evaluated to treat epilepsy. The DNMT inhibitors 5-azacytidine (5azaC) and zebularine can effectively inhibit DNA methylation in neurons and block LTP and memory formation (Levenson et al. 2006, Miller, Campbell and Sweatt 2008, Miller and Sweatt 2007), suggesting that they are good candidate drugs to evaluate in epilepsy paradigms. When both agents were applied in a Rett syndrome mouse model, treatment facilitated a significant decrease in frequency of miniature excitatory post-synaptic currents (mEPSCs) and rate of spontaneous synaptic vesicle fusion (Nelson et al. 2008). Since decreasing mEPSCs can reduce neuronal excitability, methylation inhibitors may possess anti-seizure properties, and should thus be tested in more classic epilepsy models. In addition to methylcytosine analogs, DNA methylation can be reversed pharmacologically by increasing histone acetylation through the use of HDAC inhibitors (Cervoni and Szyf 2001, Milutinovic et al. 2007), underscoring that multiple epigenetic factors work in a concerted manner to regulate gene expression and careful consideration of

Drug name	Epigenetic target	(Deutsch et al. 2008)	Outcome	Reference
Sodium Butyrate	Inhibits class 1 and II HDACs except HDAC6 and HDAC10	IECS to produce tonic hindlimb extension	Increased H3 and H4 acetylation in hippocampus and cortex and improved anti-seizure efficacy of MK-801	(Deutsch et al. 2008)
VPA	Inhibits class I HDACs and to a lesser extent class II HDACs	IBO injection (excitotoxin) to kill GABAergic and cholinergic neurons	Increased H3 acetylation in cortex and NBM and significant protection of both cholinergic and GABAergic neurons present in the injected area	(Eleuteri et al. 2009)
		Kainic Acid induced SE	No significant effect on seizure strength or frequency but inhibited seizure-induced neurogenesis in hippocampus and prevented memory impairment	(Jessberger et al. 2007)
		PTZ induced seizures	Increased thresholds to all seizure types	(Hoffmann, Czapp and Loscher 2008)
TSA	Inhibits class I and II HDACs	Kainic Acid induced SE	Prevented the down-regulation of GluR2 in hippocampus	(Jessberger et al. 2007)
		PTZ induced seizures	No dose-dependent anticonvulsant effects	(Hoffmann et al. 2008)
		Pilocarpine induced seizures	Prevented the down-regulation of GluR2 in hippocampus	(Huang et al. 2002)
		Kainic Acid induced seizures	Histone hyperacetylation of IEGs c-jun and c-fos	(Sng, Taniura and Yoneda 2005)
Zebularine	Inhibits DNMTs	Rett Syndrome (MeCP2 KO mice)	Deficits in spontaneous synaptic transmission	(Nelson, Kavalali and Monteggia 2008)

Abbreviations: HDAC=histone deacetylase. SE=status epilepticus. IECS=incremental electroconvulsive shock. VPA=valproic acid. IBO=ibotenic acid. NBM=nucleus basalis magnocellularis. TSA=trichostatin A. GluR2=glutamate receptor 2. PTZ=pentylenetetrazole. IEG=immediate early genes. DNMT=DNA methyltransferase. KO=knock out

Table 1. Epigenetic therapy in epilepsy models

undesired secondary effects of such compounds must be taken when designing a therapeutic approach.

7.2 HDAC inhibitors and treatment of epilepsy

HDAC inhibitors (HDACi) are classified into six groups based on their chemical structures: (1) hydroxamic acids, including TSA and SAHA; (2) small-molecular-weight carboxylates, including sodium butyrate, valproic acid, and sodium phenylbutyrate; (3) benzamides, including MS-275 and CI-994; (4) epoxyketones, including AOE and trapoxin B; (5) cyclic peptides, including depsipeptide and apicidin; and (6) hybrid molecules, such as CHAP31 and CHAP50 (Drummond et al. 2005 and references there in). Most HDACi are broad-spectrum within the classical HDAC family, and isoform-specific inhibitors have been difficult to design due to the high sequence homology within the catalytically-active sites of HDACs (Bieliauskas and Pflum 2008). Therefore, the majority of published studies have employed HDAC inhibitors that have multiple secondary targets within and beyond the CNS, but collectively, a compelling argument can be made to explore their efficacy in most epilepsy paradigms. Hydroxamic acids encompass the broadest set of HDACi, and primarily inhibit class I/II HDACs when used in the nanomolar range (Bieliauskas and Pflum 2008), however side effects in patients have been reported, particularly with TSA (Villar-Garea and Esteller 2004). In contrast, the carboxylates are very well tolerated in animals and humans, and have been used in dose escalating studies in the clinic (Atmaca et al. 2007). HDAC inhibitors have been extensively studied in models of neurodegenerative disease (Hahnen et al. 2008), and some agents–such as valproic acid (VPA), sodium butyrate and LBH589–are now being tested in clinical trials in patients with spinal muscular atrophy (SMA), Huntington's disease (HD), Alzheimer's disease (AD), and amyotrophic lateral sclerosis (ALS).

The most widely used HDAC inhibitor, Valproate (VPA), has been used as an anti-epileptic therapeutic agent for over 40 years, and its effects in the nervous system have recently been reviewed in detail elsewhere (MacDonald and Roskams 2009, Loscher 1999). However, VPA has primarily been used for its multitude of effects on CNS excitation pathways that have not taken into account its HDAC inhibition activity. Briefly, VPA can (1) increase the level of the inhibitory neurotransmitter γ-aminobutyric acid (GABA), (2) reduce sodium conductance through voltage-gated sodium channels, (3) suppress N-methyl-D-aspartate (NMDA) receptor-mediated excitation, (4) have teratogenic activity in both humans and mouse models.

While VPA is well tolerated and can attenuate seizure activity, evidence suggests that it is not truly antiepileptic. In other words, VPA can acutely and chronically reduce the risk of recurrent seizures, but treatment does not alter the development of epilepsy (Shinnar and Berg 1996, Haut and Shinnar 2008). One possible explanation for this dichotomy is that even though VPA augments presynaptic GABA release (reviewed in Loscher 1999), thereby conferring antiseizure properties, VPA also increases BDNF expression (Fukumoto et al. 2001) and can reduce $GABA_A$ receptor γ2 subunit, GAD65, GAD67, and KCC2 expression (Fukuchi et al., 2009), thus impairing GABAergic function over time and potentially shifting the balance of neurotransmission to a more hyperexcitable state. Furthermore, GABAergic signaling regulates neurogenesis and neuronal differentiation of immature neurons (Ben-Ari 2002), so VPA-mediated alterations in GABAergic neurotransmission could impair neurogenesis and subsequently cause cognitive impairment, particularly in children and adolescents where brain development is still very actively occurring. In fact, mice lacking MeCP2 from GABA-releasing neurons consequently have impaired GABA function, and display many of the characteristic symptoms of Rett syndrome and autism (Chao et al.). Thus, if inhibitory neurogenesis is indeed perturbed as a secondary action of this compound, treating patients with VPA to control seizures could inadvertently hasten the progression of epilepsy. However, in a recent study, treatment with VPA following kainic acid-induced seizures did inhibit hippocampal neurogenesis, but surprisingly improved cognitive impairment compared with controls who received kainic acid alone (Jessberger et al. 2007). This contradiction supports the hypothesis that seizure-induced neurogenesis can be detrimental, but the consequences of chronically inhibiting neurogenesis are likely to be harmful.

A final potential use for HDAC inhibitors in treating epilepsy is in enhancing the survival of neurons in existing circuits that might otherwise succumb to excitotoxic cell death due to hyper-excitation and the resulting ionic imbalances. A growing body of evidence places HDAC inhibition capable of mediating survival signaling, cytoskeletal stabilization in neurons, and CREB-mediated signaling following ischemia and oxidative stress (reviewed in Sleiman et al. 2009). With the development and testing of new generations of specific HDAC inhibitors that are not only CNS-permeable, but usable in short-term pulses in animal models of appropriate neurological diseases, it is possible that HDACi-mediated neuroprotection and stabilization of existing brain circuitry is a potential mechanism for preventing the spread or progression of epilepsy, and limiting the accompanying cognitive deficits that result from poorly controlled seizures in epileptic patients.

8. Conclusions

After sequencing the human genome - and the genomes of numerous other species, it is apparent that organisms with a higher order of complexity within their CNS have acquired a more complex non-coding genome. The majority of this sequence is comprised of regulatory elements that contextually modulate protein expression and function. Although a large part of development is due to the complex transcriptional regulation required of multiple members of the same gene family, it is likely that analysis of the structural organization, the regulation of the non-coding genome, and the role of epigenetics in modulating these phenomena will reveal a more in-depth understanding of our own human phenotype. Within these unique DNA modifications are clues to the origin, susceptibility, and progression of neurological disease, including epilepsy.

Epigenetic processes are certainly involved in the development and progression of epilepsy, and epilepsy, in turn, can change the epigenetic landscape of the CNS (summarized in Fig 2). Regardless of whether seizures begin early or later in life; the processes outlined above (synaptic plasticity, neuro-gliogenesis, and neuroprotection) are ongoing developmental processes that are all mediated by epigenetic changes in chromatin structure. Those same changes in chromatin--based on environment, stimulation, and developmental programs--drive the individual biology within distinct CNS cells. Thus epigenetics provides a mechanism whereby CNS cells can react to internal and external stimuli, and record the experience in both a modifiable and heritable manner. The emergence of genomic diagnostics, coupled with high resolution imaging to pinpoint functionally "normal" versus "aberrant" cellular responses to these stimuli, will allow us to identify the aberrant circuitry that leads to the progression of epilepsy and its underlying pathology.

Concurrent with this, advances in combinatorial chemistry and high throughput screening approaches will allow for the ongoing and rapid development of subtype-specific HDAC inhibitors (and drugs to modify other histone marks such as methylation and phosphorylation). Because the pharmacological manipulation of epigenetic factors is a growing target for many diseases (notably cancer), the future holds great promise in being able to evaluate the therapeutic efficacy of these agents in neurological diseases, and in particular, for the beneficial effects they may afford to patients with epilepsy.

9. Acknowledgements

This work was supported by grants from the Michael Smith Foundation for Health Research and the Canadian Institutes of Health Research.

10. References

Abramova, N., C. Charniga, S. K. Goderie & S. Temple (2005) Stage-specific changes in gene expression in acutely isolated mouse CNS progenitor cells. *Dev Biol,* 283, 269-81.

Amir, R. E., I. B. Van den Veyver, M. Wan, C. Q. Tran, U. Francke & H. Y. Zoghbi (1999) Rett syndrome is caused by mutations in X-linked MECP2, encoding methyl-CpG-binding protein 2. *Nat Genet,* 23, 185-8.

Atmaca, A., S. E. Al-Batran, A. Maurer, A. Neumann, T. Heinzel, B. Hentsch, S. E. Schwarz, S. Hovelmann, M. Gottlicher, A. Knuth & E. Jager (2007) Valproic acid (VPA) in patients with refractory advanced cancer: a dose escalating phase I clinical trial. *Br J Cancer,* 97, 177-82.

Azuara, V., P. Perry, S. Sauer, M. Spivakov, H. F. Jorgensen, R. M. John, M. Gouti, M. Casanova, G. Warnes, M. Merkenschlager & A. G. Fisher (2006) Chromatin signatures of pluripotent cell lines. *Nat Cell Biol,* 8, 532-8.

Ballas, N., C. Grunseich, D. D. Lu, J. C. Speh & G. Mandel (2005) REST and its corepressors mediate plasticity of neuronal gene chromatin throughout neurogenesis. *Cell,* 121, 645-57.

Ballas, N. & G. Mandel (2005) The many faces of REST oversee epigenetic programming of neuronal genes. *Curr Opin Neurobiol,* 15, 500-6.

Ben-Ari, Y. (2002) Excitatory actions of gaba during development: the nature of the nurture. *Nat Rev Neurosci,* 3, 728-39.

Berger, S. L., T. Kouzarides, R. Shiekhattar & A. Shilatifard (2009) An operational definition of epigenetics. *Genes Dev,* 23, 781-3.

Bernstein, B. E., M. Kamal, K. Lindblad-Toh, S. Bekiranov, D. K. Bailey, D. J. Huebert, S. McMahon, E. K. Karlsson, E. J. Kulbokas, 3rd, T. R. Gingeras, S. L. Schreiber & E. S. Lander (2005) Genomic maps and comparative analysis of histone modifications in human and mouse. *Cell,* 120, 169-81.

Bernstein, B. E., A. Meissner & E. S. Lander (2007) The mammalian epigenome. *Cell,* 128, 669-81.

Bernstein, B. E., T. S. Mikkelsen, X. Xie, M. Kamal, D. J. Huebert, J. Cuff, B. Fry, A. Meissner, M. Wernig, K. Plath, R. Jaenisch, A. Wagschal, R. Feil, S. L. Schreiber & E. S. Lander (2006) A bivalent chromatin structure marks key developmental genes in embryonic stem cells. *Cell,* 125, 315-26.

Bieliauskas, A. V. & M. K. Pflum (2008) Isoform-selective histone deacetylase inhibitors. *Chem Soc Rev,* 37, 1402-13.

Bienvenu, T. & J. Chelly (2006) Molecular genetics of Rett syndrome: when DNA methylation goes unrecognized. *Nat Rev Genet,* 7, 415-26.
Bird, A. (1992) The essentials of DNA methylation. *Cell,* 70, 5-8.
--- (2002) DNA methylation patterns and epigenetic memory. *Genes Dev,* 16, 6-21.
Bjerling, P., R. A. Silverstein, G. Thon, A. Caudy, S. Grewal & K. Ekwall (2002) Functional divergence between histone deacetylases in fission yeast by distinct cellular localization and in vivo specificity. *Mol Cell Biol,* 22, 2170-81.
Borrelli, E., E. J. Nestler, C. D. Allis & P. Sassone-Corsi (2008) Decoding the epigenetic language of neuronal plasticity. *Neuron,* 60, 961-74.
Brunson, K. L., Y. Chen, S. Avishai-Eliner & T. Z. Baram (2003) Stress and the developing hippocampus: a double-edged sword? *Mol Neurobiol,* 27, 121-36.
Cervoni, N. & M. Szyf (2001) Demethylase activity is directed by histone acetylation. *J Biol Chem,* 276, 40778-87.
Chao, H. T., H. Chen, R. C. Samaco, M. Xue, M. Chahrour, J. Yoo, J. L. Neul, S. Gong, H. C. Lu, N. Heintz, M. Ekker, J. L. Rubenstein, J. L. Noebels, C. Rosenmund & H. Y. Zoghbi Dysfunction in GABA signalling mediates autism-like stereotypies and Rett syndrome phenotypes. *Nature,* 468, 263-9.
Croll, S. D., C. Suri, D. L. Compton, M. V. Simmons, G. D. Yancopoulos, R. M. Lindsay, S. J. Wiegand, J. S. Rudge & H. E. Scharfman (1999) Brain-derived neurotrophic factor transgenic mice exhibit passive avoidance deficits, increased seizure severity and in vitro hyperexcitability in the hippocampus and entorhinal cortex. *Neuroscience,* 93, 1491-506.
Das, P. M. & R. Singal (2004) DNA methylation and cancer. *J Clin Oncol,* 22, 4632-42.
de Ruijter, A. J., A. H. van Gennip, H. N. Caron, S. Kemp & A. B. van Kuilenburg (2003) Histone deacetylases (HDACs): characterization of the classical HDAC family. *Biochem J,* 370, 737-49.
Deutsch, S. I., R. B. Rosse, K. D. Long, B. L. Gaskins, J. A. Burket & J. Mastropaolo (2008) Sodium butyrate, an epigenetic interventional strategy, attenuates a stress-induced alteration of MK-801's pharmacologic action. *Eur Neuropsychopharmacol,* 18, 565-8.
Drummond, D. C., C. O. Noble, D. B. Kirpotin, Z. Guo, G. K. Scott & C. C. Benz (2005) Clinical development of histone deacetylase inhibitors as anticancer agents. *Annu Rev Pharmacol Toxicol,* 45, 495-528.
Duan, W., B. Ladenheim, R. G. Cutler, Kruman, II, J. L. Cadet & M. P. Mattson (2002) Dietary folate deficiency and elevated homocysteine levels endanger dopaminergic neurons in models of Parkinson's disease. *J Neurochem,* 80, 101-10.
Edwards, H. E., D. Dortok, J. Tam, D. Won & W. M. Burnham (2002) Prenatal stress alters seizure thresholds and the development of kindled seizures in infant and adult rats. *Horm Behav,* 42, 437-47.
Egger, G., G. Liang, A. Aparicio & P. A. Jones (2004) Epigenetics in human disease and prospects for epigenetic therapy. *Nature,* 429, 457-63.
Ehrlich, M., M. A. Gama-Sosa, L. H. Huang, R. M. Midgett, K. C. Kuo, R. A. McCune & C. Gehrke (1982) Amount and distribution of 5-methylcytosine in human DNA from different types of tissues of cells. *Nucleic Acids Res,* 10, 2709-21.
Eleuteri, S., B. Monti, S. Brignani & A. Contestabile (2009) Chronic dietary administration of valproic acid protects neurons of the rat nucleus basalis magnocellularis from ibotenic acid neurotoxicity. *Neurotox Res,* 15, 127-32.

Fan, G., C. Beard, R. Z. Chen, G. Csankovszki, Y. Sun, M. Siniaia, D. Biniszkiewicz, B. Bates, P. P. Lee, R. Kuhn, A. Trumpp, C. Poon, C. B. Wilson & R. Jaenisch (2001) DNA hypomethylation perturbs the function and survival of CNS neurons in postnatal animals. *J Neurosci,* 21, 788-97.

Fan, G., K. Martinowich, M. H. Chin, F. He, S. D. Fouse, L. Hutnick, D. Hattori, W. Ge, Y. Shen, H. Wu, J. ten Hoeve, K. Shuai & Y. E. Sun (2005) DNA methylation controls the timing of astrogliogenesis through regulation of JAK-STAT signaling. *Development,* 132, 3345-56.

Feng, J., H. Chang, E. Li & G. Fan (2005) Dynamic expression of de novo DNA methyltransferases Dnmt3a and Dnmt3b in the central nervous system. *J Neurosci Res,* 79, 734-46.

Fischle, W., F. Dequiedt, M. J. Hendzel, M. G. Guenther, M. A. Lazar, W. Voelter & E. Verdin (2002) Enzymatic activity associated with class II HDACs is dependent on a multiprotein complex containing HDAC3 and SMRT/N-CoR. *Mol Cell,* 9, 45-57.

Forster, E., S. Zhao & M. Frotscher (2006) Laminating the hippocampus. *Nat Rev Neurosci,* 7, 259-67.

Fuks, F. (2005) DNA methylation and histone modifications: teaming up to silence genes. *Curr Opin Genet Dev,* 15, 490-5.

Fukumoto, T., S. Morinobu, Y. Okamoto, A. Kagaya & S. Yamawaki (2001) Chronic lithium treatment increases the expression of brain-derived neurotrophic factor in the rat brain. *Psychopharmacology (Berl),* 158, 100-6.

Gao, L., M. A. Cueto, F. Asselbergs & P. Atadja (2002) Cloning and functional characterization of HDAC11, a novel member of the human histone deacetylase family. *J Biol Chem,* 277, 25748-55.

Garriga-Canut, M., B. Schoenike, R. Qazi, K. Bergendahl, T. J. Daley, R. M. Pfender, J. F. Morrison, J. Ockuly, C. Stafstrom, T. Sutula & A. Roopra (2006) 2-Deoxy-D-glucose reduces epilepsy progression by NRSF-CtBP-dependent metabolic regulation of chromatin structure. *Nat Neurosci,* 9, 1382-7.

Glaze, D. G., R. J. Schultz & J. D. Frost (1998) Rett syndrome: characterization of seizures versus non-seizures. *Electroencephalogr Clin Neurophysiol,* 106, 79-83.

Goldberg, A. D., C. D. Allis & E. Bernstein (2007) Epigenetics: a landscape takes shape. *Cell,* 128, 635-8.

Goll, M. G. & T. H. Bestor (2005) Eukaryotic cytosine methyltransferases. *Annu Rev Biochem,* 74, 481-514.

Greenberg, D. A. & D. K. Pal (2007) The state of the art in the genetic analysis of the epilepsies. *Curr Neurol Neurosci Rep,* 7, 320-8.

Greenwood, R., J. Golding, E. Ross & C. Verity (1998) Prenatal and perinatal antecedents of febrile convulsions and afebrile seizures: data from a national cohort study. *Paediatr Perinat Epidemiol,* 12 Suppl 1, 76-95.

Gregoretti, I. V., Y. M. Lee & H. V. Goodson (2004) Molecular evolution of the histone deacetylase family: functional implications of phylogenetic analysis. *J Mol Biol,* 338, 17-31.

Guan, J. S., S. J. Haggarty, E. Giacometti, J. H. Dannenberg, N. Joseph, J. Gao, T. J. Nieland, Y. Zhou, X. Wang, R. Mazitschek, J. E. Bradner, R. A. DePinho, R. Jaenisch & L. H. Tsai (2009) HDAC2 negatively regulates memory formation and synaptic plasticity. *Nature,* 459, 55-60.

Guarente, L. & F. Picard (2005) Calorie restriction--the SIR2 connection. *Cell,* 120, 473-82.

Haas, C. A., O. Dudeck, M. Kirsch, C. Huszka, G. Kann, S. Pollak, J. Zentner & M. Frotscher (2002) Role for reelin in the development of granule cell dispersion in temporal lobe epilepsy. *J Neurosci,* 22, 5797-802.

Haas, C. A. & M. Frotscher (2010) Reelin deficiency causes granule cell dispersion in epilepsy. *Exp Brain Res,* 200, 141-9.

Hahnen, E., J. Hauke, C. Trankle, I. Y. Eyupoglu, B. Wirth & I. Blumcke (2008) Histone deacetylase inhibitors: possible implications for neurodegenerative disorders. *Expert Opin Investig Drugs,* 17, 169-84.

Hassan, Y. I. & J. Zempleni (2006) Epigenetic regulation of chromatin structure and gene function by biotin. *J Nutr,* 136, 1763-5.

Haut, S. R. & S. Shinnar (2008) Considerations in the treatment of a first unprovoked seizure. *Semin Neurol,* 28, 289-96.

Hoffmann, K., M. Czapp & W. Loscher (2008) Increase in antiepileptic efficacy during prolonged treatment with valproic acid: role of inhibition of histone deacetylases? *Epilepsy Res,* 81, 107-13.

Houser, C. R. (1990) Granule cell dispersion in the dentate gyrus of humans with temporal lobe epilepsy. *Brain Res,* 535, 195-204.

Hsieh, J. & F. H. Gage (2005) Chromatin remodeling in neural development and plasticity. *Curr Opin Cell Biol,* 17, 664-71.

Huang, Y., J. J. Doherty & R. Dingledine (2002) Altered histone acetylation at glutamate receptor 2 and brain-derived neurotrophic factor genes is an early event triggered by status epilepticus. *J Neurosci,* 22, 8422-8.

Huang, Y., S. J. Myers & R. Dingledine (1999) Transcriptional repression by REST: recruitment of Sin3A and histone deacetylase to neuronal genes. *Nat Neurosci,* 2, 867-72.

Humphrey, G. W., Y. H. Wang, T. Hirai, R. Padmanabhan, D. M. Panchision, L. F. Newell, R. D. McKay & B. H. Howard (2008) Complementary roles for histone deacetylases 1, 2, and 3 in differentiation of pluripotent stem cells. *Differentiation,* 76, 348-56.

Jaenisch, R. & A. Bird (2003) Epigenetic regulation of gene expression: how the genome integrates intrinsic and environmental signals. *Nat Genet,* 33 Suppl, 245-54.

Jenuwein, T. & C. D. Allis (2001) Translating the histone code. *Science,* 293, 1074-80.

Jessberger, S., K. Nakashima, G. D. Clemenson, Jr., E. Mejia, E. Mathews, K. Ure, S. Ogawa, C. M. Sinton, F. H. Gage & J. Hsieh (2007) Epigenetic modulation of seizure-induced neurogenesis and cognitive decline. *J Neurosci,* 27, 5967-75.

Jin, B., Q. Tao, J. Peng, H. M. Soo, W. Wu, J. Ying, C. R. Fields, A. L. Delmas, X. Liu, J. Qiu & K. D. Robertson (2008) DNA methyltransferase 3B (DNMT3B) mutations in ICF syndrome lead to altered epigenetic modifications and aberrant expression of genes regulating development, neurogenesis and immune function. *Hum Mol Genet,* 17, 690-709.

Jones, P. A. & S. B. Baylin (2002) The fundamental role of epigenetic events in cancer. *Nat Rev Genet,* 3, 415-28.

Juttermann, R., E. Li & R. Jaenisch (1994) Toxicity of 5-aza-2'-deoxycytidine to mammalian cells is mediated primarily by covalent trapping of DNA methyltransferase rather than DNA demethylation. *Proc Natl Acad Sci U S A,* 91, 11797-801.

Kobow, K., I. Jeske, M. Hildebrandt, J. Hauke, E. Hahnen, R. Buslei, M. Buchfelder, D. Weigel, H. Stefan, B. Kasper, E. Pauli & I. Blumcke (2009) Increased reelin promoter methylation is associated with granule cell dispersion in human temporal lobe epilepsy. *J Neuropathol Exp Neurol,* 68, 356-64.

Kouzarides, T. (2007) Chromatin modifications and their function. *Cell,* 128, 693-705.

Kruman, II, T. S. Kumaravel, A. Lohani, W. A. Pedersen, R. G. Cutler, Y. Kruman, N. Haughey, J. Lee, M. Evans & M. P. Mattson (2002) Folic acid deficiency and homocysteine impair DNA repair in hippocampal neurons and sensitize them to amyloid toxicity in experimental models of Alzheimer's disease. *J Neurosci,* 22, 1752-62.

Kuruba, R., B. Hattiangady & A. K. Shetty (2009) Hippocampal neurogenesis and neural stem cells in temporal lobe epilepsy. *Epilepsy Behav,* 14 Suppl 1, 65-73.

Ladd-Acosta, C., J. Pevsner, S. Sabunciyan, R. H. Yolken, M. J. Webster, T. Dinkins, P. A. Callinan, J. B. Fan, J. B. Potash & A. P. Feinberg (2007) DNA methylation signatures within the human brain. *Am J Hum Genet,* 81, 1304-15.

Lagger, G., D. O'Carroll, M. Rembold, H. Khier, J. Tischler, G. Weitzer, B. Schuettengruber, C. Hauser, R. Brunmeir, T. Jenuwein & C. Seiser (2002) Essential function of histone deacetylase 1 in proliferation control and CDK inhibitor repression. *EMBO J,* 21, 2672-81.

Lagrange, A. H., E. J. Botzolakis & R. L. Macdonald (2007) Enhanced macroscopic desensitization shapes the response of alpha4 subtype-containing GABAA receptors to synaptic and extrasynaptic GABA. *J Physiol,* 578, 655-76.

Laird, P. W. (2003) The power and the promise of DNA methylation markers. *Nat Rev Cancer,* 3, 253-66.

Lefevre, F. & N. Aronson (2000) Ketogenic diet for the treatment of refractory epilepsy in children: A systematic review of efficacy. *Pediatrics,* 105, E46.

Levenson, J. M., S. Qiu & E. J. Weeber (2008) The role of reelin in adult synaptic function and the genetic and epigenetic regulation of the reelin gene. *Biochim Biophys Acta,* 1779, 422-31.

Levenson, J. M., T. L. Roth, F. D. Lubin, C. A. Miller, I. C. Huang, P. Desai, L. M. Malone & J. D. Sweatt (2006) Evidence that DNA (cytosine-5) methyltransferase regulates synaptic plasticity in the hippocampus. *J Biol Chem,* 281, 15763-73.

Li, E., T. H. Bestor & R. Jaenisch (1992) Targeted mutation of the DNA methyltransferase gene results in embryonic lethality. *Cell,* 69, 915-26.

Lillycrop, K. A., J. L. Slater-Jefferies, M. A. Hanson, K. M. Godfrey, A. A. Jackson & G. C. Burdge (2007) Induction of altered epigenetic regulation of the hepatic glucocorticoid receptor in the offspring of rats fed a protein-restricted diet during pregnancy suggests that reduced DNA methyltransferase-1 expression is involved in impaired DNA methylation and changes in histone modifications. *Br J Nutr,* 97, 1064-73.

Lim, D. A., M. Suarez-Farinas, F. Naef, C. R. Hacker, B. Menn, H. Takebayashi, M. Magnasco, N. Patil & A. Alvarez-Buylla (2006) In vivo transcriptional profile analysis reveals RNA splicing and chromatin remodeling as prominent processes for adult neurogenesis. *Mol Cell Neurosci,* 31, 131-48.

Lin, S. Y., K. Wu, E. S. Levine, H. T. Mount, P. C. Suen & I. B. Black (1998) BDNF acutely increases tyrosine phosphorylation of the NMDA receptor subunit 2B in cortical and hippocampal postsynaptic densities. *Brain Res Mol Brain Res,* 55, 20-7.

Liu, H., J. Kaur, K. Dashtipour, R. Kinyamu, C. E. Ribak & L. K. Friedman (2003) Suppression of hippocampal neurogenesis is associated with developmental stage, number of perinatal seizure episodes, and glucocorticosteroid level. *Exp Neurol,* 184, 196-213.

Loscher, W. (1999) Valproate: a reappraisal of its pharmacodynamic properties and mechanisms of action. *Prog Neurobiol,* 58, 31-59.

Loscher, W. & C. Brandt (2010) Prevention or modification of epileptogenesis after brain insults: experimental approaches and translational research. *Pharmacol Rev,* 62, 668-700.

Luger, K., A. W. Mader, R. K. Richmond, D. F. Sargent & T. J. Richmond (1997) Crystal structure of the nucleosome core particle at 2.8 A resolution. *Nature,* 389, 251-60.

Lukasiuk, K., M. Dabrowski, A. Adach & A. Pitkanen (2006) Epileptogenesis-related genes revisited. *Prog Brain Res,* 158, 223-41.

MacDonald, J. L., C. S. Gin & A. J. Roskams (2005) Stage-specific induction of DNA methyltransferases in olfactory receptor neuron development. *Dev Biol,* 288, 461-73.

MacDonald, J. L. & A. J. Roskams (2008) Histone deacetylases 1 and 2 are expressed at distinct stages of neuro-glial development. *Dev Dyn,* 237, 2256-67.

--- (2009) Epigenetic regulation of nervous system development by DNA methylation and histone deacetylation. *Prog Neurobiol,* 88, 170-83.

Malenka, R. C. & M. F. Bear (2004) LTP and LTD: an embarrassment of riches. *Neuron,* 44, 5-21.

Mathern, G. W., J. P. Leite, J. K. Pretorius, B. Quinn, W. J. Peacock & T. L. Babb (1994) Children with severe epilepsy: evidence of hippocampal neuron losses and aberrant mossy fiber sprouting during postnatal granule cell migration and differentiation. *Brain Res Dev Brain Res,* 78, 70-80.

McCabe, B. K., D. C. Silveira, M. R. Cilio, B. H. Cha, X. Liu, Y. Sogawa & G. L. Holmes (2001) Reduced neurogenesis after neonatal seizures. *J Neurosci,* 21, 2094-103.

Miller, C. A., S. L. Campbell & J. D. Sweatt (2008) DNA methylation and histone acetylation work in concert to regulate memory formation and synaptic plasticity. *Neurobiol Learn Mem,* 89, 599-603.

Miller, C. A. & J. D. Sweatt (2007) Covalent modification of DNA regulates memory formation. *Neuron,* 53, 857-69.

Milutinovic, S., A. C. D'Alessio, N. Detich & M. Szyf (2007) Valproate induces widespread epigenetic reprogramming which involves demethylation of specific genes. *Carcinogenesis,* 28, 560-71.

Nelson, E. D., E. T. Kavalali & L. M. Monteggia (2008) Activity-dependent suppression of miniature neurotransmission through the regulation of DNA methylation. *J Neurosci,* 28, 395-406.

Okano, M., D. W. Bell, D. A. Haber & E. Li (1999) DNA methyltransferases Dnmt3a and Dnmt3b are essential for de novo methylation and mammalian development. *Cell,* 99, 247-57.

Ooi, L. & I. C. Wood (2007) Chromatin crosstalk in development and disease: lessons from REST. *Nat Rev Genet,* 8, 544-54.

Ottman, R., J. F. Annegers, N. Risch, W. A. Hauser & M. Susser (1996) Relations of genetic and environmental factors in the etiology of epilepsy. *Ann Neurol,* 39, 442-9.

Parent, J. M., T. W. Yu, R. T. Leibowitz, D. H. Geschwind, R. S. Sloviter & D. H. Lowenstein (1997) Dentate granule cell neurogenesis is increased by seizures and contributes to aberrant network reorganization in the adult rat hippocampus. *J Neurosci,* 17, 3727-38.

Paulsen, M. & A. C. Ferguson-Smith (2001) DNA methylation in genomic imprinting, development, and disease. *J Pathol,* 195, 97-110.

Porter, B. E. (2008) Neurogenesis and epilepsy in the developing brain. *Epilepsia,* 49 Suppl 5, 50-4.

Qureshi, I. A. & M. F. Mehler (2009) Regulation of non-coding RNA networks in the nervous system--what's the REST of the story? *Neurosci Lett,* 466, 73-80.

--- (2010) Epigenetic mechanisms underlying human epileptic disorders and the process of epileptogenesis. *Neurobiol Dis,* 39, 53-60.

Robertson, K. D. (2005) DNA methylation and human disease. *Nat Rev Genet,* 6, 597-610.

Sanchez, R. M., S. Koh, C. Rio, C. Wang, E. D. Lamperti, D. Sharma, G. Corfas & F. E. Jensen (2001) Decreased glutamate receptor 2 expression and enhanced epileptogenesis in immature rat hippocampus after perinatal hypoxia-induced seizures. *J Neurosci,* 21, 8154-63.

Scaravilli, F. 1998. *Neuropathology of epilepsy.* World Scientific.

Scharfman, H. E., J. H. Goodman & A. L. Sollas (1999) Actions of brain-derived neurotrophic factor in slices from rats with spontaneous seizures and mossy fiber sprouting in the dentate gyrus. *J Neurosci,* 19, 5619-31.

--- (2000) Granule-like neurons at the hilar/CA3 border after status epilepticus and their synchrony with area CA3 pyramidal cells: functional implications of seizure-induced neurogenesis. *J Neurosci,* 20, 6144-58.

Schuurmans, C. & F. Guillemot (2002) Molecular mechanisms underlying cell fate specification in the developing telencephalon. *Curr Opin Neurobiol,* 12, 26-34.

Seshadri, S., A. Beiser, J. Selhub, P. F. Jacques, I. H. Rosenberg, R. B. D'Agostino, P. W. Wilson & P. A. Wolf (2002) Plasma homocysteine as a risk factor for dementia and Alzheimer's disease. *N Engl J Med,* 346, 476-83.

Shea, T. B., J. Lyons-Weiler & E. Rogers (2002) Homocysteine, folate deprivation and Alzheimer neuropathology. *J Alzheimers Dis,* 4, 261-7.

Shen, S. & P. Casaccia-Bonnefil (2008) Post-translational modifications of nucleosomal histones in oligodendrocyte lineage cells in development and disease. *J Mol Neurosci,* 35, 13-22.

Shen, S., J. Li & P. Casaccia-Bonnefil (2005) Histone modifications affect timing of oligodendrocyte progenitor differentiation in the developing rat brain. *J Cell Biol,* 169, 577-89.

Shinnar, S. & A. T. Berg (1996) Does antiepileptic drug therapy prevent the development of "chronic" epilepsy? *Epilepsia,* 37, 701-8.

Siegmund, K. D., C. M. Connor, M. Campan, T. I. Long, D. J. Weisenberger, D. Biniszkiewicz, R. Jaenisch, P. W. Laird & S. Akbarian (2007) DNA methylation in the human cerebral cortex is dynamically regulated throughout the life span and involves differentiated neurons. *PLoS One,* 2, e895.

Sleiman, S. F., M. Basso, L. Mahishi, A. P. Kozikowski, M. E. Donohoe, B. Langley & R. R. Ratan (2009) Putting the 'HAT' back on survival signalling: the promises and challenges of HDAC inhibition in the treatment of neurological conditions. *Expert Opin Investig Drugs,* 18, 573-84.

Sng, J. C., H. Taniura & Y. Yoneda (2005) Inhibition of histone deacetylation by trichostatin A intensifies the transcriptions of neuronal c-fos and c-jun genes after kainate stimulation. *Neurosci Lett,* 386, 150-5.

Stafstrom, C. E. (2004) Dietary approaches to epilepsy treatment: old and new options on the menu. *Epilepsy Curr,* 4, 215-22.

Stanfield, B. B. & W. M. Cowan (1979) The morphology of the hippocampus and dentate gyrus in normal and reeler mice. *J Comp Neurol,* 185, 393-422.

Strahl, B. D. & C. D. Allis (2000) The language of covalent histone modifications. *Nature,* 403, 41-5.

Takei, N., K. Sasaoka, K. Inoue, M. Takahashi, Y. Endo & H. Hatanaka (1997) Brain-derived neurotrophic factor increases the stimulation-evoked release of glutamate and the levels of exocytosis-associated proteins in cultured cortical neurons from embryonic rats. *J Neurochem,* 68, 370-5.

Takizawa, T., K. Nakashima, M. Namihira, W. Ochiai, A. Uemura, M. Yanagisawa, N. Fujita, M. Nakao & T. Taga (2001) DNA methylation is a critical cell-intrinsic determinant of astrocyte differentiation in the fetal brain. *Dev Cell,* 1, 749-58.

Tanaka, T., H. Saito & N. Matsuki (1997) Inhibition of GABAA synaptic responses by brain-derived neurotrophic factor (BDNF) in rat hippocampus. *J Neurosci,* 17, 2959-66.

Teter, B., I. Rozovsky, K. Krohn, C. Anderson, H. Osterburg & C. Finch (1996) Methylation of the glial fibrillary acidic protein gene shows novel biphasic changes during brain development. *Glia,* 17, 195-205.

Tietjen, I., J. M. Rihel, Y. Cao, G. Koentges, L. Zakhary & C. Dulac (2003) Single-cell transcriptional analysis of neuronal progenitors. *Neuron,* 38, 161-75.

Tsankova, N. M., A. Kumar & E. J. Nestler (2004) Histone modifications at gene promoter regions in rat hippocampus after acute and chronic electroconvulsive seizures. *J Neurosci,* 24, 5603-10.

Urdinguio, R. G., L. Lopez-Serra, P. Lopez-Nieva, M. Alaminos, R. Diaz-Uriarte, A. F. Fernandez & M. Esteller (2008) Mecp2-null mice provide new neuronal targets for Rett syndrome. *PLoS One,* 3, e3669.

Vakoc, C. R., S. A. Mandat, B. A. Olenchock & G. A. Blobel (2005) Histone H3 lysine 9 methylation and HP1gamma are associated with transcription elongation through mammalian chromatin. *Mol Cell,* 19, 381-91.

Villar-Garea, A. & M. Esteller (2004) Histone deacetylase inhibitors: understanding a new wave of anticancer agents. *Int J Cancer,* 112, 171-8.

Wade, P. A. (2001) Transcriptional control at regulatory checkpoints by histone deacetylases: molecular connections between cancer and chromatin. *Hum Mol Genet,* 10, 693-8.

Weaver, I. C., N. Cervoni, F. A. Champagne, A. C. D'Alessio, S. Sharma, J. R. Seckl, S. Dymov, M. Szyf & M. J. Meaney (2004) Epigenetic programming by maternal behavior. *Nat Neurosci,* 7, 847-54.

Weaver, I. C., A. C. D'Alessio, S. E. Brown, I. C. Hellstrom, S. Dymov, S. Sharma, M. Szyf & M. J. Meaney (2007) The transcription factor nerve growth factor-inducible protein a mediates epigenetic programming: altering epigenetic marks by immediate-early genes. *J Neurosci*, 27, 1756-68.

Weinstock, M. (2001) Alterations induced by gestational stress in brain morphology and behaviour of the offspring. *Prog Neurobiol*, 65, 427-51.

Yang, X. J. & E. Seto (2008) The Rpd3/Hda1 family of lysine deacetylases: from bacteria and yeast to mice and men. *Nat Rev Mol Cell Biol*, 9, 206-18.

Zempleni, J., Y. C. Chew, Y. I. Hassan & S. S. Wijeratne (2008) Epigenetic regulation of chromatin structure and gene function by biotin: are biotin requirements being met? *Nutr Rev*, 66 Suppl 1, S46-8.

Zhao, X., T. Ueba, B. R. Christie, B. Barkho, M. J. McConnell, K. Nakashima, E. S. Lein, B. D. Eadie, A. R. Willhoite, A. R. Muotri, R. G. Summers, J. Chun, K. F. Lee & F. H. Gage (2003) Mice lacking methyl-CpG binding protein 1 have deficits in adult neurogenesis and hippocampal function. *Proc Natl Acad Sci U S A*, 100, 6777-82.

13

Multimodal MRI Evaluation in Intractable Epilepsy with Pathologically Confirmed Mesial Temporal Sclerosis

Jai Jai Shiva Shankar
QE II Hospital, Dalhousie University
Halifax
Canada

1. Introduction

Medial temporal lobe epilepsy (MTLE) is a common syndrome. Many of the cases of medial temporal lobe epilepsy often remain resistant to drug therapy. Surgical resection of the affected temporal lobe is often final option to control/reduce the seizure frequency. Mesial temporal sclerosis which can be unilateral or bilateral is the most common cause of medial temporal lobe epilepsy. Accurate preoperative lateralization of the mesial temporal lobe sclerosis is essential, because the surgical strategy and outcome is distinctive in this group of patients. Currently many non-invasive methods like MRI, EEG and neuropsychological assessment are used to achieve this goal.

Number of studies have shown role of various MRI techniques in lateralizing the seizure focus in cases of mesial temporal sclerosis (1-8). Newer quantitative MRI along with qualitative MR techniques has improved the overall sensitivity of MRI for the detection of MTS (9-12). We planned to examine the relative sensitivity of specific MRI sequences in patients with pathologically confirmed MTS.

2. Materials and methods

We reviewed results of MRI scans of 44 patients who were subjected to anterior temporal lobectomy and had pathological confirmation of MTS. The definition of intractable epilepsy is taken when patient is having at least two episodes of seizures per month even after being on at least two antiepileptic drugs for at least two years. We compared each combination of test results to resected tissue pathology to determine the association with MTS. Patients were excluded if imaging revealed other pathologies such as tumors or vascular lesions. Epileptogenic temporal lobe was identified by detailed physiological studies (EEG, VEEG) and neuropsychological studies in all patients.

MRI studies- MRI studies were performed using a standard protocol in a Siemens Magnetom Vision 1.5 T magnet in all patients.

Following images were obtained in the temporal lobe protocol- T1(TR-650 ms;TE-14 ms; slice thickness-3 mm), PD-T2(TR-2300ms;TE-17 & 102 ms; slice thickness-3mm) and FLAIR(TR-9000 ms;TE-105 ms;TI-1800ms;slice thickness-3 mm) images in a plane parallel and perpendicular to the long axis of hippocampus (fig 1) and 3D volume acquisition of the entire brain using T1 W MPRAGE sequence(TR-9.7 ms;TE-4 ms; flip angle- 12;FOV-250;slice thickness-1 mm).

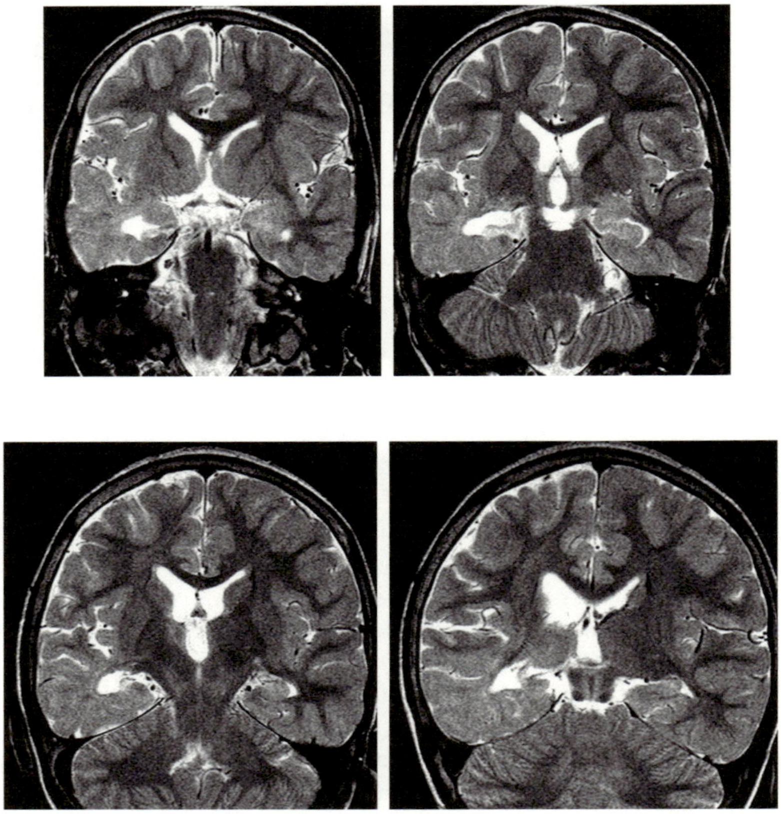

Fig. 1. T2 W images perpendicular to long axis of hippocampus showing Right mesial temporal sclerosis

Demographic variable	Measure
No of patients	44
Male	30
Female	14
Mean age of the patients	28 yrs(11- 45 yrs)
Mean age of seizure onset	12 yrs(3 mth-32 yrs)
Mean duration of seizure	17 yrs(3-37 yrs)
Lt temporal resection	22
Rt temporal resection	22

Table 1. Demography of patient population-

Quantitative analysis: This included T2 relaxometry and volumetry.
T2 relaxometry was calculated in a multiple coronal slices from dual echo sequences obtained at TEs of 17 and 102 ms with a slice thickness of 3 mm. Hippocampal T2 relaxometry maps were generated manually from the measured image intensities in the hippocampal structures. T2 values were obtained from a predetermined region of interests. Measurements were taken from each ROI inside the hippocampus excluding the temporal horn CSF (fig 2).

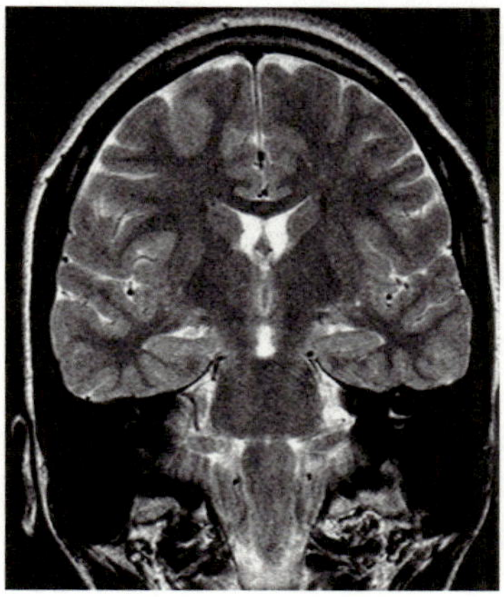

A

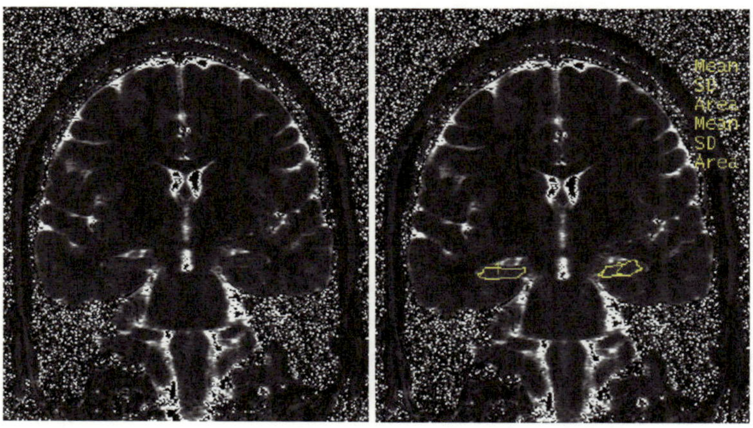

B C

Fig. 2. *A*- T2 W image perpendicular to the long axis of hippocampus. *B*- T2 relaxometry map of the same image. *C*- Outline of hippocampus in cross section on a T2 relaxometry map.

For volumetric analysis images were transferred to Siemens Magnetom vision workstation. Volumetric measurements were performed by outlining the region of interest (ROIs) manually on a magnified image (fig 3). Anatomical guidelines for outlining the hippocampal formation followed previous protocols (9, 13).

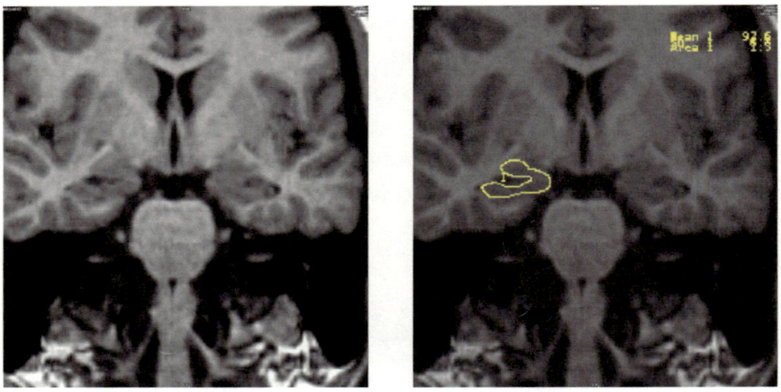

A B

Fig. 3. A-T1W MPRAGE 1mm thick image perpendicular to the long axis of hippocampus. B- Outline of hippocampus in cross section.

Qualitative MR analysis: included three parameters signal changes, loss of internal architecture and volume loss.

Visual analysis was performed on T1, T2 and FLAIR images to assess following

Surgical technique and histological tissue analysis- All surgical procedure was performed by neurosurgeon. The resection included a standard neocorticotomy of anterior temporal lobe, sparing the superior temporal gyrus. Amygdala and anterior half to two-third of hippocampus were resected and sent for pathological analysis.

The diagnosis of mesial temporal sclerosis was based on the presence of hippocampal neuronal loss and gliosis.

Statistical analysis-Sensitivity of each tests were calculated individually and in multiple combinations. The results of each technique are then compared with the outcome results of the surgery.

3. Results

Visual analysis

Atrophy: Unilateral hippocampal atrophy was detected in 36 of 44 patients (81%). Bilateral atrophy was noted in 2 patients and 6 were normal.

Signal changes: 39 of 44 patients (88.6%) had signal changes which correspond to the site of surgery. 2 patients had bilateral signal changes and lateralization was not possible by signal changes.

Quantitative analysis

Of the 44 patients only 20 patients could be analysed by the quantitative MR analysis because of the non-availability of the raw data.

T2 relaxometry: Higher abnormal T2 values were noted in 16 of 20 patients (85 %) on the side of surgery performed. Normal mean value was taken as 100.2 ± 4.18 msec (right-100.5 msec; left-98.9 msec). The cutoff was set 2 SD above the average and was 109 msec (14). Of these 16 patients 13 had unilateral abnormality and 3 had bilateral abnormality. In patients with bilateral abnormality T2 values were higher on the affected side than the contralateral side.

Volumetric analysis: 18 of 20 patients (90%) showed decreased volume corresponding to the resected side(normal mean value taken as 3571 ± 311 cmm for left and 3696 ± 310 cmm for right)(7). Of these 15 were unilateral and correctly lateralized. The remaining 3 had significant bilateral atrophy with the smaller size corresponding to the affected side in all the patients. Using the right/left volumetric ratio of hippocampal formation, 19 of 20 patients (95%) showed marked differences, with the ratio correctly lateralizing the affected side. The volumetric analysis was normal in one patient.

MRI sequences	Sensitivity
Qualitative	80 %
T2 relaxometry	85 %
Volumetry	90 %

Modality correlation

Visual analysis which took into account both the FLAIR signal changes and visual qualitative atrophy led to correct lateralization in 39 of 44 patients(88.6%). Remaining 5 patients did not have either volume loss or signal changes.

Of the 20 patients in which we had quantitative data only 16 (80%) could be correctly lateralized by the visual qualitative analysis. Of the remaining four patients 2 patients had higher T2 relaxation values with correct lateralization and 3 had smaller volume lateralizing to the affected side. With combined visual analysis and T2 relaxometry analysis 18 patients (90%) were lateralized correctly. When we combined the results of visual analysis and volumetric analysis 19 patients (95 %) were lateralized correctly. On combining all the three modalities all the 20 patients (100%) patients were lateralized correctly; one patient who had normal volume bilaterally was showing high T2 values on the surgery side.

MRI sequences	Sensitivity
Qualitative	80 %
Qualitative + T2	90 %
Qualitative + volumetry	95 %
Qualitative+ T2 + volumetry	100%

4. Discussion

We compared the sensitivity and relative utility of different MR sequences in patients with MTS. This study was specifically designed to assess the sensitivity of the MRI sequences in population of highly selected patients with histologically confirmed MTS. Similar to previous studies we found that qualitative and quantitative analysis are both highly reliable in experienced hands with individual sensitivity ranging from 85-95%.

This study shows that the use of multiple MR techniques in the investigation of patients with intractable mesial temporal lobe sclerosis offers advantages over individual modalities. The combined sensitivity of all the MR techniques together was 100% for correct lateralization of the epileptogenic temporal lobe.

Visual analysis of FLAIR sequences and T1 W sequences for atrophy demonstrated abnormalities in 88.6%. Other published studies show similar results (11). Jack et al reported identification of atrophy by visual analysis in 83 % and by signal changes on T2 W images in 79% of patients of MTS (15). A more recent study using FLAIR found abnormalities in 97% of the patients with MTS (16). This suggests that with current MRI techniques the sensitivity of visual identification across different centers is relatively reliable.

However the identification of bilateral hippocampal atrophy by visual analysis may be difficult. Only 2 of the 4 patients with bilateral hippocampal atrophy by absolute hippocampal volumes demonstrated visually detected bilateral atrophy. The FLAIR sequence detected bilateral signal changes in only 2 of these patients. Therefore visual analysis is accurate in detecting unilateral MTS but may not be adequate to identify bilateral hippocampal atrophy in some patients.

However visual analysis correctly lateralized the most abnormal hippocampus in most of those with volumetric based bilateral hippocampal atrophy. In 3 of the 4 patients with bilateral hippocampal atrophy, the more affected side was localized by visual analysis. Though our results were influenced by the selection of the patients (only operated patients) previous study by Jack et al demonstrated that even in those patients with bilateral symmetric hippocampal changes, lateralization and successful surgery is possible (17).

Some studies have reported that T2 relaxometry is a reliable method to detect MTS. Jackson et al originally reported that T2 relaxometry maps were abnormal in all patients with MTS (18). However other groups have reported relatively lesser sensitivity (19), in our study the sensitivity of T2 relaxometry to identify the affected side is only 85 % similar to other study.

Majority of the patients who had loss of volume also had longer T2 relaxation. This result indicates a strong relationship between the volumetry and T2 relaxometry. However literature shows discrepancy between the two techniques (7).

The different results of T2 relaxometry across studies may be considered to be due to different technical reasons. Previously published studies had used multi-echo sequences using 8-16 different TEs (7, 18) whereas we have used only dual echo sequences. Other point of difference is that earlier studies have used shorter TR (1500 ms) while we have used TR of 2300 ms (11).

Convergence of all MRI findings in MTS increases the likelihood of a correct diagnosis. Correct lateralization was possible in majority of the patients by qualitative visual analysis; quantitative techniques may provide useful information in the rest. Volumetric measurements using differential right -left volumes provided localization in 90 % of patients, compared to T2 relaxometry which was abnormal in only 85%. Visual analysis failed to recognize the signal changes in only one patient who had abnormal T2 relaxation.

The results of this study suggest that visual qualitative analysis is sensitive in the detection of MTS in most patients. Although quantitative techniques increase the sensitivity of lateralization these are technically demanding and time consuming with the exception of T2 relaxometry. So for routine clinical purpose simple strategy will be to use visual analysis and T2 relaxometry to lateralize the MTLE first. If this is not successful then volumetry can be used as an additional technique.

5. References

[1] Bronen RA, Cheung G, Charles JT, et al. Imaging findings in hippocampal sclerosis: correlation with pathology. AJNR 1991; 12: 933-940.

[2] Kujniecky R, De La Sayette V, Ethier R, et al. Magnetic resonance imaging in temporal lobe epilepsy: pathological correlations. Ann Neurology 1987; 22: 341-347.

[3] Jackson GD, Berkovic SF, Duncan JS, Connelly A. Optimizing the diagnosis of hippocampal sclerosis using magnetic resonance imaging. AJNR 1993; 14: 753-762.

[4] Jack CRJ, Sharbrough FW, Cascino GD, Hirschorn KA, et al. Magnetic resonance image based hippocampal volumetry: correlation with outcome after temporal lobectomy. Ann Neurol 1992; 31: 138-146.

[5] Cascino GD, Jack JCR, Parisi JE, et al. Magnetic resonance image based volume studies in temporal lobe epilepsy: pathological correlations. Ann Neurol 1991; 30:31-36.

[6] Spencer SS, McCarthy G, Spencer DD. Diagnosis of medial temporal lobe seizure onset: relative specificity and sensitivity of quantitative MRI. Neurology 1993; 43: 2117-2124.

[7] Kuzniecky RI, Bilir E,Gilliam F, et al. Multimodality MRI in mesial temporal sclerosis: relative sensitivity and specificity. Neurology 1997; 49: 774-778.

[8] Kilpatrick C, O'Brien T, Matkovic Z, Cook M, Kaye. A Preoperative evaluation for temporal lobe surgery. J Clin Neurosci. 2003 Sep; 10(5):535-9.

[9] Cendes F, Andermann F, Gloor P, et al. MRI volumetric measurement of amygdala and hippocampus in temporal lobe epilepsy. Neurology 1993; 43:718-725.

[10] Jack JC. MRI based hippocampal volume measurements in epilepsy. Epilepsia 1994; 35: S21-S29.

[11] Jackson G. New techniques in MR. Epilepsia 1994; 35: S2-S13.

[12] Tien RD, Felsberg GJ, Campi de Castro C, et al. Complex partial seizures and mesial temporal sclerosis: evaluation with fast spin-echo MR imaging. Radiology 1993; 189: 835-842.

[13] Bathia S, Brookheim S, Gaillard W, Theodore W. Measurement of whole temporal lobe and hippocampus for MR volumetry:normative data. Neurology 1993; 43: 1793-1799.

[14] Briellmann RS, Jackson GD, Kalnins R, Berkovic SF. Hemicranial volume deficits in patients with temporal lobe epilepsy with and without hippocampal sclerosis. Epilepsia. 1998 Nov; 39(11):1174-81.

[15] Jack C, Mullen B, Sharbrough F, et al. Intractable non-lesional epilepsy of temporal lobe origin: lateralization by interictal SPECT versus MRI. Neurology 1994; 44: 829-836.

[16] Jack C, Rydberg C, Krecke K, et al. Mesial temporal sclerosis diagnosis with FLAIR versus spin-echo MR imaging. Radiology 1996; 199: 367-373.

[17] Jack C, Trenerry M, Cascino G, Shanbrough F, So E et al. Bilaterally asymmetric hippocampi and surgical outcome. Neurology 1995; 45: 1353-1358.
[18] Jackson GD, Connelly A, Duncan JS, et al. Detection of hippocampal pathology in intractable partial epilepsy: increased sensitivity with quantitative magnetic resonance T2 relaxometry. Neurology 1993; 43: 1793-1799.
[19] Van Paesschen W, Sisdiya S, Connelly A, et al. Quantitative hippocampal MRI and intractable temporal lobe epilepsy. Neurology 1995; 45: 2233-2240.

Part 3

Therapeutic Regimes and Side Effects

14

The Gingival Fibromatoses

Sofia Douzgou[1] and Bruno Dallapiccola[2]
[1]*Department of Genetics, Institute of Child Health*
"Aghia Sophia" Children's Hospital, Athens
[2]*Division of Medical Genetics, "Bambino Gesù" Pediatric Hospital IRCCS, Rome*
[1]*Greece*
[2]*Italy*

1. Introduction

1.1 Definition

Gingival fibromatosis (GF) is a slowly progressive, benign, non-bleeding, painless, localized or generalized overgrowth of the maxillary and mandibular keratinized gingiva (Baptista, 2002). It is also recognized as congenital hypertrophy of the gums, gingivae elephantiasis, gingival gigantism, symmetrical fibroma of the palate, gingival hyperplasia, gingival overgrowth (GO), and congenital macrogengiva (Emerson, 1965). The condition occurs both in isolated and syndromic forms, and results from either genetic or acquired mechanisms. The most common causes accounting for the isolated forms include the effect of a systemic drug treatment and single gene mutations (hereditary GF or HGF). In addition GF can manifest within a systemic disease (Häkkinen and Csiszar, 2007).

1.2 Clinical presentation

Gingival overgrowth's dimensions are classified in three grades: grade I: growth confined to the interdental papilla, grade II: growth involving both papilla and marginal gingiva, grade III: growth which covers three quarters or more of the dental crown (Bökenkamp et al., 1994). In referral to the period of onset, the overgrowth can be classified as: pre-eruptive (<6 months of age), during the deciduous dentition (from 6 months to 6 years), during the mixed dentition period (6 to 12 years) and during the permanent dentition periods, before (12 to 20 years) and after adolescence (age 20 or later). The overgrowth results in dental defects, including diastemata, malocclusion, delayed eruption of permanent dentition or prolonged retention of primary dentition, causing aesthetic and functional problems. Treatment with functional gingivectomy is often followed by recurrence of the overgrowth. Given the rarity of HGF, available information about its clinical presentation is based on individual observations. The phenotypic spectrum is considerably wide and varies both for the number of teeth involved and the degree of clinical expression. The localized forms of HGF usually involve the maxillary tuberosities and labial gingiva around the mandibular molars. However, the symmetric, generalized form of HGF, involving the labial, lingual and palatal gingiva is the most common. Males and females are equally affected. Hyperplastic gums may be normal or erythematous and consist of dense, fibrous tissue that feels fixed and nodular on palpation. Although the alveolar bone is not usually involved, gingival hyperplasia causes periodontal problems because of difficult oral hygiene. The overgrowth can also result in functional and aesthetic problems, create diastemata, prevent or slow the growth of teeth and determine facial changes as a result of lip protrusion. The overgrowth can also lead to serious speech and chewing problems and may prevent the normal closure of the lips (Baptista, 2002).

The onset of GO usually coincides with the eruption of the permanent incisors, or, sometimes, with the eruption of primary dentition. In very rare cases, it can also be congenital (Anderson et al., 1969). Since HGF has never been observed in edentulous patients, it seems that the presence of dentition is necessary for the development of GO.

1.3 Histology

Histological characterization and differentiation has not been possible, to date, for all forms of HGF, especially for the syndromic ones. The various forms of HGF have similar histological features, suggesting that the pathogenic mutations affect different levels of the same cellular or molecular pathway. Hereditary gingival fibromatosis is characterized by moderate hyperplasia of the hyperkeratotic epithelium, comprised a network of elongated ridges. The epithelial hyperplasia may also be secondary to acanthosis, which has, however, only been found in areas of chronic inflammation. Fibrosis occurs with accumulation of collagen and elastic and oxytalan fibers in the connective tissue, comprised a few fibroblasts and blood vessels. Fibroblasts seem to alternate with thin or thick collagen fibrils. Unlike the characteristic "woven basket" arrangement of collagen fibers in the normal gingiva, the ones of fibrotic gingiva appear parallel. Rarely, osseous calcifications may be present as well as many neurovascular bundles (Kelekis-Cholakis et al., 2002, Doufexi et al., 2005).

The diagnosis of HGF is based on the collection of clinical history and on clinical examination, since no specific immunohistochemical markers have been identified, to date.

2. Isolated gingival fibromatosis

2.1 Drug-induced gingival fibromatosis

The most common cause of isolated GO involves anticonvulsant drug therapy, the use of calcium channel blockers for treating angina and hypertension or cyclosporine A for preventing the rejection of organs transplanted in subjects affected by autoimmune diseases.

Anticonvulsants	Calcium channel blockers	Antibiotics
Phenytoin	Nifedipine	Cyclosporin A
Carbamazepine	Amlodipine	
Etosuximide	Bepridil	
Sodium valproate	Felodipine	
Primidone	Nitrendipine	
Fenoprofen	Nicardine	
Felbamate	Verapamil	
Mephenytoin	Nimodipine	
Mesuximide		
Phenobarbital		
Phensuximide		

Table 1. Drugs that may induce gingival fibromatosis (Doufexi et al., 2005)

Among the first two drugs' categories, phenytoin and nifedipine are responsible for the most frequent forms of GF. The prevalence of GF secondary to drug treatment ranges in different studies, from 0 to 100% following long term phenytoin therapy, 0.5 to 83% after nifedipine and 8 to 81% following treatment with cyclosporin A (Kataoka et al ., 2005). The variability of these figures, which reflects heterogeneity of investigated cases, does not allow at present to suggest any empiric risk of developing an adverse reaction to these medications. In addition, to date, a correlation between the administered dose and the prevalence and severity of GF cannot be established. Nevertheless, it has been found that the combined regimen of nifedipine and cyclosporine in children undergoing organ transplants increases both the prevalence and severity of GF (Somacarrera et al., 1994). The development of GF after drug exposure has been related to an underlying individual genetic susceptibility. Possible candidate risk factors have been considered the polymorphic mutations in genes affecting the activity of cytochrome P450, which is responsible for the hepatic metabolism of drugs implicated in GF (Seymour et al., 2000).

2.2 Hereditary gingival fibromatosis

Hereditary gingival fibromatosis is a rare disorder (about one in 750,000 individuals), transmitted either as an autosomal dominant or, rarely, an autosomal recessive trait (Jorgenson and Cocker, 1974, Takagi et al., 1991). Different inheritance patterns, ages at onset and severity of the clinical manifestations in these patients, along with the presence of both isolated and syndromic forms reflect the underlying genetic heterogeneity. To date, four loci for isolated HGF have been identified, on chromosomes 2p21 (GINGF1, MIM # 135300), 5q13-q22 (GINGF2, MIM 605544), 2p23.3-p22.3 (GINGF3, MIM 609955) and 11p15 (GINGF4, MIM 611010). An additional locus has been assigned to chromosome 2p16-p13. Sequencing of the 16 known genes, which mapped...GINGF1, in the critical region of GINGF1 disclosed a heterozygous frameshift mutation in Son-of-Sevenless-1 (SOS-1) gene, which co-segregated with the disease in a Brazilian family (Hart et al., 2002).
Emerson described in 1965, the segregation of isolated GF in a family, for 4 generations. The disease was transmitted to the children from an affected parent, with the exception of a woman who, though not affected, transmitted the disease to subsequent generations through affected children, down to her great-grandchildren. The only affected male did not have children (Emerson, 1965). The transmission of the disease through an unaffected woman may be related to a lack of penetrance of the mutation or to mutations of an imprinted gene that is expressed only if maternally transmitted.
Linkage analysis of the entire genome in a Brazilian family with isolated, autosomal dominant GF, led to the identification of a locus on chromosome 2p21-p22, named GINGF1. Among the 32 family members identified, 12 had GF of varying severity; the youngest patient was 4 years old (Hart et al., 1998). Shashi et al have extended linkage analysis to more members of the family previously described and characterized the duplication 2p13-p21, already observed in a child by Fryns et al. (1989). This study restricted the disease-locus to a region of 8 Mb on chromosome 2p21, while the chromosomal region found duplicated in the child, was proximal to the first, on 2p13-p16 (Fryns et al., 1989, Shashi et al., 1999). Genotyping of four Chinese families with the same method, localized the disease-locus in a region of 8.7 cM on chromosome 2p21, which overlaps with that found in the Brazilian family, by 3.8 cM (Xiao et al., 2000). The sequencing of the 16 known genes present in the candidate region, has led to the identification of a heterozygous frameshift mutation, the insertion of a cytosine (g.126.142-126.143insC) in the Son-Of-Sevenless gene, 1 (SOS-1). The

mutation causes premature termination of the protein and the formation of a chimeric product, that consists of 1,105 amino acids, 1,083 amino of which are preserved, towards the NH2-terminal, followed by 22 new ones. The premature termination eliminates four functional domains near the COOH- terminal, rich in proline, that are necessary for binding with wild type Grb2 (Hart et al., 2002).

Wild type SOS protein consists of three functional segments: the catalytic segment, consisting of the Cdc25 domain and the domain of exchange with Ras (REM), a regulatory NH2-terminal segment that contains the histone domain, the DH domain and the PH domain (homologous to plecstrin) that interacts with PIP2 phosphatidic acid, and the COOH-terminal segment that contains binding sites for various proteins including Grb2.

SOS1 protein acts as a guanine exchange factor (GEF), which links receptor tyrosine kinases to the Ras pathway and controls, therefore, cell proliferation, differentiation, vescicle trafficking and regulation of the cytoskeleton's actin. Under the supervision of two classes of regulatory proteins, the GEF and those activating the GTPase, the Ras protein functions as a molecular switch in the cycle of GDP/GTP. Three Ras-GEFs have been characterized, SOS, the guanine nucleotide-releasing factor and the guanylate nucleotide-releasing protein. All three control the activity of Ras by catalyzing the release of GDP and the association with GTP. Two regulatory regions determine the GEF activity of SOS1: a catalytic site that interacts with the nucleotide-free form of Ras and an allosteric site that enhances the exchange activity when linked to the nucleotide-bound form of Ras. Growth factors induce a rapid dimerization and self-phosphorylation of their receptors. Phosphotyrosine residues in the catalytic region of the receptors act as binding sites for the SH2 domains of various proteins that function as intracellular messengers. By stimulating the growth factor, SOS is recruited from the cytoplasm to the cell membrane as a result of its interaction with Grb2, which is linked to the tyrosine residues of the phosphorylated receptor through its SH2 domain. In this way the interaction between Grb2 and SOS causes the translocation of the complex to the cell membrane, where GDP is exchanged with GTP and Ras is activated. Although the complex Grb2-SOS1 functions exclusively as a Ras activator, SOS1 may also function as a GEF that is specific to the Rac1 GTPase.

Further studies of the mechanism of Ras activation evidenced the following: after growth factor stimulation, SOS translocates to the cell membrane through at least two independent sites, the Grb2 binding site located near the COOH-terminal and the lipid-binding domain, PH. In addition to facilitate the anchor to the membrane, the interaction with the Grb2 protein overcomes the negative self-regulation of SOS mediated by its COOH terminal. The contact of the PH domain with the membrane phospholipids induces conformational changes that allow the binding of Ras.GDP to the allosteric site of SOS, lowering SOS activity. The Ras.GTP generated during the low activity period of SOS binds to the same allosteric site, carrying this way SOS to its maximum activity. This model explains the mechanism of translocation to the cell membrane in association with the regulation of the catalytic activity of SOS. Moreover, the interaction of SOS with Ras.GDP or Ras.GTP further its position on the membrane (Gureasko et al., 2008). It has also been demontsrated that after stimulation with growth factor, Ras is activated both at the Golgi apparatus level and at the cell membrane. Activation of Ras at the cell membrane is transitory, while its action at the Golgi is delayed and prolonged (Buday et al., 2008).

Jang et al showed that the total level of SOS1 transcript is lower in gingival fibroblasts of patients with HGF in respect to those of normal subjects, suggesting that the mutated SOS1 transcript is significantly lower than the wild type transcript. However, the silencing of the transcript using RNA interference caused a significant reduction of cell proliferation than the one caused by the silencing of the wild type transcript. This suggests that the increased proliferation of HGF fibroblasts is mainly due to the function of mutated SOS1. The authors also noted that the mutation in the SOS1 protein did not alter its distribution on the cell membrane or at the level of organelles and that the mutated SOS1 protein was capable of maintaining the activation of the Ras/MAPK pathway, in the absence of stimulation by growth factors. Therefore, this study evidenced that the HGF mutation determined the gain of function of SOS1, which, in this way, was implicated in the proliferation of fibroblasts regardless of binding with Grb2. The authors also proposed the application of RNA interference as a method of allele-specific depletion of the HGF mutated SOS1 as a control measure of gym hyperplasia (Jang et al., 2007).

The locus 2p23.3-p22.3 (GINGF3) was identified in a Chinese family of 5 generations with autosomal dominant isolated GF, with onset between 2 and 6 years, around the period of tooth eruption. The 12 patients examined had GO that varied from mild to severe. Over 70 genes mapped in the region identified. The direct sequencing of the *GPR113* and *SEL1* genes, selected as candidates based on their functions in signal transduction and tumor suppression respectively, evidenced no mutations (Ye et al., 2005).

In 2001, the analysis of a Chinese family with autosomal dominant isolated GF segregating through 4 generations, led to the identification of the 5q13-q22 locus (GINGF2). Ten of the 20 family members examined showed GF of very early onset, on average between 1 and 6 months of age. Forty-five genes were mapped located in the region identified, some with known functions in the control of cell growth or cell cycle (*LY64, RAD17, THBS4, CETN3, GPR11, NAIP, OCLN, RASA1, EFNA5, FER*). Among these the gene encoding the protein kinase IV, calcium/calmodulin-dependent was proposed as a candidate, given the presence of the phenocopy induced by calcium channel blockers (*CAMK4*, MIM 114080) (Xiao et al., 2001).

Zhu et al observed two large Chinese families with isolated HGF. The disease occured only in the offspring of affected or carrier females, suggesting a defect of imprinting. The disease segregated, respectively, for 5 and 4 generations and manifested within the first year of life. Linkage analysis of the entire genome was positive for the 11p15 locus. The 11p15 chromosomal region contains at least 14 genes that are subject to imprinting, divided into two groups, and is a region rich in tumor suppressor genes. The authors researched possible mutations or epimutations in the 14 known genes, localized within the region, with negative results. This study did not exclude, however, the presence of small interstitial deletions in the regulatory regions of the analyzed genes, not detectable with the techniques used or in other genes with maternal expression, localized in the region but unknown so far (Zhu et al., 2007).

2.3 Leukemic gingival fibromatosis

Gingival overgrowth is frequently associated with FAB M4 and M5 subtypes of acute myelogenous leukemia and, rarely, myelodysplastic syndrome (chronic myelomonocytic leukemia). The gingival biopsy shows diffuse tumor infiltration, subepithelial. The neoplastic cells appear large with pleomorphic nuclei, large nucleoli and eosinophilic cytoplasm. Although a risk factor for the development of lesions in cases of extramedullary acute myelogenous leukemia, is the presence of cytogenetic abnormalities (t(8; 21), inv16), there is, to date, no correlation between specific cytogenetic abnormalities and gingival involvement (Vural et al., 2004).

2.4 Differential diagnosis

The drug-induced forms are clinical and histological phenocopies of the hereditary forms, which can be distinguished only based on positive family history. In addition, acquired forms can be recognized based on the presence of dental plaques and regression following elimination of the pathogenic noxa (Doufexi et al., 2005). Generalized GO may also result from local inflammation, pregnancy or leukemia. Although the leukemic forms resemble HGF, they can be differentiated based on negative family history and histological evidence of neoplastic infiltration.

3. Syndromic gingival fibromatosis

We classified GF syndromes in two large groups of known and unknown aetiology. In the first group, GF has been described as an occasional or constant sign of some syndromes of known aetiology, characterized by the fact that the causative molecular lesions affect the same cellular pathway.

The second group consists of the rare reports of GF associated with a variable constellation of signs and symptoms that, taken together, represent the group of syndromic GF of unknown aetiology. The significant phenotypic overlap of these conditions is underlined by the presence of intermediate phenotypes that, to date, cannot be classified with certainty in distinct clinical entities. This clinical heterogeneity is reflected into a genetic heterogeneity, evidenced by the presence of observations of autosomal dominant or recessive transmission. The different conditions or observations are described below, based on a range of variable expression, which extends between the association of GF with hypertrichosis up to the multi-systemic syndromes of Zimmermann-Laband and Ramon.

3.1 Definition of hypertrichosis

Hypertrichosis is defined as the excessive growth of hair, which is distributed normally according to a variable spectrum, compared to the one of individuals of the same age, sex and ethnicity. Hypertrichosis may present with localized or generalized distribution and consist of immature or terminal hair. In the case of generalized hypertrichosis (GH), facial hair is accentuated on the frontal, temporal and preauricular regions. The eyebrows may be thick or confluent. On the back, hair converges along the midline, where it often forms whirls over the spine. The distribution can also be localized, associated with nevi or a *spina bifida occulta*, a previous trauma or irritation from chemicals and some inherited conditions autosomal dominant or recessive. Hypertrichosis should be distinguished from hirsutism that is excessive hair growth with distribution of male type (upper lip, chin, chest, *linea alba*, thighs and armpits), and that can be idiopathic or associated with overproduction of androgens. In contrast to hypertrichosis, the presence of hirsutism in childhood should orient towards the exclusion of endocrine causes of virilization. Generalized hypertrichosis may be one of the signs of a syndrome or of a metabolic disease (Baumeister, 1995).

3.2 Syndromic gingival fibromatosis of known aetiology

The syndromic forms of GF of known aetiology, include some phacomatoses, such as neurofibromatosis type 1, tuberous sclerosis and certain metabolic diseases such as alpha-mannosidosis (MIM #248500), Salla disease (MIM #604369), and I cell disease (MIM #252500). In the case of the phacomatoses, the overgrowth is characterized by fibrotic changes typical of gum neurofibromas/angiofibromas. In the case of metabolic diseases, histology shows the accumulation of gum-specific molecules, identical to those identified in other tissues (Ishigami et al., 1995, Gorlin et al., 2001). Almost all patients with Robinow syndrome (MIM # 268310) have gingival hyperplasia with dental crowding (Wilkie, 2008). The gingival hyperplasia is observed in 65% of patients with Costello syndrome (Hennekam, 2003) and in patients with leprechaunism or Donohue syndrome (MIM #246200) (Gorlin et al., 2001). Gingival hyperplasia is a constant feature of the multiple osteolysis syndrome of Murray-Puretic-Drescher, while it occurs occasionally in Winchester syndrome (MIM #277950) (Gorlin et al., 2001, Mosig et al., 2008). A single epileptic patient with Bardet-Biedl syndrome manifested GF, probably secondary to carbamazepine therapy (Drugowick et al., 2007). With the exception of the phacomatoses and Costello syndrome, that are due to autosomal dominant mutations, all other known disorders with GF are inherited as autosomal recessive traits. Sun et al. (2009) demonstrated that generalized hypertrichosis terminalis with or without gingival hyperplasia is a contiguous gene disorder caused by deletion of chromosome 17q24.2-q24.3. One of the affected individuals displayed a phenotype resembling Julia Pastrana (1834-1860), the first known case of GF, hypertrichosis, macrocephaly and coarse facies (Bondeson e Miles, 1993).

3.2.1 Ras-MAPK pathway and gingival overgrowth

Gingival overgrowth may be an occasional or recurrent feature in some genetic disorders caused by alterations in the proteins of the RAS-MAPK pathway. This pathway is regulated by the action of the SOS-1 protein, which is mutated in a subset of patients with isolated GF. Hart et al., (2007) demonstrated that the overall level of SOS-1 transcript is lower in HGF1 fibroblasts. The relative level of wild-type SOS-1 transcript appeared to be higher than the mutant transcript in HGF1 fibroblasts. The targeting of mutant transcripts by methods of RNA interference produced more profound effects on reduction of cell proliferation than the targeting of the wild-type, suggesting that the increased proliferation of HGF1 fibroblasts was chiefly dependent upon the function of mutant SOS-1.

Ras proteins are enzymes associated to the cell membrane that fluctuate from the active state of binding the active guanosine triphosphate (GTP) to the inactive state of binding with guanosine bisphosphate (GDP). The Ras GTPases are key mediators in pathways that transmit extracellular stimuli, through receptors on the cell surface, to the cell nucleus. They act as molecular switches in the processes of proliferation, differentiation, survival and cell death and are activated by different types of cellular receptors or calcium channels, upstream of the pathway. The exchange reaction between GDP and GTP is triggered by guanine nucleotide exchange factors, including the SOS-1 protein. The activated form of association with the GTP interacts with a broad spectrum of effector proteins including Raf, MEK1/2 and ERK1/2, and triggers downstream pathways (Aoki et al., 2008).

The SOS-1 protein is expressed in various tissues and cells, including human gingiva, where it can be localized inside the epithelial and stromal cells. The SOS-1-Ras-ERK1/2 pathway seems to be the central switch of expression of key molecules of the fibrosis process and of HGF. In fact, the activation of this pathway increases the expression of type IV collagen, the connective tissue growth factor CTGF, growth factor TGF-b, of the collagenase inhibitors TIMP and decreases the expression of metalloprotease MMP that degrades extracellular matrix components. The loss of function of metalloprotease type 2, that causes Winchester syndrome, results, therefore, in an altered homeostasis of connective tissue with accumulation of its physiological substrates, including collagen, fibronectin and laminin. Thus, the increased activation of the Ras/MAPK pathway by mutations of the *SOS-1* gene that determine a permanently active form of the coded protein, result in the increase of the expression of all pro-fibrotic molecules mentioned above.

Drugs that induce GF disturb the metabolic pathways involved in the translation of signals on behalf of the intracellular calcium ions (Ca^{2+}). This suggests that this pathway is involved in the development of fibrosis. Several ion channels located on the cell membrane regulate the flow of Ca^{2+} ions, which, in turn, affects the signal transduction pathways, including the Ras/MAPK pathway, directly or indirectly, through proteins that bind Ca^{2+}. Among these, the best characterized to date are the calmodulins (CaM) that reduce the expression of TGF-β and the activation of ERK1/2.

Ras proteins also participate in the communication between the insulin-receptor complex on the cell surface and the activation of cytosolic proteins downstream. In particular, the insulin receptor interacts with the proteins Gab-1, p60dok, Cbl, APS and isoforms of Shc10. The phosphorylated tyrosine residues of the activated insulin receptor act as docking sites for proteins containing SH2 domains (Src-homology-2). Many of these molecules are "adaptors", including proteins PI(3)K and Grb2, which, in turn, bind to the guanine nucleotide exchange factors, including the SOS protein-1 and activate the Ras/MAPK pathway (Saltiel and Kahn, 2001). However, it is not known whether insulin receptors are expressed in gingival tissue.

In conclusion, the SOS-1-Ras-ERK1/2 pathway regulates genes whose expression is altered in HGF and are involved in the process of fibrosis. It might be suggested that a defect at any level of this signaling cascade, which increases the expression of pro-fibrotic genes, promotes the development of GF.

It is interesting to observe a gingival phenotype both in NF1, which is caused by loss of function of neurofibromin, a negative regulator of Ras activation, and in Costello syndrome, caused by gain of function mutations of the *H-Ras* gene. Although the biochemical functions of tuberin and hamartin are not known to date, coded respectively by the *TSC1* and *TSC2* genes, we know that tuberin contains a region of homology with proteins that activate small GTPases such as Ras protein. The loss of function of tuberin could lead to a continuous stimulation of the pathways triggered by Ras. The CMG2 protein, mutated in the Murray-Puretic-Drescher syndrome, which is consistently associated with gingival hyperplasia, is an integrin-like molecule of the cell membrane that regulates cell adhesion to laminin and to collagen type IV. The metabolic pathways regulated by CMG2 are not known in detail, to date, but it is known that the cell adhesion pathway transmits signals to SOS-1-Ras-ERK1/2 and therefore there is a possible link between CMG2 and this signaling cascade. The differential involvement of multiple tissues or of the gingiva exclusively seems to depend on the functional importance of each of the mutated genes in the different cells and tissues (Häkkinen and Csiszar, 2007).

Several heterozygous, gain of function mutations of the *SOS-1* gene have been associated with a distinct form of Noonan syndrome with high prevalence of ptosis and pulmonary valve stenosis, ectodermal symptoms and, generally, the absence of mental and developmental retardation. None of the affected with confirmed *SOS-1* mutations described to date, presented with GF or was predisposed to the development of tumors. Furthermore, the mutations described are not associated with any type of tumor (Tartaglia et al., 2007, Roberts et al., 2007, Zenker et al., 2007). There were no further observations of HGF due to *SOS-1* mutations. The C.3248-3249insC mutation in exon 21 of the gene, linked to HGF, has not been observed to date in people with Noonan syndrome. All SOS-1 mutations result in a gain of function but the one related to HGF is the only frameshift one, resulting in a

chimeric, truncated protein. All other *SOS-1* mutations described to date do not result in truncated proteins. The HGF mutation affects the *SOS-1* domain of binding to Grb2 correlated to its self-negative regulation, but functional studies have shown that this mutation does not alter the intracellular localization of *SOS-1* or its function of activating the Ras/MAPK pathway via ERK1/2 (Jang et al., 2007).
Mutations in key components of the MAPK pathway that cause prolonged activation of ERK are related to the formation of tumors (Aoki et al., 2005). The formation of skin tumors has been highlighted in transgenic mice for *SOS-1*, artificially constructed, with deletion of the COOH terminal (Sibilia et al., 2000). It is believed that the activity of the strong promoters used in these experiments produces high levels of expression of the mutant protein that causes significant increase of ERK activity and leads to transformation. This means, there is probably a threshold of protein expression beyond which transformation happens. It is assumed that the benign form of the overgrowth in HGF can be interpreted as follows: the low levels of mutant *SOS-1* that is partially free from self-inhibition could lead to a continuous activation of ERK that could be sufficient to cause increased proliferation but not cell transformation (Jang et al., 2007). In the presence of a cellular environment with EGFR receptor of reduced activity, transgenic mice do not form skin cancers, despite the gain of function, and thus the continued activation of the MAPK on behalf of the artificial SOS-1 protein (Sibilia et al., 2000).
In conclusion, it is not yet known why the various *SOS-1* mutations produce distinct phenotypes or why the overgrowth in HGF is confined in the gingival tissue. A specific mutation-disease correlation could be hypothesized, secondary to the specific functions of the SOS-1 protein in gingival tissue or a tolerance/compensation of the gain of function caused by the frameshift mutation, in the other tissues (Jang et al., 2007).

3.3 Syndromic gingival fibromatosis of unknown aetiology

A number of subjects with GF associated with variable signs and symptoms can be regarded as examples of GF syndromes of unknown etiology, which, in descending order of number of observations, include GF, hypertrichosis, epilepsy and/or mental retardation (MR) syndrome; Zimmermann-Laband syndrome (MIM %135500); Jones syndrome (Jones et al., 1997); Ramon syndrome (MIM 2662700); Rutherfurd syndrome (MIM %180900), GF syndrome and characteristic facies (MIM 228560). GO is an occasional feature of Sturge-Weber syndrome (MIM 185300). This anomaly is secondary to angiomatous proliferation, worsened by GF caused by treatment of the epileptic symptoms (Bhansali et al., 2008). In general, these cases are rare and mostly sporadic, with the exception of Ramon syndrome, an autosomal recessive disorder, and single reports of affected sibs pairs, born to unaffected parents, presenting with GF, hypertrichosis, epilepsy and/or MR or manifesting the Zimmermann-Laband syndrome or intermediate phenotypes (Gorlin et al., 2001).
Taking into account the GF syndromic forms of unknown aetiology mentioned above, the existence in the literature of not clearly distinct phenotypes becomes evident, given the rarity of the observations and the significant overlap of signs/symptoms. There are "wide" clinical spectrums such as Ramon and ZL syndromes, which include a set of signs/symptoms that have also been observed individually associated with GF. The constant segregation of the association of GF with acro-osteolysis or cherubism, all three very rare signs, suggests that the ZL and Ramon syndromes are distinct clinical genetic entities. The two syndromes share, with different frequencies, the observations of GF, hypertrichosis, epilepsy and MR, an association described as an isolated clinical entity,

and retinal alterations of the pigmentosum type (Koch et al., 1992, Parkin and Law, 2001). It has been suggested that the association of isolated GF with hypertrichosis is the minimum clinical expression of the phenotypic spectrum of the ZLS (Lacombe et al., 1994) but that should probably be differentiated, given the absence of any further signs/symptoms (Robertson et al., 1998). An important hallmark is the finger hypoplasia, especially of the feet, and/or of the nails with or without an underlying hypoplasia of the terminal phalanges, especially in a patient without cognitive impairment and/or organomegaly, both non-mandatory symptoms of the ZLS. Based on the observation of the association of this last sign to GF and a hyperextensibility of the small joints Bakaeen and Scully (1991) reported the recurrence of the syndrome of ZL, in the children of a couple of cousins.

The unclear distinction between the phenotype of ZL and GF, hypertrichosis, epilepsy, MR, has been highlighted by several observations of intermediate phenotypes. Vontobel et al (1973) described a sporadic patient, who presented GF, congenital generalized hypertrichosis, mild hypoplasia of the fingernails and, especially, the feet, and acromegaloid features acromegaloidi that were not due to an underlying endocrinological disorder. The patient had psychomotor retardation (she walked alone at the age of 2 years, spoke the first phrases at 3-4 years), but her IQ was normal. Göhlich-Ratman et al (2000) observed the recurrence, in two sisters, daughters of first cousins, of coarse facies, profound MR with severe language impairment, early onset gingival hyperplasia, hypertrichosis and generalized tonic-clonic seizures with onset at 2 years of age. Both also had brachydactyly type E with bilateral shortness of metacarpals III-V and brachitelephalangy of the first finger, hypoplastic toenails, and bilateral sandal gap. The authors rule out ZLS for the lack of open bite and hepatomegaly, signs, however, that are not present in all patients with ZL reported in the literature. They speculate, however, that this is a broader phenotype than that observed by Anavi et al (1989) or a distinct syndrome of autosomal recessive GF.

However, the assumption that all these clinical features are part of the same phenotypic spectrum seems validated by the observation of segregation of distinct phenotypes from a father to his two sons. The father, at the age of 45, presented with GF, hypertrichosis, hearing loss and hypotelephalangism with brachydactyly and nail hypoplasia of the thumbs. His 13-year-old son had the same clinical picture, along with hypertrichosis, in the absence of MR. A second son, of 10 months, had inherited the paternal GF and defects of the fingers. The mother and the only daughter were not affected (Haytac and Ozcelik, 2007).

Gingival overgrowth variably associated with GH, MR or epilepsy has been described as a distinct, isolated disorder, with an autosomal dominant inheritance pattern (Anderson et al., 1969, Horning et al., 1985, Cuestas-Carnero and Bornancini, 1988), or as a manifestation of more complex disorders similar to ZLS (Gorlin et al., 2001). It was suggested that the association of GO, GH, MR or epilepsy could represent the mildest expression of ZLS. Distinguishing features in the former include absence of additional features, in particular nail hypoplasia with or without hypotelephalangism, mostly affecting the hands (Lacombe et al., 1994, Robertson et al., 1998). Clinical variability between patients with GO, GH, MR or epilepsy likely reflects genetic heterogeneity is also supported by different inheritance patterns (Nevin et al., 1971, Bakaeen and Scully, 1991, Haytac and Ozcelik, 2007). All these disorders can be lumped in a continuum of increasing severity, from the mildest phenotypes displaying GO, GH, MR and epilepsy to the most complex disorders reported by Göhlich-Ratman et al (2000) and Ramon et al (1967).

4. Generalized hypetrichosis, tonic-clonic seizures with onset in the first months of life, severe mental retardation and gingival overgrowth unrelated to the antiepileptic treatment

We had the opportunity to evaluate an 8-year old girl that was referred for genetic counselling because of MR and convulsions. She was the first daughter of healthy non-consanguineous Italian parents. A younger sister was clinically normal. At birth, the mother was 24-years-old and the father 29. Family history was unremarkable. Pregnancy was complicated by threatened miscarriage during the first trimester, for which the mother was advised with bed rest and treated with isoxuprine. No exposure to teratogenic agents was reported. Serologic tests for cytomegalovirus, toxoplasmosis and rubella, and triple serum marker screening were negative. A standard ultrasound scan at 22½ weeks of gestation was normal. The patient was born at 36 weeks of gestation with the use of forceps. Birth weight was 3,130 g (50th percentile), length 47 cm (10th percentile) and OFC 34 cm (25th percentile). She presented with delayed after birth cry and there was, transitory, self-resolving cyanosis, obvious generalised hypertrichosis and jaundice, which was treated with phototherapy. Apgar scores were not recorded. Cord blood gas values were normal, no resuscitation was required and paediatric monitoring did not reveal any end-organ dysfunction. The patient developed tremors from the first days of life, that, by age of 2 years turned into recalcitrant, generalized, tonic-clonic seizures. The episodes were initially unsuccessfully treated with phenobarbital that was substituted with sodium valproate. Treatment with sodium valproate easily controlled the seizures but this was changed to topiramate after 14 months because the patient was frequently observed lethargic. Developmental milestones were delayed: she sat at 9 months and walked at 2 years. At the time of the evaluation she was undergoing psychomotricity since the last 6 years.

On physical examination she had presented excessive growth of apparently terminal hair, distributed over the upper lip, cheeks, back, arms and forearms and legs. The hair on the back converged over the midline, forming whorls over the lower spine. The face and hands were otherwise unremarkable. Oral inspection disclosed a grade III GO, covering at least threequarters of the tooth crowns (Bökenkamp et al., 1993). Enlarged gingiva was normal in colour and felt firm on palpation. The patient was mentally retarded and had not acquired yet any language skills. She was 120 cm tall and weighed 21 kg (both on the 3rd percentile). On clinical evaluation, the parents were normal.

Electroencephalography disclosed bilateral parossistic activity over the frontal and temporal regions, with a right-side prevalence. Brain computed tomography and magnetic resonance imaging, spine radiographs, heart and abdominal ultrasound were unremarkable. Auditory brainstem response test and ophthalmologic evaluation were normal. The effect of anticonvulsant therapy was monitored with computerized bone mineralometry, which showed unremarkable results. Blood levels of total and free testosterone and DHEA-S were normal. Metabolic workout including serum lactate, ammonia, amino acids, organic acids, cholesterol, very long chain fatty acids, lysosomal enzymes, transferrin isoelectric focusing and urinary mucopolisaccarides was normal. Fibroblast chromosome analysis at the 550 bands level and aCGH analysis at 125 kb of resolution yielded normal results. Parents did not give their permission to perform gum biopsy.

This latter patient presented with a unique association of GH, tonic-clonic seizures with onset in the first months of life, severe MR and GO unrelated to antiepileptic treatment, in the absence of other signs and/or symptoms (Douzgou et al., 2009). The clinical features of this patient overlapped in part those found in cases of GO associated with GH, MR, epilepsy and ZLS or related phenotypes (Araiche and Brode, 1959, Nevin et al., 1971, Vontobel et al., 1973, Bakaeen and Scully, 1991, Haytac and Ozcelik, 2007). Tonic-clonic seizures have been reported so far only in a single patient with ZLS, who did not manifest GH (Chodirker et al., 1986). Two patients with the GH of Cantu syndrome (CS) presented with GO but manifested additional features and had no seizure (Rosser et al., 1989). Following the original observation of Anavi et al (1989), concerning a brother-sister pair born to consanguineous parents, two additional patients have been reported with similar clinical characteristics, including central nervous system (CNS) anomalies and neurological features (Snyder, 1965, Kiss, 1990). CNS anomalies were not found in our patient, arguing for a different origin of her neurological manifestations. Our patient also resembled Snyder's case 2, but absence of ataxia appeared as the major distinguishing criteria.

ZLS and Ramon syndrome are considered separate disorders, characterized by the association of GO with hypotelephalangism or cherubism. GH, MR, epilepsy and retinal changes can be overlapping features (Gorlin et al., 2001, Koch et al, 2002). It seems that these two diseases represent the extreme spectrum of the phenotypes exhibiting GO, GH, MR and epilepsy. All these disorders can be lumped in a continuum of increasing severity, from the mildest phenotypes displaying GO, GH, MR and epilepsy to the most complex disorders reported by Göhlich-Ratman et al (2000) and Ramon et al (1967). The unique phenotype of our patient, displaying GO, GH, MR and epilepsy without other signs and/or symptoms overlaps, in part, with the features observed in the three autosomal recessive disorders sharing GO, GH, MR and epilepsy and seems to represent a further example of clinical variability within the occurring in GO plus conditions (**Table 2**).

4.1 Genetic counselling of gingival fibromatosis

The genetic counselling of a person with GF begins with the collection of anamnestic data such as exposure to GF-inducing drugs, the presence of systemic conditions (pregnancy, leukemia), other family members affected, presence of psychomotor retardation and/or seizures. Physical examination can evaluate a number of signs/symptoms that may orient towards the definition of the recurrence risk (RR). In the absence of other signs/symptoms associated, the *SOS-1* gene can be sequenced. In case the molecular analysis is negative, a linkage analysis of the GINGF2-4 known loci, to date, can be undertaken. The presence of hearing loss (Jones syndrome) or corneal opacities (Rutherfurd syndrome) or the association with hypertrichosis suggest an autosomal dominant segregation. The presence of cherubism confirms the diagnosis of Ramon syndrome, which is autosomal recessive. The finding of macrocephaly orients towards the clinical entities described by Canun et al. (2003) and Goldblatt and Singer (1992), with different modes of transmission, depending on the associated dysmorphisms. The recognition of a pattern of multisystemic anomalies (heart disease and/or short stature and/or genitourinary anomalies) associated to GF and hypertrichosis may point to specific, rare syndromes of defined RR. The nail hypoplasia with or without hypotelephalangism allows the diagnosis of ZL, but does not define the RR. Regarding possible patients with the combination of variable GF, hypertrichosis, epilepsy and MR, cerebral magnetic resonance imaging and X-rays of hands and/or a metacarpophalangeal profile may confirm a 25% RR in the cases, respectively, of CNS anomalies or brachydactyly/metacarpy (**Figure 1**).

Feature	GO, GH, MR or epilepsy			Intermediate phenotypes					ZLS	CS	GO, GH, MR, epilepsy and other neurological signs			GO, GH, MR, epilepsy and BDE	RS	Douzgou et al.,2009
	1	2	3	4	5	6	7	8	9	10	11, P2	12	13	14	9	
GO	+	+	+	+	+	+	+	+	+	+/-	+	+	+	+	+	+
GH	+	+	+	-	-	+	-	+/-	+/-	+	+	+	+	+	+/-	+
Tonic-clonic seizures, onset <4y	+	-	-	-	+	-	-	-	+/-	-	+	+	+	+	+	+
MR	-	+	+/-	+	+	-	-	+/-	+/-	+/-	+	+	+	+	+	+
Other	-	-	-	+	+	+	+	+	+	+	+	+	+	+	+	-
Dysmorphic face and/or cherubism	-	-	-	-	-	+	+	+/-	+	+	-	-	+	+	+	-
Neurological signs and/or CNS anomalies	-	-	-	-	-	-	-	-	-	BA/-	At	Hp, BA	SP, BA	Hp	-	-
Nail hypo/dysplasia	-	-	-	-	-	+	+	+	+	-	-	-	-	+	-	-
Brachydactyly	-	-	-	-	-	+	+	+	+	-	-	-	-	+	-	-
Contractures	-	-	-	-	+	-	-	-	-	-	-	-	-	-	+/-	-
Joint hyperextensibility	-	-	-	-	-	-	+	-	+/-	-	-	-	-	-	-	-
Skeletal dysplasia, generalised	-	-	-	-	-	-	-	-	-	+	-	-	-	-	-	-
Heart defect	-	-	-	-	-	-	-	-	+/-	+	-	-	-	+/-	-	-
Hepato/splenomegaly	-	-	-	-	-	-	-	-	+/-	+/-	-	-	-	-	-	-
Urogenital anomalies	-	-	-	-	-	-	-	-	-	-	-	-	-	+/-	+/-	-
Deafness	-	-	-	+	-	-	-	+	-	-	-	-	-	-	+/-	-
Ocular anomalies	-	-	-	-	-	-	-	-	+/-	-	-	-	-	-	+/-	-
Nevi, multiple	-	+	-	-	-	-	-	-	-	-	-	-	-	-	-	+
Growth retardation, postnatal	-	-	-	-	-	-	-	-	-	-	-	-	-	-	+	-
Segregation	-	-	AD	-	AR	-	AR	AD	AD	AD	-	AR	-	AR	AR	-

1, Horning et al. (1985); 2, Anderson et al. (1969); 3, Cuestas-Carnero and Bornancini (1988); 4, Araiche and Brode (1959); 5, Nevin et al. (1971); 6, Vontobel et al. (1973); 7, Bakaeen and Scully (1991); 8, Haytac and Oczelik (2007); 9, Gorlin et al. (2001); 10, Rosser (1998); 11, Snyder (1965); 12, Anavi et al. (1989); 13, Kiss (1990); 14, Göhlich-Ratman et al. (2000); +, present; - absent; +/-, variable; GO, gingival overgrowth; GH generalized hypertrichosis; MR, mental retardation; y, years; RS, Ramon syndrome; ZLS, Zimmermann-Laband syndrome; CS, Cantu syndrome; P2, patient 2; BDE, brachydactyly type E; CNS, central nervous system; At, ataxia; BA, brain atrophy; SP, spastic paraparesis; Hp, hypotonia; AR, autosomal recessive; AD, dominant.

Table 2. Clinical features in patients with GF syndromic disorders.

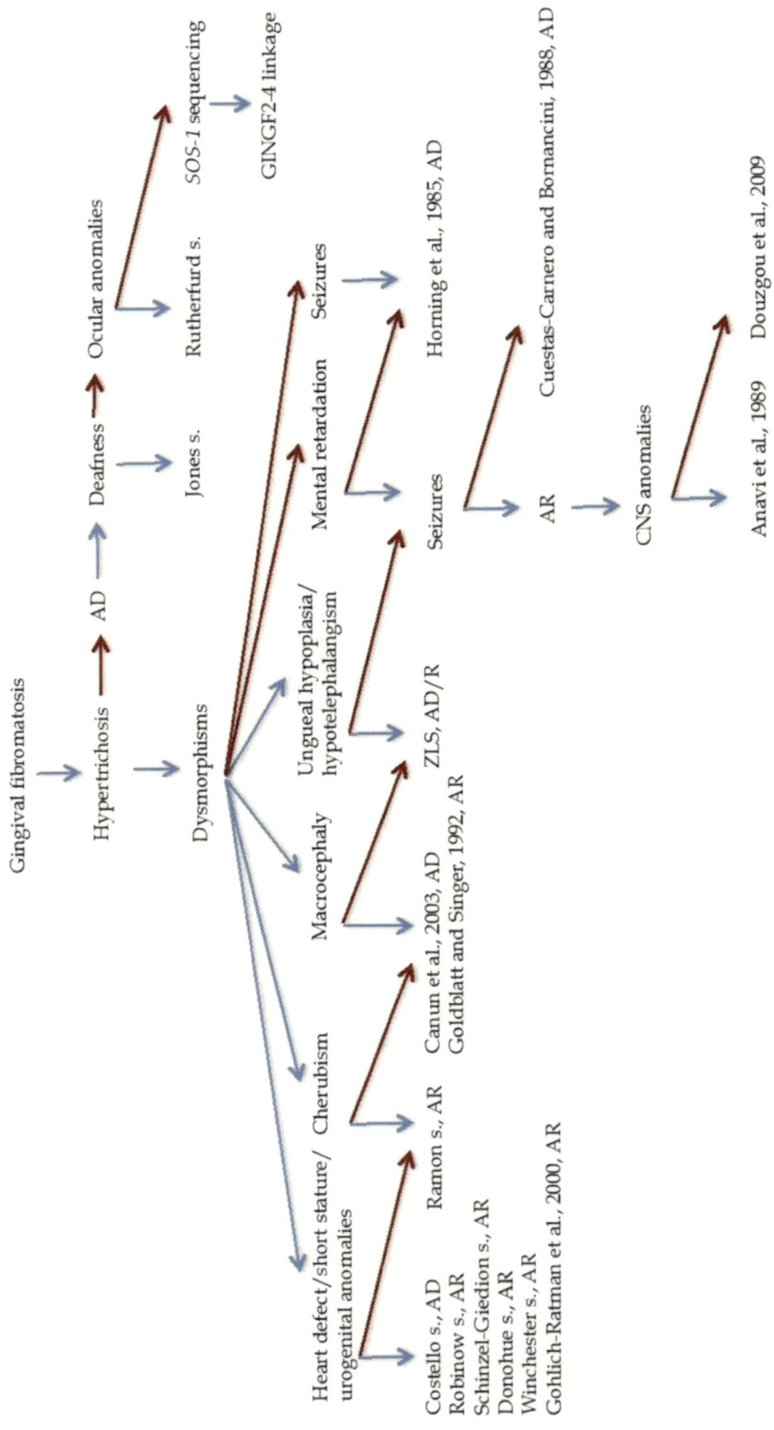

Fig. 1. HGF genetic counselling algorithm; blue arrows, presence; red arrows, absence.

The prognosis of patients with syndromic GF is related to the presence of MR, postnatal growth failure, epilepsy, heart disease and predisposition to cancer. In the specific patient that we described, given a possible diagnosis of ZLS, the monitoring of cardiorespiratory function before the age of 18 years or before embarking on exercise programs is suggested.

5. Conclusion

The patient that we observed is an example of an extremely rare developmental defect present at birth, which is not obvious to the methods currently used for prenatal diagnosis. Her condition is part of the 2-3% of congenital dysmorphisms that require genetic counselling. The absence of a known genetic lesion narrows the diagnostic approach to the clinical-observational aspect. The comparison and classification of this very rare clinical observation was essential in defining the risk of recurrence of the family and the patient's prognosis. The clinical classification of rare genetic conditions is an essential step, along with the descriptions of additional observations and the advances in research, for the discovery of their molecular causes, and thus for the care of the patients and their families.

Of all the branches of medical genetics, genetic counselling of rare congenital dysmorphisms represents the field with the greatest impact of the clinical geneticist. This is justified by such an association of factors as the high incidence of birth defects and hence the increased demand of services of genetic counselling and the rarity of the individual observations, which does not, therefore, permit the diagnosis in first level health services and/or by staff with a general training in medical genetics. The organization of the clinical genetics service in a second or third level facility allows the grouping of these observations in registers or databases that permits the comparison of clinical pictures among different patients as well as the exchange of opinions with other experts. All these processes depict the clinical geneticist as the central, decision-making figure of the genetic counselling of patients with rare dysmorphisms.

6. References

[1] Anavi Y, Lerman P, Mintz S, Kiviti S. Idiopathic familial gingival fibromatosis associated with mental retardation, epilepsy and hypertrichosis. Dev Med Child Neurol 1989;31:538-42.

[2] Anderson J, Cunliffe WJ, Roberts DF, Close H. Hereditary gingival fibromatosis. Br Med J 1969;3:218-19.

[3] Aoki Y, Niihori T, Kawame H, Kurosawa K, Ohashi H, Tanaka Y, Filocamo M, Kato K, Suzuki Y, Kure S, Matsubara Y. Germline mutations in HRAS proto-oncogene cause Costello syndrome. Nat Genet 2005;37:1038-40.

[4] Aoki Y, Niihori T, Narumi Y, Kure S, Matsubara Y. The RAS/MAPK syndromes: novel roles of the RAS pathway in human genetic disorders. Hum Mutat. 2008;29:992-06.

[5] Araiche M, Brode H. A case of fibromatosis gingivae. Oral Surg Oral Med Oral Pathol 1959;12:1307-10.

[6] Bakaeen G, Scully C. Hereditary gingival fibromatosis in a family with the Zimmermann-Laband syndrome. J Oral Pathol Med 1991;20:457-9.

[7] Baptista IP. Hereditary gingival fibromatosis: a case report. J Clin Periodontol 2002;29:871-4.

[8] Baumeister FA, Schwarz HP, Stengel-Rutkowski S. Childhood hypertrichosis: diagnosis and management. Arch Dis Child 1995;72:457-9.

[9] Bhansali RS, Yeltiwar RK, Agrawal AA. Periodontal management of gingival enlargement associated with Sturge-Weber syndrome. J Periodontol 2008;79:549-55.

[10] Bökenkamp A, Bohnhorst B, Beier C, Albers N, Offner G, Brodehl J. Nifedipine aggravates cyclosporine A-induced gingival hyperplasia. Pediatr Nephrol 1994;8:181-5.

[11] Bondeson J, Miles AE. Julia Pastrana, the nondescript: an example of congenital, generalized hypertrichosis terminalis with gingival hyperplasia. Am J Med Genet 1993;47:198-212.

[12] Buday L, Downward J. Many faces of Ras activation. Biochim Biophys Acta. 2008 May 21.

[13] Canún S, Guevara-Sanginés EG, Elvira-Morales A, Sierra-Romero Mdel C, Rodríguez-Asbun H. Hypertrichosis terminalis, gingival hyperplasia, and a characteristic face: a new distinct entity. Am J Med Genet A 2003;116A:278-83.

[14] Chodirker BN, Chudley AE, Toffler MA, Reed MH. Zimmerman-Laband syndrome and profound mental retardation. Am J Med Genet 1986;25(3):543-7.

[15] Cuestas-Carnero R, Bornancini CA. Hereditary generalized gingival fibromatosis associated with hypertrichosis: report of five cases in one family. J Oral Maxillofac Surg 1988;46:415-20.

[16] Doufexi A, Mina M, Ioannidou E. Gingival overgrowth in children: epidemiology, pathogenesis, and complications. A literature review. J Periodontol 2005;76:3-10.

[17] Drugowick RM, Da Rós Gonçalves L, Barrôso AS, Feres-Filho EJ, Maia LC. Treatment of gingival overgrowth in a child with Bardet-Biedl syndrome. J Periodontol 2007;78:1159-63.

[18] Emerson TG. Hereditary gingival hyperplasia. a family pedigree of four generations. Oral Surg Oral Med Oral Pathol 1965;19:1-9.

[19] Fryns JP, Kleczkowska A, Kenis H, Decock P, Van den Berghe H. Partial duplication of the short arm of chromosome 2 (dup(2)(p13----p21) associated with mental retardation and an Aarskog-like phenotype. Ann Genet 1989;32:174-6.

[20] Göhlich-Ratmann G, Lackner A, Schaper J, Voit T, Gillessen-Kaesbach G. Syndrome of gingival hypertrophy, hirsutism, mental retardation and brachymetacarpia in two sisters: specific entity or variant of a described condition? Am J Med Genet Part A 2000;95:241-6.

[21] Goldblatt J, Singer SL. Autosomal recessive gingival fibromatosis with distinctive facies. Clin Genet 1992;42:306-8.

[22] Gorlin RJ, Cohen MM, Hennekam RCM. Syndromes of the Head and Neck, 3rd edn. New York: Oxford University Press 2001: 847-858.

[23] Gureasko J, Galush WJ, Boykevisch S, Sondermann H, Bar-Sagi D, Groves JT, Kuriyan J. Membrane-dependent signal integration by the Ras activator Son of sevenless. Nat Struct Mol Biol 2008;15:452-61.

[24] Häkkinen L, Csiszar A. Hereditary gingival fibromatosis: characteristics and novel putative pathogenic mechanisms. J Dent Res 2007;86:25-34.

[25] Hart TC, Pallos D, Bowden DW, Bolyard J, Pettenati MJ, Cortelli JR. Genetic linkage of hereditary gingival fibromatosis to chromosome 2p21. Am J Hum Genet 1998;62:876-83.

[26] Hart TC, Zhang Y, Gorry MC, Hart PS, Cooper M, Marazita ML, et al. A mutation in the SOS1 gene causes hereditary gingival fibromatosis type 1. Am J Hum Genet 2002;70:943-954.
[27] Haytac MC, Ozcelik O. The phenotypic overlap of syndromes associated with hereditary gingival fibromatosis: follow-up of a family for five years. Oral Surg Oral Med Oral Pathol Oral Radiol Endod 2007;103:521-7.
[28] Hennekam RC. Costello syndrome: an overview. Am J Med Genet C Semin Med Genet 2003;117C:42-8.
[29] Horning GM, Fisher JG, Barker BF, Killoy WJ, Lowe JW. Gingival fibromatosis with hypertrichosis. A case report. J Periodontol. 1985;56:344-7.
[30] Ishigami T, Schmidt-Westhausen A, Philipsen HP, Baiborodin SI, Gelderblom H, Reichart PA. Oral manifestations of alpha-mannosidosis: report of a case with ultrastructural findings. J Oral Pathol Med 1995;24:85-8.
[31] Jang SI, Lee EJ, Hart PS, Ramaswami M, Pallos D, Hart TC. Germ line gain of function with SOS1 mutation in hereditary gingival fibromatosis. J Biol Chem 2007;282:20245-5.
[32] Jorgenson RJ, Cocker ME. Variation in the inheritance and expression of gingival fibromatosis. J Periodontol 1974;45:472-7.
[33] Kataoka M, Kido J, Shinohara Y, Nagata T. Drug-induced gingival overgrowth—a review. Biol Pharm Bull 2005;28:1817-21.
[34] Kelekis-Cholakis A, Wiltshire WA, Birek C. Treatment and longterm follow-up of a patient with hereditary gingival fibromatosis: a case report. J Can Dent Assoc 2002;68:290-4.
[35] Kiss P. Gingival fibromatosis, mental retardation, epilepsy and hypertrichosis. Dev Med Child Neurol 1990;32:459-60.
[36] Koch P, Wettstein A, Knauber J, Zaun H. A new case of Zimmermann-Laband syndrome with atypical retinitis pigmentosa. Acta Derm Venereol 1992;72:376-9.
[37] Lacombe D, Bioulac-Sage P, Sibout M, Daussac E, Lesure F, Manchart JP, Battin J. Congenital marked hypertrichosis and Laband syndrome in a child: overlap between the gingival fibromatosis-hypertrichosis and Laband syndromes. Genet Couns 1994;5:251-6.
[38] Mosig RA, Dowling O, Martignetti JA. MMP2 and the Multicentric Osteolysis, Nodulosis and Arthtropathy (MONA). Inborn Errors of Development: The Molecular Basis of Clinical Disorders of Morphogenesis. Oxford Monographs on Medical Genetics. 2nd edn. 2008.
[39] Parkin B, Law C. Axenfeld anomaly and retinal changes in Ramon syndrome: follow-up of two sibs. Am J Med Genet 2001;104:131-4.
[40] Perkoff D. Primary generalized hypertrophy of the gums. Lancet 1929;1:1294-7.
[41] Ramon Y, Berman W, Bubis JJ. Gingival fibromatosis combined with cherubism. Oral Surg Oral Med Oral Pathol 1967;24:435-48.
[42] Roberts AE, Araki T, Swanson KD, Montgomery KT, Schiripo TA, Joshi VA, Li L, Yassin Y, Tamburino AM, Neel BG, Kucherlapati RS. Germline gain-of-function mutations in SOS1 cause Noonan syndrome. Nat Genet 2007;39:70-4.
[43] Robertson SP, Lipp H, Bankier A. Zimmermann-Laband syndrome in an adult. Long-term follow-up of a patient with vascular and cardiac complications. Am J Med Genet 1998;78:160-4.

[44] Saltiel AR, Kahn CR. Insulin signalling and the regulation of glucose and lipid metabolism. Nature 2001;414:799-806.
[45] Seymour RA, Ellis JS, Thomason JM. Risk factors for drug-induced gingival overgrowth. J Clin Periodontol 2000;27:217-23.
[46] Sibilia M, Fleischmann A, Behrens A, Stingl L, Carroll J, Watt FM, Schlessinger J, Wagner EF. The EGF receptor provides an essential survival signal for SOS-dependent skin tumor development. Cell 2000;102:211-20.
[47] Shashi V, Pallos D, Pettenati MJ, Cortelli JR, Fryns JP, von Kap-Herr C, Hart TC. Genetic heterogeneity of gingival fibromatosis on chromosome 2p. J Med Genet 1999;36:683-6.
[48] Snyder CH. Syndrome of gingival hyperplasia, hirsutism, and convulsions; dilantin intoxication without dilantin. J Pediatr 1965;67:499-502.
[49] Somacarrera ML, Hernández G, Acero J, Moskow BS. Factors related to the incidence and severity of cyclosporin-induced gingival overgrowth in transplant patients. A longitudinal study. J Periodontol 1994;65:671-5.
[50] Takagi M, Yamamoto H, Mega H, Hsieh KJ, Shioda S, Enomoto S. Heterogeneity in the gingival fibromatoses. Cancer 1991;68:2202-12.
[51] Tartaglia M, Pennacchio LA, Zhao C, Yadav KK, Fodale V, Sarkozy A, Pandit B, Oishi K, Martinelli S, Schackwitz W, Ustaszewska A, Martin J, Bristow J, Carta C, Lepri F, Neri C, Vasta I, Gibson K, Curry CJ, Siguero JP, Digilio MC, Zampino G, Dallapiccola B, Bar-Sagi D, Gelb BD. Gain-of-function SOS1 mutations cause a distinctive form of Noonan syndrome. Nat Genet 2007;39:75-9.
[52] Vontobel F. Idiopathic gingival hyperplasia and hypertrichosis associated with acromegaloid features. Helv Paediatr Acta 1973;28:401-11.
[53] Vural F, Ozcan MA, Ozsan GH, Demirkan F, Piskin O, Ates H, Kargi A, Undar B. Gingival involvement in a patient with CD56+ chronic myelomonocytic leukemia. Leuk Lymphoma 2004;45:415-8.
[54] Wilkie AOM. ROR2 and Brachydactyly type B and Recessive Robinow Syndrome. Inborn Errors of Development: The Molecular Basis of Clinical Disorders of Morphogenesis. Oxford Monographs on Medical Genetics. 2nd edn. 2008.
[55] Xiao S, Wang X, Qu B, Yang M, Liu G, Bu L, Wang Y, Zhu L, Lei H, Hu L, Zhang X, Liu J, Zhao G, Kong X. Refinement of the locus for autosomal dominant hereditary gingival fibromatosis (GINGF) to a 3.8-cM region on 2p21. Genomics 2000;68:247-52.
[56] Xiao S, Bu L, Zhu L, Zheng G, Yang M, Qian M, et al. A new locus for hereditary gingival fibromatosis (GINGF2) maps to 5q13-q22. Genomics 2001;74:180-185.
[57] Ye X, Shi L, Cheng Y, Peng Q, Huang S, Liu J, et al. A novel locus for autosomal dominant hereditary gingival fibromatosis, GINGF3, maps to chromosome 2p22.3-p23.3. Clin Genet 2005;68:239-244.
[58] Zenker M, Horn D, Wieczorek D, Allanson J, Pauli S, van der Burgt I, Doerr HG, Gaspar H, Hofbeck M, Gillessen-Kaesbach G, Koch A, Meinecke P, Mundlos S, Nowka A, Rauch A, Reif S, von Schnakenburg C, Seidel H, Wehner LE, Zweier C, Bauhuber S, Matejas V, Kratz CP, Thomas C, Kutsche K. SOS1 is the second most common Noonan gene but plays no major role in cardio-facio-cutaneous syndrome. J Med Genet 2007;44:651-6.
[59] Zhu Y, Zhang W, Huo Z, Zhang Y, Xia Y, Li B, Kong X, Hu L. A novel locus for maternally inherited human gingival fibromatosis at chromosome 11p15. Hum Genet 2007;121:113-23.

15

Experimental Epilepsy Models and Morphologic Alterations of Experimental Epilepsy Models in Brain and Hippocampus

Ilgaz Akdogan and Nilufer Goksin Yonguc
Pamukkale University, School of Medicine, Department of Anatomy, Denizli
Turkey

1. Introduction

Epilepsy is a neurological disease arising from abnormal and uncontrollable electrical firings of a group of neurons appearing in the central nervous system. Experimental epilepsy models have been developed to assess the pathophysiology of epileptic seizures and to search for new effective anti-epileptic drugs.

This chapter is designed to describe characteristics of experimental epilepsy models and morphological and anatomical changes of brain, particularly hippocampus (Figure 1), in these models. Because of the hippocampal neuronal hyperexcitability during epileptic seizures, hippocampus has been one of the best choices in terms of target area that reveals most efficiently the effects of seizures in experimental epilepsy models.

The purpose of the study determines which model should be chosen for epilepsies. This type of studies may have three purposes: 1. Developing new drugs, 2. Exploring the mechanisms, 3. Determining the relationships between basic events and the development of events for epilepsy.

An ideal model of epilepsy should have the following characteristics: 1. Seizures should be as the spontaneous recurrent seizures, 2. Seizures should be similar to seizures in humans, 3. The EEG pattern should be similar to related type of epilepsy, and 4. The frequency of seizures should be sufficient to test acute and chronic effects of drugs. However, there is no single model that meets all these criteria.

Some researchers classify seizures according to generation of the epilepsy model, not according to seizures in humans. Experimental models are divided into three groups according to this classification: 1. experimental seizures induced by chemical convulsants or by electrical stimulation, 2. reflex epilepsies, and 3. idiopathic epilepsies.

Epileptic seizures are classified in three groups:

1. Partial seizures, which can be further subdivided into simple partial seizures and complex partial seizures. 2. Generalized seizures which can be further subdivided into tonic, clonic, tonic-clonic (grand mal), absence (petit-mal) seizures, and status epilepticus. 3. Unclassified seizures.

In experimental epilepsy studies, animal models have been developed according to this classification (Table-1).

1- Simple partial, acute
2- Simple partial, chronic
3- Complex partial
4- Generalized tonic-clonic
5- Generalized absence
6- Status epilepticus.

Animal (the experimental) models of the epilepsies:

1- Simple partial, acute	*4- Generalized tonic-clonic*	*5- Generalized absence*
	Genetic	Thalamic stimulation
Penicillin	Photosensitive boboons	Bilateral cortical foci
Bicuculline	Audiogenic seizures in mice	Systemic penicillin
Picrotoxin	Mongolian gerbil	Intraventricular opiates
Strychnine	Epilepsy mice	
	Genetically epilepsy-prone rats	
2- Simple partial, chronic		
Cortically implanted metals	Maximal electroshock	
Aluminum hydroxide	Chemical convulsants	
Cobalt	Pentylenetetrazol	
Zinc	Systemic penicillin (as a tonic-clonic model)	
Manganese	Picrotoxin	*6- Status epilepticus*
Iron	Bicuculline	Lithium-pilocarpine
Cryogenic injury	Methionine sulfoximide	Cobalt-homocystine
	Bemegride	Recurrent stimulation
	Others	
3- Complex partial	Metabolic derangements	
Kainic acid	Hypoxia	
Tetanus toxin	Hypoglycemia	
Kindling	Hyperbaric oxygen	
	Hypercarbia	
	Drug withdrawal	
	High temperature	

Table 1. Animal (the experimental) models of the epilepsies.

2. Simple partial, acute

Penicillin

The most popular method to study simple partial (focal) seizures has been by application of a topical chemical convulsant. Chemical convulsants are widely used for inducing seizures easily and rapidly. The common antibiotic, penicillin (a chemical convulsant), was discovered during neurosurgical procedures, in which it was applied to brain to prevent infection. When a cottoned pledget soaked in penicillin is placed on exposed rat or cat cortex, regionally placed electrodes record recurring interictal spikes within a few minutes. These discharges resemble human interictal spikes recorded from cortex. During the interictal spike neurons in the region of the focus tend to fire synchronously. If penicillin is injected into the neocortex, the injected cortical area becomes a source of epileptic seizures. The penicillin epilepsy (PE) model has been one of the most important model for answering questions about the neuronal basis of epilepsy. This model is also suitable for analysis of spread of seizure activity.

PE model is one of the most useful acute models in the field of experimental epilepsy studies. This model is also essential for analysis in synchronous and spread of epileptogenic seizure activity. It allows obtaining EEG records as in acute partial epilepsy by application penicillin to cortical surface. Penicillin-induced epileptic activity begins focally, but then spread and cause generalized epilepsy. In this regard, it resembles the grand-mal epilepsy.

PE model leads to neuronal loss in CA1-CA2-CA3 subfields of hippocampus and hippocampal volume decrease in rats, in proportion to the given dose.

However, there are no neuronal loss and volume decrease in dentate gyrus of penicillin epileptic rats.

Bicuculline, Picrotoxin, Strychnine

Bicuculline is an alkaloid that is used only in experimental studies. There are structural similarities between bicuculline and penicillin. Picrotoxin is a poisonous crystalline plant compound, found primarily in the fruit of the climbing plant *Anamirta cocculus*. Strychnine is a poisonous alkaloid that is obtained from seeds of the nux vomica tree (*S. nux-vomica*) and related plants of the genus *Strychnos*. Strychnine acts as a non-competitive blocker of inhibitory glycine. It was shown that topical application of 5% bicuculline to temporal cortex generates paroxysmal depolarization in cats, after a few seconds.

Bicuculline, picrotoxin and strychnine are antagonists to the action of the inhibitory neurotransmitter GABA, and generate epileptiform activity, in particular by blocking $GABA_A$ receptors. The $GABA_A$ antagonists, bicuculline or picrotoxin, greatly increase burst firing in dopaminergic neurons whereas $GABA_B$ antagonists cause a modest shift away from burst firing towards pacemaker-like firing. The three principal GABAergic inputs to nigral dopaminergic neurons arise from striatum, globus pallidus and from the axon collaterals of nigral pars reticulata projection neurons, each of which appear to act in vivo primarily on $GABA_A$ receptors.

Bicuculline induced status epilepticus with duration of 1 or 2 h leads to morphological changes in fronto-parietal cortex and hippocampus of rats. Astrocytic edema and wide-spread neuronal changes of two different kinds occur in the fronto-parietal cortex of the animals. Type 1 injured neurons are characterized by condensation of karyoplasms and cytoplasm (type 1a), which in some neurons become so intense that the nucleus can no longer be clearly discerned (type 1b). The type 2 injured neurons have slit-formed cytoplasmic vacuoles chiefly caused by dilatation of the rough endoplasmic reticulum. In the hippocampus the most conspicuous alteration is astrocytic edema which is most marked around the perikarya of pyramidal neurons in CA1-CA4 and subiculum. In the dentate gyrus the edema is less pronounced and, when present, affects particularly the hilar zone of the stratum granulosum. The nerve cell changes are less pronounced than in the cerebral cortex. The vast majority of the hippocampal pyramidal neurons in CA1-CA4 show minor configurationally and tinctorial abnormalities (incipient type 1a change). Severe nerve cell alterations (type 1b) are present but very rarely affect the pyramidal neurons of CA1-CA4 and subiculum, whereas in the dentate gyrus pyramidal basket neurons of stratum granulosum and pyramidal nerve cells in stratum polymorphic show the severe type 1b changes.

3. Simple partial, chronic

Cortically implanted metals

Alumina hydroxide

The best validated and most realistic models for the epilepsies are those employing implantation of metals in brain to generate a state of 'spontaneously' recurrent simple partial seizures. The prototype of this group of models is the alumina hydroxide gel model. In a typical preparation 4% alumina hydroxide will be injected into surgically exposed monkey neocortex at a few adjacent sites. A similar model can be produced in the cat. Spontaneous and recurrent seizures generally begin one to two months after the injection, and persist for as long as several years. The seizures themselves are similar to simple partial seizures in humans, with rhythmic jerking of an extremity or face contra lateral to the aluminum lesion, and occasional progression to secondarily generalized tonic-clonic seizures. Interictal and ictal EEGs appear similar to clinical studies. Neuropathological specimens obtained from biopsies in the region of an established alumina focus in monkeys show gliosis and distortion of dendritic neuronal trees, similar to the picture seen in human neocortical foci.

Cobalt

Cortical implantation of cobalt can produce chronic or subacute models of recurrent seizures in animals. GABA receptors have been found to be decreased in the region of cobalt foci of rat motor cortex, 2-3 weeks after establishment of the focus. Furthermore in the unilateral cobalt model, the lack of anatomic differences in the white or gray matter outside the areas of MR signal loss caused by cobalt suggests no widespread cerebral injury.

Zinc, Copper, Manganese, Iron

Intraventricular application of the metals, such as zinc, copper, manganese, iron leads seizures. These effects of these metals are thought to be occur by blocking Na,K-ATPase membrane pump.

A chronic model for experimental epilepsy can be generated by injecting 10 µl zinc sulfate into rabbit hippocampus. In this model, epileptic seizure continues for weeks and clinical or electrophysiological aspects are similar to complex partial and secondary generalized seizures in addition to simple partial seizures. Neuronal loss in both hippocampus and cerebellum has been found after intracortical zinc injection. Also, zinc model generates spontaneous epileptic seizures and generalized convulsions in rabbits but not in rats. It should be remembered that aluminum model generates spontaneous seizures in rats.

In oxygen and glucose deprivation model of trans-synaptic Zn^{2+} movement, Ca-A/K channels have been expected to play a late role in neuronal injury. It is suggested with strong presynaptic activation, basal numbers of Ca-A/K channels permit sufficient Zn^{2+}entry to mediate rapid neuronal damage in a study of oxygen and glucose deprivation model. These observations may provide new rationale for neuroprotective strategies targeting Ca-K channels and Zn^{2+} passage through them in conditions of ischemia or epilepsy, which are associated with rapid synaptic Zn^{2+}release.

Cryogenic injury

One model that doesn't require injection of exogenous drugs into brain is cryogenic or freeze exogenous drugs into brain is cryogenic or freeze lesion model for partial simple seizures. Ethylchloride lesions or cold trauma from a liquid nitrogen probe produces a highly epileptogenic lesion, giving rise to seizures within a few hours of the lesion and persisting for a few days. Substantial cerebral edema generally accompanies the lesion.

4. Complex partial

Complex partial seizures are usually arise from the limbic lobe, including amygdala, hippocampus, and less often, temporal neocortex or extratemporal structures.

Kainic acid

Kainic acid (KA) is a rigid analog of the putative excitatory neurotransmitter, glutamate and potent agonist of the AMPA/kainate class of glutamate receptors. KA has been used to induce limbic seizures. Systemic and intracerebral administration of KA initially induces a characterized pattern of seizure activity that lasts for hours, followed by a latent seizure-free period of weeks, preceding the development of spontaneous recurrent focal seizures that begin between 3 and 4 weeks. Injection of KA is followed by cytotoxic brain edema, characterized by massive swelling of perineuronal and perivascular astroglia, resulting in parenchymal necrosis of the affected region.

Primary interest in KA has derived from its ability to produce relatively selective lesions of cell bodies in brain, while sparing axons of passage. For reasons that are still incompletely understood, KA has an especially prominent toxic effect on hippocampus, even when injected systemically, or at brain sites remote from hippocampus. In doses less than those required to produce cell injury, KA can induce seizures in hippocampus. Animals given KA 4 mg/kg i.v., or 0.8-2.0 µg intra-hippocampally, will show periodic arrest of activity, masticatory movements, complex motor activity, and some times extension to generalized tonic-clonic activity. Stereo-encephalography shows major spike activity originating in the limbic system. KA is a prototype of an excitotoxic compound. KA produces an acute or substance model of seizures, lasting hours to days. The accompanying hippocampal lesions may be considered to confound the model, or alternatively, to portray the pattern of limbic cell damage which can occur with clinical status epilepticus.

KA treated rats have been found to have significantly smaller hippocampus and a significant increase in ventricular size. The histological findings were neuronal loss and neuronal degeneration in CA1 and CA3 of the hippocampus, which was accompanied by strong microglia activation. The MRI of KA treated rats showed enlarged ventricles. Volumetric analysis of MRI images demonstrated a significant reduction in hippocampal volume of experimental rats 10 days following KA injection, whereas the cingulate cortex, retrosplenial cortex, and total brain volumes of these animals were not changed. Even 10 days after the KA injection neuronal loss was still ongoing.

The dentate gyrus of epileptic KA treated rats are strikingly similar to those of reported for human temporal lobe epilepsy, so the findings of neuron loss and axon reorganization in the hippocampus of KA treated rats may be important in epileptogenesis.

The similarities in patterns of neuron loss and granule cell axon reorganization between the epileptic human dentate gyrus and that of KA treated rats and other experimental models of epilepsy suggest the existence of population of highly vulnerable neurons that can be killed by naturally occurring traumatic events (e.g., status epilepticus, head injury, cerebral infections) and experimental treatments (e.g., kainate or pilocarpine toxicity and repetitive stimulation of the perforant pathway).

There are also functional similarities in the dentate gyrus of KA treated rats and in human temporal lobe epilepsy. So, homologous regions of the dentate gyrus suffer the most severe cell loss and axon reorganization in epileptic KA treated rats and in human temporal lobe epilepsy.

In addition, administration of KA activates ionotropic glutamate receptors, and selectively induces excitotoxic cell death in the CA3 and CA1 hippocampal subfields and within the dentate gyrus, while sparing neurons in the CA2 subfield and the dentate granule cell layer. Furthermore, there is a direct relationship between the generation epileptiform activity and the extent of damage in hippocampal subfields. Many features of this rodent model, such as hippocampal sclerosis and mossy fiber sprouting, resemble human temporal lobe epilepsy. As a result the KA model replicates several phenomenological features of human temporal lobe epilepsy and can be used as an animal preparation to understand the basic mechanisms of epileptogenesis.

Following a single 9mg/kg KA injection to rats, the most important histopathological changes are occur time dependent and include neuronal degeneration, microgliosis, astrogliosis. Focus of the neuronal damage in CA1 prior to CA3 damage resembling human lesions as opposed to CA3 dominance observed in some rodent models; hilar neuronal loss; activated microgliosis; astrogliosis; and aberrant mossy fiber sprouting in the inner molecular layer of dentate gyrus. Intracerebroventricular administration of KA induces selective neuronal loss in the CA3 subfield and activates glial cells in the rat hippocampus.

Similar to rats, administration of kainic acid (KA) to mice elicits epileptic behavior in a dose-dependent manner and causes distinct neuronal degeneration in limbic structures such as the hippocampus. KA treated mice show acute neuronal loss in the CA1 and CA3 regions of hippocampus, which is followed by the activation of glial cells and delayed neural cell death. KA treated mice also observe volume decrease in dorsal and ventral hippocampus.

Also, systemic administration of KA to rodents is a widely used experimental model of epilepsy and neurodegeneration. This treatment results in the appearance of chronic, spontaneous, recurrent seizures and neurodegenerative changes in the dentate gyrus.

Tetanus toxin

A model of recurrent, chronic partial seizures can be produced by injection of tetanus toxin into rat or cat hippocampus. Categorization of the model with complex partial seizure models results from the location of the usual injection site in limbic structures, rather than the properties of the toxin itself. The tetanus toxin model resembles those produced by injection of other convulsant substances into hippocampus, but it has some intriguing idiosyncrasies.

Tetanus is a disease produced from the gram-positive bacteria, *Clostridium tetani*. In the disease state toxin is transported from the periphery to the spinal cord, where it is believed to interfere with presynaptic release of inhibitory neurotransmitter. In contrast, injection into hippocampus of a dose of toxin 3-6 times the mouse probably produces effects only locally. Seizures may occur within a day after injection and then on a chronically recurrent basis over weeks. A seizure in a rat typically begins with arrest of activity. Followed by myoclonic jerks of the front limbs, and in some animals generalized tonic-clonic seizures. Whether or not the seizure generalizes depends upon several factors, including spread to the cingulate area.

A single dose of tetanus toxin, injected unilaterally into the hippocampus, produced a time-dependent neuronal loss in the CA1 pyramidal cell layer accompanied by a reduction in the binding of gamma-[3H]aminobutyric acid ([3H]GABA) to $GABA_A$ but not $GABA_B$ sites in the pyramidal cell layer.

Kindling

Kindling is a phenomenon by which repeated shocks to various parts of brain result in enhanced electrical excitability of brain. Kindling has become one of the most popular ways to model long-term plastic changes in brain excitability. Such plastic changes are believed to participate not only in epileptogenesis, but also in memory and learning. The kindling model is conceptually related to models for long term potentiation, although kindling paradigms tend to be more chronic than those for long-term potentiation (LTP), and focus more on epileptic changes than on enhanced evoked electrical responses.

Kindling is usually initiated by electrical stimulation of the amygdala, but most regions of forebrain can be kindled. To produce the model, bipolar stimulating wires are implanted in amygdala or elsewhere in brain. The animal recovers from the surgery, than daily electrical stimulus trains are applied via the electrodes. A fairly wide range of stimulation parameters may be effective in induction of kindling. After a few days of stimulation a train of shocks begins to induce electrical after discharges, which become progressively more complex and prolonged with each kindling stimulus. At this time, the animal is said to be 'kindled'. If continued for a few weeks, rodents exhibit "spontaneous" epileptic seizures.

Rapid kindling paradigms able to model status epilepticus in rodents, within a few hours or days of kindling have been described. Repeated stimulation by excitatory chemicals can also produce kindling.

The amygdala possesses the lowest threshold for the induction of kindling, an established experimental model of temporal lobe epilepsy in which daily electrical stimulation results in a gradual progression and intensification of limbic motor seizures.

Kindling through daily administration of brief electrical stimulations to the left basolateral nucleus of the amygdala resulted in a significant impairment of LTP in both the lateral amygdala and the CA1 of rat hippocampus. In contrast to KA model, DNA fragmentation and reactive microglia in the CA1, CA3, and hilus of the dentate gyrus region do not detected in the kindling model. Neuronal death occurs as a result of DNA fragmentation in hippocampal pyramidal cells in KA model.

Dentate gyrus of kindled rats is enlarged. The increase in area associated with kindling is the result of an enlargement of the molecular layer and the hilus of the dentate gyrus. Absolute neuronal counts show no change following kindling in the hilus of the dentate gyrus.

After kindling, i.e., specific electrical stimulation of the rat ventral hippocampus, cells numbers are significantly decrease in hippocampus, the hilus, and dentate gyrus.

5. Generalized tonic-clonic seizures

Genetic

There are no good animal models for primary generalized, spontaneously recurrent tonic-clonic (grand mal) seizures. Because idiopathic grand mal epilepsy shows a genetic component, investigators have attempted to develop models from genetically aberrant strains of animals; including baboons, beagles, Mongolian gerbils, mice, and rats. Each of these models has distinctions from clinical grand mal, either in the requirement for certain types of precipitating stimuli, or other associated non-epileptic deficits.

Epilepsy mice

The 'epilepsy' (abbreviated 'El') mice exhibit seizures that are best induced by vestibular stimuli, such as tossing or spinning the mice. Manifestations of seizures in this strain may include limb and face automatisms such as chewing and salivating. Electrical discharges originate in deep limbic structures. These features are analogous to clinical complex partial epilepsy. Like human complex partial epilepsy, seizures may generalize to tonic-clonic activity. Heritability of vestibulogenic seizure tendency in El is dominant, but the gene locus or loci and neurochemical defects are unknown. EEG studies have revealed that interictal discharge originate from parietal cortex and especially from hippocampus. In other words, these rats have temporal lobe epilepsy. Degeneration of neurons in stratum pyramidale (in CA1-CA2 subfields) and increase of GABA and VIP containing neurons in stratum radiatum have been reported in the hippocampus of El mice.

Genetically epilepsy-prone rats

Genetically epilepsy-prone rat model is one of the best known genetic epilepsy model. Previously it has been known that only audiogenic stimuli can induce seizures in this strain but afterwards it has been understood that also many other physical and chemical stimuli such as hyperthermia, electroshock, pentylenetetrazol and bicuculline can easily induce seizures.

Maximal electroshock

Maximal electroshock (MES) is arguably the best studied and most useful animal model of seizures. In particular, this model is often used to study of antiepileptic drug development. A distinction is made between minimal and maximal seizures. Minimal seizures are characterized by a 'stun reaction' and clonic movements of the face and forelimbs. Maximal seizures show tonic hind-limb extension and flexion, followed by clonus. A MES seizure meets criteria if there is tonic hind-limb extension. Studies may choose to evaluate either minimal or maximal electroshock seizures.

Chemical convulsants

Numerous chemical compounds can induce generalized seizures when administered systematically. Pentylenetetrazol, penicillin, bemegride, picrotoxin, bicuculline, strychnine, allyglycine, flurothyl, homocysteine are a few of those of greatest interest for epilepsy research.

Pentylenetetrazol model

Pentylenetetrazol (PTZ) is one of the mostly used chemicals to study of antiepileptic drug development. PTZ is tetrazol derivative with consistent convulsive actions in mice, rats, cats and primates, when given by the parenteral route. PTZ initially produces myoclonic jerks, which than become sustained, and may lead to waves or polyspikes.

PTZ-treatment leads to hippocampal atrophy in rats. PTZ-treated rats show selective neuronal loss and astrocytosis in the hippocampus. MRI studies on PTZ-treated rats show decrease in cerebellum volume.

On the other hand, PTZ treatment needs repeated injections to result in cell loss in hippocampus, which might be a result of enhanced activity of glutamergic systems.

Systemic penicillin as a tonic-clonic model

Penicillin was discussed above as an agent able to produce acute seizures, when placed on cortex. Clinical experience has indicated that high systemic doses of penicillin in humans can produce myoclonus, generalized tonic-clonic seizures and encephalopathy. In the hospital setting encephalopathy occurs most commonly with i.v. dosages above 20 million units per day, especially if concurrent renal failure maintains high levels and alters the blood-brain barrier. It was shown that parenteral penicillin could produce generalized seizures in cats.

Other inhibitory antagonists

Other popular systemic convulsants include picrotoxin, bicuculline, methionine sulfoximine, bemegride, allyglycine, strychnine, and certain general anesthetics.

Bemegride (Megimide) is a glutarimide derivative similar in action to PTZ. It has been used to produce clonic or tonic-clonic seizures, or to activate focal epilepsy. Several of drugs used to produce partial seizures when focally applied, for example picrotoxin and bicuculline, will produce generalized clonic and tonic-clonic seizures, when given systemically.

Brain metabolism early in bicuculline-induced generalized tonic-clonic seizures is greatest in neocortex and synaptically linked regions, as opposed to brainstem. A potent generalized seizure model can be produced by i.v. injection of strychnine. Strychnine interacts with GABA-benzodiazepine receptors, but a more important action of strychnine is probably against glycine. Glycine is an important inhibitory neurotransmitter in brainstem and spinal cord with structural homology to the much larger strychnine molecule. Strychnine serves as a non-competitiveinhibitor of glycine receptor. Resulting seizures differ in character from those produced by primary GABA antagonists in that they are mainly extensor tonic, with little cortical EEG seizure activity.

Some convulsants apparently act by mimicry of excitatory neurotransmission. It is often difficult to induce seizures by systemic administration of glutamate, although monosodium glutamate can penetrate to brain and produce convulsions in 10-day-old rats.

Metabolic derangements

In clinical practice many metabolic derangements can lead to seizures including, hypoxia, hypoglycemia, uremia, drug withdrawal and high temperature. These conditions have not in general been useful for studying mechanisms of the epilepsies because they usually produce other central nervous system disturbances peculiar to the model employed. Three metabolic disturbances have, however, been employed in a few studies of generalized seizures; hyperbaric oxygen, and hypercarbia.

Hyperthermic seizures-but not hyperthermia alone-results in numerous argyrophilic neurons in discrete regions of the limbic system; within 24 hours of seizures, a significant proportion of neurons in the central nucleus of the amygdala and in the hippocampal CA3 and CA1 pyramidal cell layer are affected.

6. Generalized-absence seizures

Thalamic stimulation

The concept of a thalamic reticular formation is able to influence wide areas of cortex. Stimulation of midline and intralaminar thalamus can produce absence and EEG spike-waves. The role of thalamus versus cortex in the generation of absence epilepsy remains a subject of great interest and controversy. The thalamic stimulation model for petit mal is, however, infrequently used because of the need for chronic electrode implantation, and for ongoing stimulation during testing.

Bilateal cortical foci

Models of petit mal produced by bilateral cortical foci derive from the hypothesis that absence epilepsy is a result of diffuse cortical dysfunction. Application of dilute convulsants such as estrogen, PTZ, and penicillin to widespread regions of cat cortex produces bursts. A similar model can be produced in rhesus monkeys.

Systemic penicillin

Intramuscular injection of 300,000 units/kg of penicillin G into a cat results in recurrent episodes of arrested activity, staring, myoclonus, facial-oral twitching and occasional progression to generalized tonic-clonic seizures. Seizure activity begins about 1 h after injection of drug and continues intermittently for 6-8 h. The EEG shows a variety of spike-wave morphologies, emerging from a relatively normal background. These features are similar to those seen with clinical absence, except of course that clinical absence recurs apparently spontaneously for years.

Clinical absence (petit mal) epilepsy has been hypothesized to originate subcortically, with participation of brainstem and thalamic reticular formation. Absence seizures in the feline penicillin model have been difficult to reconcile with this hypothesis. Application of penicillin to wide regions of cortex, but no to thalamus, can produce SW EEG discharges. Discharges in this model probably originate cortically, but are maintained and elaborated by recurrent thalamo-cortical circuitry.

Intraventricular opiates

Low dose morphine sulfate is believed to be anticonvulsant, but high dose parenteral morphine can induce clonic convulsions in rodents. The behavioral-EEG pattern after intraventricular opiates can be classified either with the complex partial or the absence models of the epilepsies. Relation to petit mal epilepsy has been supported by ontogenetic studies of opiate-induced seizures and by thr relatively specific responsiveness of these seizures to anti-petit mal agents.

7. Status epilepticus

Status epilepticus is a condition characterized by an epileptic seizure that is sufficiently prolonged or repeated at sufficiently brief intervals. Certain research questions require models of recurrent seizures or status epilepticus. Many of the chemical convulsants able to produce seizures-for example, KA, flurothyl, bicuculline, and PTZ can also produce status epilepticus when administered in large quantities to rodents.

Lithium-pilocarpine

One recently popularized model of status epilepticus is the lithium-pilocarpine model. In this model rats are pretreated with lithium chloride. At least 20 h later the cholinergic agent pilocarpine is given. Generalize clonic or tonic-clonic seizure activity begins about 30 min after administration of pilocarpine, and continues for several hours. The EEG pattern displays a progression very similar to the stages seen in human status epilepticus. Chronic pretreatment for one month with daily lithium reduces the convulsant threshold of pilocarpine 26-fold.

In lithium-pilocarpine treated adult rats, neuronal damage and neuronal death develops mainly in the hippocampus, the hilus of the dentate gyrus, the piriform and entorhinal cortices, the amygdala, the neocortex and the thalamus. Also, lithium-pilocarpine treatment leads to hippocampal damage that is typically observed in the CA1 and CA3 pyramidal cell layers and the hilus of the dentate gyrus in mice with status epilepticus.

Cobalt-homocystine

Another drug combination able to induce status epilepticus in animals is focal cobalt in conjunction with systemic homocysteine. Homocysteine is an agent able on its own to produce powerful tonic-clonic seizures. This model also has the advantage of a "focus" for frequently recurring seizures.

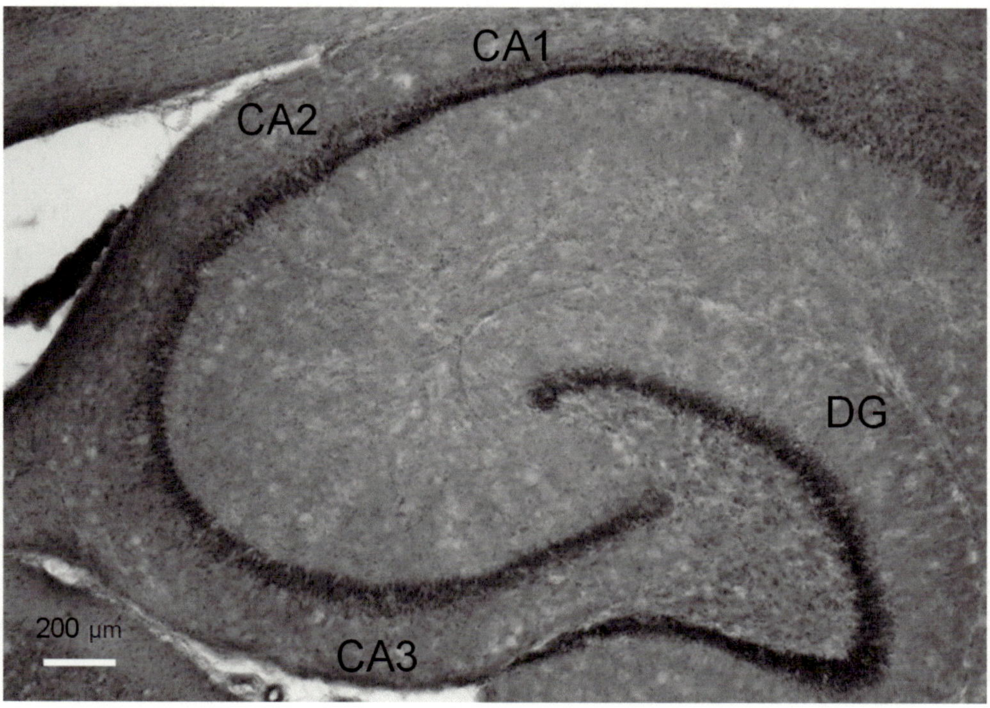

Fig. 1. A representative image for rat hippocampus CA1, CA2 and CA3 subfields. CA1: hippocampus CA field, CA2: hippocampus CA2 field, CA3: hippocampus CA3 field, DG: dentate gyrus, Hematoxylene and eosin stain, 4X magnification, scale bar = 200 μm.

Recurrent stimulation

Several electrical paradigms have been suggested as a recipe for producing status epilepticus in rats.

8. Conclusion

Epilepsy is a group of neurological disorders characterized by clinical aspects, not an only specific disease. Seizures are outward signs of epilepsy and occur from time to time. A wide variety of models have been developed in order to explore the principal mechanisms of epilepsies, develop more effective anti-epileptic drugs epilepsy and determine the pathological events underlying different types of epileptic seizures. Summary of the results so far obtained from these models:

1. There is not only one model for answering all questions about epilepsy.
2. Studies performed by using experimental models, can only explore the basic mechanisms of the model which is used.
3. Some chemical convulsants can induce more than one epilepsy model. Crystallized penicillin can induce simple partial, generalized myoclonic, generalized tonic-clonic and generalized absence epilepsy when given in different ways. Therefore, EEG and behavior should be analyzed to determine the induced model.
4. Kindling has become one of the most popular models to investigate neurochemical and structural long-term changes in brain.
5. It is not sufficient to use one or a few model in studies of epilepsy. Constantly new and better models should be developed to find the best model that answers the question.
6. Various models should be used constantly to investigate the issues such as the molecular mechanisms, genetic background, ion channels and related molecules in the cell membrane, second messenger systems.

Thus, the basic mechanisms of epilepsy will be better understood, more effective drugs and treatments will be developed for the type of epileptic seizures.

9. References

[1] Adıguzel. E., Akdogan, I., Duzcan, S.E., Tufan, A.C. (2002). Effect of penicillin induced epilepsy seizure on granulare cell layer of dentate gyrus in rat: A stereological study. *Neuroscience Research Communications*, 31(2): 101-109.

[2] Akdogan, I., Adıguzel, E., Akyer, P. (2003). Penisilinle epilepsi oluşturulan sıçanlarda gyrus dentatus granuler hücre tabakasındaki hacim değişiklikleri. *Epilepsi*, 9(2): 67-72.

[3] Akdogan, I., Adiguzel, E., Yilmaz, I., Ozdemir, M.B., Sahiner, M., Tufan, A.C. (2008). Penicillin-induced epilepsy model in rats: dose-dependant effect on hippocampal volume and neuron number. *Brain Research Bulletin*. 77(4): 172-177.

[4] Akdogan, I., Unal, N., Adıguzel, E. (2002). Estimation of the number of neurons in the hippocampus of rats with penicillin induced epilepsy. *Image Analysis and Stereology*, 21: 117-120.

[5] Andre, V., Dube C., Francois, J., Leroy, C., Rigoulot, M., Roch C., Namer I.J., Nehlig A. (2007). Pathogenesis and pharmacology of epilepsy in the Lithium-pilocarpine model. *Epilepsia*, 48: 41-47.

[6] Atillo, A., Söderfeldt, B., Kalimo, H., Olsson, Y., Siesjö, B.K. (1983). Pathogenesis of brain lesions caused by experimental epilepsy. Light- and electron-microscopic changes in the rat hippocampus following bicuculline-induced status epilepticus. *Acta Neuropathology (Berl)*. 59(1): 11-24.

[7] Azcoitia, I., Sierra, A., Garcia-Segura, L.M. (1998). Estradiol prevents kainic acid-induced neuronal loss in the rat dentate gyrus. *Neuroreport*. 9: 3075-3079.

[8] Bagetta, G., Knott, C., Nistico, G., Bowery, N.G. (1990). Tetanus toxin produces neuronal loss and a reduction in GABAA but not GABAB binding sites in rat hippocampus. *Neuroscience Letters*. 109: 7-12.

[9] Bagetta, G.,Nistico, G., Bowery, N.G. (1990). Prevention by the NMDA receptor antagonist, MK801 of neuronal loss produced by tetanus toxin in the rat hippocampus. *British Journal of Pharmacology*, 101: 776-780.

[10] Becker, A., Braun, H., Schroder, H., Grecksch, G., Hollt, V. (1999). Effects of enadoline on the development of pentylenetetrazol kindling, learning performance, and hippocampal morphology. *Brain Research*, 823: 191–197.

[11] Bertram, E.H., Lothman, E.W. (1993). Morphometric effects of intermittent kindled seizures and limbic status epilepticus in the dentate gyrus of the rat. *Brain Research*. 603(1): 25-31.

[12] Biziere, K., Chambon, J.P. (1987). Modeles Animaux D'epilepsie et Crises Experimentales, *Rev. Neurol. (Paris)*. 143: 329–340.

[13] Bolkvadze, T.A., Dzhaparidze, N.D., Zhvaniya, M.G., Bikashvili, T.Z., Chilachava, L.R. (2008). Kindling-induced hippocampal cell death in rats. *Neuroscience and Behavioral Physiology*. 38(4): 359-362.

[14] Briellmann, R.S., Wellard, R.M., Jackson, G.D. (2005). Seizure-associated abnormalities in epilepsy: evidence from MR imaging. *Epilepsia*, 46(5): 760-766.

[15] Buckmaster, P.S., Dudek, F.E. (1997). Neuron loss, granule cell axon reorganization, and functional changes in the dentate gyrus of epileptic kainate-treated rats. *Journal of Comperative Neurology*. 385: 385-404.

[16] Celada, P., Paladini, C.A., Tepper, J.M. (1999). GABAergic control of rat substantia nigra dopaminergic neurons: role of globus pallidus and substantia nigra pars reticulata. Neuroscience. 89(3): 813-825.

[17] Chang, J.H., Yang, X.F., Zempel, J.M., Rothman, S.M. (2004). The unilateral cobalt wire model of neocortical epilepsy: a method of producing subacute focal seizures in rodents. *Epilepsy Research*. 61: 153-160.

[18] Fang, F., Lei, H. (2010). Increased hippocampal T2 in a rat model of pentylenetetrazol-induced kindling correlates with seizure scores. *Journal of Neurological Sciences*. 292: 16-23.

[19] Fisher, R.S. (1989). Animal models of the epilepsies. *Brain Research Reviews*. 14: 245-278.

[20] Kienzler, F., Norwood, B.A., Sloviter, R.S. (2009). Hippocampal injury, atrophy, synaptic reorganization, and epileptogenesis after perforant pathway stimulation-induced status epilepticus in the mouse. *Journal of Comperative Neurology*.515(2): 181-196.

[21] Kim, S.W., Yu, Y.M., Piao, C.S., Kim, J.B., Lee, J.K. (2004). Inhibition of delayed induction of p38 mitogen-activated protein kinase attenuates kainic acid-induced neuronal loss in the hippocampus. *Brain Research*.1007: 188-191.

[22] Lindsay, K.W., Bone, I., Callender, R. (1997). Neurology and Neurosurgery Illustrated, Third ed., Churchill Livingstone, Edinburgh, London, Philadelphia, p. 88.

[23] Marangoz, C. (1997). Deneysel epilepsi modelleri. OMU Tıp Dergisi, 14 (3): 147-186.

[24] Matsuoka, Y., Okazaki, M., Takata, K., Kitamura, Y., Ohta, S., Sekino, Y., Taniguchi, T. (1999). Endogenous adenosine protects CA1 neurons from kainic acid-induced neuronal cell loss in the rat hippocampus. *The European Journal of Neuroscience.* 11: 3617-3625.

[25] McCord MC, Lorenzana A, Bloom CS, Chancer ZO, Schauwecker PE. (2008). Effect of age on kainate-induced seizure severity and cell death. *Neuroscience*. 154: 1143-1153.

[26] Müller, C.J., Bankstahl, M., Gröticke, I., Löscher, W. (2009). Pilocarpine vs. lithium-pilocarpine for induction of status epilepticus in mice: development of spontaneous seizures, behavioral alterations and neuronal damage. *European Journal of Pharmacology*, 619: 15-24.

[27] Schubert, M., Siegmund, H., Pape, H.C., Albrecht, D. (2005). Kindling-induced changes in plasticity of the rat amygdala and hippocampus. *Learning and Memory*. 12: 520-526.

[28] Sharma, A.K., Jordan, W.H., Reams, R.Y., Hall, D.G., Snyder, P.W. (2008). Temporal profile of clinical signs and histopathologic changes in an F-344 rat model of kainic acid-induced mesial temporal lobe epilepsy. *Toxicologic Pathology*. 36(7): 932-943.

[29] Tooyama, I., Bellier, J.P., Park, M., Minnasch, P., Uemura, S., Hisano, T., Iwami, M., Aimi, Y., Yasuhara, O., Kimura, H. (2002). Morphologic study of neuronal death, glial activation, and progenitor cell division in the hippocampus of rat models of epilepsy. *Epilepsia*, 43 (9): 39-43.

[30] Toth, Z., Yan, X.X., Haftoglou, S., Ribak, C.E., Baram, T.Z. (1998). Seizure-induced neuronal injury: vulnerability to febrile seizures in an immature rat model. *Journal of Neuroscience*.18(11): 4285-4294.

[31] Williams, P.L. (Ed.) (1995). Gray's Anatomy. Thirty eighth Edition, Churchill Livingstone, New York, Edinburgh, London, Tokyo, Madrid, Melbourne.

[32] Wolf, O.T., Dyakin, V., Patel, A., Vadasz, C., de Leon, M.J., McEwen, B.S., Bulloch, K. (2002). Volumetric structural magnetic resonance imaging (MRI) of the rat hippocampus following kainic acid (KA) treatment, *Brain Research*. 934: 87–96.

[33] Yin, H.Z., Sensi, S.L., Ogoshi, F., Weiss, J.H. (2002). Blockade of Ca2+-permeable AMPA/kainate channels decreases oxygen-glucose deprivation-induced Zn2+ accumulation and neuronal loss in hippocampal pyramidal neurons. *Journal of Neuroscience*. 22(4): 1273-1279.

16

Two Types of Epilepsy Models and Processes of Cognition: Pentylenetetrazole Kindling and Absence Epilepsy of WAG/Rij Rats Strain

A. S. Bazyan
Institute of Higher Nervous Activity and Neurophysiology
Russian Academy of Science, Moscow
Russia

1. Introduction

In many studies a fundamental difference between two types of generalized epileptic activity, convulsive epilepsy and absence non-convulsive epilepsy was described. All forms of convulsive epilepsy, both in human and animal models, are characterized by increased activity of excitatory amino acid transmitter systems (Hara et al., 2006; Leke et al., 2006; Schilling et al., 2006) and/or decreased activity of the inhibitory GABAergic system (Bazyan et al., 2001b; Quilichini et al., 2006; Laschet et al., 2007) of the brain. The main difference between absence non convulsive epilepsy and convulsive epilepsy is in a fact that pharmacological stimulation or inhibition of excitatory glutamate synaptic transmission causes relative enhancement or reduction of the severity of absence epilepsy (Ngomba et al., 2005; Citraro et al., 2006), and increased GABAergic inhibition also leads to enhanced absence epilepsy (Coenen et al., 1995; Bouwman et al., 2003; 2004).

The next fundamental difference between absence epilepsy and other generalized epilepsy forms consists in the profile of epileptic discharge. Usually, convulsive epileptic discharges appear on the wave of excitation. The gradual growth of excitation reaches the threshold level after which epileptic discharges appear. During absence epilepsy, the discharge is fundamentally different. A spike-wave discharge consists of an inhibitory phase and an action potential. The inhibitory phase is represented by a slow wave on an EEG. The spike is an indicator of cell excitation (action potential). A rebound spike appears at the end of the inhibitory period, and the cycle repeats again and again (Midzianovskaya et al., 2001).

In this paper we compared mechanisms underlying two kinds of epileptic activity, pentylenetetrazole kindling and absence epilepsy, and their interaction with processes of learning, memory, emotional and motivational states.

2. Pharmacological reminders restore benzodiazepine site density of $GABA_A$ receptors and conditioned memory: Allosteric plasticity and intraneuronal integration by the help of transduction signal

Interaction of BDZ with its own site activates slow endocellular metabolic reactions through activation of protein kinase C (Niles et al., 1997; Nomura et al., 1997; Johnston et al., 1998), induces transductional signal and modifies genes expression. In this connection $GABA_A$ receptor subunit protein expression is reduced (Johnston et al., 1998), while the c-fos gene expression is induced (Niles et al., 1997). Neuroactive steroids are analogs of steroid hormones, but unlike them they interact with somatodendritic and postsynaptic $GABA_A$ receptors (Rupprecht, Holsdoer 1999). Interaction of neuroactive steroids with $GABA_A$ receptor triggers a process of oxygenation, which transforms some endocellular metabolites into ligands of endocellular steroid receptors. After linkage of ligands with receptors an expression of genes occurs.

Thus, BDZ site of the $GABA_A$ receptor induces intracellular slow metabolic reactions via a protein kinase C-dependent mechanism (Niles et al., 1997; Nomura et al., 1997; Johnston et al., 1998; Ghori et al., 2010; Bignante et al., 2010). In the first part of our study (Bazyan et al., 2001b) we investigated long-term components, apparently metabolic components of $GABA_A$ supramolecular complex in convulsive states, specifically, long-term characteristics of [^{3}H]-diazepam binding in the cerebellar cortex after an acute injection of PTZ in convulsive doses.

Acute PTZ treatment

Male Wistar rats were used. The first series comprised the rats endogenously sensitive and resistant to the PTZ. In PTZ-sensitive animals, seizures provoked a significant decrease in the B_{max} of [^{3}H]-diazepam binding by 16% versus control and by 14% versus resistant rats at 30 minutes after the termination of seizures, with no change in the K_d. No differences in [^{3}H]-diazepam binding between the control and resistant rats at 1 hour after the PTZ treatment and the control, sensitive and resistant rats on day 7 after the PTZ treatment were found. These results show that initially the characteristics of [^{3}H]-diazepam binding to BDZ site in the sensitive and resistant rats were similar, but the PTZ treatment induced a greater response of BDZ receptors in sensitive rats versus resistant rats. It means that sensitive animals show more intensive allosteric regulation of BDZ site of $GABA_A$ receptor by PTZ than resistant rats. On day 7 the characteristics of [^{3}H]-diazepam binding came back to the initial level. This type of reaction reflected the efficiency of BDZ site allosteric regulation by PTZ as opposed to "initial activity", when the characteristics of diazepam binding are different initially.

The second series comprised the rats, in which a convulsive dose of PTZ (50 mg/kg) resulted in seizure scores of 4 to 5 points. They were sacrificed 1 hour or 48 hours later and on day 7 after the PTZ treatment. The density (B_{max}) of [^{3}H]-diazepam binding sites was significantly reduced by 19% at 1 hour after the PTZ treatment and by 16% at 48 hours with no change in the K_d. No significant changes were found on day 7.

PTZ-induced kindling. Acquired sensitivity

The third series comprised the rats, in which a subconvulsive dose of PTZ (20 mg/kg, once daily for 24 days) elicited kindled seizures scoring 4 to 5 points. They were sacrificed 1 hour or 48 hours later and on day 7 after the last injection. The rats with kindled seizures scoring 4 to 5 points were selected from the total population of animals. Daily injections of PTZ (20 mg/kg) resulted in a gradual increase in sensitivity to PTZ (Bazyan et al., 2001b) and a significant decrease in the B_{max} of [^{3}H]-diazepam binding by 19% at 1 hour after the PTZ treatment and by 16% at 48 hours after the last injection. The binding K_d was unchanged. On day 7, no significant changes were observed (Fig. 1A). These findings in the kindled rats are similar to the results found after an acute administration of the convulsive dose. Thus, kindling led to the establishment of a new level of the BDZ site allosteric regulation by PTZ, because PTZ interacts with PCT site and modifies binding of [^{3}H]-diazepam with BDZ site.

The high efficiency of the BDZ receptor allosteric regulation, which is produced by administering PTZ daily at subconvulsive doses, is termed "allosteric plasticity". This procedure induces a long-term, high sensitivity to low PTZ doses, which is determined by the decreasing of BDZ site density in the cerebellar cortex that occurs 48 hours after the termination of PTZ treatment with no change in the K_d, and subsequent normalization on day 7 (Fig. 1A), therefore, the allosteric plasticity formed the basis for the development of high sensitivity to PTZ.

It is known that kindling can lead to a long-term decrease of the $GABA_A$ receptor complex density, due to changes in the synthesis of the respective proteins. A series of 40 kindling-induced seizures (by rapid hippocampal stimulation) led to biphasic alterations of $GABA_A$ receptor subunit mRNA levels in dentate gyrus with only minor changes in CA_1-CA_3 (Kokaia et al., 1994). Up to 4 hours after the last seizure the expression of mRNA for α1 subunit was slightly decreased in dentate gyrus, whereas marked reductions were observed for β3 and γ2 subunits. Between 12 and 48 hours there were major increases of α1 (by 59%) and γ2 (by 35%) subunits mRNA levels but no significant changes of β3 subunit mRNA expression. The subunits mRNA levels returned to control values in 5 days. These results are similar to ours (Fig. 1A). The biphasic changes of $GABA_A$ receptor subunits may be related to their recombination.

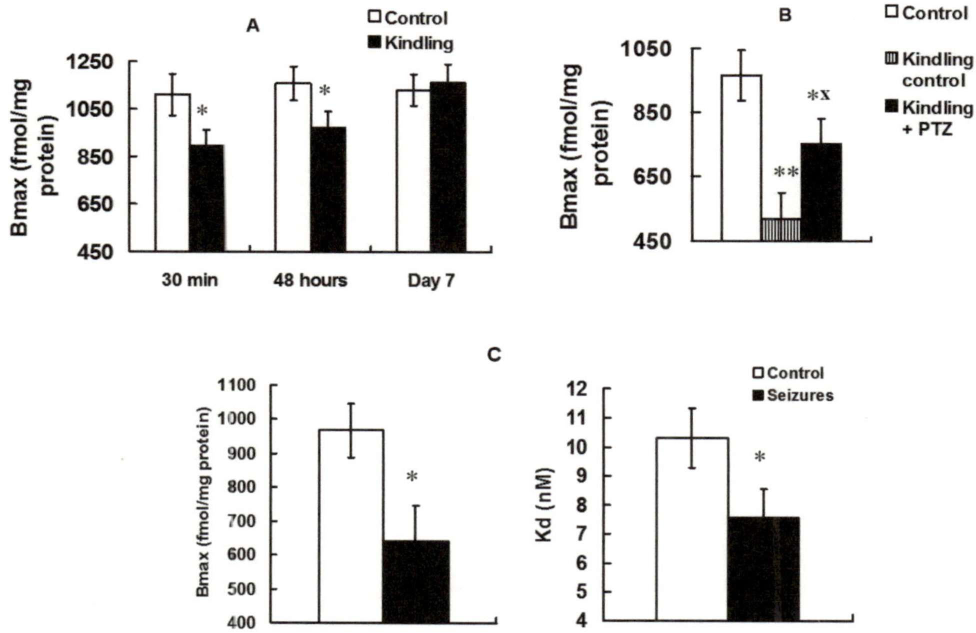

Fig. 1. Effects of chronic PTZ treatment and subsequent PTZ challenge on [^{3}H]-diazepam binding to membranes from the cerebellar cortex of 3- to 4-months and 10-months rats. **A**, BDZ site density (B_{max}) in 3- to 4-months-old rats kindled with PTZ at a dose of 20 mg/kg. *$p_t < 0.05$ versus control (n = 6 in each group). **B**, BDZ site density (B_{max}) in 10-months-old kindled rats challenged with PTZ (+ PTZ) at a dose of 30 mg/kg. **$p_t < 0.01$, kindled versus control; *$p_t < 0.05$, kindled + PTZ versus control; $^x p_t < 0.05$, kindled + PTZ versus kindled control (n = 6 in each group). **C**, BDZ site density (B_{max}) and affinity (K_d) in 10-months-old rats after acute seizures induced by PTZ at a dose of 30 mg/kg. *$p_t < 0.05$ versus control (n = 6 in each group).

After 6 months (about 10-months-old rats)

For the period of 6 months both the control and kindled rats were kept in the breeding facility. At the second stage, the persistence of kindling was studied. Two control groups and two groups of kindled rats were treated with 20 and 30 mg/kg PTZ (Bazyan et al., 2001b). The kindling response of high sensitivity to low PTZ doses was preserved through the 6-months rest period after the kindling treatment, but not completely and with some attenuation. A subconvulsive dose of PTZ (20 mg/kg) induced no seizures in the control rats but elicited seizures in 60% of the kindled rats (1 to 2 points). At the next dose of PTZ (30 mg/kg) seizures were observed in 56% of the control rats (maximal scores of 2 to 3 points) and in 100% of the kindled rats (maximal scores of 3 to 4 points).

For the study of [^{3}H]-diazepam binding four groups of animals were used (Bazyan et al., 2001b): 1) control rats, no PTZ challenge; 2) acute seizures control rats, 30 min after the termination of acute seizures (2 to 3 points) induced by a PTZ (30 mg/kg) challenge; 3) kindled control rats, no PTZ challenge, but with a history of seizures (4 to 5 points) 6 months ago; 4) kindling + PTZ challenge, 1 hour (30 min after the termination of seizures, 3 to 4 points) induced by a PTZ (30 mg/kg) challenge.

In the kindled control rats with a history of seizures (4 to 5 points) 6 months before, the B_{max} of [^{3}H]-diazepam binding was reduced to 54% with no change in K_d without a PTZ challenge (Fig. 1B). It was shown above that the development of kindling represented the development of allosteric plasticity. But 6 months later the BDZ site activity was found to be modified. We may suggest, therefore, that allosteric plasticity is an intracellular process and the decrease in BDZ site density 6 months after the kindling reflected an ongoing intracellular process.

After a PTZ challenge, the B_{max} of [^{3}H]-diazepam binding in the kindled rats was found to be enhanced to 78%, still being significantly lower than in the control rats, with no change in the K_d. This paradoxical finding can be logically explained as follows. At the time of termination of kindling (Fig. 1A), the BDZ site density is reduced to 80.97% versus the control 4-months-old rats. After a rest period of 6 months, there was a decrease in BDZ sity density to 53.57% in the kindled rats without a PTZ challenge. Acute PTZ administration to the kindled rats induced seizures and partially restored the BDZ site density, just to the level of BDZ density found in the control 10-months-old rats (77.77%, Fig. 1B), which was established 6 months before. At the same time, the K_d of BDZ site binding was unchanged in the kindled rats, whereas in the control 10-months-old rats that had seizures after a single PTZ challenge BDZ receptors density B_{max} and K_d was significantly altered. The PTZ (30 mg/kg) challenge in the ten-months-old intact rats resulted in seizures (acute seizures, scores 2 to 3 points) which were accompanied by a decrease in both indices of [^{3}H]-diazepam binding: the B_{max} to 66%, and the K_d to 73% (Fig. 1C). We suggest that the PTZ challenge acted as a reminder to the kindled animals, reproducing the modification of BDZ site acquired 6 months ago, irrespective of their current status and animal's age.

The increased density of BDZ site of $GABA_A$ receptors (versus the kindled control) can be interpreted as an enhancement of GABAergic inhibition, while it is thought that seizures are based on the process of neuronal hyperactivation accompanied by a reduction in the BDZ site density both in kindling-induced (Fig. 1A) and single-dose PTZ-induced seizures. Therefore, it is likely that at 6 months, when seizures are retrieved by a PTZ challenge and the level of GABAergic inhibition is restored, the level of glutamate receptors may also be restored, assuming that they were modified and consolidated in the process of kindling 6 months ago. The level of glutamate receptors may only be restored of neuronal GABA and glutamate receptors interact within a single integrated system interconnected through intracellular transduction signal.

The interaction and integration of neuronal GABA and glutamate receptors has been shown in several studies. Thus, in PTZ-induced kindling the reduction in GABAergic functions is blocked by MK-801, an antagonist of NMDA receptors (Corda et al., 1992). NMDA receptors are involved in the process of kindling induced by FG 7142, an inverse agonist of the BDZ receptor (Stephens & Turski, 1993). Also, the NMDA-induced long-term potentiation is found to be controlled by the intercellular metabolic systems of the $GABA_A$ receptor complex, being inhibited by BDZ site agonists (Evans & Viola-McCabe, 1996; Higashima et al., 1998) and facilitated by its antagonists (Stackman et al., 1996; Seabrook et al., 1997). Positive allosteric activation of $GABA_A$ receptors bi-directionally modulates hippocampal glutamate plasticity and behaviour (Shen et al., 2009). BDZ withdrawal anxiety is associated with potentiation of AMPA receptor currents in hippocampal CA1 pyramidal neurons attributable to increased synaptic incorporation of GluA1-containing AMPA receptors (Shen et al., 2010).

The differences in BDZ reaction between the PTZ-sensitive and PTZ-resistant rats (Bazyan 2001b) can be accounted for by differences in the intensity of allosteric regulation of the $GABA_A$ receptors, based on differences in their subunit composition. We propose, accordingly, that the acquisition of high level allosteric regulation by the kindled rats is best explained by the intracellular metabolic feedback mechanism which is schematically shown in Fig. 2. In this scheme, PTZ interacts with the PCT site of $GABA_A$ receptor and modifies the BDZ site and $GABA_A$ receptor, which in turn alter the concentration of second messengers. The second messengers can modify phosphorylation reactions by changing protein kinase activities. The cycle is closed by modifications of GABA and BDZ sites, leading to changes in density as well as some redistribution of their subunits. In the process of kindling the cycle is repeated again and again, resulting in further decreases of the $GABA_A$ receptor complex. Protein kinases can modify gene expression, acting via a secondary nuclear signal and altering the synthesis of the subunits forming the $GABA_A$ receptor complex, whereby the reduced density, redistribution of the receptor subunits and, ultimately, the acquired efficiency of allosteric regulation or allosteric plasticity are consolidated.

As indicated above, changes in cellular phosphorylation levels by protein kinases can modify glutamatergic receptors augmenting their responses to endogenous excitatory amino acids. The metabolic regulation of a glutamatergic synapse (Fig. 2) is similar to that described for hippocampal neurons (Mayford et al., 1995). We added a feedback loop for metabolic regulation controlled by NMDA receptors in the hippocampus or by mGlu1 receptors in the cerebellum, since we assume that the feedback metabolic regulation, or autoregulation of glutamatergic and GABAergic receptors, is a necessary condition for maintaining the processes of long-term potentiation and long-term depression. The regulation of AMPA receptors and autoregulation of NMDA receptors in the hippocampus have been studied experimentally (Bayazitov & Kleshchevnikov, 2000).

Thus, one can assume that plasticity is a result of cooperative activity of GABA and glutamatergic receptors integrated into interrelated system. Integration includes also automodification of receptors activity. Further, a new level of activity, produced by secondary intranuclear signals modifies genes expression and consolidates a newly developed activity of receptors.

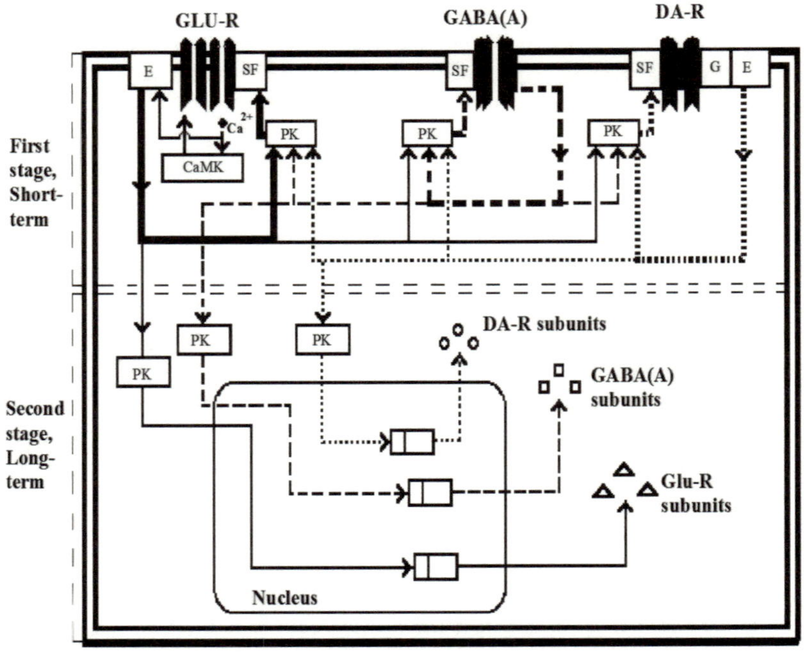

Fig. 2. A tentative model of intraneuronal metabolic integration. GLU-R, glutamatergic receptors; GABA(A), $GABA_A$ receptor; DA-R, dopamine receptor; E, second messenger synthesizing enzyme; SF, phosphorylation substrate; G, G-protein, PK, different type of protein kinases; CaMK, calcium/calmodulin-dependent protein kinase. Metabolic reactions mediated by glutamatergic receptors are shown as *solid lines*. Metabolic reactions mediated by $GABA_A$ receptor are shown as *dashed lines*. Metabolic reactions mediated by dopamine receptors are shown as *dotted lines*. Intracellular metabolic feedback loops (autoregulation) are shown as the respective *thick lines*. For other details, see in text.

Interaction of PTZ-induced seizures with learning, memory and emotional state

It is well known that a convulsive state is an amnesic state. It is also known that convulsive disorders are accompanied by mental disorders, such as anxiety and fear, or depressive states (Clement et al., 1997; Depaulis et al., 1997; Maxudova & Flesher, 1998). At the same time, anxiogenic effects of PTZ are also known [Biggio et al., 1990; Venault et al., 1992; Simon et al., 1993]. It was shown [Bazyan et al., 2000b] that haloperidol-induced catalepsy, which produces a long-term modification of DA receptors, is modified by defensive conditioning. So, the next investigation [Bazyan et al., 2001a] was designed to study the modification of seizures by learning; the facilitation of amnesic memory trace retrieval by a pharmacological reminder of the emotional state which accompanied the learning processes. Passive avoidance conditioning was performed (Bazyan et al., 2001a). The rats were divided into three groups according to their levels of learning: *group I* - high level of learning; *group II* - middle level of learning; *group III* - low level of learning. PTZ was injected 75 mg/kg and 50 mg/kg i.p. immediately after the learning session of group I and group II accordingly. Amnesia provoked by PTZ seizures was found on days 2. Unconditioned reminder acted as an unamnesic agent for group I and evoked memory retrieval on day 2. The effects of pharmacological reminder were studied in groups II and III on day 2 (Bazyan et al., 2001a).

After conditioning retrieval testing some rats in group II were treated with PTZ (30 mg/kg i.p.). The rats in which PTZ elicited seizures were excluded from further experiments. Haloperidol, a nonselective dopamine (DA) D_2 antagonist, was administered (0.25 mg/kg i.p.) to some rats in groups II and III. The amnestic effect of the convulsive PTZ dose of 50 mg/kg was canceled by a lower, subconvulsive doze of 30 mg/kg, as well as by haloperidol at a low doze of 0.25 mg/kg. The low doze of haloperidol 0.25 mg/kg facilitated memory retrieval in the animals of group III. At the same time, this doze of haloperidol had no effect on the latency of moving into the dark compartment in untrained animals. The effects of a low dose of haloperidol were studied in a separate series of experiments. Rats were treated with haloperidol (0.25 mg/kg, i.p.). Haloperidol at 0.25 mg/kg provoked "freezing". Catalepsy was not shown. Herewith, the rats showed the typical pose of fear (hunched), the number of dejections was also increased (Bazyan et al., 2001a). Thus, the amnesic memory trace is expected to be reproduced by chemicaly different anxiogens, such as haloperidol. Hence the mechanism of reflex retrieval is related to the mechanism of emotional state retrieval.

The mesocorticolimbic DA system is a reward and reinforcement system, directly involved in learning and memory (Wise, 1978, 2009; Joseph et al., 2003; Bazyan, & Grigoryan, 2006). The nigrostriatal DA system basically controls activity of GABA and glutamatergic receptors of middle spiny neurons of dorsal striatum, which regulates a motor function (Greengard, et al., 1999; Mink, 2003). Also, the DA system is involved in the modification of various epileptiform states (Al Tajir & Starr, 1991; Ogren & Pakh, 1993; Amabeoku & Chikuni, 1994). The results shown in our work (Bazyan et al., 2000b), allow us to suggest that in the process of learning the receptors of the DA system and $GABA_A$ receptors of the brain interact and become modified and integrated, thus forming a learning-depended emotional state. We suggest that this integration is accomplished by the mechanism of intracellular integration of glutamate, $GABA_A$ and DA receptors by means of transduction signal. The intracellular integration by transduction signal of glutamate, $GABA_A$ and DA receptors is schematically shown in Fig. 2. DA receptors can undergo automodification by the metabotropic feedback loop and then modify the activity of glutamate and $GABA_A$ receptors by intracellular phosphorylation [Greengard et al., 1999]. Via the same reactions of intracellular phosphorylation, glutamate and $GABA_A$ receptors can control the efficiency of DA receptors. At the second stage, the modifications established at the first stage are consolidated through the modification of expression of the respective genes. The ability of DA receptors to undergo automodifications has been demonstrated both at the level of radioligand binding and at the level of gene expression in various brain structures and various experimental procedures (Soghomonian, 1993; Qin & Weiss, 1994; Richtand et al., 2010).

Thus, PTZ induced seizures cause amnesia and dissociation state. Low subconvulsive PTZ doses restore a memory trace. Low PTZ doses have also anxiogenic effect. As active avoidance is based on anxiogenic state it may be restored by induction of the anxiogenic state by PTZ. Haloperidol, another anxiogenic compound in low subcataleptic doses is able to restore an amnesic memory trace. It seems that DA receptors are also involved in endocellular integration together with GABA and glutamatergic receptors and all rules of endocellular integration described for GABA and glutamatergic receptors are also applied for DA receptors.

3. Absence epilepsy of WAG/Rij rat's strain

Absence epilepsy in men and in WAG/Rij (Wistar Albino Glaxo, from Rijswijk) rats is a genetic animal model of generalized human absence epilepsy (Midzianovskaya et al., 2001;

Van Luitelaar & Coenen, 1997; Meeren et al., 2002), which principally differs from convulsive forms of epilepsy. For example, a number of widely used anticonvulsants enhance absence epilepsy (Coenen et al., 1995; Hosford & Wang, 1997; Bouwman et al., 2003; 2004; Maris et al., 2006; Tolmacheva & van Luijtelaar, 2007). A series of spontaneous spike-wave discharges (SWD) induced by hyperpolarization appear on a normal EEG. The SWDs in EEG of WAG/Rij rats start at about 2-3 months. At the age of six months, all rats have several hundred SWDs per day. The generalized and widespread bilaterally presented synchronous SWDs are the result of highly synchronized oscillations in the thalamocortical network. SWDs have a local cortical origin in the perioral region of the somatosensory cortex (Meeren et al., 2002; 2009; van Luijtelaar & Sitnikova, 2006). Besides, there is another strain of rats with absence epilepsy deduced GAERS (Genetic Absence Epilepsy Rats from Strasbourg) similar to WAG/Rij rats.

There are two other features, which make WAG/Rij rats as a valid model of human absence epilepsy: 1) The changed expression of genes coding low threshold Ca^{2+} channel of T - type ($I_{Ca,T}$) of WAG/Rij compared to ACI control rats (Broicher, et al., 2008) and mutation of genes coding $I_{Ca,T}$ by people with absence epilepsy (Vitko et al., 2007; Arias-Olguín, et al., 2008); 2) Local variations of $GABA_A$ receptors subunit expression in thalamo-cortical systems (Liu, et al., 2007) of WAG/Rij rats and mutation of genes coding subunits of $GABA_A$ receptors in people with absence epilepsy (Bowser, et al., 2002; Kang & Macdonald, 2004).

Chlorine conductance of the $GABA_A$ receptor at absence epilepsy and PTZ kindling

In the study [Rebrov et al., 2007], we determined the features of the functional activity of the $GABA_A$ receptor (intensity of chloride current) in WAG/Rij rats with a genetic predisposition to absence epilepsy and Wistar rats at an early stage of kindling development (absence epilepsy) and after kindling (generalized tonic–clonic seizures). Muscimol was found to dramatically increase $^{36}Cl^-$ conductivity in synaptoneurosomes of the brain cortex after its addition to the incubation medium as compared to the basal level in all groups of animals. We found a fundamental difference between the muscimol-induced $^{36}Cl^-$ conductivity of synaptoneurosomes from the brain cortex (frontal and somatosensory areas) of the convulsive PTZ-treated Wistar rats and WAG/Rij rats with absence epilepsy. Development of the tonic–clonic kindling induced a significant decrease in muscimol-induced $^{36}Cl^-$ conductivity in neocortical synaptoneurosomes as compared to the control rats. The muscimol-induced $^{36}Cl^-$ conductivity of synaptoneurosomes from the somatosensory and frontal cortex of the control WAG/Rij rats was considerably higher than in the control Wistar rats.

The high muscimol-induced $^{36}Cl^-$ conductivity in the neocortical synaptoneurosomes of the WAG/Rij rats corresponds to the hyperpolarization-induced nature of spike-wave discharges in absence epilepsy (Inoue et al., 1993; Midzianovskaya et al., 2001; Meeren et al., 2002; 2009; Maris et al., 2006) and the presence of a cortical focus in the somatosensory cortex (Meeren et al., 2002; 2009; van Luijtelaar & Sitnikova, 2006). This proposal agrees with the pharmacological results that describe regulation of spike-wave discharges by activation or inhibition of WAG/Rij rats GABA system (Peeters et al., 1989; 1990; Coenen et al., 1995; Hosford & Wang, 1997; Bouwman et al., 2003; 2004; Maris et al., 2006; Tolmacheva, van Luijtelaar, 2007). Our results, obtained in animals with nonconvulsive kindling, which is an experimental model of absence epilepsy (Caddick & Hosford, 1996; Snead 1996; 1998), also point to an increase in the activity of the $GABA_A$ receptor via intensification of the chlorine current.

Thus, two types of generalized seizures are accompanied by opposing changes in the $GABA_A$-mediated $^{36}Cl^-$ conductivity inside neocortical synaptoneurosomes. $^{36}Cl^-$ conductivity decreased in rats with PTZ-induced convulsive kindling and increased in rats with a genetic predisposition to nonconvulsive absence epilepsy.

Cognitive processes in WAG/Rij rats

Learning and memory

It is known that SWDs are controlled by the DA-ergic system of the brain. Antagonists of D2 DA receptors increase and agonists decrease of SWDs (De Bruin et al., 2000; Deransart et al., 2000; Midzianovskaya et al., 2001). It is possible the opioid system of brain also controls SWDs (Lason et al., 1990; 1992; 1994a; 1994b; 1995; Przewlocka et al., 1995). It is very well known that the mesocorticolimbic DA-ergic system is the system of reinforcement; it actualizes an emotional positive state and is also involved in processes of learning and memory (Wise, 1978, 2009; Joseph et al., 2003; Bazyan, & Grigoryan, 2006). The opioid system controls the threshold of pain sensitivity and actualizes the motivation of escape and avoidance of pain (Baranauskas, & Nistri, 1998; Bazyan, et al., 2000a;). An infringement of WAG/Rij rat's behavior was shown (Bazyan et al., 2000c; Sarkisova and Kulikov, 2000). The decrease of memory reproduction, spontaneous catalepsy, low threshold of haloperidol-induced catalepsy and the actualization of depression were found in WAG/Rij rats. All these data can be explained by a DA deficit of WAG/Rij rat brain. The goal of the investigation (Getsova et al., 2003; 2004) was to study the possibility of WAG/Rij rat's behavior correction by pharmacological activation of DA-ergic system.

The procedure of passive avoidance is described above. The defensive conditioned reflex of two-way avoidance was established in a shuttle-box. There were three series of experiments. First series: disulfiram (25 mg/kg i.p.), inhibitor of dopamine-β-hydroxylase, was administered to Wistar and WAG/Rij rats 4 hours before the 1st day learning session. Second series: L-DOPA (25 mg/kg i.p.) was administered to Wistar and WAG/Rij rats 4 hours before the 1st learning session. In the 3rd series of experiment disulfiram (25 mg/kg i.p.) was administered immediately after 1st learning session in Wistar and WAG/Rij rats. Saline was administered i.p. in the same number of control Wistar and WAG/Rij rats. An amnesic reaction in control WAG/Rij rats versus control Wistar rats was found in day 2 of the passive avoidance conditioning procedure. The administration of disulfiram before as well as after passive avoidance conditioning increased the reflex reproduction on the next day after learning both in Wistar and WAG/Rij rats. The reproduction of passive avoidance memory was increased 1,34 and 1,41 times in Wistar rats and 4,21 and 4,89 times in WAG/Rij rats accordingly.

The administration of disulfiram 4 hours before establishment of active avoidance conditioning changed the learning processes in the first day. It was shown that control WAG/Rij rats realized 2,23 times more avoidance reactions than control Wistar rats in the first day of learning. Disulfiram administration before learning decreased the number of avoidance responses in the first day: in Wistar rats 1,47 times and in WAG/Rij rats 6,45 times. In the second day of learning an amnestic effect in control WAG/Rij rats versus control Wistar rats was found. The index of memory trace storage of WAG/Rij rats was 2,11 times lower than in Wistar rats. The administration of disulfiram increased the memory trace storage of Wistar rats in 1,44 times and in WAG/Rij rats 7,33 times. The other inductor of DA system activation, L-DOPA, a precursor of DA synthesis, was used for comparison. Synergic effects of disulfiram and L-DOPA administered 4 hours before learning were found. The administration of L-DOPA 4 hours before learning decreased the number of avoidances in the first day of learning in Wistar rats 1,76 times and in WAG/Rij rats 7,65 times. Herewith, the index of memory trace storage was increased in Wistar rats 1,82 times and in WAG/Rij rats 7,70 times. The high number of avoidances in WAG/Rij rats on the first day of active avoidance conditioning was found earlier (Bazyan et al., 2000c; 2001). We explain this reaction by the low efficiency of opioid system in WAG/Rij strain (Lason et al., 1990; 1992; 1994a; 1994b; 1995; Przewlocka et al., 1995) and as a consequence a low pain threshold and a high level of escape and avoidance motivation. It is shown (Altier & Stewart, 1998; 1999; Calabrese 2001) that activation of the DA-ergic system evokes analgesic reaction including activation of the opioid system (Suaudeau & Costentin, 1995; Cook et al., 2000; Magnusson & Fisher, 2000; Gao et al., 2001; Trekova et al., 2001). It was suggested that a deficit of dopaminergic system in WAG/Rij rats is the biological correlate of these behavioural deficits and that an enhanced sensitivity to DA-ergic agents is the consequence of this deficit.

DA activity in WAG/Rij rats

Further we studied some parameters of DA activity in WAG/Rij rats in attempt to find their deficiency. The goal of our first experiment (Midzianovskaya et al., 2004) was to investigate DA and its metabolites, DOPAC and HVA concentration in the following brain structures of Wistar and WAG/Rij rats: frontal cortex, parietal cortex, medulla, striatum, thalamus and cerebelum. Concentrations of DA and its metabolites have been defined by method of high performer's liquid chromatography. There was no difference in dopamine concentration in WAG/Rij versus to Wistar rats. But the changes of dopamine metabolites concentration and relation HVA/DA in some structures were substantially different for WAG/Rij and Wistar rats. There was a significant reduction of DOPAC concentration in striatum, and of HVA concentration in thalamus in SWDs rats. Reduction of metabolites concentration in the thalamus and striatum is related to enhancement of DA activity in these structures. The strengthening of DA activity may occur as compensation for DA deficiency at behavioural level. The deficiency of dopaminergic activity is likely to be linked with changes of DA receptors. In order to test such probability we compared (Birioukova et al., 2006) D_1 and D_2/D_3 DA receptors binding sites in some brain areas of WAG/Rij rats. DA receptors-binding sites were analysed using *in vitro* autoradiography.
A significant reduction of [^{3}H] SCH 23390 binding sites density with D_1 DA receptors of WAG/Rij rats compared to ACI rats in the shell of nucleus accumbens and in the head of caudate nucleus is seen. In other structures the significant changes are not observed. A significant increase of [^{3}H] spiperone binding sites density with D_2/D_3 DA receptors of WAG/Rij rats compared to ACI in motor, somatosensory and parietal cortex is seen. In the head of caudate nucleus and in the hippocampal CA3 area of WAG/Rij rats the [^{3}H] spiperone binding sites density with D_2/D_3 DA receptors is substantially lower than in the same structures of ACI rats. In the other structures there are no signifint differences on these measures. Our results show a deficiency of mesolimbic (NAcb shell) and mesocortical (motor, somatosensory and parietal cortex) DAergic activity at the level of somatodentritic D1- up-regulated and D2-like down-regulated DA receptors in WAG/Rij versus to ACI rats. At the same time a deficiency of nigrostriatal DAergic system in the head of caudate nucleus caused by reduction of D1-like DA receptors density is compensated by reduction of D2-like DA receptors density. The deficiency of mesocorticolimbic DA systems corresponds to behavioral features of WAG/Rij rats. During active and passive avoidance a

deficit of reinforcement in WAG/Rij rats has been revealed (Getsova et al., 2003; Getsova et al., 2004) which was eliminated by administration of the DA precursor, or a low doze of disulfiram, inhibitor of dopamine-β-hydroxylase, by increase of DA concentration in brain. Besides, there was shown that WAG/Rij rats have a higher level of depression than control Wistar rats without of absence epilepsy (Sarkisova et al., 2003; Sarkisova & Kulikov 2006). Depression of WAG/Rij rats has a DA-ergic nature (Sarkisova et al., 2008). The high depression of WAG/Rij rats may be explained by deficiency of the DA mesocorticolimbic system.

The question arises then. If the absence epilepsy is related with disturbance or mutation of $GABA_A$ receptor and low-threshold Ca^{2+} channel of T-type then what is a role of DA receptors in it. Why there is a functional deficiency of these receptors seen? We suggest that diminished activity of DA receptors and DA system deficit occur due to disruption of intracellular integration triggered by transductional signal (Fig. 2). The initial disruption of $GABA_A$ receptor activity disrupts transductional signal on the first stage induced by this receptor. Disruption of transductional signal changes modification of other receptors and their activity. On the second stage the disrupted activity of receptors is consolidated and stored by expression of genes. It should be noted that we did not practically see the changes of DA concentrations in structures investigated but could see the changes of receptors activity. So, a process of intracellular integration may disrupt activity of other neurotransmitter and neuromodulatory systems, for instance activity of opioide system disrupted in WAG/Rij rats (Lason et al., 1990; 1992: 1994a; 1994b; 1995; Przewlocka et al., 1995).

Our results (Birioukova et al., 2006; Rebrov et al., 2007) confirm the idea that absence epilepsy is connected with function of the hyperpolarization-induced cyclic nucleotide-gated pacemaker I_h channel, which subunits are expressed in thalamic neurons (Clapham, 1998). Recent studies have shown (Strauss, 2004) that subunits of I_h channel are expressed in neurons of the somatosensory cortex of WAG/Rij rats.

Hyperpolarization-activated *I*h pacemaker channel during absence epilepsy

Hyperpolarization-activated cyclic nucleotide-gated cationic I_h pacemaker channels maintain spontaneous periodic activation, which was discovered in the brain. In all, four isoforms of this channel are known (HCN1-HCN4, hyperpolarization-activated and cyclic nucleotide-gated) (Bazyan & Segal, 2010). The HCN channel is open at an average membrane potential of -80 mV. However, different subunits of the HCN channel possess different functional properties. For example, HCN1 channels become activated five to ten times faster than HCN2 channels. Also, HCN1 channels become activated at a membrane potential that is 20 mV more positive than the potential required for HCN2 activation. The HCN1 channel demonstrates minimal response to cAMP binding (+4 mV) to the cAMP-binding domain on the C-terminus (see Bazyan & Segal, 2010), whereas the HCN2 channel demonstrates a clear response (+17 mV). Coexpressed heteromultimeric channels demonstrate a relatively larger shift in response to cAMP (+14 mV).

The literature reviewed suggests that the I_h channel and low-threshold T-type Ca^{2+} channel ($I_{Ca2+,\ T}$) work in tandem (Bazyan, Segal, 2010). Hyperpolarization opens the I_h channel, and cationic current depolarizes the membrane to the threshold and induces a spike. Hyperpolarization also opens the $I_{Ca2+,\ T}$ channels. The entrance of Ca^{2+} ions into the cell induce Ca^{2+}-dependent cAMP synthesis, and cAMP dramatically increases channel activity through binding to the CNBD locus of HCN subunits. The HCN1 subunit responds weakly to cAMP binding, therefore, a decrease in the proportion of HCN1 subunits in the channel increases pacemaker activity and an increase in the proportion of HCN1 subunits in the channel decreases pacemaker activity.

Several studies have focused on I_h channel activity during absence epilepsy. The fast component of I_h activation in neurons of WAG/Rij rats was significantly reduced (a 50% decrease in the current density), and was four time slower than in the neurons of nonepileptic Wistar or ACI rats (Strauss et al., 2004). The results of Western blot and PCR analysis corresponded to a decreased I_h current. A decrease by 34% was found in the level of the HCN1 subunit protein in the cerebral cortex of WAG/Rij rats as compared to Wistar rats but HCN1 mRNA had stable expression. The protein and mRNA levels of the other three I_h channel subunits (HCN2-HCN4) were not altered (Strauss et al., 2004). These results suggest that there are substantially fewer HCN1 subunits in the combined complex of the I_h channel in WAG/Rij rats than in rats of the control strains. This fact allows one to make the assumption that these channels work substantially more slowly but possess higher activity than the I_h channels of Wistar and ACI rats. High activity is defined, for example, by insignificant modification of the HCN1 subunit after cAMP binding, whereas modification of the HCN2 subunit is stronger. This means that the increase in the proportion of the HCN1 subunit in the channel complex decreases its response to cAMP binding, and, in contrast, the channel with more HCN2 subunits and less HCN1 subunits in its composition functions better.

It has been already shown that neonatal handling and mother deprivation in the early childhood of WAG/Rij rats (during postnatal 1-21days) result in reduced seizures and decreased interspike interval and frequency spectrum power of spike-wave discharges of adult WAG/Rij rats (Schridde & van Luijtelaar, 2005). Whole cell patch-clamp recordings from the cells of the fifth pyramidal layer, in situ hybridization, and Western blot analysis of the cortex of adult WAG/Rij rats (Schridde et al., 2006) showed an increase in the HCN1 protein level in the somatosensory cortex of handled and mother-deprived rats as compared to control rats. This increase was selective for the HCN1 subunit and did not affect the expression of HCN2-HCN4 subunit proteins, neither did expression of the mRNA of any subunit (HCN2, HCN3, HCN4). These results indicate that relatively mild changes in the environment of neonatal rats have long-lasting consequences for paroxysm activity and suggest that increased concentration of the HCN1 subunit in I_h channel composition is related to reduced absence epileptic activity. It was demonstrated that genetic absence epilepsy is highly susceptible to early interventions that lead to increased I_h current and higher concentrations of the HCN1 subunit as compared to control rats. However, the level of mRNA and protein of HCN2, HCN3 and HCN4 subunits did not differ in control and WAG/Rij rats (Schridde et al., 2006). These results indicate that the I_h channel plays an important role in the generation of seizures in a specific small area of the somatosensory cortex, and may be simply explained by alterations in the subunit composition of I_h channel, namely, an increased proportion of HCN1 subunits.

4. Conclusion

We have described that efficiency of allosteric regulation depends on subunits structure of $GABA_A$ receptor. We came to conclusion that the subunits composition of $GABA_A$ receptor in sensitive and resistant rats is different. The results assume that allosteric plasticity of

$GABA_A$ receptor and its consolidation are related with modification of subunits expression which finally lead to modification of $GABA_A$ receptor subunits structure. PTZ induced seizures cause amnesia and dissociation state. Low subconvulsive PTZ doses restore a memory trace. Low PTZ doses have also anxiogenic effect. Haloperidol, another anxiogenic compound in low subcataleptic doses is able to restore an amnesic memory trace. The process of plasticity represents a cooperation and integration of GABA, glutamate and DA receptors into interdependent systems. Its integration includes automodification of receptors activity. On the second stage, a new level of activity, by means of secondary intranuclear signals induce modification of genes expression, which consolidates a newly developed activity of receptors.

Two types of generalized seizures are accompanied by opposing changes in the muscimol-indused $GABA_A$-mediated $^{36}Cl^-$ conductivity. GABA reaction decreased in rats with PTZ-induced convulsive kindling and increased in WAG/Rij rats with a genetic predisposition to nonconvulsive absence epilepsy. In the shell of nucleus accumbens the lower density of D1-like DA receptors was found. The results specify deficiency of mesolimbic dopaminergic system activity of WAG/Rij rat brain that corresponds to specific behavioral characteristics of WAG/Rij rats and to pharmacological experimental data. It has been assumed that the source of spike-wave discharges was the I_h pacemaker channel that is localized in the thalamic reticular nucleus and in the pyramidal neurons of the somatosensory cortex layers three, four, and five. The analysis of the experimental data shows that one of the basic mechanisms for the long-term regulation of I_h pacemaker activity is the modification of the number of HCN1 subunits in the pacemaker channel of WAG/Rij rats strain.

5. Acknowledgements

This work was supported by Russian-Netherlands cooperative grants, NWO-RFBR grant 005-RUS99/2; and Russian Foundation of Fundamental Investigations grant № 09-04-01283-a.

6. References

Al Tajir, G. & Starr, M. S., (1991) Anticonvulsant effect of striatal dopamine D2 receptor stimulation: dependence on cortical circuits? *Neurosci.* 43(1): 51-57.

Altier, N. & Stewart, J. (1998) Dopamine receptor antagonists in the nucleus accumbens attenuate analgesia induced by ventral tegmental area substance P or morphine and by nucleus accumbens amphetamine. *J. Pharmacol. Exp. Ther.* 285(2): 208-215.

Altier, N. & Stewart, J. (1999) The role of dopamine in the nucleus accumbens in analgesia, *Life Sci.* 659(22): 2269-2287.

Amabeoku, G. & Chikuni, O. (1994) GABAergic and dopaminergic systems may be involved in seizures induced by pyrimethamine in mice, *Gen. Pharmacol.* 25(6): 1269-1277.

Arias-Olguín, I.I., Vitko, I., Fortuna, M., Baumgart, J.P., Sokolova, S., Shumilin. I.A., Van Deusen, A., Soriano-García, M., Gomora. J.C. & Perez-Reyes E. (2008) Characterization of the gating brake in the I-II loop of Ca(v)3.2 T-type Ca(2+) channels, *J Biol Chem.* 283(13): 8136-8144.

Baranauskas, G. & Nistri, A. (1998) Sensitization of pain pathways in the spinal cord: cellular mechanisms. *Progr. Neurobiol.* 54(3): 349-365.

Bayazitov, I.T. & Kleshchevnikov, A.M., (2000) Afferent high strength tetanizations favours potentiation of the NMDA vs AMPA receptor-mediated components of field EPSP in CA1 hippocampal slices of rats, *Brain Res.* 866(1): 15-23.

Bazyan, A.S., Orlova, N.V. & Getsova, V.M. (2000a) Modification of rats brain monoaminergic system efficiency and emotional states during development of emotional resonance reaction by dalargin, *Zur. Vissh. Nervn. Dejatel.* 50(3): 500-508.

Bazyan, A.S., Getsova, V.M. & Orlova, N.V., (2000b) Haloperidol catalepsy consolidation in the rat as a model of neuromodulatory integration, *Neurosci.* 99(2): 279-288.

Bazyan, A.S., Orlova, N.V. & Getsova V.M. (2000c) Characterisation of learning and memory in the WAG/Rij rats prone to absence epilepsy, *in* Kuznetsova, G.D., Coenen, A.M.L., Chepurnov S.A., van Luijtelaar, E.L.J.M., (eds) *The WAG/Rij rats model of absence epilepsy: the Nijmegen - Moscow research.* Nijmegen University Press, Nijmegen, 99-104.

Bazyan A.S., Getsova V.M. & Orlova N.V. (2001a) Pharmacological reminders of emotional state facilitate the retrieval of traces from amnesiac memory, *Neurosci Behav Physiol.* 31(5): 509-515.

Bazyan A.S., Zhulin V.V., Karpova M.N., Klishina N.Y. & Glebov R.N., (2001b) Long-term reduction of benzodiazepine receptor density in the rat cerebellum by acute seizures and kindling and its recovery six months later by a pentylenetetrazole challenge, *Brain Res.* 888(2): 212-220.

Bazyan, A.S., Midzianovskaya, I.S., Kuznetsova, G.D., Sarkisova, K.Y., Orlova, N.V., Getsova, V.M. & Lushkin, A.A. (2001c) Possible mechanisms of WAG/Rij rats strain typological behavior actualization. *Zur. Vissh. Nervn. Dejatel.* 51(6): 720-727.

Bazyan A.S., & Grigoryan G.A. (2006) Molecular and chemical bases of emotional states and reinforcement, *Usp. Fiziol. Nauk.* 37(1): 68–83.

Bazyan A.S. & Segal O.L. (2010) Hyperpolarization–activated I_h pacemaker channel in the mammalian brain, *Neurochemical Journal* 4(4): 241–251.

Biggio, G., Concas, A., Corda, M. G., Giorgi, O., Sanna, E. & Serra M. (1990) GABAergic and dopaminergic transmission in the rat cerebral cortex: effect of stress, anxiolytic and anxiogenic drugs, *Pharmac. Ther.* 48(2): 121-142.

Bignante E.A., Paglini G. & Molina V.A. (2010) Previous stress exposure enhances both anxiety-like behaviour and p35 levels in the basolateral amygdala complex: modulation by midazolam, *Eur Neuropsychopharmacol.* 20(6): 388-397.

Birioukova, L.M., Midzyanovskaya, I.S., Lensu, L. Tuomisto S.,, van Luijtelaar G. & Bazyan A.S. (2006) Distribution D1- and D2-like dopamine receptors of WAG/Rij and ACI rats brain regions with and without absence epilepsy accordingly, *Neurokhimia* 23(3): 234-239.

Bowser D.N., Wagner D.A., Czajkowski C., Cromer B.A., Parker M.W., Wallace R.H., Harkin L.A., Mulley J.C., Marini C., Berkovic S.F., Williams D.A., Jones M.V. & Petrou S. (2002) Altered kinetics and benzodiazepine sensitivity of a GABAA receptor subunit mutation [γ2(R43Q)] found in human epilepsy, *PNAS* 99(23): 15170–15175.

Bouwman B.M., van den Broek P.L., van Luijtelaar G. & van Rijn C.M. (2003) The effects of vigabatrin on type II spike wave discharges in rats, *Neurosci. Lett.* 338(3): 177-180.

Bouwman B.M., Heesen E. & van Rijn C.M. (2004) The interaction between vigabatrin and diazepam on the electroencephalogram during active behaviour in rats: an isobolic analysis, *Eur. J. Pharmacol.* 495(2-3): 119-128.

Broicher T., Kanyshkova T., Meuth P., Pape H.C. & Budde T. (2008) Correlation of T-channel coding gene expression, IT, and the low threshold Ca2+ spike in the thalamus of a rat model of absence epilepsy, *Mol Cell Neurosci.* 39(3): 384-399.

Caddick S.J. & Hosford D.A. (1996) The role of GABAB mechanisms in animal models of absence seizures, *Mol Neurobiol.* 13(1): 23-32.

Calabrese, E.J. (2001) Dopamine: biphasic dose responses. *Crit. Rev. Toxicol.* 31(4-5): 563-583.

Citraro, R., Russo, E., Gratteri, S., Di Paola, E.D., Ibbadu, G.F., Curinga, C., Gitto, R., Chimirri, A., Donato, G. & De Sarro, G. (2006) Effects of non-competitive AMPA receptor antagonists injected into some brain areas of WAG/Rij rats, an animal model of generalized absence epilepsy, *Neuropharmacol.* 51(6): 1058-1067.

Clapham D.E. (1998) Not so funny anymore: pacing channels are cloned, *Neuron* 21(1): 5-7.

Clement, Y., Bondoux, D., Launay, J.M. & Chapouthier, G. (1997) Convulsive effects of a benzodiazepine receptor inverse agonist: are they related to anxiogenic processes? *J. Physiol. Paris.* 91(1): 21-29.

Coenen A.M.L., Blezer E.M.H. & van Luijtelaar E.L.J.M. (1995) Effects of the GABA-uptake inhibitor tiagabine on electroencephalogram, spike-wave discharges and behaviour of rats, *Epilepsy Res.* 21(2): 89-94.

Cook, CD., Barrett, A.C., Syvanthong, C & Picker, M.J. (2000) Modulatory effects of dopamine D3/2 agonists on kappa opioid-induced antinociception and diuresis in the rat, *Psychopharmacol. (Berl).* 152(1): 14-23.

Corda, M. G., Orlandi, M., Lecca, D. & Giorgi, O. (1992) Decrease in GABAergic function induced by pentylenetetrazole kindling in rats: antagonism by MK-801, *J. Pharmacol. Exptl. Therap.* 262(2): 792-800.

De Bruin, N.M.W.J., Luijtelaar, E.L.J.M., Jansen, S.J., Cools, A.R. & Ellenbroek, B.A. (2000) Dopamine characteristics in different rat genotypes: the relations to absence epilepsy, *Neurocsi. Res.* 38(2): 165-173.

Depaulis, A., Helfer, V., Deransart, C. & Marescaux, C. (1997) Anxiogenic-like consequences in animal models of complex partial seizures, *Neurosci. Biobehav. Rev.* 21(6): 767-774.

Deransart C., Landwehrmeyer G.B., Feuerstein T.J. & Lucking C.H. (2001) Up-regulation of D3 dopaminergic receptor mRNA in the core of nucleus accumbens accompanies the development of seizures in a genetic model of absence-epilepsy in the rat, *Mol. Brain Res.* 94(1-2): 166-177.

Evans, M. S. & Viola-McCabe K. E. (1996) Midazolam inhibits long-term potentiation through modulation of GABAA receptors, *Neuropharmacol.* 35(3): 347-357.

Fisher, J.L., Zhang, J., & MacDonald, R.L. (1997) The role of alphal and alpha6 subtype amino-terminal domains in allosteric regulation of gamma-aminobutyric acida receptors, *Mol. Pharmacol.* 52(4): P. 714-724.

Gao, X., Zhang, Y. & Wu, G. (2001) Effects of dopaminergic agents on carrageenan hyperalgesia after intrathecal administration to rats, *Eur. J. Pharmacol.* 418(1): 73-77.

Getsova V.M., Orlova N.V., Folomkina A.A. & Bazyan A.S. (2003) Low doses of disulfiram and L-DOPA evokes synergic modifications in behavior of two rat strains Wistar and WAG/Rij, *Zur. Vissh. Nervn. Dejatel.* 53(5): 674-680.

Getsova V.M., Orlova N.V., Folomkina A.A. & Bazyan A.S. (2004) The behavioural correlates of dopamine deficit by WAG/Rij rats strain, *in* G. van Luijtelar, G.D. Kuznetsova, A. Coenen, S.A. Chepurnov, (eds) *The WAG/Rij model of absence epilepsy: The Nijmegan – Russian Federation papers*, Nijmegan Institute for Cognition and Information: The Netherlands, 293-304.

Ghori K, O'Driscoll J & Shorten G. (2010) The effect of midazolam on neutrophil mitogen-activated protein kinase, *Eur J Anaesthesiol.* 27(6): 562-565.

Greengard, P., Allen, P.B. & Nairn, A.C. (1999) Beyond the dopamine receptor: the DARPP-32/protein phosphatase-1 cascade, *Neuron* 23(3): 435-447.

Hara, H., Yamada, N., Kodama, M., Matsumoto, Y., Wake, Y. & Kuroda, S. (2006) Effect of YM872, a selective and highly water-soluble AMPA receptor antagonist, in the rat kindling and rekindling model of epilepsy, *Eur J Pharmacol.* 531(1-3): 59-65.

Higashima, M., Kinoshita, H. & Koshino Y. (1998) Differences in the effects of zolpidem and diazepam on recurrent inhibition and long-term potentiation in rat hippocampal slices, *Neurosci. Lett.* 245(2): 77-80.

Hosford, D.A. & Wang, Y. (1997) Utility of the lethargic (lh/lh) mouse model of absence seizures in predicting the effects of lamotrigine, vigabatrin, tiagabine, gabapentin, and topiramate against human absence seizures, *Epilepsia* 38(4): 408–414.

Inoue, M., Duysens, J., Vossen, J.M.H. & Coenen, A.M.L. (1993) Thalamic multiple-unit activity underlying spike-wave discharges in anesthetized rats, *Brain Res.* 612(1-2) 35-40.

Johnston J. D., Price S. A. & Bristow D. R. (1998) Flunitrazepam rapidly reduces GABA(A) receptor subunit protein expression via a protein kinase C-dependent mechanism, *Br. J. Pharmacol.* 124(7): 1338-1340.

Joseph M.H., Datla K. & Young A.M. (2003) The interpretation of the measurement of nucleus accumbens dopamine by in vivo dialysis: the kick, the craving or the cognition? *Neurosci Biobehav Rev.* 27(6): 527-541.

Kang J. & Macdonald R.L. (2004) The GABAA receptor γ2 subunit R43Q mutation linked to childhood absence epilepsy and ebrile seizures causes retention of α1β2γ2S receptors in the endoplasmic reticulum, *J. Neurosci.* 24(40): 8672-8677

Kokaia, M., Pratt, G. D., Elmer, E., Bengzon, J., Fritschy, J. M., Kokaia, Z., Lindvall, O. and Mohler, H. (1994). Biphasic differential changes of GABAA receptor subunit mRNA levels in dentate gyrus granule cells following recurrent kindling-induced seizures, *Mol. Brain Res.* 23(4): 323-332.

Laschet, J.J., Kurcewicz, I., Minier, F., Trottier, S., Khallou-Laschet, J., Louvel, J., Gigout, S., Turak, B., Biraben, A., Scarabin, J.M., Devaux, B., Chauvel, P. & Pumain R. (2007) Dysfunction of GABAA receptor glycolysis-dependent modulation in human partial epilepsy, *PNAS* 104(9): 3472-3477.

Lason, W., Przewlocka, B., Przewlocki, R., Coenen, A.M.L. & van Luijtelaar, E.L.J.M. (1990) The role of opioid mechanisms in non-convulsive seizures in WAG/Rij rats. *in* van Ree, J.M., Mulder, A.H., Weigamt, V.M., Wimersma Greidadanus, Tj.B. (eds.), *New leads in opioid research*, Excerpta Medica, Amsterdam, 350-352.

Lason, W., Przewlocka, B., Coenen, A.M.L., van Luijtelaar, E.L.J.M. & Przewlocki, R. (1992) Endogenous opioid peptide in brain and pituitary of rats with absence epilepsy, *Neuropeptid.* 21(3): 147-152;

Lason, W., Przewlocka, B., Coenen, A.M.L., Przewlocki, R. & van Luitelaar, E.L.J.M. (1994a) The effect of μu and delta receptor agonists and antagonists of absence epilepsy in WAG/Rij ruts, *Neuropharmacol* 33(2): 161-166.

Lason, W., Przewlocka, B., van Luijtelaar, E.L.J.M. & Coenen, A.M.L. (1994b) Proenkerphalin and prodynorphin mRNA level in brain of rats with absence epilepsy, *Neuropeptid.* 27(6): 343-347.

Lason, W., Przewlocka, B., Coenen, A.M.L., Przewlocki, R. & van Luijtelaar, E.L.J.M. (1995) The role of opioid system in absence epilepsy in rats. In: Duncan J.S., Panayiotupolos C.P. eds. *Typical absences and related epileptic syndromes,* Churchill Communications Europe, London, 161-166.

Leke R., Oliveira D.L., Schmidt A.P., Avila T.T., Jorge R.S., Fischer A., Wofchuk S., Souza D.O. & Portela L.V. (2006) Methotrexate induces seizure and decreases glutamate uptake in brain slices: prevention by ionotropic glutamate receptors antagonists and adenosine, *Life Sci.* 80(1): 1-8.

Liu X.B., Coble J., van Luijtelaar G. & Jones E.G. (2007) Reticular nucleus-specific changes in alpha3 subunit protein at GABA synapses in genetically epilepsy-prone rats, *PNAS* 104(30):12512-12517.

Magnusson, J.E. & Fisher, K. (2000) The involvement of dopamine in nociception: the role of D(l) and D(2) receptors in the dorsolateral striatum, *Brain Res.* 855(2): 260-266;

Maris, E., Bouwman, B.M., Suffczynski, P. & van Rijn, C.M. (2006) Starting and stopping mechanisms of absence epileptic seizures are revealed by hazard functions, *J. Neurosci. Methods* 152(1-2): 107–115.

Mayford, M., Abel, T. & Kandel, E. R. (1995) Transgenic approaches to cognition. Cur. Opin. Neurobiol. 5, 141-148.

Maxudova, A. & Flesher, V. (1998) Psychopharmacology of epilepsy. Blackwell Vissenshafts Ferlag, Berlin- Vein, 180 pp.

Meeren, H.K.M., Pijn J.P.M., van Luijtelaar E.L.J.M., Coenen A.M.L. & Lopes da Silva F.H. (2002) Cortical focus drives widespread corticothalamic networks during spontaneous absence seizures in rats, *J. Neurosci.* 22(4): 1480–1495.

Meeren, H.K., Veening, J.G., Möderscheim, T.A., Coenen, A.M. & van Luijtelaar, G. (2009) Thalamic lesions in a genetic rat model of absence epilepsy: dissociation between spike-wave discharges and sleep spindles, *Exp Neurol.* 217(1): 25-37.

Midzianovskaya, I.S., Kuznetsova, G.D., Coenen, A.M.L., Spiridonov, A.M. & van Luijtelaar E.L.J.M. (2001) Electrophysiological and pharmacological characteristics of two types of spike-wave discharges in WAG/Rij rats, *Brain Res.* 911(1): 62-70.

Midzianovskaya I. S., Kuznetsova G. D., Tuomisto L., MacDonald U., Kulikov M. A. & Bazyan A. S. (2004) The dopamine and it metabolites concentration in the different structures of WAG/Rij and Wistar rats strains' brain: the comparative analysis of audiogenic, absence and mixed form epilepsy, *Neurokimia,* 21(4): 264-270/

Mink, J.W. (2003) The basal ganglia // Fundamental neuroscience. 2nd ed. Scuire L.R., Bloom F.T., McConnell S.C., Roberts J.L., Spitzer N.C., Zigmond M.J. eds. Elsevier Science.: Academic Press. P. 815-839.

Ngomba, R.T., Biagioni, F., Casciato, S., Willems-van Bree, E., Battaglia, G., Bruno, V., Nicoletti, F. & van Luijtelaar, E.L. (2005) The preferential mGlu2/3 receptor antagonist, LY341495, reduces the frequency of spike-wave discharges in the WAG/Rij rat model of absence epilepsy, *Neuropharmacol.* 49(Suppl 1): 89-103.

Niles, L.P., Smith, L.J. & Tenn, C.C. (1997) Modulation of c-fos expression in the rat striatum by diazepam, *Neurosci. Lett.* 236(1): 5-8.

Nomura, Y., Kitamura, Y., Ohnuki, T., Arima, T., Yamanaka, Y., Sasaki, K. & Oomura, Y. (1997) Alterations in acetylcholine, NMDA, benzodiazepine receptors and protein kinase C in the brain of the senescence-accelerated mouse: an animal model useful for studies on cognitive enhances, *Behav. Brain Res.* 83(1-2): 51-55.

Ogren, S.O. & Pakh, B. (1993) Effects of dopamine D1 and D2 receptor agonists and antagonists on seizures induced by chemoconvulsants in mice, *Pharmacol. Toxicol.* 72(4-5): 213-220.

Peeters, B.W.M.M., van Rijn, C.M., Vossen, J.M.H. & Coenen, A.M.L. (1989) Effects of GABA-ergic agents on spontaneous non-convulsive epilepsy, EEG and behaviour, in the WAG/RIJ inbred strain of rats, *Life Sci.* 45(13): 1171-1176.

Peeters, B. W. M. M., van Rijn, C. M., Nutt, D. J., Titulaer, M. N. G., Vossen, J. M. H. & Coenen, A. M. L. (1990) Diazepam and Ro 15-1788 increase absence epilepsy in WAG/Rij rats chronicaly exposed to diazepam, *Eur. J. Pharmacol.* 178(1): P. 111-114.

Przewlocka, B., Lason, W., Machelska, H., van Luijtelaar, E.L.J.M., Coenen, A.M.L. & Przewlocki, R. (1995) Kappa opioid receptor agonists suppress absence seizures in WAG/Rij rats, *Neurosci. Let.* 186(2-3): 131-134.

Qin, Z. H. & Weiss B. (1994) Dopamine receptor blockade increases dopamine D2 receptor and glutamic acid decarboxylase mRNAs in mouse substantia nigra, *Eur. J. Pharmacol.* 269(1): 25-33.

Quilichini, P.P., Chiron, C., Ben-Ari, Y. & Gozlan, H. (2006) Stiripentol, a putative antiepileptic drug, enhances the duration of opening of GABA-A receptor channels, *Epilepsia* 47(4): 704-716.

Rebrov, I.G., Karpova, M.N., Andreev, A.A., Klishina, N.Yu., Kuznetsova, G.D., van Luijtelaar, G., & Bazyan, A.S. (2007) Chlorine conductance of the GABAA receptor of synaptoneurosomes from the brain cortex of WAG/Rij rats with absence epilepsy and Wistar rats at an early period in the development of nonconvulsive or tonic–clonic kindling, *Neurochemical Journal*, 1(4):. 293–298.

Richtand, N.M., Liu, Y., Ahlbrand, R., Sullivan, J.R., Newman, A.H. & McNamara, R.K. (2010) Dopaminergic regulation of dopamine D3 and D3nf receptor mRNA expression. *Synapse* 64(8):634-643.

Rupprecht, R. & Holsdoer F. (1999) Neuroactive steroids: mechanisms of action and neuropsychofarmacological perspectives, *Trends in Neurocsi.* 22(9): 410-416.

Sarkisova, K.Y. & Kulikov M.A. (2000) WAG/Rij rats: a new genetically - based model of depression, *in* Kuznetsova, G.D., Coenen, A., Chepurnov S.A., van Luijtelar E.L.J.M. (eds) *The WAG/Rij rats model of absence epilepsy: the Nijmegen – Moscow research.* Nijmegen University Press, Nijmegen, 105-112.

Sarkisova, K.Yu., Midzianovskaia, I.S. & Kulikov, M.A. (2003) Depressive–like behavioral alterations and *c-fos* expression in the dopaminergic brain regions in WAG/Rij rats with genetic absence epilepsy, *Behav. Brain Res.* 144.(1-2): 211–226.

Sarkisova, K.Yu. & Kulikov, M.A. (2006) Behavioral characteristics of WAG/Rij rats susceptible and non– susceptible to audiogenic seizures, *Behav. Brain Res.* 166(1): 9–18.

Sarkisova, K.Y., Kulikov, M.A., Midzyanovskaya, I.S. & Folomkina, A.A. (2008) Dopamine-dependent nature of depression-like behavior in WAG/Rij rats with genetic absence epilepsy, *Neurosci Behav Physiol.* 38(2):119-28.

Seabrook, G. R., Easter, A., Dawson, G. R. & Bowery B. J., 1997. Modulation of long-term potentiation in CA1 region of mouse hippocampal brain slices by $GABA_A$ receptor benzodiazepine site ligands, *Neuropharmacol.* 36(6): 823-830.

Schilling, M., Wetzel, W., Grecksch, G. & Becker, A. (2006) Pentylenetetrazole kindling affects sleep in rats, *Epilepsia* 47(12): 2075-2082.

Schridde, U. & van Luijtelaar, G. (2005) The role of the environment on the development of spike-wave discharges in two strains of rats, *Physiol. Behav.* 84(3): P. 379-386.

Schridde, U., Strauss, U., Brauer, A. & van Luijtelaar, G. (2006) Environmental manipulation early in development alters seizure activity, Ih and HCN1 protein expression later in life, *Eur. J. Neurosci.* 23(12): P. 3346–3358.

Shen, G., Mohamed, M.S., Das, P. & Tietz, E.I. (2009) Positive allosteric activation of GABAA receptors bi-directionally modulates hippocampal glutamate plasticity and behaviour, *Biochem Soc Trans.* 37(Pt 6):1394-1398.

Shen, G., Van Sickle, B.J. & Tietz, E.I. (2010) Calcium/calmodulin-dependent protein kinase II mediates hippocampal glutamatergic plasticity during benzodiazepine withdrawal, *Neuropsychopharmacol.* 35(9):1897-1909.

Simon, P., Panissaud, C. & Costentin, J. (1993) Anxiogenic-like effects induced by stimulation of dopamine receptors, *Pharmac. Biochem. Behav.* 45(3): 685-690.

Snead O.C. 3rd. (1996) Antiabsence seizure activity of specific $GABA_B$ and gamma-Hydroxybutyric acid receptor antagonists *Pharmacol. Biochem. Behav.* 53(1): 73-79.

Snead O.C. 3rd. (1998) Ganaxolone, a selective, high-affinity steroid modulator of the gamma-aminobutyric acid-A receptor, exacerbates seizures in animal models of absence, *Ann. Neurol.* 44(4): 688-691.

Soghomonian, J.J. (1993) Effects of neonatal 6-hydroxydopamine injections on glutamate decarboxylase, preproenkephalin and dopamine D2 receptor mRNAs in the adult rat striatum, *Brain Res.* 621(2): 249-259.

Stackman, R.W., Walsh, T.J., Brucato, F.H. & Swartzwelder H.S. (1996) Medial septal benzodiazepine receptors modulate hippocampal evoked responses and long-term potentiation, *Brain Res.* 717(1-2): 12-21.

Stephens, D. N. & Turski, L., (1993) Kindling to the benzodiazepine receptor inverse agonist, FG 7142: evidence for involvement of NMDA, but not non-NMDA, glutamatergic receptors, *Neuropharmacol.* 132(10): 1011-1817.

Strauss U., Kole M.H., Bräuer A.U., Pahnke J., Bajorat R., Rolfs A., Nitsch R. & Deisz R.A. (2004) An impaired neocortical Ih is associated with enhanced excitability and absence epilepsy, *Eur J Neurosci.* 19(11): 3048-3058.

Suaudeau, C & Costentin, J. (1995) Analgesic effect of the direct D2 dopamine receptor agonist RU 24926 and cross tolerance with morphine, *Fundam. Clin. Pharmacol.* 9(2): 147-152.

Tolmacheva, E.A. & van Luijtelaar, G. (2007) Absence seizures are reduced by the enhancement of GABA-ergic inhibition in the hippocampus in WAG/Rij rats, *Neurosci. Lett.* 416(1): 17–21.

Trekova, N.A., Vetrilin, L.A., Basharova, L.A., Mikovskaya, O.I. & Khlopushina, T.G. (2001) Anti-dopamine antibodies: effects on behavior in an "open field", pain sensitivity, CNS monoamine content, and functional activity of immunocytes in C57B1/6 mice, *Neurosci. Behav. Physiol.* 31(1): 7-13.

Van Luitelaar, E.L.J.M. & Coenen, A.M.L. (1997) The WAG/Rij Model of Absence Epilepsy: Ten Years of Research. A Computation of Papers. Nijmegen University Press. Nijmegan. The Netherlands. 433 pp.

van Luijtelaar, G. & Sitnikova, E. (2006) Global and focal aspects of absence epilepsy: The contribution of genetic models, *Neurosci. Biobehav. Rev.* 30(7): 983–1003.

Venault, P., Chapouthier, G., Prado-de-Carvalho, L. & Rossier, J., (1992). Effects of convulsant ligands of the GABA-benzodiazepine receptor complex in conflict and learning tasks in mice, *Encephalon* 18(6): 655-660.

Vitko, I., Bidaud, I., Arias, J.M., Mezghrani, A., Lory, P. & Perez-Reyes, E. (2007) The I–II loop controls plasma membrane expression and gating of Cav3.2 T-Type Ca2+ channels: A paradigm for childhood absence epilepsy mutations, *J. Neurosci.* 27(2): 322-330.

Wise, R.A. (1978) Catecholamine theories of reward: a critical review *Brain Res.* 152(2): 215-247.

Wise, R.A. (2009) Roles for nigrosriatal–not just mesocorticolimbic–dopamine in reward and addiction *Trends Neurosci.* 32(10): 517–524.

17

Monoamines and Sleep: Effects of Oxcarbazepine

Alfonso Alfaro-Rodríguez[1], Emilio Arch-Tirado[2] and Rigoberto González-Piña[3]
[1]*Laboratorio de Neuroquímica*
[2]*Laboratorio de Bioacústica*
[3]*Laboratorio de Neuroplasticidad*
Departamento de Neurofisiología, Instituto Nacional de Rehabilitación, SSA
México

1. Introduction

Oxcarbazepine (OXC) is a second generation antiepileptic drug (AED) whose chemical structure resembles carbamazepine but has a different metabolism. OXC is rapidly reduced to 10, 11-dihiydro-10-hydroxy-carbamazepine (monohydroxy derivative, MHD), the clinically relevant metabolite of OXC (Kalis & Huff, 2001).

OXC is used for the treatment of partial seizures as a monotherapy or as an adjunctive therapy in adults and children aged 4 to 16 years. OXC Is also sometimes used to treat acute mania in adults, as well as bipolar disorder, a disease that causes episodes of depression, episodes of frenzied, abnormal excitement, and neuropathic pain (Landmark, 2007, Tidwell & Swims; 2003). The mechanism of action for OXC is not completely understood. Electrophysiological studies suggest that the presence of the active MHD metabolite results in the blockage of voltage-sensitive sodium channels, possibly through the modulation of high-voltage calcium channels and an increase in K^+ channel conductance (Mclean et al., 1994). The ability of OXC and MHD to limit repetitive high-frequency firing of sodium-dependent action potentials on neurons can contribute to inhibition of the spread of seizure activity from a focal point (Kalis & Huff; 2001, Landmark; 2007).

On the other hand, Clinckers (2005) showed that hippocampal DA and 5-HT levels are critically involved in the anticonvulsant activity of OXC. These anticonvulsant effects were restricted to a well-defined anticonvulsant concentration range and were proven to be mediated by D_2 and 5-HT_{1A} receptor stimulation (Clinckers et al., 2004). The lack of effect after systemic administration might originate from pharmacodynamic interactions with other brain areas suppressing increases in hippocampal monoamines.

The neurobiological relationships between epilepsy and sleep are receiving increased experimental attention. A key role for limbic monoamines in epilepsy has been established, and recently some studies showed the importance of hippocampal monoamines in limbic seizure control (Wójtowicz, et al. 2009).

Epileptic phenomena may provoke sleep modifications, such as those that have been observed in idiopathic generalized epilepsies, in partial epilepsy with or without seizures, and in secondarily generalized seizures, as well as in animal models of temporal lobe epilepsy that is induced by kainic acid (KA) (Ben-Ari, 1985; Sperk, 1994). Because seizures that are induced by systemic administration of KA arise in the limbic system and remain largely confined therein, they may serve as a model for complex partial seizures in humans. One of the uses of such a model would be as a test system for analyzing the effects of limbic seizures on sleep pattern organization.

However, after kainic acid (KA) administration, animals currently display a complex pattern of behavior known as "head and body shakes", which has been related to the serotoninergic system. Serotonin (5-HT) plays an important role in the central nervous system by controlling posture and movements, as well as behavior (Ben-Ari, et al. 1981; Osorio-Rico, 2003). The normothymic effects of OXC may be related to its impact on neurotransmitter systems because the GABA-ergic, serotoninergic and dopaminergic systems are all related to sleep functions (Ben-Ari, et al. 1981).

OXC may also exert effects on the brain's neurotransmitter systems and on structures related to the sleep cycle at both the cellular and molecular levels.

Therefore, the aim of this work was to analyze the effects of OXC on sleep patterns, "head and body shakes", and the participation of 5-HT and DA in the hippocampus in a model of kainic-induced seizures.

2. Materials and methods

2.1 Animals

Sixty male Wistar rats weighing 280-300 g were used. They were fed with a standard chow diet (Purina, México City) and drank water *ad libitum*. Animals were maintained under controlled conditions, with a temperature of 25°C, a relative humidity of 40% and a 12 h:12h light-dark cycle, with lights on at 08:00 h.

The rats were separated into acrylic box cages, with five animals per cage, until they were treated with each experimental condition. All experimental protocols were approved by the Research Committee of the National Institute of Rehabilitation, SSA México. The rats were treated according to the Guide for the Care and Use of Experimental Animals (Olfert et al. 1993).

2.2 Surgeries

To perform sleep recordings, animals were implanted with electrodes. To this end, animals were anesthetized with sodium pentobarbital (40 mg/kg i.p.) and mounted in a stereotaxic frame (David Kopff Instruments, Munich, Germany). The rats were implanted with bipolar stainless steel electrodes (Bore 0.010 in., Coated 0.013 in., A-M Systems, Inc., Carlsborg, WA) in the right sensorimotor cortex (2 mm length) for electroencephalographic recording (EEG) and in the neck muscles (50 mm length) for electromyographic recording (EMG). A screw was implanted on the skull to serve as a reference. Electrodes were then soldered to miniconnectors and secured to the skull with dental acrylic. After seven days of postoperative recovery, the rats were placed in a soundproofed recording cage and given free access to food and water under controlled light-dark conditions (08:00-20:00 h light, 20:00-08:00 h dark) without any movement restrictions. 7 days after the surgery, a basal polysomnographic study for 10 h (8:00-18:00 h) was performed and later used as a control. Subsequently, rats were allocated to one of three experimental groups: the KA group (n=10), which was administered KA (10 mg/kg, i.p.); the Oxcarbazepine group (n=10), which was administered OXC (50 mg/kg, i.p, dissolved in ethanol (5%) and carboxymethylcellulose); and the OXC+KA group (n=10), which was administered KA 30 minutes after OXC-treatment. A new session of polygraphic recordings were performed for 10 h over 3 days. The rats were then returned to the animal facility, where the veterinarians would care for them.

2.3 Behavioral assessment

Three additional groups of rats that were administered either saline solution (n=7), KA (n=11) or OXC+KA (n=12) were used to assess the frequency of head and body shakes in each condition. There was no need for an OXC group since it is widely known that this substance does not elicit seizures. Head and body shakes were visually recorded for a total period of two hours (8:30-12:30 h) by an observer who was unaware of the drug treatment, according to the protocol of Altagracia et al. (1994).

2.4 Analysis of serotonin (5-HT), 5-hydroxy-indol-acetic acid (5-HIAA), dopamine (DA), noradrenaline (NA) and Homovanilic acid (HVA)

The levels of serotonin and its metabolite were studied, because KA induces seizures that are promoted by elevated levels of serotonin. It was found that pretreatment with OXC increased the levels of serotonin and its metabolite in the brain, which was consistent with the finding that OXC reduced the frequency of head and body shakes. After 4 hours of behavioral assessment, rats from all three groups were sacrificed by decapitation. The hippocampus was dissected out according to the techniques of Glowinski and Iversen (Glowinski & Iversen 1996). The tissues were immediately placed into Teflon tubes that were kept on ice, sonicated in 0.4 N of percloric acid with 0.1% (w/v) of sodium metabisulfite followed by 10 min of centrifugation at 15,000 rpm at 4°C. The supernatants were kept frozen at 70°C until chromatographic analysis. The contents of 5-HT, its metabolite 5-HIAA, and catecholamines (DA, NA and HVA), were analyzed by high-performance liquid chromatography (HPLC) with an electrochemical detector according to the protocol of Alfaro-Rodríguez et al. (2006). A Perkin-Elmer LC-250 liquid chromatograph with a metrohm electrochemical detector was used. Calibration curves for monoamines were constructed using known concentrations of standards prepared in percloric metabisulfite solution that were injected into the 20 µl loop of chromatograph. Peaks were integrated with the Perkin Elmer LC 1020 program. The concentration of indolamine in the samples was obtained by interpolation of their respective standard curves.

We used an Alltech adsorbosphere catecholamine 3U analytical column (particle size= 3 µm). The mobile phase consisted of an aqueous phosphate buffer solution (0.1 M, pH 3.2) that contained 0.2 mM sodium octyl sulfate, 0.1mM of EDTA and 14% v/v methanol. The flow rate was 1.2 ml/min, and the potential was fixed at 0.80 V against an Ag/AgCl reference electrode.

2.5 Analysis of sleep and statistical analysis of results

Each of the printed polygraphic recordings was analyzed visually, according to Alfaro-Rodríguez and Gonzalez-Pina (2005). Briefly, they were classified as follows: Wakefulness (W), which was characterized by the desynchronization of the EEG and the presence of muscle tone (EMG) that was accentuated during movements; Slow Wave Sleep (SWS), which was characterized by the presence of sleep spindles, slow waves with voltage higher than 75 µV, and a decrease in EMG voltage; and Paradoxical Sleep (PS), which was

characterized by the desynchronization of the EEG and an absence of EMG voltage. Mean duration values (mean ± S.E.M.) of each EEG state were statistically compared by a one-way analysis of variance (ANOVA), and subsequent comparisons within groups were performed using a Tukey test, with $p \leq 0.01$.
Results from the counting of the head and body shakes were analyzed by ANOVA followed by Dunnett's test. Values of $P<0.01$ were considered to be significant.
Monoamine concentration and metabolite/neurotransmitter rate values were analyzed statistically by ANOVA, and subsequent comparison within groups were carried out by a Tukey test.

3. Results

3.1 Effects of kainic acid on sleep

Table 1 shows the results that were obtained from the sleep recordings. A single dose of KA (10 mg/kg) affected the organization of the sleep patterns. Kainic acid induced animals to stay awake for the whole initial 10 hours of electroencephalographic recording. During the follow-up on the next day, the W increased its total duration, and therefore, the SWS and PS decreased their respective total durations. The mean duration of the SWS and PS did not show any significant changes. On the second day, all parameters returned to control levels, suggesting that the rats did recovered from the effects of KA on the sleep-wake cycle 48hrs after treatment.

3.2 Effect of oxcarbazepine on sleep

OXC had a strong and immediate effect on the sleep-wake cycle. On the treatment day, the animals in the OXC group increased their sleep behavior throughout the recording period, remaining in sleep posture most of the time, only moving to eat or drink. OXC induced a significant decrease in W (21.5%), with a concomitant increase in total sleep time (SWS: 12.56% and PS: 28.7%). The sleep-wake cycle returned to their control values by day 1, and remained unchanged on day 2 (table 1).

3.3 Effect of oxcarbazepine + kainic acid on sleep

The animals treated with OXC 30 min before KA injection showed significant changes in almost all the sleep-wake parameters that were measured. The latency of SWS increased to 289.98 min ($p<0.001$) and that of PS to 304.45 min ($p<0.01$). There was also a significant increase in total time of W ($p<0.05$). However, these changes were much less dramatic than those observed under treatment with kainic acid alone. The present results suggested that there was an anticonvulsive effect of OXC on the KA-induced changes in the sleep patterns and a protective activity on seizures. During the following days of recordings, the amount of wakefulness progressively decreased, returning to control values by day 1 (Table 1).

3.4 Effects of KA and OXC+KA on the head and body shakes

KA administration produced a significant increase in the frequencies of the head and body shakes during the first two hours following drug administration (Table 2). Administration of OXC 30 min prior to kainic acid treatment reduced the frequency of head and body shakes to 42% of those of the KA group. The increase in head and body shakes observed seemed to be related to sleep behavior. The frequency of head and body shakes in animals began to decrease after the second hour (Table 2).

3.5 Total 5-HT and 5-HIAA content in hippocampus

When the average concentration of monoamines (μg/g of tissue) was analyzed, the contents of 5-HT increased in KA group ($p<0.05$), but there was a more significant increase in the KA+OXC group ($p<0.001$; Fig. 1). In addition, there was a significant increase in the 5-HIAA content in the same group ($p<0.01$). The increase in serotonin and its metabolite levels was correlated to sleep behavior ($p< 0.01$, Fig 1).

	Kainic Acid			
	Control	Day 0	Day 1	Day 2
W (min)	246.33± 8.1	600±0	401.01± 20.56*	246.96±20.17
SWS (min)	298.58±9.9	0±0	184.07±9.2*	292.05±10.3
SWS (mean duration; min)	8.60±0.90	0±0	7.51±0.90	8.90± 0.8
SWS (Latency; min)	61.89±6.5	0±0	110.21±10.5 **	61.36± 8.3
PS (min)	54.50 ±4.99	0±0	14.05±4.5 **	60.90± 7.2
PS (Frequency)	56.0±4.0	0+0	30.80±9.0	57.07±3.6
PS (mean duration; min)	2.72±0.9	0±0	2.81±0.9	2.51± 0.89
PS (Latency; min)	79.31±7.5	0±0	120.50±7.5 *	67.72± 8.1
	Oxcarbazepine			
W (min)	246.33± 8.1	193.60± 9.15*	252.80± 8.7	249.95± 8.8
SWS (min)	298.58±9.9	336.10±10.42*	289.91±9.2	297.55±10.3
SWS (mean duration; min)	8.60±0.90	9.35± 0.65	8.21±0.90	8.40± 0.8
SWS (Latency; min)	61.89±6.5	30.52±23.53**	59.21±8.5	58.36± 8.3
PS (min)	54.50 ±4.99	70.16± 5.42*	56.92±4.5	52.02± 5.2
PS (Frequency)	56.0±4.0	70.10 ±7.4*	55.2 ± 3.5	54.8±3.59
PS (mean duration; min)	2.72±0.9	3.52± 0.92	2.80±0.92	2.79± 0.89
PS (Latency; min)	79.31±7.5	39.36± 2.42*	71.50±7.5	77.72± 8.4
	Oxcarbazepine + Kainic Acid			
W (min)	246.33± 8.1	305.12± 9.1*	248.90± 9.9	246.95± 9.3
SWS (min)	298.58±9.9	259.12± 11.20*	292.91±9.5	293.99±10.3
SWS (mean duration; min)	8.60±0.90	10.45±1.43*	8.27±0.96	8.40± 0.8
SWS (Latency; min)	61.89±6.5	289.98±22.01**	56.21±8.8	58.36± 8.3
PS (min)	54.50 ±4.99	35.43± 4.89*	57.92±4.7	59.02± 5.2
PS (Frequency)	56.0±5.90	65.93±4.99	51.2 ± 3.9	55.8±3.5
PS (mean duration; min)	2.72±0.9	2.90± 0.54	2.81±0.98	2.82± 0.81
PS (Latency; min)	79.31±7.5	304.45± 28.90**	73.50±7.5	74.72± 8.8

Table 1. Sleep parameters (mean ± S.E.M.) recorded over 10 h in rats treated with kainic acid (KA; 10 mg/Kg; n=10), with oxcarbazepine (OXC; 50 mg/kg, n=10) and with OXC+KA (n=10) for the treatment day and the two subsequent days. Data of the control group were obtained from the basal recordings in all the rats (n= 30). It is observed that animals treated with KA remained awake over the 10 hours of initial recording, immediately following drug administration. Abbreviations: W, total time spent in waking state; SWS, total time spent in slow wave sleep; PS, total time spent in paradoxical sleep. Statistical analysis was performed with one way ANOVA followed by Tukey´s test. Statistically different from control; *$p\leq0.01$, ** $p\leq0.001$.

Treatments	Frequency of head and body shakes (counts per 2 hr)	Frequency of head and body shakes (counts per 3 hr)	Frequency of head and body shakes (counts per 4 hr)	Number of independent experiments
Saline + Saline	0	0	0	7
Kainic acid (10 mg/kg)	130 ± 21	138 ± 29	128 ± 25	11
Oxcarbazepine (50 mg/kg) + Kainic acid	75 ± 18*	29 ± 9**	0	12

Table 2. Effects of oxcarbazepine + kainic acid on the frequency of head and body shakes induced by kainic acid. Behavioral results are expressed as mean ± S.E.M. of n=7-12 independent experiments. *P<0.05, **p<0.01, statistically different from the kainic acid group. ANOVA followed by Dunnet´s test.

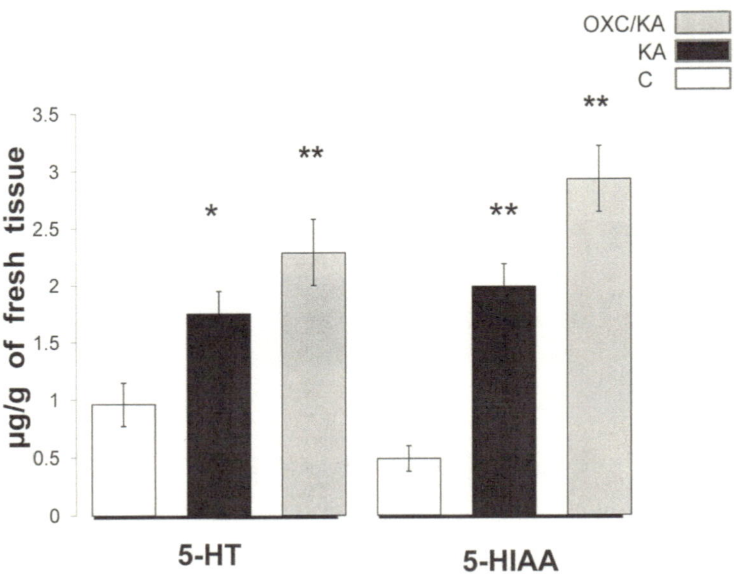

Fig. 1. Total content of serotonin (5-HT) and its metabolite 5-hydroxy-indol-acetic acid (5-HIAA) in the hippocampus. There was a significant increase in the concentrations of both 5-HT and 5-HIAA in the kainic acid (KA) and oxcarbazepine /KA-treated (OXC/CA) rats, in comparison with control (C). One-way ANOVA and *pos hoc* Tukey test *p≤0.05 **p≤0.01.

The 5-HIAA/5-HT ratio revealed that the metabolite 5-HIAA increased more than its precursor in both, the KA alone and the OXC+KA conditions (Fig 2).

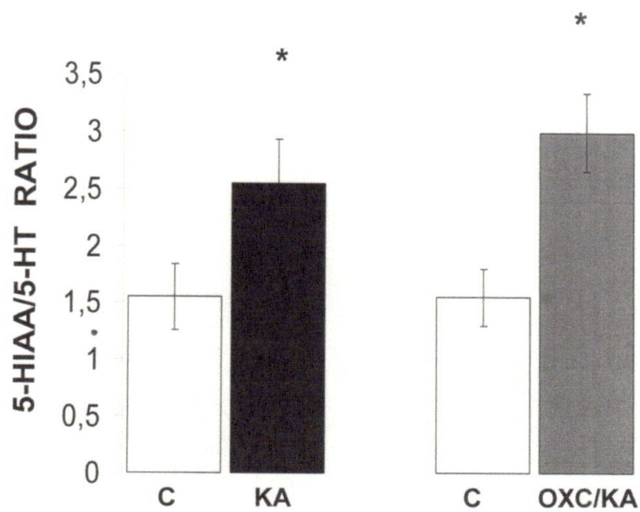

Fig. 2. 5-HIAA/5-HT ratio estimated in the hippocampus. The 5-HIAA/5-HT ratio was significantly increased in the kainic acid (KA) and oxcarbazepine /KA-treated (OXC/CA) rats compared to control (C). One-way ANOVA and *pos hoc* Tukey test *p≤0.05.

3.6 Total DA, NA and HVA content in hippocampus

When the average concentration of monoamines (μg/g of tissue) was examined, a significant increase in DA and HVA was observed for both the KA (DA, HVA: $p<0.05$) and the KA+OXC groups (DA: $p<0.01$, HVA: $p<0.05$). Moreover, this increase in catecholamine levels is related to sleep behavior. By contrast, the metabolite NA decreased significantly in both the KA and KA+ OXC groups ($p<0.05$) (Fig. 3).

4. Discussion

4.1 Effects on sleep

As described previously in the rat model of temporal lobe epilepsy, we observed a significant KA-induced disorganization of the sleep-wakefulness cycle that involved both the SWS and PS phases (Alfaro et al. 2009). This suggests that such sleep inhibition and longtime insomnia is not only due to a physical effect of the immediate pharmacological action of KA, but also to an action that is exercised on the neurophysiological mechanisms that regulate the sleep-wakefulness cycle. It is also interesting, from a pathophysiological point of view, that the reduction of sleep that is induced by epileptic seizures did not produce a compensatory increase, as is normally observed with sleep inhibition that is produced by other means (Frank et al. 1997). Whereas our findings showed that OXC induces an increase in both sleep phases, CBZ has an inhibitory effect on PS (Alfaro-Rodríguez et al. 2002; Alfaro et al. 2009, Ayala-Guerrero et al. 2002).

In contrast to CBZ, which had no effects on the sleep-wake cycle (Alfaro et al. 2009), animals treated with OXC adopted a sleep behavior through the observation period. Time sleep initiation (latency) decreased and mean duration and frequency are increased significantly in OXC treated animals. On the other hand, in OXC-pretreated animals, the frequency and duration of behavioral and electrophysiological manifestations of KA-evoked seizures decreased.

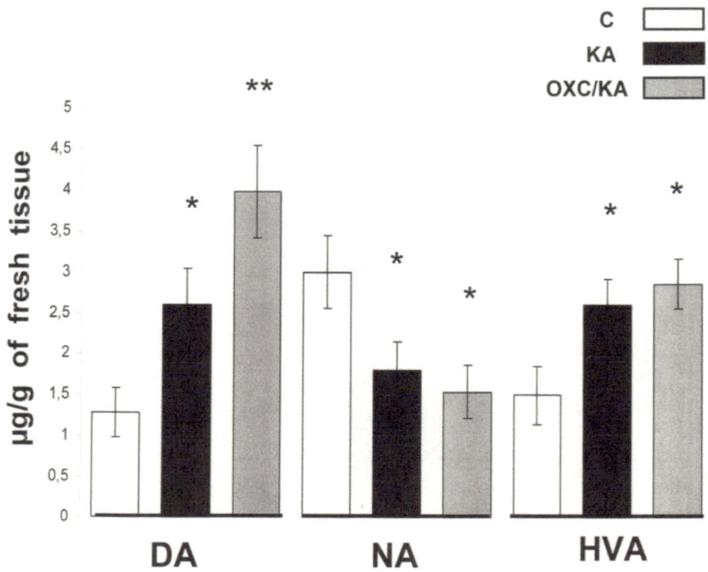

Fig. 3. Total content of dopamine (DA), noradrenaline and the dopamine metabolite, homovanilic acid (HVA) in the hippocampus. An increase in both the DA and HVA concentration was observed in the kainic acid (KA) and oxcarbazepine /KA-treated (OXC/CA) rats, when these groups were compared with Control (C). In contrast, NA was significantly decreased in both experimental groups. One-way ANOVA and *pos hoc* Tukey test $^*p \leq 0.05$ $^{**}p \leq 0.01$.

The neurochemical mechanisms of OXC might be mediated by promoting the activation of the monoaminergic systems, which contribute to the anticonvulsant activity of OXC. OXC activates endogenous DA and 5-HT leading to the activation of D_1 and 5-HT_{1A} receptors in the hippocampal region (Clinckers et al. 2005). This information is important because sleep is believed to contribute preferentially to the consolidation of explicit memories, which are thought to be encoded within the prefrontal-hippocampal circuit. Hippocampus-dependent declarative memory beneficiates particularly from SWS, whereas PS seems to benefit procedural aspects of memory (Kalia; 2006).}

Several researchers are currently trying to unravel the neurobiological relationships between epilepsy and sleep. After all, these phenomena often develop in the same vulnerable brain regions, and the importance of comorbid of sleep- wake cycle and epilepsy is an active area of research. Facilitation of central serotonin, dopamine and noradrenaline release seems to be associated with both anticonvulsant and sleep disorders effects (Shouse et al. 2001).

4.2 Effects of kainic acid on the hippocampus

The hippocampal formation is one of the most seizures-prone structures in the brain due to its defining characteristic; the presence of a tri-synaptic circuit of fibers. The reverberation of impulse activity in the hippocampal loop is suggested to cause and maintain epileptiform-like activity patterns (Stringer and Lothman, 1992). Hippocampal cells are endowed with several voltage and ligand-gated conductances, which play a major role in the cells´ excitability. Blockage of GABAergic transmission has been consistently proven to precipitate seizures. It has thus been assumed that abnormal GABAergic neurotransmission may be related to epilepsy (Prince, 1978). However, *in vivo* epilepsy can also be induced with exposure to an agonist of glutamate receptors, in a manner that may not be directly related to GABAergic mechanisms. One such agent is kainic acid, whose induced seizures are a well-established model of temporal lobe epilepsy, and KA-induced epileptic seizures reliably occur at the systemic dose of 10mg/kg used in this study. Khazipov & Holmes (2003) implicate GABA inhibitory mechanisms in the KA- induced emergence of synchronized epileptiform-like activity patterns in the hippocampus.

4.3 Relationship between monoamines and OXC and their effects on sleep and seizures

Clinckers (2005) provided evidence that OXC and MHD led to an increase in the release of monoamines to the extracellular space. Thus, their anticonvulsant effects seem to depend upon the enhancement of endogenous DA and 5-HT transmission and the subsequent activation of D_2 and $5HT_{1A}$ receptors. In recent studies, OXC and its active metabolite (MHD) have been shown to exert important dopamine- and serotonin-promoting effects in the limbic area (Kovacs, 2008). Therefore, in our study, we assumed that the OXC-induced decrease in seizures and increase in sleep was mediated by serotonergic and dopaminergic system.

In a previous study (Clinckers, et al. 2005), it was shown that hippocampal DA and 5-HT levels are critically involved in the anticonvulsant activity of OXC. Furthermore, this study suggested that the lack of effect after systemic administration might originate from the pharmacodynamic interactions with other brain areas which result in the suppression of hippocampal monoamine increases. In addition, it was also shown that the selective block of either the D_2 receptor or the 5-HT_1 receptor was able to completely abolish the anticonvulsant effects of OXC and MHD. These results indicate that activation of both receptor types is necessary for the anticonvulsant effects of OXC and MHD.

We also found that 5-HT, 5-HIAA and DA were also increased, an effect possibly exerted by the alteration of the excitation-inhibition balance. In our results the increase of 5-HIAA suggests the active participation of 5-HT metabolism in the pattern of changes by KA and KA+OXC. Excitatory and inhibitory actions of DA have been reported in hippocampus (Barone, et al. 1991 Starr, 1996). High DA concentrations enhance glutamate release via D_1/D_5 receptor stimulation, while low concentrations reduce excitatory responses via D_2 receptors. Both excitatory and inhibitory hippocampal transmission can be reduced via receptor 5-HT_3 activation (Dorostkar & Boehm, 2007). Additionally, hippocampal 5-HT reduces glutamate release by acting on presynaptic 5-HT_{1A} receptors (Mauler et al. 2001). During selective 5-HT_{1A} blockade, 5-HT produces fast excitation probably mediated by 5-HT_{2C} receptors (Beck 1992). Moreover, 5-HT inhibits GABA-ergic hippocampal interneurons via presynaptic 5-HT_{1A} receptors (Schmitz et al.1995a). The inhibitory effect of 5-HT on glutamatergic transmission may therefore be partially counterbalanced by a 5-HT-mediated disinhibition of the principal hippocampal output cells (Schmitz et al.1998).

However, in our results we found that the levels of catecholamines such as NA were decreased from the control values in both KA and KA+OXC groups. In contrast, HVA was a significantly increased in both groups. These results suggested an effect of OXC on the metabolism of catecholamines.

4.4 Effects of KA and KA/OXC on limbic seizures

It's known that KA produces neurochemical changes in monoamines (Bourne et al. 2001). KA also produces alterations in the complex behavioral pattern known as "limbic seizures".

One of the components of this pattern, the head and body shakes, is frequently associated with the intensity of seizures (Sperk 1994), increased levels of amine metabolites for both 5-HT and DA and the NA content after KA administration (Ben-Ari, 1981). Other studies have demonstrated that 5HT is involved in the development of the wet dog-shakes, which is a response in rats and some other models that involves central 5HT activity (Osorio-Rico, 2003). In these cases, the participation of 5HT that is induced by KA may cause toxic effects. Another report has shown the participation of D_2 dopamine receptors in the susceptibility of mice to kainic acid-evoked hippocampal cell death (Bozzi et al. 2000).
In our results we found that neurochemical changes produced as a consequence of KA administration involved increases in the levels of 5-HT, 5-HIAA and DA, HVA, and a decrease in the levels of NA. With the addition of OXC (KA/OXC group), there was an ever larger increase in all these systems, except for NA, which remained decreased. The increment in 5-HT and its metabolite together with the DA increment in the KA/OXC treatment mediate disinhibition of the principal hippocampal output cells probably induced by MHD, the active metabolite of OXC. The anti-convulsive effects of OXC are achieved by 5HT and other neurotransmitters, such as NA and DA, which generate SWS and the first minutes of PS. OXC significantly reduced motor seizures. The 50 mg/kg dose of OXC was also able to diminish the kainic acid-evoked body and head shakes (47%), as has been previously shown in studies (Landmark, 2007; Mclean et al. 1994).
These results explain why, KA-induced seizures disappear within the third hour of OXC treatment, while in previous study using CBZ (Alfaro, et al. 2009) the seizures disappeared six hours after administration of treatment.
Several anti-epileptic drugs such as OXC increase extracellular levels of DA and/or 5-HT in brain areas involved in epileptogenesis (Biggs et al. 1995; Southam et al.1998; Murakami et al. 2001). It is not clear whether these increases in monoamine levels have a direct anticonvulsant effect, contribute to the total anticonvulsant effect, or are just a drug side-effect.

4.5 Mechanisms of action of OXC on ionic channels

Like CBZ, OXC and MHD are considered to exert their pharmacological effects by stabilization of Na^+ channels in a voltage-, frequency-, and time-dependent manner (Mclean et al. 1994; Malow et al. 1998). They also block high-threshold Ca^{2+} current (Akaike et al. 2001) and increase K^+ channel conductance (Malow et al. 1998). The mechanism of action of OXC has been proposed to differ that of CBZ by the modulation of the Ca^{2+} channels (Calabresi, 1995; Wellinton & Goa, 2001), although the study by Sitges, et al. (2007) does not show remarkable differences between the inhibition exerted by the older and newer anticonvulsants on channel-mediated release of glutamate evoked by high K^+.
The effect of OXC appears to be related to the dose and to the serum concentrations of MHD. In general, daily fluctuations in MHD concentration are relatively slight, smaller than would be expected from the elimination half-life of the compound. Therapeutic monitoring may help to decide whether adverse effects are dependent on MHD concentrations (May, et al., 2003).

5. Conclusions

We, therefore, believe that the effects of OXC and MHD on hippocampal monoaminergic transmission are contributors to the anticonvulsive effects of these compounds.

These results are clinically relevant as hippocampus plays a significant role in seizures in many diseases. These results also offer a better understanding of the mechanisms by which anticonvulsants affect the seizures along with the origin of seizures.

6. References

Akaike, K., Tanaka, H., Tojo, S., Fukumoto, S., Imamura,S. & Takigawa, M. (2001) Kainic acid-induced dorsal and ventral hippocampal seizures in rats. *Brain Res.* Vol. 900, No. 1, (May 2001), pp. 65-71, ISSN 0006-8993

Alfaro-Rodríguez, A., González-Piña, R., Arch-Tirado, E., Carrasco-Portugal, M., Pérez-Guillé, B., Soriano-Rosales, R. E., Padilla-Martin, K., Uribe-Escamilla, R. & Labra-Ruiz, N. (2009) Neuro-protective effects of carbamazepine on sleep patterns and head and body shakes in kainic acid-treated rats. *Chem. Biol. Interact.* Vol. 180, No. 3, (August, 2009), pp. 376-82, ISSN 0009-2797

Alfaro-Rodríguez, A., González-Piña, R., González-Maciel, A. & Arch-Tirado, E. (2006) Serotonin and 5-hydroxy-indole-acetic acid contents in dorsal raphe and suprachiasmatic nuclei in normal, malnourished and rehabilitated rats under 24 h of sleep deprivation. *Brain Res.* Vol. 1110, No. 1, (September 2006), pp. 95-101, ISSN 0006-8993

Alfaro-Rodríguez, A. & González-Piña, R. (2005) Ozone-induced paradoxical sleep decrease is related to diminished acetylcholine levels in the medial preoptic area in rats. *Chem. Biol. Interact.* Vol. 151, No. 3, (February 2005), pp. 151-158, ISSN 0009-2797

Alfaro-Rodríguez, A., Labra-Ruiz, N., Carrasco-Portugal, M., Gonzalez-Maciel, A., Perez-Guille, B &, Soriano-Rosales, R. (2002) Effect of Carbamazepine on sleep patterns disturbed by epilepsy. *Proc. West. Pharmacol. Soc.* Vol. 45, (December 2002), pp. 62-64, ISSN 0083-8969

Altagracia, M., Kravzov, J., Santamaría, A., Ríos, C., Ordaz, H. & Gonzalez, L. (1994) Dapsone administration prevents quinolinate-induced neurotoxicity in rats. *Proc. West. Pharmacol. Soc.* Vol.37, (December 1994), pp. 63, ISSN 0083-8969

Ayala-Guerrero, F., Alfaro-Rodríguez, A., Martínez, C., Campos-Sepúlveda, E., Vargas, L. & Mexicano G. (2002) Effect of kainic acid-induced seizures on sleep patterns. *Proc. West. Pharmacol. Soc.* Vol 45, (December 2002) pp. 178-180, ISSN 0083-8969

Barone, P., Palma, V., DeBartolomeis, A., Tedeschi, E., Muscettola, G. & Campanella, G. (1991) Dopamine D1 and D2 receptors mediate opposite functions in seizures induced by lithium-pilocarpine. *Eur. J. Pharmacol.* Vol. 195, No. 1, (March 1991), pp. 157-62, ISSN 0014-2999

Bazil, C. W., Castro, L. H. & Walczakt, T. S. (2000) Reduction of rapid eye movement sleep by diurnal and nocturnal seizures in temporal lobe epilepsy. *Arch Neurol.* Vol. 57, No. 3, (March 2000), pp. 363-368, ISSN 0003-9942

Bazil, C. W. & Walczak, T. S. (1997) Effects of sleep and sleep stage on epileptic and nonepileptic seizures. *Epilepsia.* Vol. 38, No. 1, (January 1997), pp. 56-62, ISSN 1528-1167

Beck, S. G. (1992) 5-Hydroxytryptamine increases excitability of CA1 hippocampal pyramidal cells. *Synapse,* Vol. 10, No. 4, (April 1992), pp. 334-340, ISSN 1098-2396

Bedard, P. & Pycock, C. J. (1977) "Wet-dog" shakes behaviour in the rat: a possible quantitative model of central 5-hydroxytryptamine activity. *Neuropharmacology,* Vol. 16, No. 10, (October 1977), pp. 663-670, ISSN 0028-3908

Ben-Ari, Y. (1985) Limbic seizure and brain damage produced by kainic acid: mechanisms and relevance to human temporal lobe epilepsy. *Neuroscience*, Vol. 14, No. 2, (February 1985), pp. 375-403, ISSN 0306-4522

Ben-Ari, Y., Tremblay, E., Riche, D., Ghilini, G. & Naquel, R. (1981) Electroencephalographic, clinical and pathological alterations following systemic administration of kainic acid, bicuculine or pentetrazole: metabolic mapping using the deoxyglucose method with special reference to the pathology of epilepsy. *Neuroscience*, Vol. 6, No. 7, pp. 1361-1391, ISSN 0306-4522

Clinckers, R., Smolders, I., Meurs, A., Ebinger, G. & Michotte, Y. (2005). Hippocampal dopamine and serotonin elevations as pharmacodynamic markers for the anticonvulsant efficacy of oxcarbazepine and 10,11-dihydro-10-hydroxycarbamazepine. *Neurosci. Lett.*, Vol. 390, No. 1, (December 2005), pp. 48-53, ISSN 0304-3940

Clinckers, R., Smolders, I., Meurs, A., Ebinger, G. & Michotte, Y. (2004) Anticonvulsant action of hippocampal dopamine and serotonin is independently mediated by D and 5-HT receptors. *J. Neurochem.*, Vol. 89, No. 4, (May 2004), pp. 834-43, ISSN 1471-4159.

Crespel, A., Coubes P. & Baldy-Molulinier, M. (2000) Sleep influence on seizures and epilepsy effects on sleep in parcial frontal and temporal lobe epilepsias. *Clin. Neurophysiol.*, Vol. 111, No. Suppl 2, (September 2000), pp. S54-59, ISSN 0736-0258

Degen, R. & Rodin, E. A. (1991) *Epilepsy, sleep and sleep deprivation* (Eds.) Amsterdam, Elsevier 1991.

Dorostkar, M. M. & Boehm, S. (2007) Opposite effects of presynaptic 5-HT3 receptor activation on spontaneous and action potential-evoked GABA release at hippocampal synapses. *J. Neurochem.*, Vol 100, No. 2, (January 2007), pp. 395-405, ISSN 1471-4159.

Frank, M. G., Page, J. & Helle, H. C. (1997) The effects of REM sleep-inhibiting drugs in neonatal rats: evidence for a distinction between neonatal active sleep and REM sleep. *Brain Res.*, Vol 778, No. 1, (December 1997), pp. 64-72, ISSN 0006-8993

Gigli, G. L., Placidini, F., Diomedi, M., Maschio, M., Silvestre, G., Scalise, A. & Marciani, M. G. (1997) Nocturnal sleep and daytime somnolence in untreated patiens with temporal lobe epilepsy: Changes after treatment with controlled-release carbamazepine. *Epilepsia*, Vol. 38, No. 6, (June 1997), pp. 696-701, ISSN 1528-1167

Glowinski, J. & Iversen, L. L. (1966) Regional studies of catecholamines in the rat brain. I. The disposition of (3H)norepinephrine, (3H)dopamine and (3H)dopa in various regions of the brain. *J. Neurochem.*, Vol. 13, No. 8, (August 1966), pp. 655-669, ISSN 1470-4159

Grabenstatter, H. L., Clark, S. & Dudet, F. E. (2007) Anticonvulsivant effects of carbamazepine on spontaneous seizures in rats with kainite-induced epilepsy: comparison of intraperitoneal injections with drug-in-food protocols. *Epilepsia*, Vol. 48, No. 12, (December 2007), pp. 2287-2295, ISSN 1528-1167

Halász, P. (1984) Sleep arousal and electroclinical manifestations of generalized epilepsy with spike wave pattern. In: Degen, R., Niedermeyer, E., (Eds.) Epilepsy, sleep and sleep deprivation. Amsterdam, Elsevier, pp. 97-107.

Landmark, C.J. (2007) Targets for antiepileptic drugs in the synapse. *Med. Sci. Monit.*, Vol 13, No. 1, (January 2007), pp. RA1-7, ISSN 1234-1010

Kalia, M. (2006) Neurolobiology of sleep. *Metabolism*, Vol. 55, No. 10Suppl 2, (October 2006), pp. S2-6, ISSN 0026-0495

Kalis, M. M. & Huff, N.A. (2001) Oxcarbazepine, an antiepileptic agent. *Clinical therapeutics*, Vol. 23, No. 5, (May 2001), pp. 680-700, ISSN 0149-2918

Khazipov, R. & Holmes, G. L. (2003) Synchronization of kainate-induced epileptic activity via GABAergic inhibition in the superfused rat hippocampus in vivo. *J. Neurosci.*, Vol. 23, No. 12, (June 2003), pp. 5337-41, ISSN 0270-6474

Lerma, J., Paternain, A. V., Rodríguez-Moreno, A. & Lopez Garcia, J. C. (2001) Molecular physiology of Kainate receptors. *Physiol. Rev.*, Vol. 81, (July 2001), pp. 971-978, ISSN 0031-9333

Lothman, E. W. & Collins, R. C. (1981) Kainic acid induced limbic seizures: metabolic, behavioral, electroencephalographic and neuropathological correlates. *Brain Res.*, Vol. 218, No. 1-2, (August, 1981), pp. 299-318, ISSN 0006-8993

Malow, B. A., Lin, X., Kushwaha, R. & Aldrich, M. S. (1998) Interictal spiking increases with sleep depth in temporal lobe epilepsy. *Epilepsia*, Vol. 39, No. 12, (December 1998), pp. 1309-1316, ISSN 1528-1167

Mauler, F., Fahrig, T., Horvath, E. & Jork, R. (2001) Inhibition of evoked glutamate release by the neuroprotective 5-HT (1 A) receptor agonist BAY x 3702 in vitro and in vivo. *Brain Res.*, Vol. 888, No. 1, (January 2001), pp. 150-157, ISSN 0006-8993

May, T. W., Korn-Merker, E. & Rambeck, B. (2003) Clinical pharmacokinetics of oxcarbazepine. *Clin. Pharmakinet.*, Vol. 42, No. 12, (December 2003), pp. 1023-1042, ISSN 0312-5963

McLean, M. J., Schmutz, M. & Wamil, A. W. (1994) Oxcarbazepine: Mechanism of action. *Epilepsia*, Vol. 35, No. Suppl. 3, (June 1994), pp. S5-9, ISSN 1528-1167

Shin, C. & McNamara, J. O. 1994. Mechanism of epilepsy. *Annu. Rev. Med.*, Vol. 45, (February 1994), pp. 379-389.

Min, M. Y., Meyland, Z. & Kullmann, D. M. (1999) Synaptically released glutamate reduces gamma-aminobutyric acid (GABA)ergic inhibition in the hippocampus via kainate receptors. *Proc. Natl. Acad. Sci. U. S. A.*, Vol. 96, No. 17, (August 1999), pp. 9932-9937, ISSN 1091-6490

Olfert, E. D., Cross, B. M. & McWilliam, A. A. (1993) Guide for the care and use of experimental animals. Can. Council Anim. Care 1-211.

Osorio-Rico, L., Mancera-Flores, M. & Ríos, C. (2003) Changes in brain serotonin turnover, body and head shakes in kainic acid-treated rats. *Pharmacol and Toxicol.*, Vol. 92, No. 3, (March 2003), pp. 143-147, ISSN 0901-9928

Placidi, F., Marciani, M. G., Diomedi, M., Sauri, F., Giacomini, P. & Gigli, G. L. (2000) Effects of lamotrogine on nocturnal sleep, daytime somnolence and cognitive functions in focal epilepsy. *Acta Neurol. Scand.*, Vol. 102, No. 2, (August 2000), pp. 81-86, ISSN 1600-0404

Prince, D. A. (1978) Neurophysiology of epilepsy. *Annu. Rev. Neurosci.*, Vol. 1, (March 1978), pp. 395-415, ISSN 0325-0395

Roberts, R. (1998) Differential diagnosis of sleep disorders, non-epileptic attacks and epileptic seizures. *Curr. Opin. Neurol.*, Vol. 11, No. 2, (april 1998), pp. 135-139, ISSN 1350-7540

Sammaritano, M. & Sherwin, A. (2000) Effect of anticonvulsants on sleep. *Neurology.*, Vol. 54, No 5 Suppl 1 ,(March 14, 2000), S16-24, ISSN 0028-3878

Schliebs, R., Zilvin, M., Steinbach, J. & Rothe, T. (1989) Changes in cholinergic but not in GABAergic markers in amygdale, piriform cortex and nucleus basalis of the rat brain following systemic administration of kainic acid. *J. Neurochem.*, Vol. 53, No. 1, (July 1989), pp. 212-218, ISSN 1471-4159

Shouse, M. N., Staba, R. J., Saquib, S. F &, Farber, P. R. (2001) Long-lasting effects of feline amygdala kindling on monoamines, seizures and sleep. *Brain Res.*, Vol. 892, No. 1, (February 2001), pp. 147-65, ISSN 0006-8993

Schmitz, D., Empeson, R. M. & Heinemann, U. (1995) Serotonin reduces inhibition via 5-HT1A receptors in area CA1 of rat hippocampal slices in vitro. *J. Neurosci.*, Vol. 15, No. 11, (November 1995), pp. 7217-7225, ISSN 0270-6474

Schmitz, D., Gloveli, T., Empeson, R. M. & Heinemann, U. (1998) Comparison of the effects of serotonin in the hippocampus and the entorhinal cortex. *Mol. Neurobiol.*, Vol. 17, No. 1-3, (December 1998), pp. 59-72, ISSN 0893-7648

Sitges, M., Guarneros, A. & Nekrassov V. (2007) Effects of carbamazepine, phenytoin, valproic acid, oxcarbazepine, lamotrogine, topiramate and vinpocetine on the presynaptic Ca2+ channel-mediated release of (3H) glutamate: Comparison with the Na+ channel-mediated release. *Neuropharmacology*, Vol. 53, No. 7, (December 2007), pp. 854-862, ISSN 0028-3908

Sloviter, R. S. & Damiano, B. P. (1981) Sustained electrical stimulation of the perforant path duplicates kainite induced electrophysiologic effects and hippocampal damage in rats. *Neurosci. Lett.*, Vol. 24, No. 3), (July 1981), pp. 229-284, ISSN 0304-3940

Sperk, G. (1994) Kainic acid seizures in the rat. *Prog. Neurobiol.*, Vol. 42, No. 1, (August 1994), pp. 1-3,. ISSN 0301-0082

Stewart, R. M., Growdon, J. H., Cancian, D. & Baldessarini, R. J. (1976) 5-hydroxitryptophan-induced myoclonus: increased sensitivity to serotonin after intracranial 5,7-dihydroxytryptamine in the adult rat. *Neuropharmacol.*, Vol. 15, No. 8, (August 1976), pp. 449-455, ISSN 0028-3908

Stringer, J. L. & Lothman, E. W. (1992) Reverberatory seizure discharges in hippocampal-parahippocampal circuits. *Exp. Neurol.*, Vol. 116, No. 2, (May 1992), pp. 198-203, ISSN 0014-4886

Tidwell, A. & Swims, M. (2003) Review of the newer Antiepileptic drugs. *Am. J. Manag. Care*, Vol. 9, No. 3, (March 2003), pp. 253-276, ISSN 1936-2692

Wang, L., Zuo, C. H., Zhao, D. Y. & Wu, X. R. (2000) Brain distribution and efficacy of carbamazepine in kainic acid induced seizure in rats. *Brain Dev.*, Vol. 22, No. 3, (May 2000), pp. 154-157, ISSN 0387-7604

Wójtowicz, A. M., van den Boom, L., Chakrabarty, A., Maggio, N., Haq, R. U., Behrens, C. J. & Heinemann, U. (2009) Monoamines block kainate- and carbachol-induced gamma-oscillations but augment stimulus-induced gamma-oscillations in rat hippocampus in vitro. *Hippocampus*, Vol. 19, No. 3, (March 2009), pp. 273-288, ISSN 1098-1063

18

Medicinal Herbs and Epilepsy: A Two Edged Sword

Mahyar Janahmadi, Sahar Farajnia, Zahra Ghasemi and Ali Rastqar
Neuroscience Research Centre and Department of Physiology, Medical School
Shahid Beheshti Medical Sciences University, Tehran
Iran

1. Introduction

Epilepsy is one of the most serious neurological disorders affecting about 0.5-1% of the world population. There is no definite radical therapy against epilepsy; however, actual therapy includes simple inhibition of epileptic activity. Apart from effective drugs against epilepsy, plant extracts as well as essential oils, which have been used for generations by humans to treat the disease, are considered nowadays as potential bioactive agents that can interfere and alter cellular physiological processes involved in epileptogenesis. However, the exact underlying mechanisms and the electrophysiological consequences of action of most medicinal herbs are still not known.

Recently, we have reported that the essential oil of Anise, *Pimpinella anisum* L. (Apiaceae), which is one of the oldest known and highly used spice plants in the folk medicine, causes hyperexcitability at the cellular level and changes the neuronal firing pattern from a regular tonic discharge to an irregular and then to bursting mode in normal cells or potentiates the burst firing and the steepness of the paroxysmal shift induced by PTZ treatment (Janahmadi et al., 2008). However, we have also shown that some herbs, including *Cuminum cyminum* (Janahmadi et al, 2006) and *Artemisia drancunculus* (Farajnia et al., 2011), can inhibit the epileptiform activity induced by PTZ, a well known convulsant agent. This sort of contradictory effect of herbal essential oils and extracts *is* one reason why a certain caution is needed when medicinal herbs are used to treat patients suffering from epilepsy. The present work is focused on comparison of the electrophysiological consequences of essential oil and extract of Tarragon on PTZ-induced neuronal hyperexcitability in snail for the first time. In addition, the effect of anethole, *the chief ingredient* of many aromatic herbs, including anise and tarragon, on normal neuronal excitability is also tested.

Tarragon or dragon's-wort (*Artemisia dracunculus*) is a perennial herb in the family Asteraceae related to wormwood that exerts radical-scavenging activities (Parejo et al., 2002), antifungal and antitumor effects (Zani et al., 1991; Meepagala et al., 2002) and antiepileptic activities (Sayyah et al., 2004; Farajnia et al., 2011). In Iranian traditional medicine, the dried aerial parts of this plant were mentioned as a treatment for epilepsy (Aqili Khorasani, 1992). The composition of the essential oil of Iranian *A. dracunculus* was reported to include *trans*-anethole and α-*trans*-ocimene as the major constituents (21.1% and 20.6%, respectively). More recently, we demonstrated the dual effects of anethole on Ca^{2+}-dependent excitability in snail neurons: at low concentration anethole caused a significant reduction in the firing frequency and enhancement of AHP amplitude, but at high concentration it significantly increased the firing frequency and also decreased the AHP amplitude (Ghasemi et al., 2011). Anethole (1-methoxy-4-(1-propenyl)-benzene), which is largely used in industry as a flavor or as a odorant, possess several potential pharmacological activities such as depressive action on motor system (Boissier et al., 1967), anticarcinogenic (Al-Harbi et al., 1995), antioxidant (Freire et al., 2005), anti-inflammatory, (Chainy et al., 2000) and anesthetics activity (Ghelardini et al., 2001). It was suggested that some of the essential oils (e.g. anise) containing monoterpenoids especially *trans*-anethole exert anticonvulsant activity (Sayyah et al., 2004). *Pimpinella anisum* is another aromatic herb which contains anethole as its main constituent. Anise is native to the eastern Mediterranean and is a plant rich in volatile oils, which are employed in traditional Asian folk medicine. Water and ethanol extracts of *Pimpinella anisum* seed have several potent therapeutic effects including antioxidant and antimicrobial activities (Gülçin et al., 2003). The essential oil of anise has also been reported to exert both fungicidal and antibacterial actions (Soliman and Badeaa, 2002; Singh et al., 2002) and anticonvulsant activity (Pourgholami et al., 1999). In contrast, we have recently shown that the essential oil of anise produces neuronal hyperexcitability and potentiates PTZ-induced epileptiform activity in snail by enhancing the Ca^{2+} channels activity or inhibition of voltage and /or Ca^{2+} dependent K^+ channels function (Janahmadi et al., 2008). We believe that this effect might be due to anethole, the chief constituent of the essential oil of anise. Thus, the main aims of this study are: (1) to compare the electrophysiological effect of Tarragon extract with that of its essential oil, (2) to test the cellular effect of anethol on neuronal excitability, using intracellular recording method under current clamp condition.

2. Materials and methods

Electrophysiological recording was performed on the soma membrane of neurons from sub-oesophageal ganglia of *Helix aspersa* (Iranian garden snail). The snail brain consists of a circum-oesophageal ring of nine ganglia. Two are dorsal supra-esophageal (the cerebral ganglia) and the remaining seven constitute the suboesophageal ganglia (Kerkut et al., 1975). Snail neurons are often large and located peripherally. It is therefore possible to work on a specific neuron from on preparation to another because they can be consistently identified on the basis of their size and location. In the present study, we will focus on F1, the largest neuron located in right parietal ganglion (Fig.1).

Adult Iranian garden snails were collected from north of Iran and were kept in a dormant state until they were used. The day before experimentation, animals were activated by wetting and then they were anaesthetized by injecting them with 2 ml of 50 mM $MgCl_2$. The shell was removed with bone forceps and the snail with its head extended was pinned out on a cork board. Next, the circum-oesophageal ganglia were removed from the animal, keeping the nerves and aorta attached to the ganglia as long as possible. Then, the ganglionic mass with its main peripheral nerves and aorta was placed in a recording chamber, lined with Sylgard 170 (Dow corning Midland, MI, USA) containing normal snail Ringer solution (in mM): NaCl 80, KCl 4, $CaCl_2$ 10, $MgCl_2$ 5, Glucose 10, Hepes 5 (Taylor, 1987). In order to expose F1 neuron, the connective tissue overlying the ganglia were gently torn using two pairs of fine forceps without any pre-treatment with proteolytic enzymes. F1 cell was visually identified by its size, color and location within the right parietal ganglion (Kerkut et al., 1975). These procedures were in accordance with the guidelines of the Institutional Animal Ethics Committee at Shahid Beheshti University of Medical Sciences.

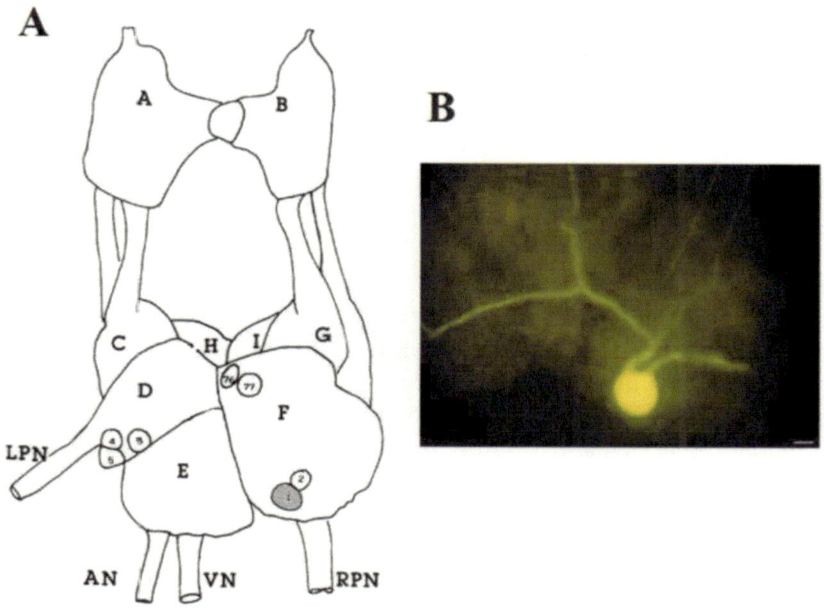

Fig. 1. (A) Scheme redrawn from Kerkut et al. (1975) showing the nine ganglia of the *H. aspersa* circum-oesophogeal ganglia and the four main peripheral nerves. The cell body of F1 (in grey colour) is located in the RPG (*A* left cerebral ganglion, *B* right cerebral ganglion, *C* LPlG, *D* LPG, *E* VG, *F* RPG, *G* RPlG, *H* left pedal ganglion, *I* right pedal ganglion, *LPN* left pallial nerve, *RP right* pallial nerve, *VN* visceral nerve, *AN* anal nerve). (B) F1 neuron was stained intracellularly by the injection of *Lucifer* Yellow (5nA hyperpolarizing current pulses of 500ms duration).

2.1 Intracellular electrophysiological recording

Sharp intracellular recording was done using Axoclamp 2B amplifier (Axon instrument, Foster City, CA, USA) at room temperature (22-25^{0}C) in snail Ringer. Each cell was impaled with single electrode (5-7MΩ). Electrode was filled with 3MKCl and in some cases with Lucifer Yellow. The reference electrode in all experiments was a silver-silver chloride wire within an agar bridge (%4 agar in snail Ringer). The above set-up and recording equipment were kept in a Faraday's cage.

Intrinsic spontaneous neuronal activity was recorded under conventional current clamp in real time by testing, before (control), and after application of drugs. Five sets of experiments were done. The first and second sets of experiments were conducted in order to examine the cellular and antiepileptic effects of essential oil of Tarragon alone or on the PTZ-induced epileptiform activity, respectively. In the third and fourth sets of experiments, the cellular and antiepileptic actions of Tarragon extract alone or against the epileptogesis induced by PTZ were assessed, respectively. The sixth set of experiment was performed to evaluate the electrophysiological effect of anethole on normal neuronal excitability in snail. Data were filtered at 30 kHz, voltage records were sampled at 20 kHz and digitized online using a 16 bit A/D converter (ADInstrument Pty Ltd., Sydney, Australia) and stored for further analysis using Chart 5 and MATLAB softwares. The following electrophysiological parameters of spikes were considered in particular: The firing pattern, the firing frequency, the resting membrane potential (RMP), the half-width of action potential (AP), The AHP amplitude, the AP amplitude. AP amplitude was defined as the change in voltage from the RMP to the peak of AP and its duration was measured at mid amplitude. The AHP amplitude was measured from the RMP to the peak negativity after an AP and the duration was measured as the time required declining to 80% of its peak value. The firing regularity was assessed using the coefficient of variation (CV) of interspike intervals (ISI) of spontaneous activity ($CV = ISI_{S.D} / _{mean} ISI$).

2.2 Plant material and drugs

The aerial parts of *Artemisia dracunculus* were collected from the north of Iran in April (2006). *A. dracunculus* was authenticated by M. Kamalinejad and a voucher specimen (no. 861) was deposited in the herbarium of Faculty of Pharmacy, Shahid Beheshti University of Medical Sciences, Tehran. The plant materials were dried, far from direct sunlight. Then 1000ml of ethanol (96%) was added to the dried leaves and kept at room temperature for 48h. Thereafter, it was filtered and the alcohol was evaporated using rotary evaporator and dried extract was obtained.

2.3 Isolation of the essential oil

The aerial parts of *A. dracunculus* were subjected to hydrodistillation for 3 h using a clevenger apparatus. The plant yielded 4% (v/w) essential oil. The essential oil was kept protected from light at 4°C (Sayyah et al., 2004). The final concentrations of 0.1% and 0.005%, required to influence the neuronal excitability for Tarragon extract and its essential oil, respectively, were chosen on the basis of the preliminary experiments.

Anethole (0.99%) was purchased from Sigma (St. Louis, MO, USA), dissolved in Ringer solution and was applied at final concentrations of 0.5% and 2%. Then the diluted anethole solution prepared in normal Ringer was perfused into the experimental chamber at a rate of approximately 2.5ml/min.

Pentylenetetrazol (PTZ, Sigma) was applied (25mM) into the bathing solution. Extract of *Artemisia dracunculus was* dissolved in absolute ethanol at a final concentration of 1% and 3% (the final concentration of vehicle in the perfusion solutions was 0.3% (v/v). The same concentration of vehicle had no effect on bioelectrical activity of neurons. The pH of solutions was adjusted to 7.8 with either Trizma hydrochloride or Trizma base (Sigma). Each solution was superfused into the experimental chamber at a rate of approximately 2.5 ml/min.

2.4 Statistical analysis

Numerical results are given as mean ± S.E.M., with n being the number of cells on which the measurement was done. Significant differences between the groups were evaluated using a student *t*-test or one way ANOVA and $P < 0.05$ was considered to be significant.

3. Results

3.1 Tarragon essential oil altered the neuronal excitability more robust than its extract

In normal Ringer, neurons showed spontaneous regularly spaced action potentials (Fig. 2) with a frequency of 0.9 ± 0.05 Hz and a mean duration of 8.02 ± 0.05 ms (n=6, Fig.3).

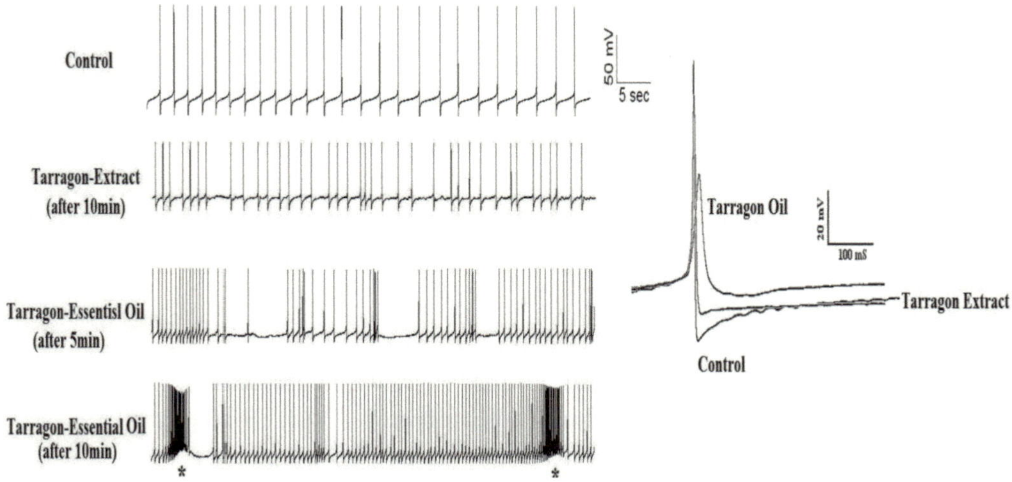

Fig. 2. Tarragon essential oil and its extract affect differentially F1 neuronal firing activity. (A) Spontaneous regular tonic firing activity in control condition. Application of Tarragon extract (0.1%) caused an increase in the firing rate associated with an irregular discharge activity after 10 min (B). However, Tarragon essential oil alone led to a neuronal hyperexcitability after 5min (C) followed by a distinct PDS (asterisk) after 10min of application (D). The inset shows superimposed action potentials recorded in control and after treatment with either Tarragon essential oil or its extract alone.

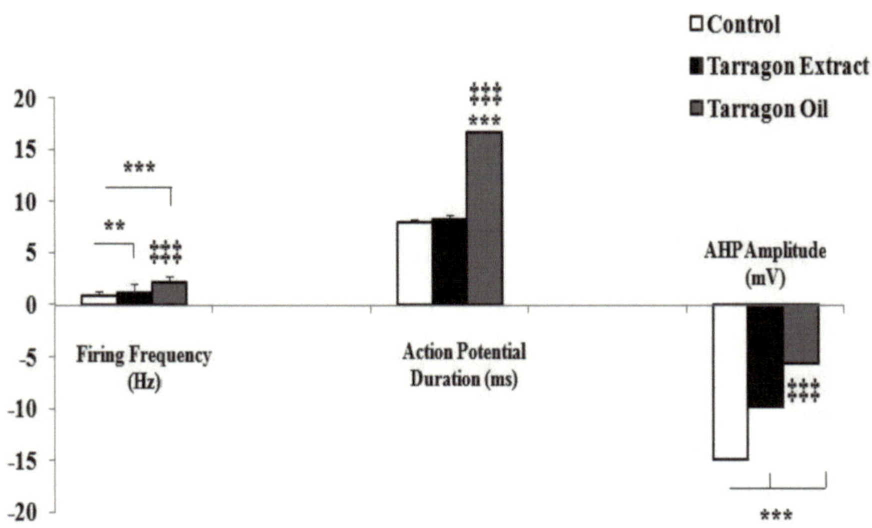

Fig. 3. Electrophysiological consequences of Tarragon application on action potential parameters in F1 neurons. Tarragon essential oil and its extract altered the AP configuration, as the essential oil profoundly increased the firing frequency and AP duration, but decreased the AHP amplitude. Tarragon extract also increased the firing rate and decreased the AHP, but to a lesser extent than did its essential oil. **, ***, significantly differences (P<0.01, P<0.001) from controls and ‡‡‡, significant difference (p<0.001) from Tarragon extract treated group.

Single action potentials were followed by AHP with mean amplitude of -14.75 ± 0.21mV (Fig. 3). When Tarragon essential oil was applied alone in the normal recording solution, within 10min caused a significant increase in the firing frequency (2.24±0.58Hz) compared to control and Tarragon extract (1.28±0.3 Hz, P<0.001), although exposure to the extract alone also produced a significant (P<0.01) increase in the excitability when compared to the normal excitability (Fig.3). Following addition of essential oil to normal Ringer solution, F1 neurons displayed a clear paroxysmal depolarization shift (PDS; Fig.2).Treatment with essential oil, furthermore, significantly resulted in a prolongation of action potentials (16.61±0.11ms, P<0.001) both compared to control and extract alone (8.35±0.14ms). However, there was no significant difference between the AP duration measured in control condition and after application of Tarragon extract (Fig. 3). Exposure to both Tarragon extract and essential oil caused a significant reduction in the AHP amplitude; however, this inhibitory effect was more profound in essential oil-treated neurons (Fig.3). Neither essential oil nor extract affected significantly the resting membrane potential of F1 cells (-43.63±0.6mV in control; -42.99±0.56mV and -42.16±1.88mV in the presence of essential oil and extract, respectively).

3.2 Tarragon extract, but not essential oil, attenuated the PTZ-induced hyperexcitability

In order to investigate and compare the potential antiepileptic effects of Tarragon essential oil and its extract, PTZ (25mM) was added to the normal Ringer solution. Neuronal exposure to PTZ resulted in a significant increase in the spontaneous firing activity associated with a paroxysmal depolarization shift and bursting (Figs.4&5A-A′). In addition, PTZ significantly increased the AP duration and decreased the AHP amplitude (Figs. 5B-B′ and 5C-C′). When, the essential oil of Tarragon was added to the Ringer solution containing PTZ , the firing frequency remained almost unchanged and even worsen the bursting activity, however the duration of AP and the amplitude of AHP were further significantly increased and decreased, respectively (Figs.4&5A).

In contrast to these effects, treatment with Tarragon extract following PTZ application did not significantly affect the AP half-width (Fig. 5B′), but significantly decreased the firing frequency and the AHP amplitude (Figs.5A′ &C′). Tarragon extract also caused the PTZ-induced PDS to be disappeared and changed the burst activity into almost regular firing interrupted occasionally by a silent period associated with inhibitory postsynaptic potentials (IPSPs) (Fig.4).

3.3 Anethole, one of the major components of the essential oil of Iranian *A. dracunculus,* had differential effects on normal neuronal firing excitability

To characterize the electrophysiological consequences of neuronal exposure to anethole on normal excitability, a low (0.5%) and a high (2%) concentrations were chosen on the basis of our previous work (Ghasemi et al., 2011).

Application of 0.5% anethole did not significantly change the RMP, but at its higher concentration (2%) hyperpolarized the cell resting membrane potential (data not shown) and altered the neuronal firing pattern from a regular spiking observed in control or in the presence of extract to an irregular hyperexcitable pattern often followed by a PDS (Fig.6).

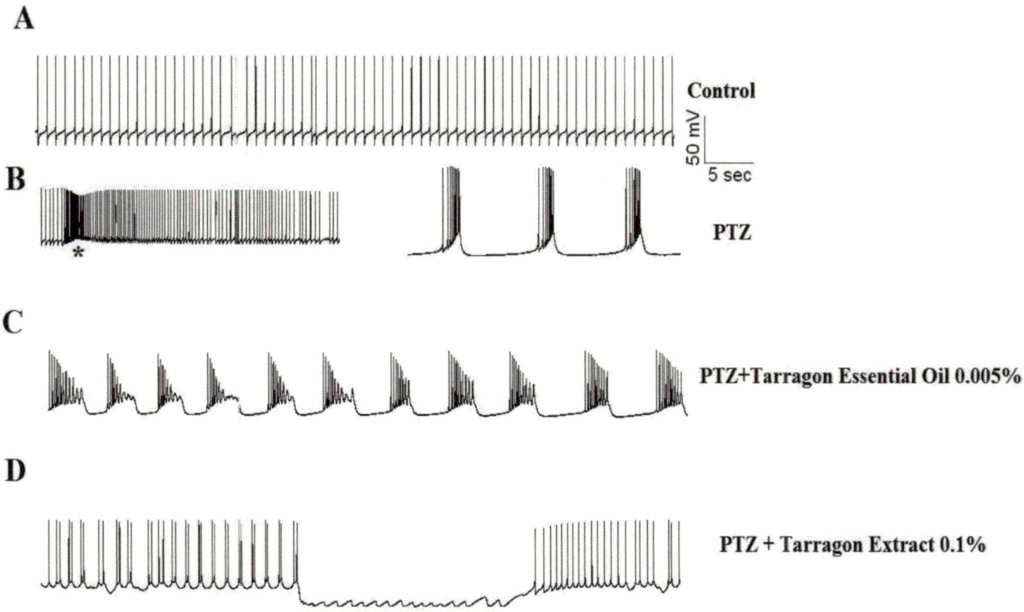

Fig. 4. Effects of Tarragon extract and essential oil on PTZ-induced epileptiform activity. (A) Spontaneous regular activity of a representative neuron under control condition. Following PTZ application, the cell became hyperexcitable and a PDS (asterisk) was appeared (B, left trace) and later the firing pattern was changed from tonic spiking to burst firing (B, right trace). Addition of Tarragon essential oil (0.005%) in the presence of PTZ worsened the PTZ-induced hyperexcitability and in this condition cell continued to exhibit burst firing *(C). Tarragon extract at concentration of 0.1%, however, decreased the PTZ-induced epileptiform activity* and caused disappearance of PDS observed in the presence of PTZ alone. Neuronal firing was interrupted by IPSPs when normal Ringer containing PTZ+Tarragon extract was perfused.

Anethole at both concentrations resulted in a significant increase in the firing frequency, but to a much greater extent after 2% anethole (from 0.8±0.03Hz in control condition to 3.11±0.09Hz and 4.13±0.03Hz after exposure to 0.5% and 2% anethole, respectively, Fig.7A). However, anethole at concentrations of 0.5% and 2% affected differently the discharge regularity, as evidenced by coefficient of variations (CV) measured in different condition. Perfusion of normal Ringer containing anethole 0.5% slightly increased the firing irregularity (CV= 0.22 after anthole 0.5% versus 0.19 in control condition), whereas 2%

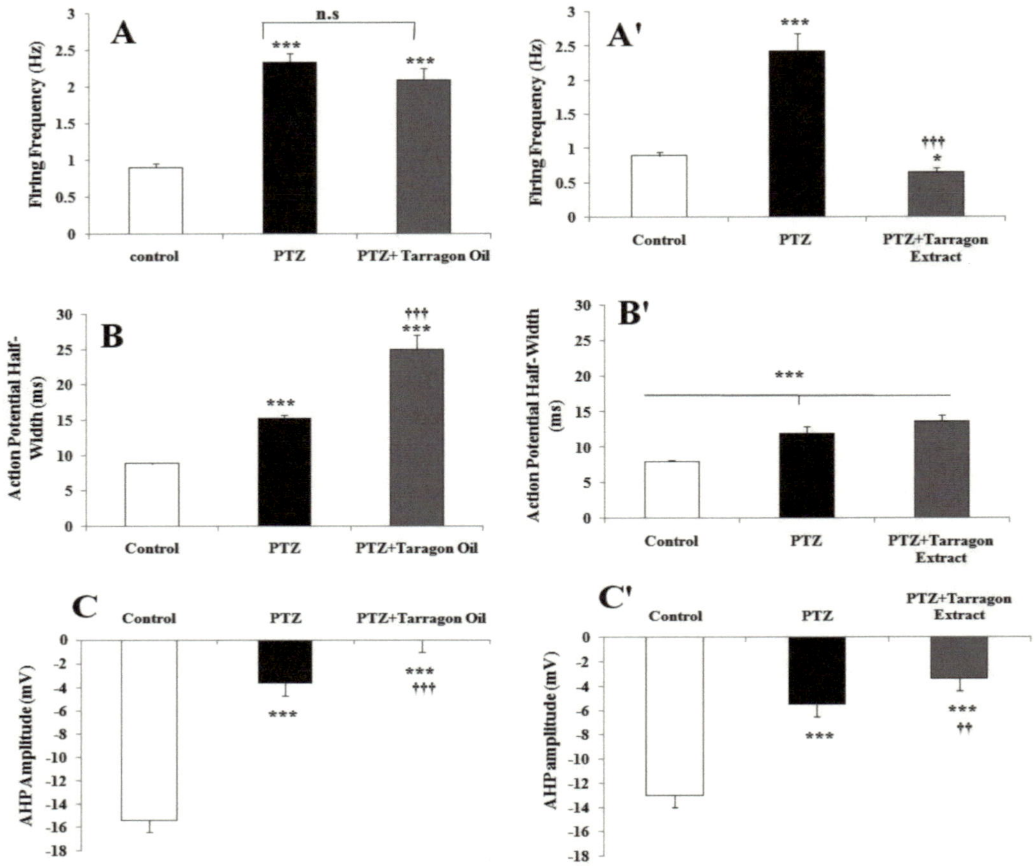

Fig. 5. The effect of anethole, the main constituent of Iranian *A. Dracunculus,* on firing activity of F1 neurons. Somatic conventional intracellular recording of spontaneous intrinsic firing F1 neuron in normal Ringer (A),after application of anethole at concentration of 0.5% (B) and following treatment with anethole 2% (C). Application of anethole at higher concentration clearly caused a neuronal excitability and elicited a PDS (asterisk).

anethole increased the firing precision as defined by smaller CV (0.03). Furthermore, anethole induced differential effect on the AHP that followed AP. At concentration of 0.5% it caused a significant reduction in the AHP amplitude, but at 2% produced a significant increase in the AHP, both compared to control and anethole 0.5% (Fig. 7C). Both high and low concentrations of anethole caused also a significant shortening of AP compared to control group, although this effect was more potent in 2% anethole-treated group when compared with 0.5% anethole (Fig.7B).

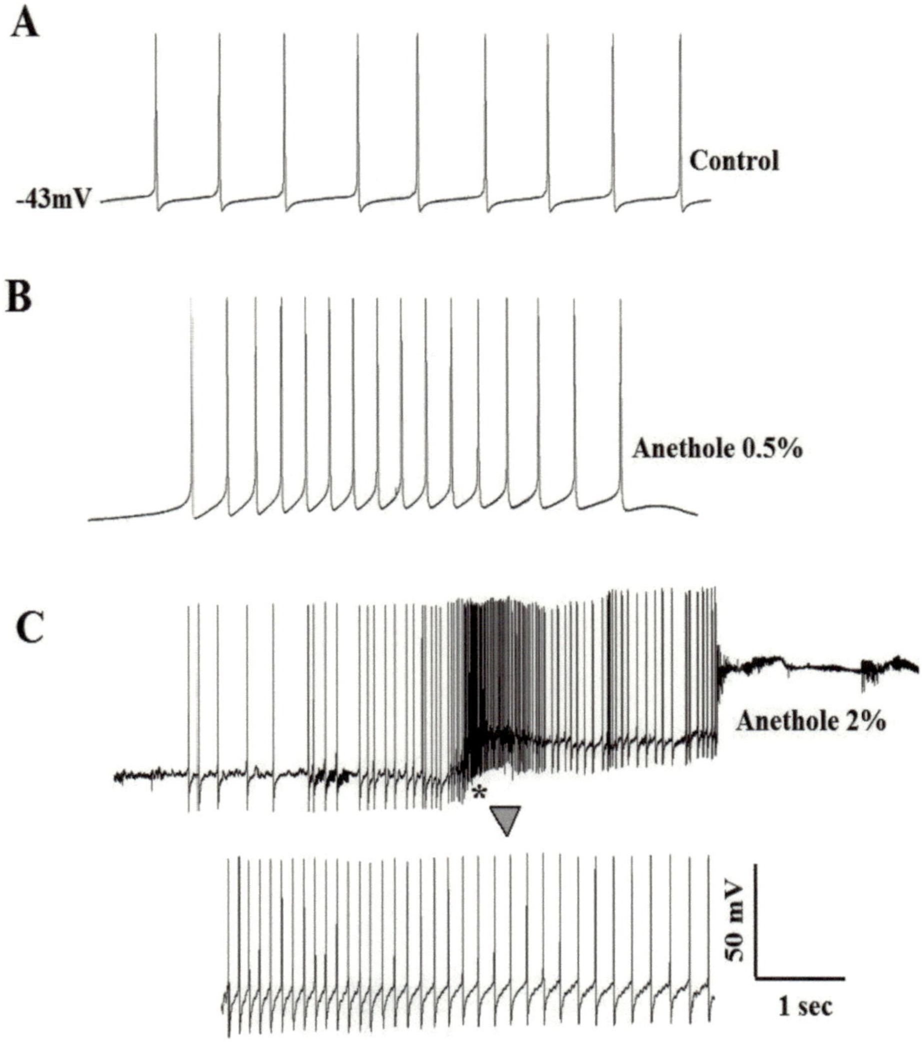

Fig. 6. The effect of anethole, the main constituent of Iranian *A. Dracunculus,* on firing activity of F1 neurons. Somatic conventional intracellular recording of spontaneous intrinsic firing F1 neuron in normal Ringer (A),fter application of anethole at concentration of 0.5% (B) and following treatment with anethole 2% (C). Application of anethole at higher concentration clearly caused a neuronal excitability and elicited a PDS (asterisk).

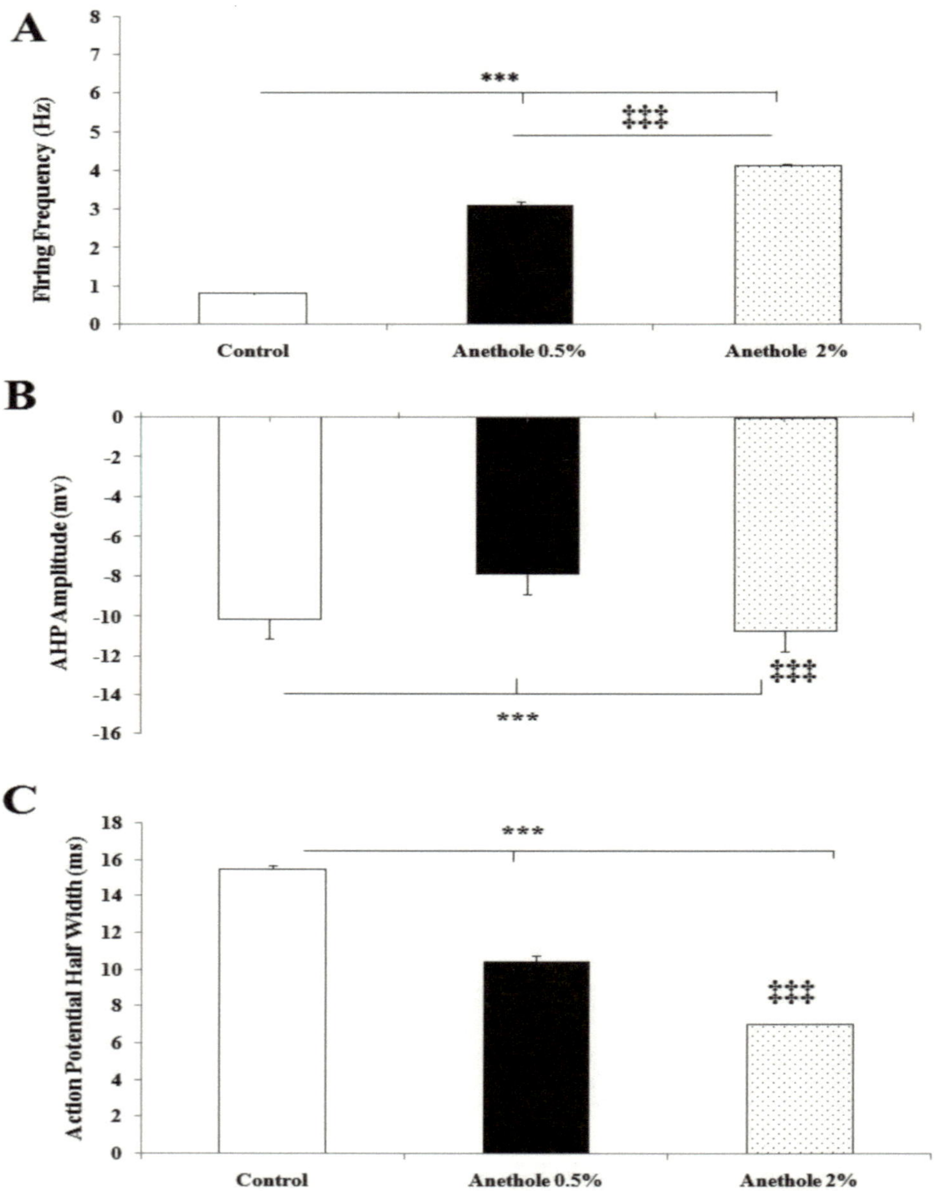

Fig. 7. Effects of anethole treatment on action potential characteristics. Effects of anethole treatment on (A) firing frequency, AHP amplitude (B) and on the AP duration (C). ***, significantly different ($P<0.001$) from control; ‡‡‡, significant different ($P<0.001$) from the 0.5% anethole- treated group.

4. Discussion

Invertebrates have often been used as an experimental model for investigating the cellular mechanisms of the effect of many convulsant and anticonvulsant agents. It has been reported that convulsant drugs such as PTZ induces a potential pattern in molluscan neurons which closely resembles the epileptic activity of mammalian neurons, called PDS (Goldensohn and Pupura, 1963; Matsumoto and Ajmone Marsan, 1964; Sugaya et al., 1973). In invertebrate neurons, following application of PTZ, the endogenous mechanisms are so pronounced that PDS may still be recorded even after complete inhibition of synaptic inputs (Faugier-Grimaud, 1974; Speckmann and Caspers, 1973). Ion channel currents underlying action potentials have been shown to participate in the generation of epileptic discharges as well as in the actions of antiepileptic drugs. Among these channels, calcium and voltage-dependent K+ channels play a crucial in the repolarization and hyperpolarization that follows PDSs. The knowledge of the cellular mechanisms of action of the medicinal plants with antiepileptic potential is allowing the design of new therapeutic approaches possibly with fewer side effects. Aromatic spice plants have been used traditionally as food and for medicinal purposes in the therapy of some diseases for a long time in the world. Essential oils and extracts in these plants are used extensively in medicine and in the food and cosmetic industries. Although, there is a distinct difference between pure essential oils and simple plant extracts, the mechanisms of these at the cellular level have not been completely elucidated yet. As an aromatic plant, Tarragon (*A. dracunculus anisum L.*) is a perennial herb in the family Asteraceae that exerts several therapeutic effects.

In traditional medicine, the fruit and dried aerial parts of Tarragon were used as a treatment for epilepsy, toothache and diarrhea (Zargari, 1989). The plant is mildly sedative (Sayyah et al., 2004) and has been taken to aid sleep (Chevallier, 1996). Recently, the anticonvulsive activity of essential oil of *Artemisia dracunculus* in a rat model of epilepsy has been shown. It is reported that the monoterpenoids especially *trans*-anethole, pinene and methyl eugenol present in the essential oil, mediates its anticonvulsant activity (Sayyah et al., 2004).

The present study compared the electrophysiological consequences of Tarragon essential oil and its extract alone and on the PTZ-induced epileptiform activity. Moreover, alterations in the parameters of the action potentials upon application of anethole as a major component of Iranian Tarragon on neuronal cells were also investigated. In our previous work we reported that the fruit essential oil of *Pimpinella anisum* L. (Umblliferae), which contains anethole, not only did not show antiepileptic activity but also induced neuronal hyperexcitability (Janahmadi et al., 2008). On the other hand, we have also showed that both the essential oil of *cuminum cyminum* and low concentration (0.05%) of Tarragon extract exhibit antiepileptic activity (Janahmadi et al., 2006; Farajnia et al., 2011).

The results obtained here showed that the essential oil of Tarragon not only does not show any antiepileptic activity at concentration of 0.005%, but also worsened the epileptiform activity induced by PTZ. Whereas, Tarragon extract, at even higher concentration (0.1%) than that we have reported more recently, can reduce and modulate PTZ-induced neuronal hyperexcitability. Furthermore, the finding showed that anethole affects the normal neuronal excitability in a concentration manner. The neuronal excitability and the firing patterns are balanced by the activity of many ion channels, including voltage and Ca^{2+}-activated K^{+} (SK and BK) channels (Faber et al., 2005; Crest and Gola, 1993; Arai et al., 2004).

Here, it was found that both essential oil and extract of *A. dracunculus* led to a decrease in the amplitude of AHPs and the essential oil, but not extract prolonged the AP duration. In snail neurons, spike duration and AHP amplitude are determined by a set of potassium channels which underlie fast and delayed outward K^+ currents (Bal et al. 2000; Sakakibara et al. 2005; Solntseva 1995; Thompson 1977). There are also two classes of Ca^{2+} activated K^+ channels (K_{Ca}); the large conductance Ca^{2+} activated K^+ channels (BK channels) and the small conductance Ca^{2+} activated K^+ channels (SK) (Crest and Gola 1993; Hermann and Erxleben 1987). SK channels mediate a Ca^{2+}-activated afterhyperpolarizing current, I_{AHP}, in most nerve cells, whereas large conductance Ca^{2+}-activated K^+ (BK) channels are responsible for the fast afterhyperpolarization (fAHP). Both types of channels are activated during the action potential causing a transient hyperpolization of the cell membrane. This produces the AHP which in turn inhabits further AP firings. Therefore, the decrease in AHP and the increase in the firing rate particularly in the presence of Tarragon essential oil could be partly related to the possible inhibition of K_{Ca} channels. However, the increase in the duration of AP following Tarragon oil treatment might be due to the inhibition of Na^+ and/or voltage-gated K^+ channels. It has now been reported that very small influxes of Na^+ through voltage-gated Na^+ channels activate a K^+ conductance which play an important role in determining AP duration in both vertebrate and invertebrate neurons (Bader et al.,1985; Hartung, 1985; Dryer et al., 1989; Budelli et al., 2009).

On the other hand, the results of the second sets of the experiments suggest that Tarragon extract has a potential antiepileptic effect. The decrease in the PTZ-induced hyperexcitability, the unchanged AP duration and the pause between active periods clearly indicate that the crude extract of Tarragon can alleviate the epileptiform activity partly through the activation of K^+ channels or receptor dependent ion channels.

It has been reported that epileptic activity can be suppressed by drugs that enhance gamma amino butyric acid-type A ($GABA_A$) receptor-mediated inhibitory neurotransmission, such as benzodiazepines and phenobarbital (Macdonald and Kelly, 1995). The presence of anticonvulsant benzodiazepines in alcoholic extract of A. *dracunculus* supports the antiepileptic potential of extract (Kavvadias et al., 2000). The appearance of IPSPs during quiescence period recorded between firing activity in the presence of Tarragon extract, therefore, could be due to the activation of $GABA_A$ receptors. However, Tarragon essential oil worsened the PTZ-induced profound hyperexcitability, as evidenced by a significant increase in the firing frequency and reduction in the AHP amplitude. The stronger antiepileptic activity of Tarragon alcoholic extract than its own essential oil could be attributed to the benzodiazepine in the extract (Kavvadias et al., 2000), as we have more recently reported that picrotoxin, a GABA antagonis, eliminates the IPSPs-induced by Tarragon extract at concentration of 0.05% (Farajnia et al., 2011). However, potentiation of PTZ-induced epileptiform activity possibly could be due, in part, to the existence of some active component, such as anethole. In the present study, we found that anethole at higher concentration (2%), but not at lower concentration (0.5%) produces hyperexcitability and paroxysmal depolarization shift very similar to that of induced by PTZ in Na^+ Ringer solution. We have more recently demonstrated that anethole affects the Ca^{2+}-dependent excitability and Ca^{2+} spike characteristics in a concentration manner (Ghasemi et al., 2011). Therefore, it can be speculated that anethole 2% increases the neuronal hyperexcitability directly or in directly through activation of outward K^+ channels, including K_{Ca}, as evidenced by a significant increase and decrease in the AP duration and AHP amplitude, respectively.

The stronger antiepileptic activity of alcoholic extract of Tarragon than its own essential oil could be attributed to the benzodiazepine in the extract (Kavvadias et al., 2000), as we have more recently reported that picrotoxin, a GABA antagonist, eliminates the IPSPs-induced by 0.05% Tarragon extract (Farajnia et al., 2011). However, potentiation of PTZ-induced epileptiform activity by essential oil possibly could be due to the existence of some active component, such as anethole. In the present study, we found that anethole at higher concentration (2%), but not at lower concentration (0.5%) produces hyperexcitability and paroxysmal depolarization shift very similar to that of induced by PTZ in Na^+ Ringer solution. Anethole treatment at concentration of 2% enhances the AHP amplitude which in turn hyperpolarizes the cell membrane and thereby removes sodium channels inactivation and increases the availability of these channels. The availability of Na^+ channel, which is strongly regulated by AHP-induced hyperpolarization, is known to regulate the firing regularity and increases the firing excitability (Patlak, 1991; Vervaeke et al., 2006; Mecer et al., 2007).

It is likely the augmentation of the amplitude of AHP following treatment with anethole 2% could be caused by activation of voltage and/or particularly calcium dependent potassium channels, which play an important role in neuronal discharge regularity. it is generally accepted that AHP amplitude is reversely correlated with the firing frequency (Madison and Nicoll, 1984; Hallworth et al., 2003; Vatanparast and Janahmadi, 2009) and blockade of these channels disrupts the precision of firing and produces less regularity in firing (Haghdoust et al., 2007; Hallworth et al., 2003; Sausbier et al., 2004; Walter et al., 2006). Therefore, increasing the firing precision and regularity, as evidenced by a significant increase in the AHP amplitude and a decrease in CV following exposure to 2% anethole here in F1 cells, could be possibly attributed to the opening of K_{Ca} channels.

We have more recently demonstrated that anethole affects the Ca^{2+}-dependent excitability and Ca^{2+} spike characteristics in a concentration manner (Ghasemi et al., 2011).

In conclusion, findings of the study suggest that herbal medicine may be considered a s a two-edged sword since some of the medicinal essential oils (such as anise and Tarragon oils) and the compounds isolated from them (e.g. anehole) have potential capacity to induce neuronal hyperexcitability and epileptiform activity or alternatively their own crude extracts may possess antiepileptic activity. Therefore, when they are used for treating patients suffer from epilepsy, a certain caution is needed.

5. References

Al-Harbi MM, Qureshi S, Raza M, Ahmed MM, Giangreco AB, Shah AH. (1995). Influence of anethole treatment on the tumour induced by Ehrlich ascites carcinoma cells in paw of Swiss albino mice. *Eur J Cancer Prev* 4 : 307-318.

Aqili Khorasani, MH. (1992). Makhzan al adviah. Safa publication, Tehran, pp 583–584.

Arai H, Kubo T, Nagahama T. (2004). Modulation of a feeding neural circuit by microinjection of K+ channel expression genes into a single identified neuron in Aplysia kurodai. *Zoolog Sci* 21(4):369-373.

Bader CR, Bernheim L, Bertrand D. (1985). Sodium-activated potassium current in cultured avian neurones. *Nature* 317: 540-542.

Bal R , Janahmadi M , Green GGR, Sanders DJ. (2000). Effect of calcium channel blockers on transient outward current of F76 and D1 neuronal soma membrane in the subesophageal ganglion of *Helix aspersa. J Membr Biol* 173:179-185.

Boissier JR, Simon P, Le Bourhis B. (1967). Experimental psychotropic action of cis and trans isomers of anethol. *Therapie* 22 : 309–323.

Budelli G, Hage TA, Wei A, Rojas P, Jong YJ, O'Malley K, Salkoff L. (2009). Na^+-activated K^+ channels express a large delayed outward current in neurons during normal physiology. Nat Neurosci 12(6):745-570.

Chainy GB, Manna SK, Chaturvedi MM, Aggarwal BB. (2000). Anethole blocks both early and late cellular responses transduced by tumor necrosis factor: effect on NF-kB, AP-1, JNK, MAPKK and apoptosis. *Oncogene* 19 (25) : 2943–2950.

Chevallier, A. (1996). *The Encyclopedia of Medicinal Plants* Dorling Kindersley, London.

Crest M , Gola M. (1993). Large conductance Ca^{2+}-activated K^+ channels are involved in both spike shaping and firing regulation in *Helix* neurones. *J Physiol* 465:265–287.

Dryer SE, Fujii JT, Martin AR. (1989). Na^+-activated K^+ current in cultured brain stem neurones from chicks. *J Physiol* 410:283–296.

Faber ESL, Delaney AJ, Sah P. (2005). SK channels regulate excitatory synaptic transmission and plasticity in the lateral amygdala. *Nat Neurosci* 8:635–641.

Farajnia S, Janahmadi M, Vatanparast J, Abbasipour H, Kamalinejad M. (2011). The Electrophysiological Consequences of *Artemisia dracunculus* L. (Tarragon) Extract on Pentylenetetrazol-Induced Epileptiform Activity in Snail Neurons. *Cell J (Yakhteh)*, 12 (4): 495-502.

Faugier-Grimaud S. (1974). Extrasynaptic mechanisms of cardiazol-induced epileptiform activity of invertebrate neurons. *Brain Res* 69: 354–360.

Freire RS, Morais SM, Catunda-Junior FE, Pinheiro DC. (2005). Synthesis and antioxidant, anti-inflammatory and gastroprotector activities of anethole and related compounds. Bioorg *Med Chem*13 (13): 4353–4358.

Ghasemi Z, Hassanpour-Ezatti M, Kamalinejad M, Janahmadi M. (2011). Functional involvement of Ca(2+) and Ca(2+)-activated K(+) channels in anethol -induced changes in Ca(2+) dependent excitability of F1 neurons in Helix aspersa. *Fitoterapia.* 82 (5):750-756.

Ghelardini C, Galeotti N, Mazzanti G. (2001).Local anaesthetic activity of monoterpenes and phenylpropanes of essential oils. *Planta Medica* 67 : 564–566.

Goldensohn ES, Pupura DP. (1963). Intracellular potentials of cortical neurons during focal epileptogenic discharges. *Science* 139: 840–842.

Gülçın I, Oktay M, Kıreçcı E, Küfrevıoğlu ÖI. (2003). Screening of antioxidant and antimicrobial activities of anise (*Pimpinella anisum* L.) seed extracts. *Food Chem* 83:371–382.

Haghdoust H, Janahmadi M, Behzadi G. (2007). Physiological role of dendrotoxin-sensitive K^+ channels in the rat cerebellar Purkinje neurons. *Physiol Res* 56: 807-813.

Hallworth N E , Wilson C J , Bevan M D. (2003). Apamin-sensitive small conductance calcium-activated potassium channels, through their selective coupling to voltage-gated calcium channels, are critical determinants of the precision, pace, and pattern of action potential generation in rat subthalamic nucleus neurones *in vitro. J Neurosci* 23:7525–7542.

Hartung K. (1985). Potentiation of a transient outward current by Na+ influx in crayfish neurones. *Pfluigers Archiv* 404: 41-44.

Hermann A, Erxleben C. (1987). Charybdotoxin selectively blocks small Ca-activated K channels in Aplysia neurons. *J Gen Physiol* 90:27-47.

Janahmadi M, Niazi F, Danyali S, Kamalinejad M. (2006). Effects of the fruit essential oil of Cuminum cyminum Linn. (Apiaceae) on pentylenetetrazol-induced epileptiform activity in F1 neurones of Helix aspersa. *J Ethnopharmacol* 104(1-2):278-282.

Janahmadi M, Farajnia S, Vatanparast J, Abbasipour H, Kamalinejad M. (2008). The fruit essential oil of Pimpinella anisum L. (Umblliferae) induces neuronal hyperexcitability in snail partly through attenuation of after-hyperpolarization. J Ethnopharmacol 120(3):360-365.

Kavvadias D, Abou-Mandour AA, Czygan FC, Beckmann H, Sand P, Riederer P, Schreier P. (2000). Identification of benzodiazepines in Artemisia dracunculus and Solanum tuberosum rationalizing their endogenous formation in plant tissue. *Biochem Biophys Res Commun* 5;269(1):290-295.

Kerkut GA, Lambert JDC, Gayton RJ, Loker JE, Walker RJ. (1975). Mapping of nerve cells in the sub-oesophageal ganglia of *Helix aspersa*. *Comp Biochem Physiol* (A) 50:1–25.

MacDonald RL, Kelly KM. (1995). Antiepileptic drug mechanisms of action. *Epilepsia* 36: 502–512.

Madison DV, Nicoll RA. (1984). Control of the repetitive discharge of rat CA 1 pyramidal neurones in vitro. *J Physiol* 354:319-331.

Matsumoto H , Ajmone Marsan C. (1964). Cortical cellular phenomen in experimental epilepsy: interictal manifestations. *Exp Neurol* 9: 286–304.

Meepagala KM, Sturtz G, Wedge DA. (2002). Antifungal constituents of the essential oil fraction of *Artemisia dracunculus* L. Var. dracunculus. *J Agr Food Chem* 50: 6989–6992.

Parejo I, Viladomat F, Bastida J, Rosas-Romero A, Flerlage N, Burillo J, Codina C. (2002). Comparison between the radical scavenging activity and antioxidant activity of six distilled and nondistilled. Mediterranean herbs and aromatic plants. *J Agr Food Chem* 50: 6882–6890.

Patlak, J B. (1991) Molecular kinetics of voltage-dependent Na^+ channels. *Physiol Rev* 71:1047-1080

Sakakibara M, Okuda F, Nomura K, Watanabe K, Meng H, Horikoshi T, Lukowiak K. (2005) Potassium currents in isolated statocyst neurons and RPeD1 in the pond snail, Lymnaea stagnalis. *J Neurophysiol* 94:3884-92.

Sausbier M, Hu H, Arntz C, Feil S, Kamm S, Adelsberger H, Sausbier U, Sailer CA, Feil R, Hofmann F, Korth M, Shipston MJ, Knaus HG, Wolfer DP, Pedroarena CM, Storm JF, Ruth P. (2004), Cerebellar ataxia and Purkinje cell dysfunction caused by Ca^{2+}-activated K^+ channel deficiency. Proc Natl Acad Sci U S A. 101:9474-9478.

Sayyah M, Nadjafnia L, Kamalinejad M .(2004). Anticonvulsant activity and chemical composition of *Artemisia dracunculus* L. essential oil. *J Ethnopharmcol* 94: 283–287.

Singh G, Kapoor IPS, Pandey SK, Singh UK, Singh RK. (2002). Studies of essential oils. Part 10. Antibacterial activity of volatile oils of some spices. *Phytother Res* 16 (7), 680–682.

Soliman KM, Badeaa RI. (2002). Effect of oil extracted from some medicinal plants on different mycotoxigenic fungi. *Food ChemToxicol* 40 (11): 1669–1675.

Solntseva EI (1995). Properties of slow early potassium current in neurons of snail Helix pomatia. *Gen Pharmacol* 26:1719-1726.

Speckmann EJ, Caspers H. (1973). Proxysmal depolarization and changes in action potentials induced by pentylenetetrazol in isolated neurons of *Helix pomatia. Epilepsia* 14: 397–408.

Sugaya A, Sugaya E, Tsujitani M. (1973). Pentylenetetrazol-induced intracellular potential changes of the neuron of the Japanese land snail *Euhadra peliomphala. Jpn J Physiol* 23: 261–274.

Taylor PS (1987) Selectivity and patch measurements of A-current channels in *Helix aspersa* neurones. *J Physiol* 388:437–447.

Thompson SH.(1977).Three pharmacologically distinct potassium channels in molluscan neurones. *J Physiol* 265:465-488.

Vatanparast J, Janahmadi M. (2009). Contribution of apamin-sensitive SK channels to the firing precision but not to the slow afterhyperpolarization and spike frequency adaptation in snail neurons. *Brain Res* 1255: 57-66.

Vervaeke K, Hu H, Graham LJ, Storm JF. (2006). Contrasting effects of the persistent Na+ current on neuronal excitability and spike timing. *Neuron* 49: 257–270.

Walter JT, Alviña K, Womack MD, Chevez C, Khodakhah K. (2006). Decreases in the precision of Purkinje cell pacemaking cause cerebellar dysfunction and ataxia. *Nat Neurosci* 9:389-397.

Zani F, Massimi G, Benvenuti S, Bianchi A, Albasini A, Melegari M, Vampa G, Bellotti A, Mazza P. (1991). Studies on the genotoxic properties of essential oils with Bacillus subtilis re-assay and Salmonella/microsome reversion assay. *Planta Medica* 57: 237–241.

Zargari A. (1989). Medicinal Plants, 2. Tehran University, Tehran.

19

In-Situ Release of Antiepileptic Drugs from Nanostructured Reservoirs

Tessy Lopez, Anna Kozina, Emma Ortiz-Islas, Karla A. Espinoza and Richard Gonzalez

Laboratorio de Nanotecnología para Medicina, Instituto Nacional de Neurología y Neurocirugía 'MVS'; Departamento de Atención a la Salud, Universidad Autónoma Metropolitana Xochimilco; Departamento de Química, Instituto Nacional de Investigaciones Nucleares; Department of Chemical and Bimolecular Engineering, Tulane University

Mexico, USA

1. Introduction

The interest to 'in situ' drug delivery systems has been sparked by the advantages of these systems, such as ease of application, localized delivery for a site-specific action, prolonged delivery periods, decreased body drug dosage with concurrent reduction in possible undesirable side effects common to most forms of systemic delivery, and improved patient compliance and comfort. There are different materials that can be potentially used as the implants, each of which has its advantages and disadvantages. Emulsion, liposomes, microcapsules and micells may be potentially used for certain applications Collins-Gold et al. (1990); Sharma (1997); Chen et al. (1997); Zhang et al. (1996), however, they still have some room for improvement. They are not the best systems for long-time delivery because of the stability, sterilization and low drug entrapment problems, as well as, in some cases, difficulty of manufacturing procedure or in control of the properties Hatfia & Amsdena (2002). As alternative, 'in situ' setting semi-solid drug depots are being developed. These implants are made of biodegradable polymers that solidify once injected into the site. Together with all the advantages, the main minus of these systems is the initial burst in the drug release connected with the release of the drug during the solidification time of the matrix. Also, some of the polymers require high temperature for injection or usage of organic solvents, which may result in necrosis or toxicity. Another polymer matrix (ethylene-vinyl acetate) was successfully used as an implant to deliver phenytoin into the brain Tamargo et al. (2002), however, the material manufacturing time is quite long, more than one month, which makes it difficult to apply routinely.

The recently developed sol-gel technology offers new possibilities for incorporating biologically active agents within inorganic titania or silica xerogels at room temperature, and for controlling their release kinetics from the gel matrix Chiriac et al. (2010); Quintar-Guerrero et al. (2010); Lopez et al. (2006); Lopez & Quintana et al. (2007); Lopez et al. (2007). This sol-gel technique is inexpensive, versatile and simple and provides easily reproducible xerogel properties. Thus, such materials are good candidates to create 'in situ' delivery systems.

2. State of the art

Phenytoin (5,5-diphenyl hydantoin) is one of the major first-line antiepileptic drugs used in the treatment of generalized and partial (with or without secondary generalization) seizures. Also, it is used acutely in the management of life threatening status epilepticus and in the treatment of serial seizures. The mechanism of action is not definitely known but extensive research strongly suggests that its main mechanism is to block frequency-, use- and voltage-dependent neuronal sodium channels and, therefore, limit repetitive firing of action potentials. In chemical structure, phenytoin is related to the barbiturates. However, the use of phenytoin clinically is problematic for several reasons. Firstly, phenytoin has a low therapeutic index so that therapeutic and toxic doses are close to each other. Secondly, because of its saturable metabolism, the relationship between plasma concentration and dose is non-linear and difficult to predict Richens & Dunlop (1975). Thirdly, it has a long term toxicity profile, including adverse cosmetic effects Reynolds (1989), which is undesirable. Also, chronic drug administration can lead to many side effects, among which language and memory problems, intellectual decline and psychiatric illness. This occurs because only a certain amount of the drug overcomes the hematoencephalic barrier, which requires its higher dosage Lolin et al. (1994). Considering this, 'in situ' prolonged drug delivery represents an alternative that has excellent therapeutic benefits.

3. Sol-gel derived materials

The encapsulation of a drug inside an inorganic nanostructured matrix is a promising way to deliver the drug. The matrix is usually some metal oxide such as Titanium or Silicon dioxides or aluminosilicates of different structures. The structure may vary from highly organized (crystals, microtubes) to an amorphous one. Such a matrix has a high surface area and porosity allowing to accommodate rather large amounts of the drug. The drug may be incorporated either by adsorption into already existing structure or during the structure formation, namely the synthesis of the matrix. The latter method is more efficient because it allows encapsulation of larger amounts of the drug and its release during a longer period. The synthesis conditions of conventional chemical processes do not always allow addition of the drug during the synthesis, since many drugs are quite sensitive to the change of the synthesis parameters such as temperature, pH, etc. Also, the solubility of the drug influences the possibility of its encapsulation. However, in this case, the sol-gel method may overcome these difficulties and become a good option, since it allows the drug encapsulation under the mild conditions. In the typical sol-gel process the synthesis starts with a solution containing metal precursors, such as metal alkoxides, water as a hydrolysis agent, and alcohol as a solvent. The reacting mixture may also include acid or base as a catalyst. Metal alkoxides undergo hydrolysis and polycondensation at near room temperature forming a sol, in which polymers or fine particles are dispersed without precipitation. Further reaction connects the particles solidifying the sol into a wet gel, which still contains water and solvents. Vaporization of the solvent and water produces a dry gel, which is a porous material. Since the sol-gel process starts with a well mixed solution, the reaction may take place at lower temperatures as compared to

conventional mixtures. This enables incorporation of otherwise decomposing compounds such as many drugs. The drug is usually added to the initial mixture and during the process accommodates within the pores. Usually amorphous material has a distribution of the pore sizes. Thus, on release, firs, the drug situated inside the large pores comes out, then the one inside the mesopores, and, finally, the one inside the micropores. This permits reaching a desired level of the drug and then to have its prolonged liberation.
The release profile of the drug incorporated into titania matrix is expected to depend on the following factors: the reservoir surface properties affecting drug-matrix interactions, the morphology of the matrix, the degree of crystallinity, drug dissolution and diffusion, and the method of incorporation of the drug into the matrix. Since the majority of these factors may be controlled by the parameters of the sol-gel synthesis, the drug release kinetics, therefore, may be tuned by tailoring the processing parameters during the sol-gel reaction. Thus, one specific parameter of the synthesis can be varied in order to change the drug release profile. In the following sections we will discuss what are the main parameters influencing the release profile and how they affect the release kinetics 'in vitro'.

4. Phenytoin-titania reservoirs

In the particular case of the drug incorporated into the sol-gel titania, there are two principal questions that one should address: (i) does the synthesis process affect the structure-activity relation and the stability of the drug and (ii) what functional groups of the matrix and the drug participate in the interaction? There are different types of interactions that can be found in the modern drug delivery systems: electrostatic (Coulombic), hydrophobic, or hydrogen-type. Sol-gel titania, if it is not calcinated, has a surface covered with hydroxyl groups with the average density of 5 OH/nm^2. These terminal hydroxyls can interact with a heteroatom of the drug molecule serving as adsorption sites favoring the drug distribution inside the matrix. Naturally, the number of OH groups capable of binding the drug would define the amount of the drug that can be carried by the matrix, whereas the strength of the interaction would influence the drug diffusion out of the reservoir. The two parameters together will influence the release profile. Thus, the surface coverage by OH groups determines the adsorption behavior and the surface reactivity.

4.1 Phenytoin-titania interactions

The solid state ^{13}C NMR study allowed us to determine that phenytoin is attached to the matrix without any changes in the structure and to establish what part of the molecule couples to the titania hydroxyl groups Lopez et al. (2010). The comparison of the two spectra for pure phenytoin and the one encapsulated into the titania matrix (Figs. 1) revealed that the same signals are present in both cases with the only difference of the peaks in the aliphatic region of the spectrum for phenytoin within titania. These peaks correspond to the nonhydrolyzed butyl radicals attached to titania. The slight shift of the signals for encapsulated phenytoin as compared to pure phenytoin implies that the structure of the phenytoin molecule in the matrix is more rigid than 'free' phenytoin. Due to the largest shifts for the two carbons of the hydantoin ring it becomes clear that the hydantoin ring in the phenytoin molecule is the system that interacts with OH groups of the titania matrix. To answer the question how exactly the interaction takes place, we suggested the possible complexes between the hydantoin ring

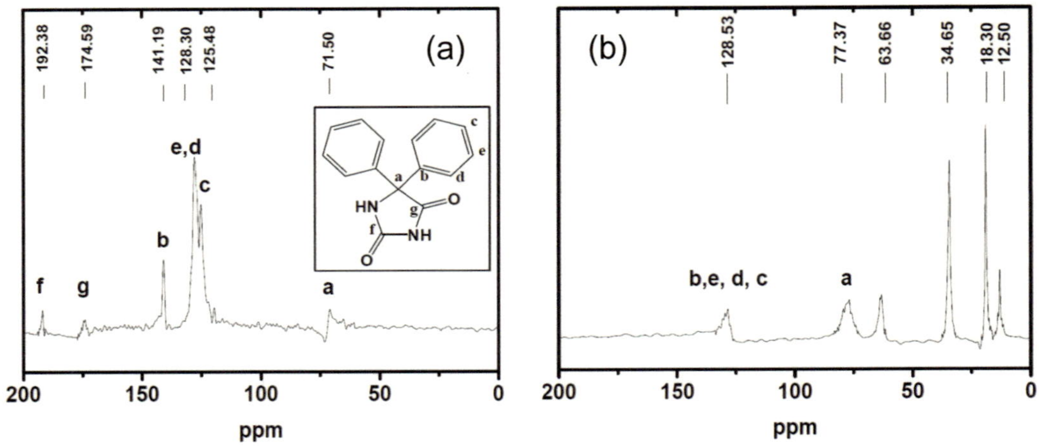

Fig. 1. Solid state ^{13}C NMR spectra of (a) pure and (b) titania encapsulated phenytoin. The peak letters indicate corresponding atoms in the phenytoin structure given on the right in (a).

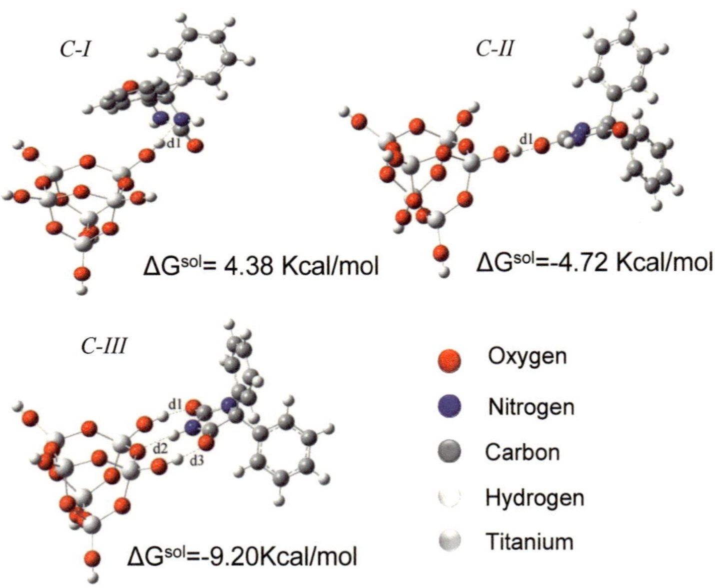

Fig. 2. Optimized geometries of phenytoin-titania complexes: $C - I$ and $C - II$ are monodentate complexes, and $C - III$ is the tridentate complex. The corresponding corrected free Gibbs energies on formation of each complex are given below.

and titania hydroxyl groups, calculated using the *Gaussian 03* Frisch et al. (2004) package of programs within the Density Functional Theory (DFT) formalism, and shown in Fig. 2.
The last complex proposed (tridentate C-III) has three simultaneous weak hydrogen-type interactions: two hydroxyl groups of titania interact with two oxygen atoms (of carbonyl groups) of phenytoin and there is an oxygen bridge from titania to a proton of the amine group of phenytoin. The calculated Gibbs energies show that C-III is more favorable in comparison to C-I and C-II. Since hydroxyl groups of titania participate in the complex

formation, phenytoin adsorption on titania should significantly depend on the hydroxylation degree of titania. The experimental evidence of the presence of C-III complex was obtained by comparison of carbonyl region of IR-spectra calculated for different complexes with the experimental IR-spectrum. Even though the carbonyl group signals do not disappear completely, as suggested in an 'ideal' theoretical system, a significant reduction of the signals suggests the presence of rather large amounts of C-III, though it is hard to conclude in what proportion to C-II and unbound phenytoin it is formed. Since the amount of hydroxyl groups on the titania surface is crucial for the phenytoin load in titania reservoirs, the hydroxylation degree was analyzed by IR and TGA/DSC analyses. It was found that with increase of water/alkoxide ratio r_w, the hydroxylation degree increases up to $r_w = 16$ and then decreases for $r_w = 24$. Water/alkoxide ratio $r_w = 16$ was concluded to be the most favorable to bind the largest amount of the drug because of the highest hydroxyl group coverage. The next step in the research was to study how different r_w would affect the phenytoin release 'in vitro'.

4.2 Water-alkoxide ratio

As it was mentioned above, titania reservoirs were synthesized by the sol-gel method. Titanium(IV) tetrabutoxide was continuously added to the mixture of deionized Millipore filtered water, filtered ethanol and sodium phenytoin at 25°C under constant stirring. The molar ethanol/alkoxide ratio was kept constant and equal to 8. The sodium phenytoin/alkoxide ratio was fixed to 7.5 mg per 1 g of alkoxide. The molar ratio of water/alkoxide r_w was taken as 4, 8, and 16. The resulting homogeneous sol was then left to gelate for 24 h under constant stirring and after that was dried at room temperature. The white powder was then dried at 40°C in a vacuum for 24 h. The surface properties were characterized by the Brunauer-Emmett-Teller (BET) method, crystallinity - by High Resolution Transmission Electron Microscopy (HRTEM), hydroxyl group coverage - by IR spectroscopy combined with a homemade vacuum heating cell under nitrogen atmosphere Lopez et al. (2011). These parameters were considered in the connection with the drug release 'in vitro'.

To give an idea about the structure and morphology of the prepared materials, it is important to notice that the structure of the reservoirs is rather complex. The primary particles formed during the polycondensation are of the size of about 3 - 5 nm (Fig. 3a). The primary particles almost immediately aggregate, forming the primary aggregates of about 50 nm size Heredia et al. (2009). Slitlike micropores of 2.5 nm are formed as a result of aggregation of the primary aggregates with the formation of the secondary aggregates. The secondary aggregates are much larger but they also can aggregate between them during the sample drying, forming the structure shown in Fig. 3b with macropores comparable to the aggregate sizes. The agglomerates have different sizes ranging from 0.1 up to 0.8 μm, building up a porous structure with large distribution of pore sizes.

Interestingly, it was found that the specific surface area increases with the addition of phenytoin to the reaction due to difference in the particle growth at larger pH (pH=10 for the solution of phenytoin sodium in water). In the case of different r_w, it was observed that the surface area first increases and then decreases, while crystallization degree decreases with the increase of water content in the reaction. Titania synthesized in this way is mainly amorphous, however, when the samples were observed under a high resolution electron microscope (HRTEM), the regions with the crystalline structures corresponding to anatase titania were observed (Fig. 4). Thus, there is an indication of a small degree of crystallinity on the nano

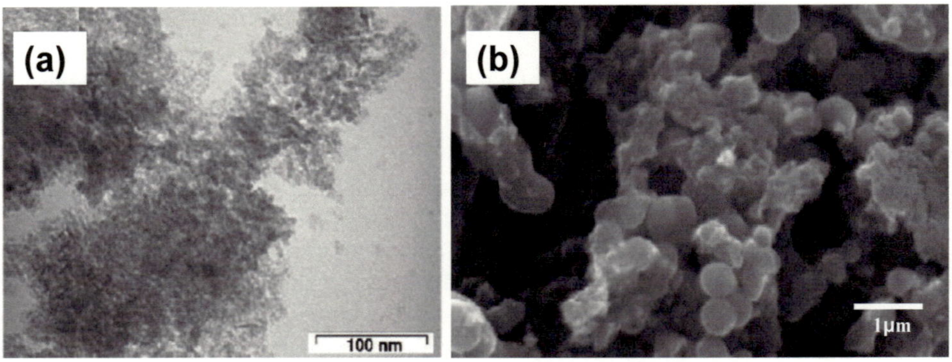

Fig. 3. (a) TEM image showing nanoparticle agglomeration and (b) SEM image showing the spherical morphology.

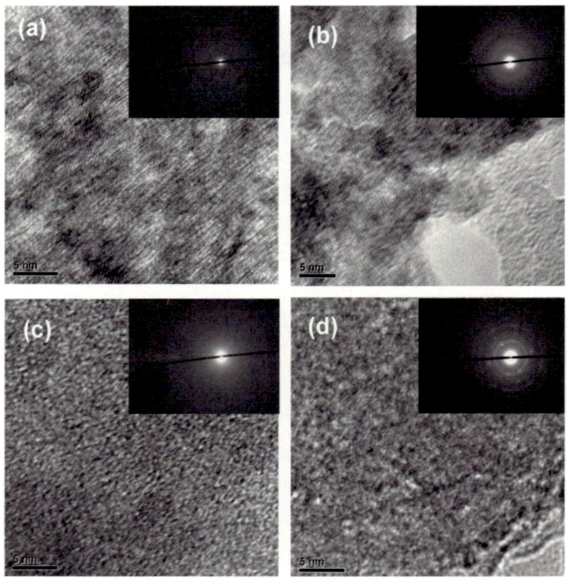

Fig. 4. HRTEM micrographs with corresponding diffraction patterns of phenytoin-titania reservoirs synthesized with different water/alkoxide ratios r_w: (a) $r_w = 4$, (b) $r_w = 8$, (c) $r_w = 16$, and (d) $r_w = 16$ titania reference (without phenytoin).

scale in the material. Moreover, the degree of crystallinity depends on the water/alkoxide ratio r_w and decreases with the increase of r_w Lopez et al. (2011).

It was possible to characterize the OH group coverage in an accurate way, excluding the contribution of the sample humidity and physically adsorbed water. The results showed that the hydroxyl group coverage increases with increase of r_w from 4 to 16. Fig. 5 shows the drug release kinetics of phenytoin from the reservoirs synthesized with different water/alkoxide ratios r_w.

For all three samples the release profiles are similar in shape and characterized by the two regimes: the initial fast release described by the short-time (ST) release rate followed by the long-time sustained release with lower release rate (LT). The initial release rate increases with

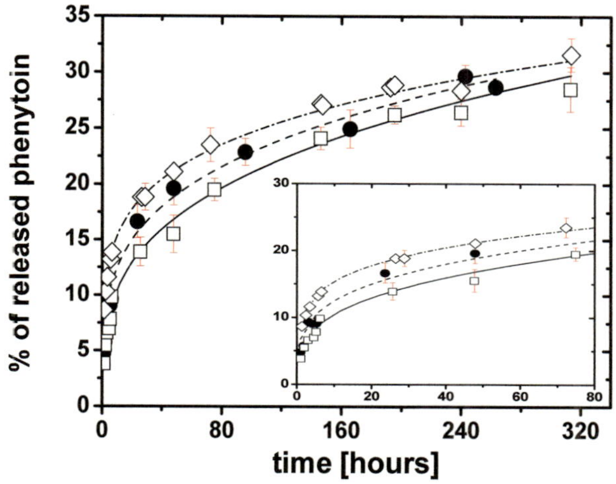

Fig. 5. Release kinetics of phenytoin to buffer from 50 mg of titania reservoirs synthesized with different water/alkoxide ratios r_w: squares $r_w = 4$, circles $r_w = 8$ and diamonds $r_w = 16$. The lines indicate the Fick's second law fits: solid for $r_w = 4$, dashed for $r_w = 8$ and dash-dotted for $r_w = 16$. The inset shows closer look to the initial release stage.

the increase of water content in the reaction. It is correlated with the size of macropores formed between the secondary aggregates of titania nanoparticles. The size of the secondary aggregates grows with increase of r_w, thus, during the initial release period, there is a drug discharge with the highest release rate and drug amount for $r_w = 16$. Then, the initial discharge slows down with the decrease of r_w.

The constant long-time release rate is affected mainly by the following factors: reservoir morphology on the surface (surface area, porosity and pore size) and in bulk (crystalline or amorphous), interactions between the matrix and the drug, and the diffusion of the molecules within the matrix. These parameters interplay in such a way that LT release rate first slightly increases with increase of water content from 4 to 8 and then decreases for $r_w = 16$. The combination of morphology, degree of hydroxylation, and crystallinity allows sample $r_w = 8$ to liberate faster than other samples during the long-term stage.

There are different empirical and semiempirical approaches that have been developed to interpret the release mechanisms. One of the simplest empirical equation is the so-called power law equation based on Fick's second law of diffusion:

$$M_t/M_\infty = kt^n, \tag{1}$$

where M is the amount of drug released after an instant t and infinite times, k is the constant that correlates with the diffusion coefficient and n is the exponent characterizing the release mechanism. If the Fickian diffusion takes place, n is equal to 0.5, 0.45 and 0.43 for a thin film, a cylinder and a sphere, respectively. For porous matrix n is expected to take lower values Peppas (1985); Peppas & Korsmeyer (1986). However, given the simplifications introduced for this model, the analysis based on the power law should be taken with precaution. The values of parameter n are very low ($n < 0.45$ for all the samples) and vary from 0.2 to 0.3. This

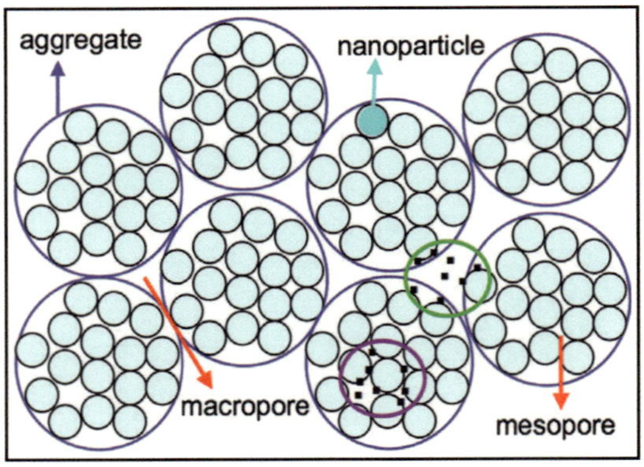

Fig. 6. (Schematic illustration of the morphology of the titania reservoirs, consisting of nanoparticles, aggregates, and macro- and mesopores. The green and purple encircled regions show phenytoin present in macropores and mesopores, respectively.

suggests that the release process is controlled by non-Fickian diffusion. The titania matrix has the pores quite heterogeneous in length, surface roughness and fractality, which may be the reason for the complex transport behavior.

4.3 Thermal treatment

With the purpose to determine the influence of the surface characteristics such as the effective surface area, porosity, and the average pore size of titania on the release kinetics of phenytoin, various titania-phenytoin reservoirs were prepared by the sol-gel method combined with the hydrothermal treatment of titanium (IV) isopropoxide in 1 M acetic acid. Control over the particle size was achieved by using the hydrothermal treatment at 220°C for different times: 1, 3, 8, 20 and 42 hours. The reservoirs were loaded with 5 wt% of phenytoin Heredia et al. (2009).

The obtained material consisted of pure anatase crystal phase independent of the heat treatment time. It was found that the average particle size defined from XRD measurements grows with the increasing treatment time. As it was previously mentioned, most nanoparticles are clustered in aggregates. The average aggregate size determined by dynamic light scattering was found to be in the range between 20 and 60 nm for the shortest and longest treatment time, respectively. The average number of nanoparticles per aggregate was found to be about 15-40 suggesting the development of porosity as shown in Fig.6.

The drug release kinetics were determined by measuring the UV-vis spectra of the buffer solution with the immersed reservoir as a function of time for a period of up to two months in a closed glass bottle. Fig. 7 shows the results of the release studies of five materials hydrothermally treated for different periods of time. It was found that the reservoirs are able to release phenytoin for more than 45 days, and the release kinetics are characterized by two regimes: an initial fast release and a subsequent slow release, similar to that observed in Fig.5. The duration of the initial fast release regime was found to depend on the hydrothermal treatment time, and decreases with nanoparticle and aggregate size. Unfortunately, the initial release rate was not quantified due to a generally non-linear behavior and insufficient data points. The slow release rate is independent of time and showed a weak dependence on the morphology of the nanomaterial. The phenytoin constant release rate was found to be

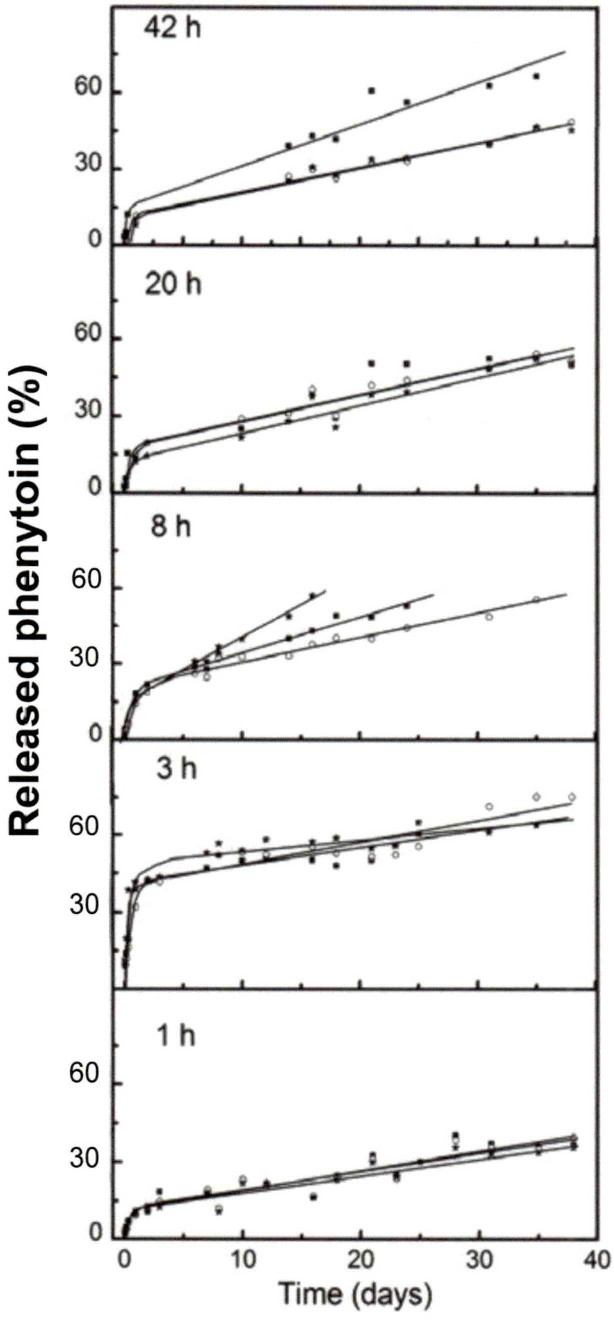

Fig. 7. Release kinetics for the titania reservoirs with different morphological properties. The released phenytoin is shown as a percentage of the initially incorporated amount of phenytoin. The kinetics were determined for three samples of each hydrothermal treatment duration. The straight lines correspond to linear fits after allowing for the initial fast release period to end.

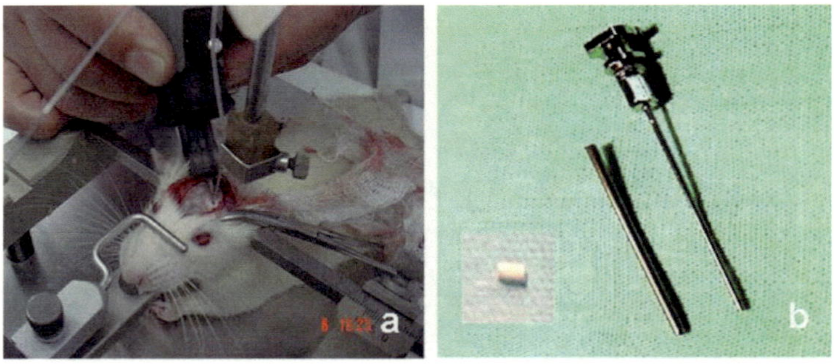

Fig. 8. (a) Stereotactic surgery is used to introduce the implant; (b) Cannula used for compressing the material to a cylinder and 1x1.5 mm titania cylinder implant.

between 0.017 mg/day and 0.030 mg/day, depending on the properties of reservoirs. One could distinguish between two main release rates: for the two smallest particles (1 and 3 h of thermal treatment) the rate is about 0.017 mg/day, while for the three largest particles (8, 20 and 42 h), the rate is about 0.030 mg/day. This trend follows the size of the mesopores, however, the dependence is remarkably weak. Taking into account that the pore size is at least a factor of two larger than the phenytoin molecules (varies from 4.3 to 12.6 nm for 1 and 42 h of treatment, respectively), the release rate is expected to be mainly related to the phenytoin-titania surface interaction. For strong interactions, the difference in specific surface area for the smaller mesopore and the larger mesopore nanomaterials would be expected to result in significantly different release rates. However, as it was shown, the release rate can be tuned to between 0.017 mg/day and 0.030 mg/day by control over the properties of the materials.

5. In vivo tests

Male Wistar rats (180-250 g) were used to study biocompatibility and effectiveness of the materials Lopez et al. (2006; 2007; 2009). All rats were induced epileptic convulsions following the Kindling model, where the rats were intraperitoneally injected with an aqueous solution of a subconvulsive dose of Pentilentetrazole (PTZ) (35 mg/kg). After each injection, observations were made for 20 min and the resulting seizures classified based on Racine's description for motor seizure activity in rats Racine (1972) as follows: 0 - normal activity; 1 - mouth and facial movements; 2 - head nodding; 3 - forelimb clonus; 4 - rearing; 5 - rearing and falling, loss of postural control, or full motor seizure activity. The animals were considered epileptics after exhibiting at least three consecutive phase 4 or 5 seizures. The material with or without phenytoin was then compressed to the form of a small cylinder with 1 mm diameter and 1.2 mm of height and stereotactically implanted into the temporal lobe of the rats (Fig. 8).

After the surgery, the animals were allowed to recover in their home cages with food and water. The effect of the implants were evaluated by further initiation of the seizure with PTZ on the rats with the reference and drug loaded reservoirs (six for each group). For the reference group of rats with a drugless TiO2 reservoir, all six rats kept on having epileptic events (Crisis-Tonic-Clonic-Generalized CTCG), thus, no curative effect was observed for these implants. The group of rats with implants showed a reduction of the intensity and frequency of the seizures, however, only about 45% of effectiveness of shielding was observed. One of the possible reasons for that may be a very small size of the implant, which results in

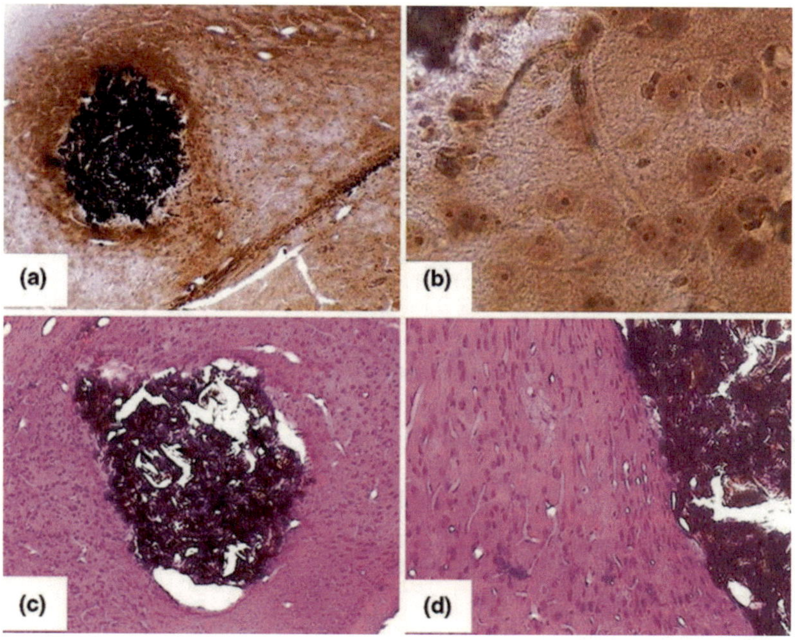

Fig. 9. Comparative histological study: (a) overall view of an histological section with the reservoir (20X); (b) The same as (a) at 100X; (c) Glial response to inflammation of the tissue in the neighborhood of the reservoir (20X); (d) Amplified limiting zone in (c) at 100X.

the release of phenytoin with the concentration lower than its terapeutic threshold. Another reason is that the release 'in vivo' may differ from 'in vitro', which requiers additional information to be able to really design the material. Our next steps would be to change the parameters of the matrix in order to find the best conditions for the reservoir to work 'in vivo'. Also, the size of the implant may be varied up to 4-5 mm in diameter Tamargo et al. (2002), which also may result in better protection.

A group of rats was sacrificed using an overdose of sodium phenobarbital administered by an intraperitoneal injection after 6 months following the implant. After that, they were perfused using a saline solution of 3.7% formaldehyde. The brains were extracted and conserved in 3.7% formaldehyde solution. The brain specimens were microtomed and conserved in a 4% formaldehyde solution for a period of 15 days. Sections (10 μm) were embedded in paraffin and viewed using an optical microscope. The sections were dyed using the Bielchowsky technique, which enables examination of the neuronal microfibrils and cell soma integrity. Implant position did not vary after 6 months in the basolateral amygdala, meaning that the reservoir was highly compatible with the nervous tissue. To confirm the lack of glial response to the implant, sections were taken of the implant zone for histological analysis and neuronal damage evaluation.

A comparative histological study Fig. 9 shows that the nerve cells are not adversely affected by the presence of the reservoir. The interfacial area between the implant and the surrounding tissue is devoid of inflammatory areas. This observation suggests that these ceramic implants can safely be used to deliver drugs to the damaged areas of the brain.

6. Outlook and prospects

An anticonvulsant drug phenytoin can be encapsulated into the sol-gel biocompatible titania and can be successfully implanted into the temporal lobe of the brain by low invasion stereotactic surgery. The implantation process is such that the damage of the surrounding tissue is minimal. The drug release from the implants is controlled by the parameters of the matrix such as its morphology, drug-matrix interaction strength, etc. Depending on the parameters of the synthesis, the release profile may be designed according to the necessities in terms of release rate and the amount of the released drug.
The first experiments 'in vivo' indicate that there is a certain degree of protection on the epileptic rats, even though no sharp fall of the seizure type was observed. Also, the biocompatibility tests revealed a good affinity between the material and the brain tissue. Thus, the first results are quite promising for the future application of the reservoirs.
One of the main prospects of the study is to achieve better protection 'in vivo' for longer time. Also, one needs to find a correlation between the drug release 'in vitro' and its effect and release profile 'in vivo'. This would allow generalization of design of the materials for different types of epilepsy patients and their needs. A very firm clinical stage is required before any commercialization of the materials.

7. References

Collins-Gold, L. C.; Lyons, R. T.; Batholow, L. C. (1990). Parenteral emulsions for drug delivery. *Adv. Drug Deliv. Rev.*, 5, (1990) 189–208.

Sharma, A. (1997) U.S. Sharma. Liposomes in drug delivery: progress and limitations. *Int. J. Pharm.*, 154, (1997) 123-140.

Chen, L.; Apte, R.N.; Cohen, S. (1997). Characterization of PLGA microspheres for the controlled delivery of IL-I for tumor immunotherapy. *J. Control. Release*, 43, (1997) 261–272.

Zhang, X.; Jackson, J. K.; Bert, H. M. (1996). Development of amphiphilic diblock copolymers as micellar carriers of taxol. *Int. J. Pharm.*, 132, (1996) 195-206.

Hatefia, A.; Amsdena, B. (2002). Biodegradable injectable in situ forming drug delivery systems. *J. Control. Release*, 80, (2002) 9–28.

Tamargo, R. J.; Rossell, L. A.; Kossoff, E. H.; Tyler, B. M.; Ewend, M. G.; Aryanpur, J. J. (2002).The intracerebral administration of phenytoin using controlled-release polymers reduces experimental seizures in rats. *Epilepsy Research* 48, (2002) 145–155.

Chiriac, A. P.; Neamtu, I.; Nita, L. E.; Nistor, M. T. (2010). Sol gel method performed for biomedical products implementation. *Mini-Rev. Med. Chem.* 10, 11, (2010) 990–1013.

Quintanar-Guerrero, D.; Ganem-Quintanar, A.; Nava-Arzaluz, M. G.; Pinon-Segundo, E. (2010). Silica xerogels as pharmaceutical drug carriers. *Expert Opin. drug deliv.*, 6, 5, (2010) 485–498.

Lopez, T.; Navarrete, J.; Conde, R.; Ascencio, J. A.; Manjarrez, J.; Gonzalez, R. D. (2006). Molecular vibrational analysis and MAS-NMR spectroscopy study of epilepsy drugs encapsulated in TiO_2-sol-gel reservoirs. *J. Biomed. Mater. Res.*, 78A, (2006) 441–448.

Lopez, T.; Quintana, P.; Ortiz-Islas, E.; Vinogradova, E.; Manjarrez, J.; Aguilar, D. H.; Castillo-Ocampo, P.; Magana, C.; Azamar, J. A. (2007). Characterization of sodium phenytoin co-gelled with titania for a controlled drug-release system. *Mat. Char.*, 58, (2007) 823-828.

Lolin, Y. I.; Ratnaraj, N.; Hjelm, M.; Patsalos, P. N. (1994). Antiepileptic drug pharmacokinetics and neuropharmacokinetics in individual rats by repetitive withdrawal of blood and cerebrospinal fluid. *Phenytoin Epilepsy Res.*, 19, 2, (1994) 99.

Lopez, T.; Espinoza, K; Kozina, A.; Galano, A. & Alexander-Katz, R. (2010). Role of hydrolysis degree in the drug-matrix interactions of nanosized sol-gel titania reservoirs for epilepsy treatment. *J. Phys. Chem. C*, 114, 47, (2010) 20022–20027.

Gaussian 03, Frisch, M. J.; Trucks, G. W.; Schlegel, H. B.; Scuseria, G. E.; Robb, M. A.; Cheeseman, J. R.; Montgomery, J. A., Jr.; Vreven, T.; Kudin, K. N.; Burant, J. C.; Millam, J. M.; Iyengar, S. S.; Tomasi, J.; Barone, V.; Mennucci, B.; Cossi, M.; Scalmani, G.; Rega, N.; Petersson, G. A.; Nakatsuji, H.; Hada, M.; Ehara, M.; Toyota, K.; Fukuda, R.; Hasegawa, J.; Ishida, M.; Nakajima, T.; Honda, Y.; Kitao, O.; Nakai, H.; Klene, M.; Li, X.; Knox, J. E.; Hratchian, H. P.; Cross, J. B.; Bakken, V.; Adamo, C.; Jaramillo, J.; Gomperts, R.; Stratmann, R. E.; Yazyev, O.; Austin, A. J.; Cammi, R.; Pomelli, C.; Ochterski, J. W.; Ayala, P. Y.; Morokuma, K.; Voth, G. A.; Salvador, P.; Dannenberg, J. J.; Zakrzewski, V. G.; Dapprich, S.; Daniels, A. D.; Strain, M. C.; Farkas, O.; Malick, D. K.; Rabuck, A. D.; Raghavachari, K.; Foresman, J. B.; Ortiz, J. V.; Cui, Q.; Baboul, A. G.; Clifford, S.; Cioslowski, J.; Stefanov, B. B.; Liu, G.; Liashenko, A.; Piskorz, P.; Komaromi, I.; Martin, R. L.; Fox, D. J.; Keith, T.; Al-Laham, M. A.; Peng, C. Y.; Nanayakkara, A.; Challacombe, M.; Gill, P. M. W.; Johnson, B.; Chen, W.; Wong, M. W.; Gonzalez, C.; Pople, J. A. (2004). *Gaussian, Inc.*, Wallingford CT, Revision D.01.

Lopez, T.; Espinoza, K. A.; Kozina, A.; Castillo, P.; Silvestre-Albero, A.; Rodriguez-Reinoso, F. & Alexander-Katz, R. (2011). Influence of water/alkoxide ratio in the synthesis of nanosized sol-gel titania on the release of phenytoin. *Langmuir*, 27(7), (2011) 4004–4009.

Peppas, N. A. (1985). Analysis of fickian and non-fickian drug release from polymers. *Pharm. Acta Helv.* 60, 4, (1985) 110–111.

Peppas, N. A.; Korsmeyer, R. W. (1986). Dynamically swelling hydrogels in controlled released applications, In: *Hydrogels in Medicine and Pharmacy*, Peppas, N. A., (Ed.) In *Medicine and Pharmacy* 3, 109–136, CRC Press, Boca Raton.

Richens, A. and Dunlop, A. (1975). Serum phenytoin levels in management of epilepsy. *Lancet*, 11, 7928, (1975) 247–248.

Reynolds, E. H. (1989). Phenytoin toxicity, In: *Antiepileptic Drugs*, Levy, R. H.; Dreifuss, F. E.; Mattson, R. H.; Meldrum, B. C. & Penry, J. K. (Eds.), 241, Raven Press, New York.

Lopez, T.; Basaldella, E. I.; Ojeda, M. L.; Manjarrez, J.; Alexander-Katz, R. (2006). Encapsulation of valproic acid and sodic phenytoin in ordered mesoporous SiO_2 solids for the treatment of temporal lobe epilepsy. *Optical Materials*, 29, (2006) 75–81.

Lopez, T.; Quintana, P.; Ascencio, J.; Gonzalez, R. D. (2007). The determination of dielectric constants of mixtures used in the treatment of epilepsy and the encapsulation of phenytoin in a titania matrix. *Colloids and Surfaces A: Physicochem. Eng. Aspects* 300, (2007) 99-105.

Lopez, T.; Alexander-Katz, R.; Castillo, P.; Gonzalez, M.; Manjarrez, J.; Gonzalez, R. D.; Ilharco, L.; Fidalgo, A.; Rieumont, J. (2009). Kinetic study of controlled release of VPA and DPH antiepileptic drugs using biocompatible nanostructured sol-gel TiO_2. *J. Mater. Sci.* 44, (2009) 5459–5468.

Racine, R. J. (1972). Modification of seizure activity by electrical stimulation: II. Motor seizure. *Electroencephalogr. Clin. Neurophysiol.* 32, (1972) 281–294.

Heredia-Cervera, B. E.; Gonzalez-Azcorra, A. A.; Rodriguez-Gattorno, G.; Lopez, T.; Ortiz-Islas, E. and Oskam, G. (2009). Controlled release of phenytoin from nanostructured TiO_2 reservoirs. *Sci. Adv. Mater.* 1, (2009) 63.

20

Quality of Life and Psychiatric Aspects in Epilepsy

Ayşe Kutlu[1] and Halil Ünalan[2]
[1]*Department of Neurology, Faculty of Medicine, Kocaeli University, Kocaeli*
[2] *Department of Physical Medicine and Rehabilitation İstanbul University, Cerrahpaşa Medical Faculty, İstanbul*
Turkey

1. Introduction

Epilepsy is a chronic disorder characterized by a spontaneous tendency for recurrent seizures which affects major aspects of a patient's life, including cognitive, behavioral, psychological and social functioning (Foldwary & Wyllie, 1999). It has been reported that cumulative lifetime risks for epilepsy and for any unprovoked seizure are 3.1% and 4.1% respectively in industrialized countries. Estimates of annual incidence of epilepsy are reported as high as 43 cases per 100,000 of the population in so-called developed countries, and are almost double this figure in the developing world (McHugh & Delanty, 2008). Another estimation points out that there are 50 million people who have epilepsy in the world (WHO 2001, Leonardi & Ustun, 2002). It was suggested that more than 80% of people with epilepsy live in developing countries, where the condition remains largely untreated (ILAE/IBE/WHO Annual Report, 1999; Meinardi et al., 2001).

2. Quality of life and psychiatric aspects in epilepsy

The science of health related quality of life (HRQOL) measurement rapidly evolved during the 1980s and 1990s within general health and in all medicine disciplines. (Tulsky & Rosenthal 2002). Despite a substantial increase in the number of published articles in recent years, research in the literature regarding the quality of lives of epileptic patients is relatively limited (Aydemir et al., 2004; Birbeck 2002). One of the most important reasons why HRQOL has become so important for those who engaged in epilepsy is related with well known characteristics of this disorder. Its chronic nature, presence of unexpected, intractable and/or frequent seizures, stigma and side effects of the antiepileptic drugs are some of these characteristics among others.

Epileptic patients experience various problems due to this disorder which will result in a lower quality of life. Seizure frequency, side effects of the antiepileptic drugs, psychological comorbidity and stigma are the factors which are associated with the severity of the disease and these factors may cause an important impact on life quality of epileptic patients.

Previous researches regarding quality of life (QOL) in epilepsy yielded contradictory results (Jacoby 1994; Leidy et al., 1999). Although most reports in this field share a common message emphasizing the negative effects of epilepsy on patients' HRQOL, there are still some other

studies which reported that this disease has little or no effect on epileptic patients' QOL (Jacoby 1994; Leidy et al., 1999). Some authors suggested that the impact of epilepsy might be minimal if the disease is well controlled and HRQOL of patients in this condition would be nearly the same as those of healthy controls (Jacoby 1994; Leidy et al.,1999). On the other hand, epileptic patients living in Europe and North America were reported to have significant impairment in HRQOL(Stavem et al., 2000; Buck et al., 1999). This discrepancy in reported results may well be related to methodological issues and/or cultural differences. However, one can easily notice that especially in studies conducted with larger samples it was found that HRQOL is decreased in patients with epilepsy (Baker et al., 2005; Baker et al., 1997).
Baker et al. reported that epilepsy has the potential to negatively affect different aspects of what is called "quality of life" (Baker et al., 2005). The authors collected data from 3889 patients with epilepsy from 10 different countries. In this multicenter survey it was concluded that the most commonly reported complaints interfering with daily living activities were nervousness, headaches and tiredness. Respondents in this study reported that their disease and its treatment had a significant impact on their HRQOL. Short Form-36 (SF-36) was used in Baker et al.'s study and patients scored significantly lower in domains such as physical and social functioning, energy and vitality (Baker et al., 2005).
In another multicenter (European) study again conducted by Baker et al. in 15 countries in Europe, data from more than 5000 patients were investigated and it was concluded that epilepsy had a negative effect on patients' social and psychological well-being (Baker et al., 1997). Argyriou et al. studied the impact of epilepsy on the psychological health and HRQOL of patients suffering from mild epilepsy in a rural area of southeastern Greece and reported that HRQOL of their patient sample was obviously affected while their psychological health remained nearly unaffected (Argyriou et al., 2004). Kutlu et al, investigated the HRQOL, anxiety and depression states of patients with epilepsy (PWE) (Kutlu et al., 2010). The SF-36 health survey scores were significantly lower in all subscales in PWE compared with the control group. Total scores for Beck Depression Inventory (BDI) were significantly higher in epilepsy patients. Hamilton anxiety scale were also found to be significantly increased in the epilepsy group. It was concluded that epilepsy significantly interferes with QOL and psychologic health of patients. In the patient group relationship between the seizure frequency and vitality was found to be statistically significant (Kutlu et al., 2010).
Women with epilepsy of childbearing age were reported to be at high risk of depression. Factors associated with depression include lack of occupation, the presence of an underlying disabling condition (with treatment), and the severity of epilepsy. Compared with the general population depressed women have greater impairment of HRQOL with epilepsy, which reflects the physical, social and emotional implications of the disease (Beghi et al., 2004).
Several comorbid psychiatric problems accompany the clinical picture in epilepsy. According to Kanner depression is the most common comorbid psychiatric disorder in patients with epilepsy though it remains underrecognized and undertreated (Kanner, 2003). According to Devinsky, seizures by definition change behaviour (Devinsky, 2004). Behavioural disorders are perhaps the most common and serious complications in epilepsy. For patients with difficult to control epilepsy, depression makes a greater contribution to impaired quality of life than seizure frequency (Devinsky, 2004). In an extended review reported by Gaitatzias et al. it was pointed out that 6% of people with epilepsy in the general population appears to suffer from a psychiatric disorder while this rate increases to 10-20% in patients with temporal lobe and/or refractory epilepsy (Gaitatzis et al., 2004). In general 30% of PWE suffer from depression, 10-20% from anxiety, 2-7% psychosis, 1-2% from personality disorders (Gaitatzis et al., 2004). On

the other hand, fear of seizures seems to play a very important role in psychiatric aspects of this disease. Newsom-Davis et al, stated that after an experience of a generalized epileptic seizure, a subsequent and anticipatory fear may well be seen in the sufferer (Newsom-Davis et al.,1998). Authors also underlined that there is a sufficient evidence in the literature suggesting that epileptic patients commonly fear death and or brain damage resulting from their seizures (Newsom-Davıs et al.,1998). Furthermore there is a strong association between the degree of psychopathology and the intensity of patients fears.

To qualify as a specific phobia, the Diagnostic and Statistical Manual IV requires that the following criteria are met: (a) a marked and persistent fear is excessive or unreasonable and cued by the presence or anticipation of a specific object or situation; (b) exposure to the phobic stimulus provokes an immediate anxiety response; (c) the person recognizes that the fear is excessive or unreasonable; (d) the phobic situation is avoided or endured with intense anxiety or distress; and (e) avoidance, anxious anticipation, or distress in the feared situation interferes significantly with the person's normal routine, occupational functioning or social activities or relationships (Newsom-Davıs et al.,1998; DSM-IV, 1994).

It is very well known that one of the most important features of epilepsy is stigma. De Boer et al. reviewed the global burden and stigma of epilepsy (De Boer et al., 2008). The authors stated that people with disabilities are among the most vulnerable in any society. Hidden disabilities such as epilepsy leads to even a greater vulnerability. Epileptic people may fear going outside their homes unaccompanied and they also fear what people might think of them if they were to have a seizure in public. Inevitably this leads to social isolation and participation restriction in the community.

In a recent study reported by Kanner et al. it was demonstrated that patients with subsyndromic depressive episodes (SSDEs), major depressive episodes (MDEs), anxiety disorders, and mixed MDEs (or SSDEs) with anxiety disorder(s) have a significantly worse quality of life than asymptomatic patients (Kanner et al., 2010). Authors also suggested that the comorbid occurrence of mixed MDE/anxiety disorders (particularly in the presence of more than one type of anxiety disorder) and SSDE/anxiety disorder yielded a worse impact on HRQOL than the occurrence of anxiety disorders alone. Another important finding of this study was that the comorbid occurrence of depressive and anxiety disorders have been found to have significant clinical implications beyond their impact on HRQOL which include:

1. An increased suicidal risk.
2. A worse course and poorer response to treatment of a depressive disorder
3. An increased risk of MDE recurrence. types of anxiety increased the probability of a new depressive episode.
4. An increased risk of failure to achieve a seizure-free state following an anterotemporal lobectomy in patients with pharmacoresistant temporal lobe epilepsy (Kanner et al., 2010).

Literature survey reveals enough evidence regarding the negative impact of mood disorders and anxiety symptoms on the quality of life of patients with epilepsy (PWEs) (Perrine et al., 1995; Gilliam, 2002; Cramer et al., 2003; Boylan et al., 2004; Johnson et al., 2004; Loring et al., 2004; Tracy et al., 2007). Symptoms of depression and anxiety are independently associated with reduced HRQOL; psychiatric comorbidity explains more variance in HRQOL than the combined groups of clinical seizure or demographic variables (Johnson et al., 2004). A study with a large sample included 435 PWEs aiming to investigate the relative impact of mood and anxiety symptoms as well as social and seizure related variables on HRQOL (Tracy et al., 2007); the presence of depressive symptoms was the strongest predictor of the composite and subscales of the Quality of Life in Epilepsy instrument used (QOLIE-31). In none of the cases did the severity of symptoms of depression interact significantly with the other variables, suggesting that its effect on HRQOL was direct and not mediated by other factors. In other studies conducted on patients with pharmacoresistant temporal lobe epilepsy (TLE), symptoms of depression were found to be the strongest independent predictors of poor quality of life but (unexpectedly) not the seizure frequency or severity (Perrine et al., 1995; Gilliam, 2002; Boylan et al., 2004). All of the mentioned studies relied on screening instruments identifying symptoms of depression and anxiety, but did not generate psychiatric diagnoses of mood or anxiety disorders, based on predetermined diagnostic criteria, such as those suggested by the Diagnostic and Statistical Manual of Mental Disorders, Fourth Edition (DSM-IV-TR, 2000). The lack of a DSM-IV-TR diagnosis does not invalidate the significance of the data cited earlier. Studies on primary mood disorders emphasised the relatively high prevalence and significant clinical impact of subsyndromic forms of depressive disorders (Van Praag et al.,2004). Whether subsyndromic depressive episodes (SSDEs) differ from major depressive episodes (MDEs) or anxiety disorders in their impact on HRQOL of PWEs is yet to be established. The purpose of van Praag et al.'s study was to test the following four hypotheses:

1. Patients with SSDEs, MDEs, and anxiety disorders have worse HRQOL than asymptomatic patients,
2. The more severe forms of depressive episodes (e.g., MDEs) have a greater negative impact on HRQOL measures than SSDEs,
3. Depressive and anxiety disorders do not differ in their impact on HRQOL,
4. Comorbidity of MDEs and anxiety disorders, but not of SSDEs and anxiety disorders, has a worse impact on HRQOL than MDEs and anxiety disorders alone (Van Praag et al.,2004).

According to Winter, self-esteem is the most important part of the ego, which is also the most important factor contributing to psychosocial well-being (35). The most important determinants of self-esteem are (1) what we think of ourselves, as a reflection of what the people we care about think of us; (2) how we evaluate ourselves in comparison to other people; and (3) our ability to reach a positive outcome concerning issues that are important to us (Winter, 1996). Literature survey reveals contradictory data regarding the correlation between epilepsy and self-esteem (Winter, 1996; Reeve & Lincoln, 2002; Lee et al., 2008). Gauffin et al. studied self-esteem, and sense of coherence in a group of young adults wtih epilepsy and compared the results with those obtained five years earlier (Gauffin et al., 2010). The authors found that there was a decline in both sense of coherence and self-esteem overtime in young adults with epilepsy. On the other hand Lee et al. reported that epilepsy in general has little impact on overall self-esteem in adolescents (Gauffin et al., 2010).

As it was mentioned above several comorbid psychiatric problems such as depression, anxiety, psychosis and personality disorders accompany the clinical picture in epilepsy. One should also bear in mind the important role of antiepileptic drugs (AEDs) in psychopathology of epilepsy (Mula & Monaco, 2009). Mula and Monaco have drawn attention to the risk benefit ratio of AED usage in epilepsy. Possible adverse effects of AEDs include behavioural problems and psychiatric disorders. According to the authors it is often difficult to determine which pyshopathological manifestations are due to the drug therapy and which may be due to the characteristics of epilepsy disease itself. Mula and Monaco concluded that the most commonly reported psychiatric adverse effects of AEDs are non-specific behavioral problems (Mula & Monaco, 2009). Among specific psychiatric diagnoses, depression is the most commonly reported. Psychosis is much less frequent.

In a study which investigated the sociodemographic and clinical factors associated with depression in epilepsy it was reported that, depressed subjects with epilepsy were significantly less likely to be married or employed and more likely to report comorbid medical problems and active seizures in the past 6 months (Thompson et al., 2009). Another important conclusion of this study was, when adjusted for all other variables, subjects with epilepsy reporting lamotrigine use were significantly less likely to be depressed compared to those not reporting lamotrigine use (Thompson et al., 2009).

In a review covering 35 years of research specifically devoted to QOL in adult epilepsy, Leone et al. classified the questionnaires used in epilepsy according to validation, diffusion of use and spesificity of domains characteristics (Leone et al., 2005). The authors concluded that questionnaires covering all three aspects (Washington Psychosocial Seizure Inventory (WPSI), Epilepsy Surgery Inventory 55 Survey (ESI-55), Quality of Life in Epilepsy Inventory (QOLIE-89), QOLIE-31, QOLIE-10, Liverpool Batteries) should be preferred when planning a QOL study in epilepsy. However those covering only two aspects (SF-36, The Side Effect and Life Satisfaction (SEALS) inventory, Epilepsy Psychosocial Effects Scale (EPSES), Performance, Sociodemographic aspects, Subjective evaluation/estimation questionnaire (PESOS), Quality of Life Assessment Schedule (QOLAS) could also be useful in selected situations or may become a first-choice instrument in the future, after more widespread use or complete validation (Leone et al., 2005). On the other hand Wiebe et al. aimed to determine the minimum clinically important change, and small medium, and large changes in broadly used epilepsy specific and generic HRQOL instruments and found that QOLIE-89, QOLIE-31, SF-36, SF-36 physical composite score and HUI-III (health utility index mark III) differentiated between no change and minimum important change with precision (Wiebe et al., 2002). Birbeck et al. in their study evaluating ability of HRQOL measures to detect change overtime in people with epilepsy, suggested that SF-36 yielded responsiveness indices comparable to those of the epilepsy targeted (specific) measures (Birbeck et al., 2000).

In a randomized controlled study May and Pfäfflin emphasized the efficacy of an educational treatment program for PWE. Modular service package epilepsy (MOSES) which was developed to improve patients' knowledge and understanding about their epilepsy, its treatment and psychosocial consequences, was used in the study. The study clearly indicated the need for patient education. Even patients with a long history of epilepsy and with additional handicaps or diseases benefitted from the MOSES program (May & Pfäfflin 2002).

Psychologically, persons with epilepsy may have feelings of worthlessness, fear, stigma, anger, and hopelessness, and may exhibit passive behavior (Chen et al., 2010). Stigmatization leads to discrimination, and people with epilepsy have been the target of prejudicial behavior in many aspects of life, over many centuries and in many cultures (De Boer et al., 2008; Pahl & De Boer, 2005). These factors decrease their psychosocial function, self efficacy, and quality of life (Chen & Tsai , 2003; Pramuka et al., 2007) and even increase the suicide rate (Bell et al., 2009).

Evidence shows that there is a spectrum of cognitive, behavioural and psychiatric disorders that accompany many forms of epilepsy. New discoveries may contribute to the development of therapies and management techniques that will better enable physicians to treat the full spectrum of disorders that epilepsy and tails (Berg , 2011).

ILAE recently recommended that the term "benign" no longer be used to describe epilepsy, precisely because of the large number of disorders often seen in association with even relatively uncomplicated epilepsy (Berg et al., 2010). Berg suggested that any patient with epilepsy should be viewed as someone who is at risk of encountering a variety of consequences including cognitive problems, behavioural disorders, depression, suicide and also sudden death (Berg , 2011).

3. Conclusion

Epilepsy, with its rich clinical features, is particularly important for HRQOL research. Despite a substantial increase in the number of published articles in recent years, research in the literature regarding the quality of lives of epileptic patients is relatively limited (Aydemir et al., 2008; Birbeck et al., 2002). Most of the current reports in this field share a common message emphasizing the negative effects of epilepsy on patients' HRQOL. Epileptic patients may experience various problems which will result in a lower quality of life. Seizure frequency, side effects of the antiepileptic drugs, psychological comorbidity and stigma are important factors associated with the severity of the disease and these factors may cause an important impact on life quality of epileptic patients. Stemming from a thorough review of the current literature, we can conclude that there is still a need for further scientific research with further validated instruments to find out more clear relation between epilepsy and HRQOL.

4. References

[1] Foldwary N & Wyllie E (1999). Epilepsy, In: *Textbook of Clinical Neurology*, Goetz G.C, Pappert E.J, pp. 1059-1088, W.B. Saunders Company, Philedelphia.

[2] McHugh JC & Delanty N (2008). Epidemiology and classification of epilepsy: *Int Rev Neurobiol*, 83, pp.11-26.

[3] World Health Organization. International Classification of Functioning Disability and Health: ICF. Geneva: (2001), WHO.

[4] Leonardi M & Ustun TB (2002). The global burden of epilepsy. *Epilepsia*, 43(Suppl. 6), pp. 21–25.

[5] ILAE/IBE/WHO. "Out of the shadows": global campaign against epilepsy. ILAE/IBE/WHO Annual Report (1999), Geneva: WHO.

[6] Meinardi H, Scott RA, Reis R & Sander JW (2001). The treatment gap in epilepsy: the current situation and ways forward. *Epilepsia*, 42, pp.136–49.

[7] Tulsky DS & Rosenthal M (2002). Quality of life measurement in rehabilitation medicine: Building an agenda for the future. *Arch Phys Med Rehabil*, 83(Suppl 2), pp. 1-3.

[8] Aydemir N, Özkara C, Canbeyli R & Tekcan A (2004). Changes in quality of life and self-perspective related to surgery in patients with temporal lobe epilepsy. *Epilepsy & Behavior*, 5, pp.735-742.

[9] Birbeck GL, Hays RD, Cui X & Vickrey BG (2002). Seizure reduction and quality of life improvements in people with epilepsy. *Epilepsia* 43, 5, pp. 535-8.

[10] Jacoby A (1994). Felt versus inacted stigma: a concept revisited. *Soc Sci Med*, 38, pp. 269-74.

[11] Leidy NK, Elizhauser A, Vickrey B & et al., (1999). Seizure frequency and health-related quality of life in adults with epilepsy. *Neurology*, 53, pp.162-6.

[12] Stavem K, Loge JH & Kaasa S (2000). Health status of people with epilepsy compared with a general reference population. *Epilepsia*, 41, pp. 85-90.

[13] Buck D, Jacoby A, Baker GA & et al., (1999). Cross-cultural differences in health-related quality of life of people with epilepsy: findings from a European study. *Quality Life Res*, 8, pp. 675-685.

[14] Baker GA, Jacoby A, Gorry J, Doughty J &Ellina V; on Behalf of the SIGN Group (2005). Quality of Life of People with Epilepsy in Iran, the Gulf, and Near East. *Epilepsia* 2005; 46, 1, pp. 132–140.

[15] Baker GA, Jacoby A, Buck D, Stalgis C & Monnet D (1997). Quality of life in people with epilepsy: A European Study. *Epilepsia* 38, 3, pp.353-362.

[16] Argyriou A.A, Papapetropoulos S, Polychronopoulos P & et al (2004). Psychosocial effects and evaluation of the health-related quality of life in patient suffering from well-controlled epilepsy. *J Neurol*, 251, pp. 310-313.

[17] Kutlu A, Başaran S, Altun NS, Unalan H & Komsuoğlu SS (2010). Quality of Life, Depression and Anxiety in Patients with Epilepsy: Controlled Study with Short Form 36 Questionnaire, Beck Depression Inventory and Hamilton Anxiety Scale. *Neurosurgery Quarterly*, 20,2, pp. 95-99.

[18] Beghi E, Roncolato M & Visona G (2004). Depression and Altered Quality of Life in Women with Epilepsy of Childbearing Age. *Epilepsia* 45, 1, pp. 64–70.

[19] Kanner AM (2003). Depression in epilepsy: prevalence, clinical semiology, pathogenic mechanisms and treatment. *Biol Psychiatry*, 54, pp. 388–398.

[20] Devinsky O (2004). Preface. *Epilepsia*, 45, (Suppl. 2), pp. 3–4.

[21] Gaitatzis A, Trimble MR & Sander JW (2004). The psychiatric comorbidity of epilepsy. *Acta Neurol Scand* 110, pp. 207–220.

[22] Newsom-Davıs I, Goldsteın LH & Fıtzpatrıck D (1998). Fear of seizures: an investigation and treatment. *Seizure*, 7, pp. 101-106.

[23.] Diagnostic and Statistical Manual of Mental Disorders,4th edn. Washington, DC, American Psychiatric Association, (1994).

[24] De Boer HM, Mula M & Sander JW (2008). The global burden and stigma of epilepsy. *Epilepsy & Behavior*, 12, pp. 540–546.

[25] Kanner AM, Barry JJ, Gilliam F, Hermann B & Meador KJ (2010). Anxiety disorders, subsyndromic depressive episodes, and major depressive episodes: Do they differ on their impact on the quality of life of patients with epilepsy? *Epilepsia*, 51,7, pp. 1152–1158.

[26] Perrine K, Hermann BP, Meador KJ, Vickrey BG, Cramer JA, Hays RD & Devinsky O (1995). The relationship of neuropsychological functioning to quality of life in epilepsy. *Arch Neurol*, 52, pp. 997–1003.

[27] Gilliam FG (2002). Optimizing Health Outcomes in Active Epilepsy. *Neurology,* 58(suppl 5), pp. 9–19.

[28] Cramer JA, Blum M, Reed M & Fanning K (2003). Epilepsy Impact Project. The influence of comorbid depression on quality of life for people with epilepsy. *Epilepsy & Behavior*, 4, pp. 515–521.

[29] Boylan LS, Flint LA, Labovitz DL, Jackson SC, Starner K & Devinsky O (2004). Depression but not seizure frequency predicts quality of life in treatment-resistant epilepsy. *Neurology*, 62, pp. 258–261.

[30] Johnson EK, Jones JE, Seidenberg M & Hermann BP (2004). The relative impact of anxiety, depression, and clinical seizure features on health related quality of life in epilepsy. *Epilepsia*, 45, pp. 544–550.

[31] Loring DW, Meador KJ & Lee GP (2004). Determinants of quality of life in epilepsy. *Epilepsy & Behavior*, 5, pp. 976–980.

[32] Tracy JI, Dechant V, Sperling MR, Cho R & Glosser D (2007). The association of mood with quality of life ratings in epilepsy. *Neurology*, 68, pp. 1101–1107.

[33] American Psychiatric Association (2000). *Diagnostic and Statistical Manual of Mental Disorders IV-TR*. American Psychiatric Press, Washington, DC.

[34] Van Praag HM, deKloet R, van Os J (2004). Diagnosing Depression. In van Praag HM, deKloet R, van Os J (Eds) Stress, the Brain and Depression. *Cambridge University Press*, Cambridge, pp. 1–8.

[35] Winter DG (1996). Personality, analysis and interpretations of lives. New York: McGraw–Hill.

[36] Baker GA, Spector S, McGrath Y & Soteriou H (2005). Impact of epilepsy in adolescence: a UK controlled study. *Epilepsy & Behavior*, 6, pp. 556–562.

[37] Reeve DK & Lincoln NB (2002). Coping with the challenge of transition in older adolescents with epilepsy. *Seizure*, 11, pp. 33–39.

[38] Lee A, Hamiwka LD, Sherman EM & Wirrell EC (2008). Self-concept in adolescents with epilepsy: biological and social correlates. *Pediatr Neurol*, 38, pp. 335–339.

[39] Gauffin H, Landtblom AM & Räty L (2010). Self-esteem and sense of coherence in young people with uncomplicated epilepsy: A 5-year follow-up. *Epilepsy & Behavior*, 17, pp. 520–524.

[40] Mula M & Monaco F (2009). Antiepileptic drugs and psychopathology of epilepsy: an update. *Epileptic Disord*, 11, pp.1-9.

[41] Thompson AW, Miller JW, Katon W, Chaytor N & Ciechanowski P (2009). Sociodemographic and Clinical Factors Associated with Depression in Epilepsy. *Epilepsy & Behavior*, 14, 4, pp. 655–660.

[42] Leone MA, Beghi E, Righini C, Apolone G & Mosconi P (2005). Epilepsy and quality of life in adults: A review of instruments. *Epilepsy Research*, 66, pp. 23–44.

[43] Wiebe S, Matijevic S, Eliasziw M & Derry PA (2002). Clinically important change in quality of life in epilepsy. *J Neurol Neurosurg Psychiatry*, 73, pp. 116–120.

[44] Birbeck GL, Kim S, Hays RD & Wickrey BG (2000). Quality of life measures in epilepsy: How well can they detect change overtime? *Neurology*, 54, pp. 1822-1827.

[45] May TW & Pfäfflin M (2002). The efficacy of an educational treatment program for patients with epilepsy (MOSES): results of a controlled, randomized study. Modular Service Package Epilepsy. *Epilepsia* 43, 5, pp. 539-49.

[46] Chen HF, Tsai YF, Lin YP, Mo-Song Shih MS & Chen JC (2010). The relationships among medicine symptom distress, self-efficacy, patient-provider relationship, and medication compliance in patients with epilepsy. *Epilepsy & Behavior*, 19, pp. 43–49.

[47] Pahl K & de Boer HM (2005). Epilepsy and rights. In: *Atlas: epilepsy care in the world*. Geneva: WHO; pp. 72–73.

[48] Chen HF & Tsai YF (2003). The psychosocial responses and coping strategies in the epilepsy. *Chang Gung Nursing*, 14, pp. 21–30.

[49] Pramuka M, Hendrickson R, Zinski A & Van Cott AC (2007). A psychosocial self management program for epilepsy: a randomized pilot study in adults. *Epilepsy & Behavior*, 11, pp. 533–45.

[50] Bell GS, Gaitatzis A, Bell CL, Johnson AL & Sander JW (2009). Suicide in people with epilepsy: how great is the risk? *Epilepsia*, 50, pp. 1933–1942.

[51] Berg AT (2011). Epilepsy, cognition, and behavior: The clinical picture. *Epilepsia*, 52(Suppl. 1), pp. 7–12.

[52] Berg AT, Berkovic SF, Brodie MJ, Buchhalter J, Cross JH, van Emde Boas W, Engel J, French J, Glauser TA, Mathern GW, Mosh SL, Nordli DR, Plouin P & Scheffer IE (2010). Revised terminology and concepts for organization of seizures and epilepsies: report of the ILAE Commission on Classification and Terminology, 2005–2009 (2010). *Epilepsia*, 51, pp. 676–685.